DR MADELEI

S0-BSY-717

Tarascon Pocket Pharmacopoeia®
2008 Deluxe Lab-coat Pocket Edition

"Desire to take medicines ... distinguishes man from animals."   *Sir William Osler*

A cell 407-223-6246. The hospitalist Group

CONTENTS

FOR TARASCON BOOKS/SOFTWARE, VISIT: WWW.TARASCON.COM

Tarascon Pocket Pharmacopoeia®
- Classic Shirt-Pocket Edition
- Deluxe Labcoat Pocket Edition
- PDA software for Palm® / Pocket PC® / BlackBerry®

Other Tarascon Pocketbooks
- Tarascon Pediatric Outpatient Pocketbook
- Tarascon Internal Medicine & Critical Care Pocketbook
- Tarascon Adult Emergency Pocketbook
- Tarascon Pediatric Emergency Pocketbook
- Tarascon Primary Care Pocketbook
- Tarascon Pocket Orthopaedica®
- How to be a Truly Excellent Junior Medical Student

See order form
on last page

"It's not how much you know, it's how fast you can find the answer."®

Important Caution – Please Read This! The information in the *Pocket Pharmacopoeia* is compiled from sources believed to be reliable, and exhaustive efforts have been put forth to make the book as accurate as possible. The *Pocket Pharmacopoeia* is edited by a panel of drug information experts with extensive peer review and input from more than 50 practicing clinicians of multiple specialties. Our goal is to provide health professionals focused, core prescribing information in a convenient, organized, and concise fashion. We include FDA-approved dosing indications and those off-label uses that have a reasonable basis to support their use. *However the accuracy and completeness of this work cannot be guaranteed.* Despite our best efforts this book may contain typographical errors and omissions. The *Pocket Pharmacopoeia* is intended as a quick and convenient reminder of information you have already learned elsewhere. The contents are to be used as a guide only, and health care professionals should use sound clinical judgment and individualize therapy to each specific patient care situation. This book is not meant to be a replacement for training, experience, continuing medical education, studying the latest drug prescribing literature, raw intelligence, good karma, or common sense. This book is sold without warranties of any kind, express or implied, and the publisher and editors disclaim any liability, loss, or damage caused by the contents. *If you do not wish to be bound by the foregoing cautions and conditions, you may return your undamaged and unexpired book to our office for a full refund.* Tarascon Publishing is independent from and has no affiliation with pharmaceutical companies. Although drug companies purchase and distribute our books as promotional items, the Tarascon editorial staff alone determine all book content.

Tarascon Pocket Pharmacopoeia® 2008 Deluxe Edition

HOW TO USE THE TARASCON POCKET PHARMACOPOEIA

The *Tarascon Pocket Pharmacopoeia* arranges drugs by clinical class with a comprehensive index in the back. Trade names are italicized and capitalized. Drug doses shown in mg/kg are generally intended for children, while fixed doses represent typical adult recommendations. Each drug entry is divided as follows:

WARNING – Black-box warnings, if any, with lower level warnings in the "notes" section.

ADULT – Selected adult FDA-approved indications & doses listed in typical frequency of use.

PEDS – Selected peds FDA-approved indications & doses listed in typical frequency of use.

UNAPPROVED ADULT – Selected adult non-FDA-approved (ie, "off-label") indications and doses listed in typical frequency of use.

UNAPPROVED PEDS – Selected pediatric non-FDA-approved (ie, "off-label") indications and doses listed in typical frequency of use.

FORMS – Formulations available from manufacturers (eg, tabs, caps, liquid, susp, cream, lotion, patches, etc), including specification of trade, generic, and over-the-counter forms. Scored pills are designated as such. Not all pharmacies stock all items, of course.

NOTES – Selected notes, additional warnings, major adverse drug interactions, dosage adjustment in renal/hepatic insufficiency, therapeutic levels, etc.

Each drug entry contains the following codes:

▶ **METABOLISM & EXCRETION: L** = primarily liver, **K** = primarily kidney, **LK** = both, but liver>kidney, **KL** = both, but kidney>liver, **LO** = liver & onions

♀ **SAFETY IN PREGNANCY: A** = Safety established using human studies, **B** = Presumed safety based on animal studies, **C** = Uncertain safety; no human studies and animal studies show an adverse effect, **D** = Unsafe - evidence of risk that may in certain clinical circumstances be justifiable, **X** = Highly unsafe - risk of use outweighs any possible benefit. For drugs which have not been assigned a category: **+**Generally accepted as safe, **?**Safety unknown or controversial, **-**Generally regarded as unsafe.

▶ **SAFETY IN LACTATION: +**Generally accepted as safe, **?**Safety unknown or controversial, **-**Generally regarded as unsafe. Many of our "**+**" listings are taken from the AAP policy "The Transfer of Drugs and Other Chemicals Into Human Milk" (see www.aap.org) and may differ from those recommended by manufacturers.

© **DEA CONTROLLED SUBSTANCES: I** = High abuse potential, no accepted use (eg, heroin, marijuana), **II** = High abuse potential and severe dependence liability (eg, morphine, codeine, hydromorphone, cocaine, amphetamines, methylphenidate, secobarbital). Some states require triplicates. **III** = Moderate dependence liability (eg, *Tylenol #3, Vicodin*), **IV** = Limited dependence liability (benzodiazepines, propoxyphene, phentermine), **V** = Limited abuse potential (eg, *Lomotil*).

$ **RELATIVE COST**: Cost codes used are "per month" of maintenance therapy (eg, antihypertensives) or "per course" of short-term therapy (eg, antibiotics). Codes are calculated using average wholesale prices (at press time in US$) for the most common indication & route of each drug at a typical adult dosage. For maintenance therapy, costs are calculated based upon a 30 day supply or the quantity that might typically be used in a given month. For short-term therapy (≤10 days), costs are calculated on a single treatment course. When multiple forms are available (eg,

Code	Cost
$	< $25
$$	$25 to $49
$$$	$50 to $99
$$$$	$100 to $199
$$$$$	≥ $200

generics), these codes reflect the least expensive generally available product. When drugs don't neatly fit into the classification scheme above, we have assigned codes based upon the relative cost of other similar drugs. *These codes should be used as a rough guide only*, as (1) they reflect cost, not charges, (2) pricing often varies substantially from location to location & time to time, and (3) HMOs, Medicaid, and buying groups often negotiate quite different pricing. Your mileage may vary. Check with your local pharmacy if you have any question.

🍁 **CANADIAN TRADE NAMES**: Unique common Canadian trade names not used in the USA are listed after a maple leaf symbol. Trade names used in both nations or only in the USA are displayed without such notation.

PAGE INDEX FOR TABLES

ABBREVIATIONS IN TEXT

AAP - American Academy of Pediatrics
ac - before meals
ADHD - attention deficit & hyperactivity disorder
AHA - American Heart Association
ANC - absolute neutrophil count
ASA - aspirin
bid - twice per day
BP - blood pressure
BPH - benign prostatic hyperplasia
CAD - coronary artery disease
cap - capsule
CMV - cytomegalovirus
CNS - central nervous system
COPD - chronic obstructive pulmonary disease
CrCl - creatinine clearance

CVA – stroke
d - day
D5W - 5% dextrose
DPI - dry powder inhaler
elem - elemental
ET - endotracheal
EPS - extrapyramidal symptoms
g - gram
gtts - drops
GERD - gastroesophageal reflux dz
GU - genitourinary
h - hour
HAART - highly active antiretroviral therapy
HCTZ - hydrochlorothiazide
HSV - herpes simplex virus
HTN - hypertension
IM - intramuscular
INR - international normalized ratio
IU - international units
IV - intravenous

JRA - juvenile rheumatoid arthritis
kg - kilogram
LFTs - liver fxn tests
LV - left ventricular
mcg - microgram
MDI - metered dose inhaler
mEq - milliequivalent
mg - milligram
MI - myocardial infarction
min - minute
mL - milliliter
mo - months old
ng - nanogram
NHLBI – National Heart, Lung, and Blood Institute
NS - normal saline
NYHA - New York Heart Association
N/V -nausea/vomiting
OA - osteoarthritis
pc - after meals
PO - by mouth
PR - by rectum

prn - as needed
q - every
qhs - at bedtime
qid - four times/day
qod - every other day
q pm - every evening
RA - rheumatoid arthritis
SC - subcutaneous
soln - solution
supp - suppository
susp - suspension
tab - tablet
TB - tuberculosis
TCAs - tricyclic antidepressants
TIA - transient ischemic attack
tid - 3 times/day
TNF - tumor necrosis factor
tiw - 3 times/week
UTI - urinary tract infection
wk - week
yo - years old

THERAPEUTIC DRUG LEVELS

Drug	Level	Optimal Timing
amikacin peak	20-35 mcg/ml	30 minutes after infusion
amikacin trough	<5 mcg/ml	Just prior to next dose
carbamazepine trough	4-12 mcg/ml	Just prior to next dose
cyclosporine trough	50-300 ng/ml	Just prior to next dose
digoxin	0.8-2.0 ng/ml	Just prior to next dose
ethosuximide trough	40-100 mcg/ml	Just prior to next dose
gentamicin peak	5-10 mcg/ml	30 minutes after infusion
gentamicin trough	<2 mcg/ml	Just prior to next dose
lidocaine	1.5-5 mcg/ml	12-24 hours after start of infusion
lithium trough	0.6-1.2 meq/l	Just prior to first morning dose
NAPA	10-30 mcg/ml	Just prior to next procainamide dose
phenobarbital trough	15-40 mcg/ml	Just prior to next dose
phenytoin trough	10-20 mcg/ml	Just prior to next dose
primidone trough	5-12 mcg/ml	Just prior to next dose
procainamide	4-10 mcg/ml	Just prior to next dose
quinidine	2-5 mcg/ml	Just prior to next dose
theophylline	5-15 mcg/ml	8-12 hrs after once daily dose
tobramycin peak	5-10 mcg/ml	30 minutes after infusion
tobramycin trough	<2 mcg/ml	Just prior to next dose
valproate trough (epilepsy)	50-100 mcg/ml	Just prior to next dose
valproate trough (mania)	45-125 mcg/ml	Just prior to next dose
vancomycin trough	5-20 mcg/ml	Just prior to next dose

Tarascon Publishing is proud to partner with the following organizations in bringing you the top-quality PDA edition of the *Pocket Pharmacopoeia*: USBMIS, Inc (software production and support), Drugstore.com (exact drug pricing information), and NeedyMeds.com (patient assistance program data).

PEDIATRIC DRUGS		Age	2m	4m	6m	9m	12m	15m	2y	3y	5y
		Kg	5	6½	8	9	10	11	13	15	19
		Lbs	11	15	17	20	22	24	28	33	42
med	*strength*	*freq*	*teaspoons of liquid per dose (1 tsp= 5 ml)*								
Tylenol (mg)		q4h	80	80	120	120	160	160	200	240	280
Tylenol (tsp)	160/t	q4h	½	½	¾	¾	1	1	1¼	1½	1¾
ibuprofen (mg)		q6h	-	-	75†	75†	100	100	125	150	175
ibuprofen (tsp)	100/t	q6h	-	-	¾†	¾†	1	1	1¼	1½	1¾
amoxicillin or	125/t	bid	1	1¼	1½	1¾	1¾	2	2¼	2¾	3½
Augmentin	200/t	bid	½	¾	1	1	1¼	1¼	1½	1¾	2¼
(not otitis media)	250/t	bid	½	½	¾	¾	1	1	1¼	1¼	1¾
	400/t	bid	¼	½	½	½	¾	¾	¾	1	1
amoxicillin,	200/t	bid	1	1¼	1¾	2	2	2¼	2¾	3	4
(otitis media)‡	250/t	bid	¾	1¼	1½	1½	1¾	1¾	2¼	2½	3¼
	400/t	bid	½	¾	¾	1	1	1¼	1½	1½	2
Augmentin ES‡	600/t	bid	⅜	½	½	¾	¾	¾	1	1¼	1½
azithromycin*§	100/t	qd	¼†	½†	½	½	½	½	¾	¾	1
(5-day Rx)	200/t	qd	--	¼†	¼	¼	¼	¼	½	½	½
Bactrim/Septra	---	bid	½	¾	1	1	1	1¼	1½	1½	2
cefaclor*	125/t	bid	1	1	1¼	1½	1½	1¾	2	2½	3
"	250/t	bid	½	½	¾	¾	¾	1	1	1¼	1½
cefadroxil	125/t	bid	½	¾	1	1	1¼	1¼	1½	1¾	2¼
"	250/t	bid	¼	½	½	½	¾	¾	¾	1	1
cefdinir	125/t	qd	--	¾†	1	1	1	1¼	1½	1¾	2
cefixime	100/t	qd	½	½	¾	¾	¾	1	1	1¼	1½
cefprozil*	125/t	bid	--	¾†	1	1	1¼	1½	1½	2	2¼
"	250/t	bid	--	½†	½	½	¾	¾	¾	1	1¼
cefuroxime	125/t	bid	--	¾	¾	1	1	1	1½	1¾	2¼
cephalexin	125/t	qid	--	½	¾	¾	1	1	1¼	1½	1¾
"	250/t	qid	--	¼	¼	½	½	½	¾	¾	1
clarithromycin	125/t	bid	½†	½†	½	½	¾	¾	¾	1	1¼
"	250/t	bid	--	--	--	¼	½	½	½	½	¾
dicloxacillin	62½/t	qid	½	¾	1	1	1¼	1¼	1½	1¾	2
nitrofurantoin	25/t	qid	¼	½	½	½	½	¾	¾	¾	1
Pediazole	---	tid	½	½	¾	¾	1	1	1	1¼	1½
penicillin V**	250/t	bid-tid	--	1	1	1	1	1	1	1	1
cetirizine	5/t	qd	-	-	½	½	½	½	½	½	½
Benadryl	12.5/t	q6h	½	½	¾	¾	1	1	1¼	1½	2
prednisolone	15/t	qd	¼	½	½	¾	¾	¾	1	1	1¼
prednisone	5/t	qd	1	1¼	1½	1¾	2	2¼	2½	3	3¾
Robitussin	---	q4h	-	-	¼†	¼†	½	½	¾	¾	1
Tylenol w/ codeine		q4h	-	-	-	-	-	-	-	1	1

* Dose shown is for otitis media only; see dosing in text for alternative indications.
† Dosing at this age/weight not recommended by manufacturer.
‡ AAP now recommends high dose (80-90 mg/kg/d) for all otitis media in children; with Augmentin used as ES only.
§Give a double dose of azithromycin the first day.
**AHA dosing for streptococcal pharyngitis. Treat for 10 days.

PEDIATRIC VITAL SIGNS AND INTRAVENOUS DRUGS

Age		Pre-matr	New-born	2m	4m	6m	9m	12m	15m	2y	3y	5y
Weight	*(Kg)*	2	3½	5	6½	8	9	10	11	13	15	19
	(Lbs)	4½	7½	11	15	17	20	22	24	28	33	42
Maint fluids	*(ml/h)*	8	14	20	26	32	36	40	42	46	50	58
ET tube	*(mm)*	2½	3/3½	3½	3½	3½	4	4	4½	4½	4½	5
Defib	*(Joules)*	4	7	10	13	16	18	20	22	26	30	38
Systolic BP	*(high)*	70	80	85	90	95	100	103	104	106	109	114
	(low)	40	60	70	70	70	70	70	70	75	75	80
Pulse rate	*(high)*	145	145	180	180	180	160	160	160	150	150	135
	(low)	100	100	110	110	110	100	100	100	90	90	65
Resp rate	*(high)*	60	60	50	50	50	46	46	30	30	25	25
	(low)	35	30	30	30	24	24	20	20	20	20	20
adenosine	*(mg)*	0.2	0.3	0.5	0.6	0.8	0.9	1	1.1	1.3	1.5	1.9
atropine	*(mg)*	0.1	0.1	0.1	0.13	0.16	0.18	0.2	0.22	0.26	0.30	0.38
Benadryl	*(mg)*	-	-	5	6½	8	9	10	11	13	15	19
bicarbonate	*(meq)*	2	3½	5	6½	8	9	10	11	13	15	19
dextrose	*(g)*	1	2	5	6½	8	9	10	11	13	15	19
epinephrine	*(mg)*	.02	.04	.05	.07	.08	.09	0.1	0.11	0.13	0.15	0.19
lidocaine	*(mg)*	2	3½	5	6½	8	9	10	11	13	15	19
morphine	*(mg)*	0.2	0.3	0.5	0.6	0.8	0.9	1	1.1	1.3	1.5	1.9
mannitol	*(g)*	2	3½	5	6½	8	9	10	11	13	15	19
naloxone	*(mg)*	.02	.04	.05	.07	.08	.09	0.1	0.11	0.13	0.15	0.19
diazepam	*(mg)*	0.6	1	1.5	2	2.5	2.7	3	3.3	3.9	4.5	5
fosphenytoin*	*(PE)*	40	70	100	130	160	180	200	220	260	300	380
lorazepam	*(mg)*	0.2	0.3	0.5	0.6	0.8	0.9	1.0	1.1	1.3	1.5	1.9
phenobarb	*(mg)*	30	60	75	100	125	125	150	175	200	225	275
phenytoin*	*(mg)*	40	70	100	130	160	180	200	220	260	300	380
ampicillin	*(mg)*	100	175	250	325	400	450	500	550	650	750	1000
ceftriaxone	*(mg)*	-	-	250	325	400	450	500	550	650	750	1000
cefotaxime	*(mg)*	100	175	250	325	400	450	500	550	650	750	1000
gentamicin	*(mg)*	5	8	12	16	20	22	25	27	32	37	47

*Loading doses; fosphenytoin dosed in "phenytoin equivalents".

If you obtained your *Pocket Pharmacopoeia* from a bookstore, please send us your address (info@tarascon.com). This allows you to be the first to hear of updates! (We don't sell or distribute our mailing lists, by the way.) The cover woodcut is *The Apothecary* by Jost Amman, Frankfurt, 1574. Congratulations to those who knew what relationship took flight at Disneyland to the beat of a different drum. In 1971 Linda Ronstadt (for whom "Different Drum" was an early big hit) had a Magic Kingdom gig; when her back-up band fell apart some hasty recruiting assembled for the first time together on stage Don Henley, Glenn Frey, and Randy Meisner. Their sound worked, and the Eagles were born. We will send a free copy of next year's edition to the first 25 who know what sliding gliding splotchy blotch should be feared.

CONVERSIONS	*Liquid:*	*Weight:*
Temperature:	1 fluid ounce = 30 ml	1 kilogram = 2.2 lbs
F = (1.8) C + 32	1 teaspoon = 5 ml	1 ounce = 30 g
C = (F - 32)/(1.8)	1 tablespoon = 15 ml	1 grain = 65 mg

INHIBITORS, INDUCERS, AND SUBSTRATES OF CYTOCHROME P450 ISOZYMES

The cytochrome P450 (CYP) inhibitors and inducers below do not necessarily cause clinically important interactions with substrates listed. Underlined drugs have shown potential for important interactions in human case reports or clinical studies. We exclude in vitro data which can be inaccurate. Refer to the *Tarascon Pocket Pharmacopoeia* drug interactions database (PDA edition) or other resources for more information if an interaction is suspected based on this chart. A drug that inhibits CYP subfamily activity can block the metabolism of substrates of that enzyme and substrate accumulation and toxicity may result. CYP inhibitors are classified by how much they increase the area-under-the-curve (AUC) of a substrate: weak (1.25-2 fold), moderate (2-5 fold), or strong (≥5 fold). A drug is considered a sensitive substrate if a CYP inhibitor increases the AUC of that drug by ≥5-fold. While AUC increases of >50% often do not affect patient response, smaller increases can be important if the therapeutic range is narrow (e.g. theophylline, warfarin, cyclosporine). A drug that induces CYP subfamily activity increases substrate metabolism and reduced substrate efficacy may result. This table may be incomplete since new evidence about drug interactions is continually being identified.

CYP 1A2

Inhibitors. *Strong:* fluvoxamine. *Moderate:* ciprofloxacin, mexiletine, propafenone, zileuton. *Weak:* acyclovir, cimetidine, famotidine, norfloxacin, verapamil. *Unclassified:* amiodarone, atazanavir, citalopram, clarithromycin, erythromycin, estradiol, ipriflavone, isoniazid, paroxetine, peginterferon alfa-2a, tacrine, ziprasidone.
Inducers: barbiturates, carbamazepine, charcoal-broiled foods, phenytoin, rifampin, ritonavir, smoking.
Substrates. *Sensitive:* alosetron, duloxetine, tizanidine. *Unclassified:* acetaminophen, amitriptyline, bortezomib, caffeine, cinacalcet, clomipramine, clozapine, cyclobenzaprine, estradiol, fluvoxamine, haloperidol, imipramine, lidocaine, mexiletine, mirtazapine, naproxen, olanzapine, ondansetron, propranolol, ramelteon, rasagiline, riluzole, ropinirole, ropivacaine, R-warfarin, tacrine, theophylline, verapamil, zileuton, zolmitriptan.

CYP 2C8

Inhibitors. *Strong:* gemfibrozil. *Weak:* trimethoprim.
Inducers: barbiturates, carbamazepine, rifabutin, rifampin.
Substrates. *Sensitive:* repaglinide. *Unclassified:* amiodarone, carbamazepine, ibuprofen, isotretinoin, loperamide, paclitaxel, pioglitazone, rosiglitazone, tolbutamide.

CYP 2C9

Inhibitors. *Moderate:* amiodarone, fluconazole, oxandrolone. *Weak:* ketoconazole. *Unclassified:* atazanavir, capecitabine, chloramphenicol, cimetidine, cotrimoxazole, delavirdine, disulfiram, fenofibrate, fluorouracil, fluvoxamine, imatinib, isoniazid, leflunomide, metronidazole, sulfamethoxazole, voriconazole, zafirlukast.
Inducers: aprepitant, barbiturates, bosentan, carbamazepine, phenytoin, rifampin, rifapentine, St John's wort.
Substrates. *Sensitive:* Flurbiprofen. *Unclassified:* alosetron, bosentan, celecoxib, chlorpropamide, diclofenac, fluoxetine, flurbiprofen, fluvastatin, formoterol, glimepiride, glipizide, glyburide, ibuprofen, irbesartan, isotretinoin, losartan, mefenamic acid, meloxicam, montelukast, naproxen, nateglinide, phenytoin, piroxicam, ramelteon, rasagiline, rosiglitazone, rosuvastatin, sildenafil, tolbutamide, torsemide, valsartan, vardenafil, voriconazole, S-warfarin, zafirlukast, zileuton.

CYP 2C19

Inhibitors. *Strong:* omeprazole. *Weak:* citalopram. *Unclassified:* delavirdine, esomeprazole, felbamate, fluconazole, fluoxetine, fluvoxamine, isoniazid, letrozole, modafinil, omeprazole, oxcarbazepine, telmisartan, voriconazole.
Inducers: rifampin, St John's wort.
Substrates. *Sensitive:* omeprazole. *Unclassified:* amitriptyline, arformoterol, bortezomib, carisoprodol, cilostazol, citalopram, clomipramine, desipramine, diazepam, escitalopram, esomeprazole, formoterol, imipramine, lansoprazole, nelfinavir, pantoprazole, phenytoin, progesterone, proguanil, propranolol, thioridazine, voriconazole, R-warfarin.

CYP 2D6

Inhibitors. *Strong*: cinacalcet, <u>fluoxetine</u>, <u>paroxetine</u>, <u>quinidine</u>. *Moderate*: duloxetine, terbinafine. *Weak*: <u>amiodarone</u>, citalopram, escitalopram, sertraline. *Unclassified*: bupropion, chloroquine, <u>cimetidine</u>, clomipramine, delavirdine, <u>diphenhydramine</u>, fluphenazine, <u>fluvoxamine</u>, haloperidol, hydroxychloroquine, imatinib, perphenazine, <u>propafenone</u>, <u>propoxyphene</u>, quinacrine, ritonavir, tolterodine, <u>thioridazine</u>, venlafaxine.

Inducers: None

Substrates. *Sensitive*: <u>desipramine</u>. *Unclassified*: almotriptan, amitriptyline, arformoterol, <u>aripiprazole</u>, atomoxetine, <u>carvedilol</u>, cevimeline, chlorpheniramine, chlorpromazine, cinacalcet, clomipramine, clozapine, <u>codeine</u>*, darifenacin, delavirdine, <u>dextromethorphan</u>, dihydrocodeine*, dolasetron, donepezil, doxepin, duloxetine, flecainide, fluoxetine, formoterol, galantamine, <u>haloperidol</u>, hydrocodone*, <u>imipramine</u>, loratadine, maprotiline, <u>methadone</u>, methamphetamine, <u>metoprolol</u>, mexiletine, <u>mirtazapine</u>, morphine, nortriptyline, ondansetron, oxycodone, palonosetron, paroxetine, perphenazine, procainamide, promethazine, propafenone, propoxyphene, <u>propranolol</u>, quetiapine, risperidone, ritonavir, tamoxifen, <u>thioridazine</u>, timolol, tolterodine, tramadol*, trazodone, venlafaxine.

CYP 3A4

Inhibitors. *Strong*: atazanavir, <u>clarithromycin</u>, <u>indinavir</u>, <u>itraconazole</u>, <u>ketoconazole</u>, <u>nefazodone</u>, nelfinavir, <u>ritonavir</u>, <u>saquinavir</u>, <u>telithromycin</u>, <u>voriconazole</u>. *Moderate*: amprenavir, <u>aprepitant</u>, <u>diltiazem</u>, <u>erythromycin</u>, <u>fluconazole</u>, <u>grapefruit juice</u> (variable), <u>verapamil</u>. *Weak*: cimetidine. *Unclassified*: amiodarone, conivaptan, cyclosporine, <u>danazol</u>, darunavir, delavirdine, ethinyl estradiol, fluoxetine, <u>fluvoxamine</u>, imatinib, miconazole, posaconazole, sertraline, quinupristin/dalfopristin, <u>troleandomycin</u>, zafirlukast.

Inducers. barbiturates, bexarotene, bosentan, <u>carbamazepine</u>, dexamethasone, ✣efavirenz, ethosuximide, <u>griseofulvin</u>, modafinil, <u>nafcillin</u>, ✣<u>nevirapine</u>, oxcarbazepine, <u>phenytoin</u>, primidone, rifabutin, ✣<u>rifampin</u>, rifapentine, ritonavir, <u>St Johns wort</u>.

Substrates. *Sensitive*: budesonide, <u>buspirone</u>, conivaptan, eletriptan, eplerenone, <u>felodipine</u>, <u>fluticasone</u>, <u>lovastatin</u>, <u>midazolam</u>, <u>saquinavir</u>, <u>sildenafil</u>, <u>simvastatin</u>, <u>triazolam</u>, vardenafil. *Unclassified*: acetaminophen, <u>alfentanil</u>, alfuzosin, aliskiren, almotriptan, alosetron, alprazolam, amiodarone, amlodipine, <u>amprenavir</u>, aprepitant, argatroban, <u>aripiprazole</u>, atazanavir, atorvastatin, bexarotene, bortezomib, bosentan, bromocriptine, buprenorphine, <u>carbamazepine</u>, cevimeline, cilostazol, cinacalcet, <u>cisapride</u>, citalopram, clarithromycin, clomipramine, clonazepam, clopidogrel, <u>colchicine</u>, <u>clozapine</u>, corticosteroids, cyclophosphamide, <u>cyclosporine</u>, <u>dapsone</u>, darifenacin, darunavir, dasatinib, <u>delavirdine</u>, desogestrel, dexamethasone, <u>diazepam</u>, dihydroergotamine, <u>diltiazem</u>, <u>disopyramide</u>, docetaxel, dofetilide, dolasetron, donepezil, doxorubicin, dutasteride, <u>efavirenz</u>, <u>ergotamine</u>, erlotinib, <u>erythromycin</u>†, esomeprazole, eszopiclone, <u>ethinyl estradiol</u>, etoposide, escitalopram, <u>fentanyl</u>, finasteride, galantamine, <u>gefitinib</u>, glyburide, haloperidol, hydrocodone, ifosfamide, <u>imatinib</u>, imipramine, <u>indinavir</u>, <u>irinotecan</u>, isotretinoin, isradipine, <u>itraconazole</u>, ketoconazole, lansoprazole, lapatinib, letrozole, lidocaine, loperamide, lopinavir, loratadine, losartan, maraviroc, <u>methadone</u>, methylergonovine, mifepristone, mirtazapine, modafinil, mometasone, montelukast, <u>nateglinide</u>, nefazodone, <u>nelfinavir</u>, nevirapine, nicardipine, <u>nifedipine</u>, nimodipine, <u>nisoldipine</u>, ondansetron, oxybutynin, oxycodone, paclitaxel, pantoprazole, <u>pimozide</u>, pioglitazone, <u>praziquantel</u>, quetiapine, <u>quinidine</u>, quinine, ranolazine, repaglinide, <u>rifabutin</u>, risperidone, ritonavir, ropivacaine, sertraline, sibutramine, sirolimus, solifenacin, sorafenib, sufentanil, sunitinib, <u>tacrolimus</u>, tadalafil, tamoxifen, telithromycin, testosterone, theophylline, tiagabine, tinidazole, tipranavir, tolterodine, toremifene, tramadol, trazodone, trimetrexate, troleandomycin, venlafaxine, <u>verapamil</u>, vinblastine, <u>vincristine</u>, vinorelbine, voriconazole, R-warfarin, zaleplon, zileuton, <u>ziprasidone</u>, <u>zolpidem</u>, zonisamide.

✣potent inducer

* Metabolism by CYP2D6 required to convert to active analgesic metabolite; analgesia may be impaired by CYP2D6 inhibitors.

† Risk of sudden death may be increased in patients receiving erythromycin concurrently with CYP 3A4 inhibitors like ketoconazole, itraconazole, fluconazole, diltiazem, verapamil, and troleandomycin (*NEJM* 2004;351:1089).

Alveolar-arterial oxygen gradient = A-a = $148 - 1.2(PaCO2) - PaO2$
    [normal = 10-20 mmHg, breathing room air at sea level]

Calculated osmolality = $2Na + glucose/18 + BUN/2.8 + ethanol/4.6$
    [norm 280-295 meq/L. Na in meq/L; all others in mg/dL]

Pediatric IV maintenance fluids (see table on page 7)
    4 ml/kg/hr **or** 100 ml/kg/day for first 10 kg, plus
    2 ml/kg/hr **or** 50 ml/kg/day for second 10 kg, plus
    1 ml/kg/hr **or** 20 ml/kg/day for all further kg

$$mcg/kg/min = \frac{16.7 \times drug\ conc\ [mg/ml] \times infusion\ rate\ [ml/h]}{weight\ [kg]}$$

$$Infusion\ rate\ [ml/h] = \frac{desired\ mcg/kg/min \times weight\ [kg] \times 60}{drug\ concentration\ [mcg/ml]}$$

Fractional excretion of sodium =
[Pre-renal, etc <1%; ATN, etc >1%] $\left[\dfrac{urine\ Na\ /\ plasma\ Na}{urine\ creat\ /\ plasma\ creat} \right] \times 100\%$

Anion gap = $Na - (Cl + HCO3)$ [normal = 10-14 meq/L]

$$Creatinine\ clearance = \frac{(lean\ kg)(140 - age)(0.85\ if\ female)}{(72)(stable\ creatinine\ [mg/dL])}$$
    [normal >80]

Glomerular filtration rate using MDRD equation (ml/min/1.73 m^2)
= $186 \times (creatinine)^{-1.154} \times (age)^{-0.203} \times (0.742\ if\ ♀) \times (1.210\ if\ African\ American)$

Body surface area (BSA) = square root of: $\left[\dfrac{height\ (cm) \times weight\ (kg)}{3600} \right]$
    [in m^2]

DRUG THERAPY REFERENCE WEBSITES (selected)

Professional societies or governmental agencies with drug therapy guidelines		
AHRQ	Agency for Healthcare Research and Quality	www.ahcpr.gov
AAP	American Academy of Pediatrics	www.aap.org
ACC	American College of Cardiology	www.acc.org
ACCP	American College of Chest Physicians	www.chestnet.org
ACCP	American College of Clinical Pharmacy	www.accp.com
AHA	American Heart Association	www.americanheart.org
ADA	American Diabetes Association	www.diabetes.org
AMA	American Medical Association	www.ama-assn.org
ATS	American Thoracic Society	www.thoracic.org
ASHP	Amer. Society Health-Systems Pharmacists	www.ashp.org
CDC	Centers for Disease Control & Prevention	www.cdc.gov
CDC	CDC bioterrorism and radiation exposures	www.bt.cdc.gov
IDSA	Infectious Diseases Society of America	www.idsociety.org
MHA	Malignant Hyperthermia Association	www.mhaus.org
NHLBI	National Heart, Lung, & Blood Institute	www.nhlbi.nih.gov
Other therapy reference sites		
Cochrane library		www.cochrane.org
Emergency Contraception Website		www.not-2-late.com
Immunization Action Coalition		www.immunize.org
Int'l Registry for Drug-Induced Arrhythmias		www.qtdrugs.org
Managing Contraception		www.managingcontraception.com
Nephrology Pharmacy Associates		www.nephrologypharmacy.com

Tarascon Pocket Pharmacopoeia Editorial Staff*

ANALGESICS: Antirheumatic Agents – Gold Compounds

NOTE: Gold toxicity may manifest as marrow suppression, proteinuria, hematuria, pruritus, rash, stomatitis or persistent diarrhea. Monitor CBC and urinary protein q 4-12 weeks (oral) or q 1-2 weeks (injectable) due to the risk of myelo-suppression and proteinuria.

auranofin (*Ridaura*) ▶K ♀C ▶+ $$$$$
ADULT - RA: Initial 3 mg PO bid or 6 mg PO daily. May increase to 3 mg tid after 6 months.
PEDS - RA: 0.1-0.15 mg/kg/day PO. Max dose 0.2 mg/kg/day. May be given daily or divided bid.
UNAPPROVED ADULT - Psoriatic arthritis: 3 mg PO bid or 6 mg PO daily.
FORMS - Trade only: Caps 3 mg.
NOTES - Contraindicated in patients with a history of any of the following gold-induced disorders: anaphylactic reactions, necrotizing enterocolitis, pulmonary fibrosis, exfoliative dermatitis, bone marrow suppression. Not recommended in pregnancy. Proteinuria has developed in 3%-9% of patients. Diarrhea, rash, stomatitis, chrysiasis (gray-to-blue pigmentation of skin) may occur. Minimize exposure to sunlight or artificial UV light. Auranofin may increase phenytoin levels.

gold sodium thiomalate (*Myochrysine*) ▶K ♀C ▶+ $$$$$
ADULT - RA: weekly IM injections: 1st dose, 10 mg. 2nd dose, 25 mg. 3rd & subsequent doses, 25-50 mg. Continue the 25-50 mg dose weekly to a cumulative dose of 0.8-1g. If improvement seen w/o toxicity, 25-50 mg every other week for 2-20 weeks. If stable, lengthen dosing intervals to q 3-4 weeks.
PEDS - JRA: test dose 10 mg IM, then 1 mg/kg, not to exceed 50 mg for a single injection. Continue this dose weekly to a cumulative dose of 0.8-1g. If improvement seen w/o toxicity, dose every other week for 2-20 weeks. If stable, lengthen dosing intervals to q 3-4 weeks.
NOTES - Administer only IM, preferably intraglu-teally. Have patient remain recumbent for approximately 10 minutes after injection. Contra-indicated in pregnancy & in patients who have uncontrolled DM, severe debilitation, renal disease, hepatic dysfunction or hepatitis, marked HTN, uncontrolled heart failure, SLE, blood dyscrasias, patients recently radiated & those with severe toxicity from previous exposure to gold or other heavy metals, urticaria, eczema & colitis. Arthralgia & dermatitis may occur.

ANALGESICS: Antirheumatic Agents – Immunomodulators – TNF Inhibitors

NOTE: Death, sepsis, and serious infections (eg, TB) have been reported. Do not start if current serious infection, discontinue if serious infection develops, and closely monitor for any new infection. Screening for latent TB infection is recommended. Use caution in those with a history of recurring infections or with underlying conditions (eg, DM) that predispose to infections.

abatacept (*Orencia*) ▶Serum ♀C ▶? $$$$$
WARNING - Do not use with TNF-blockers such as adalimumab, etanercept or infliximab or the IL-1 receptor antagonist anakinra.
ADULT - RA: Specialized dosing.
PEDS - Not approved in children.
NOTES – Monitor for COPD exacerbations and pulmonary infections. Avoid live vaccines.

adalimumab (*Humira*) ▶Serum ♀B ▶- $$$$$
WARNING - Hypersensitivity. Combination use with anakinra increases the risk of serious infections. Aplastic anemia, thrombocytopenia & leukopenia. Rare CNS disorders (eg, multiple

sclerosis, myelitis, optic neuritis) have been reported. May worsen heart failure; monitor signs /symptoms of heart failure.
ADULT - RA, psoriatic arthritis, ankylosing spondylitis: 40 mg SC q2 weeks, alone or in combination with methotrexate or other disease-modifying antirheumatic drugs (DMARDs). May increase frequency to q week if not on methotrexate. Crohn's disease: 160 mg SC at week 0, 80 mg at week 2, then 40 mg every other week starting with week 4.
PEDS - Not approved in children.
FORMS - Trade only: 40 mg pre-filled glass syringes or vials with needles, 2 per pack.
NOTES - Monitor CBC. Refrigerate & protect from light. Avoid live vaccines. Do not use in combination with anakinra.

etanercept (*Enbrel*) ▶Serum ♀B ▶- $$$$$
WARNING - Rare nervous system disorders (eg, multiple sclerosis, myelitis, optic neuritis) have been reported.

ADULT - RA, psoriatic arthritis, ankylosing spondylitis: 50 mg SC q week, alone or in combination with methotrexate. Plaque psoriasis: 50 mg SC twice weekly x 3 months, then 50 mg SC q week.

PEDS - JRA 4-17 yo: 0.8 mg/kg SC q week, to max single dose of 50 mg.

FORMS - Supplied in a carton containing 4 dose trays and as single-use prefilled syringes. Each dose tray contains one 25 mg single-use vial of etanercept, one syringe (1 mL sterile bacteriostatic water for injection, containing 0.9% benzyl alcohol), one plunger, and two alcohol swabs. Single-use syringes contain 50 mg/mL.

NOTES - Appropriate SC injection sites are thigh, abdomen & upper arm. Rotate injection sites. Refrigerate. Avoid live vaccines. The needle cover contains latex; caution if allergy.

infliximab (Remicade) ▶Serum ♀B ▶? $$$$$
WARNING - May worsen heart failure; monitor signs/symptoms of heart failure. May increase risk of lymphoma; caution if history of malignancy or if malignancy develops during treatment. Hypersensitivity reactions may occur. Rare CNS disorders (eg, multiple sclerosis, myelitis, optic neuritis) have been reported.

ADULT - RA: 3 mg/kg IV in combination with methotrexate at 0, 2 and 6 weeks. Give q8 weeks thereafter. May increase up to 10 mg/kg or q4 weeks if incomplete response. Ankylosing spondylitis: 5 mg/kg IV at 0, 2 and 6 weeks. Give q6 weeks thereafter. Plaque psoriasis; psoriatic arthritis; moderately to severely active Crohn's disease, ulcerative colitis, or fistulizing disease: 5 mg/kg IV infusion at 0, 2, and 6 weeks, then every 8 weeks.

PEDS - Moderately to severely active Crohn's disease or fistulizing disease: 5 mg/kg IV infusion at 0, 2 and 6 weeks then every 8 weeks.

UNAPPROVED ADULT - Moderate to severe ulcerative colitis: Same dose as for Crohn's disease.

NOTES - Headache, dyspnea, urticaria, nausea, infections, abdominal pain, & fever. Avoid live vaccines. 3 cases of toxic optic neuropathy reported. Refrigerate.

ANALGESICS: Antirheumatic Agents – Immunomodulators – Other

anakinra (Kineret) ▶K ♀B ▶? $$$$$
WARNING - Increased incidence of serious infections. Do not use in active infection or with TNF-blocking drugs such as adalimumab, etanercept or infliximab.

ADULT - RA: 100 mg SC daily, alone or in combo with other disease-modifying antirheumatic drugs (DMARDs) except TNF inhibitors.

PEDS - Not approved in children.

FORMS - Trade only: 100 mg pre-filled glass syringes with needles, 7 or 28 per box.

NOTES - Monitor for neutropenia. Refrigerate & protect from light. Avoid live vaccines.

leflunomide (Arava) ▶LK ♀X ▶- $$$$$
WARNING - Hepatotoxicity, interstitial lung disease. Rare reports of lymphoma, pancytopenia, agranulocytosis, thrombocytopenia, Stevens-Johnson Syndrome, cutaneous necrotizing vasculitis & severe HTN. Exclude pregnancy before starting. Women of childbearing potential must use reliable contraception.

ADULT - RA: 100 mg PO daily x 3 days. Maintenance: 10-20 mg PO daily.

PEDS - Not approved in children.

UNAPPROVED ADULT - Psoriatic arthritis: Initial: 100 mg PO daily x 3 days. Maintenance: 10-20 mg PO daily.

FORMS - Generic/Trade: Tabs 10, 20 mg. Trade only: Tab 100 mg.

NOTES - Avoid in hepatic or renal insufficiency. Monitor LFTs, CBC & creatinine monthly until stable, then q 1-2 months. Avoid in men wishing to father children or with concurrent live vaccines. May increase INR if on warfarin; check INR within 1-2 days of initiation, then weekly for 2-3 weeks & adjust the dose accordingly. Rifampin increases and cholestyramine decreases leflunomide levels. Give charcoal or cholestyramine in cases of overdose or drug toxicity. Cholestyramine: 8 g PO tid for up to 11 days. Administration on consecutive days is not necessary unless rapid elimination desired.

ANALGESICS: Antirheumatic Agents – Other

azathioprine (Azasan, Imuran, ✦Immunoprin, Oprisine) ▶LK ♀D ▶- $$$
WARNING - Chronic immunosuppression with azathioprine increases neoplasia risk. May cause marrow suppression or GI hypersensitivity reaction characterized by severe N/V.

ADULT - Severe RA: Initial dose 1 mg/kg (50-100 mg) PO daily or divided bid. Increase by 0.5 mg/kg/day at 6-8 weeks; if no serious toxicity and if initial response is unsatisfactory can then increase thereafter at 4-week intervals. Max dose 2.5 mg/kg/day. In patients with clinical response, use the lowest effective dose for maintenance therapy.

PEDS - Not approved in children.

UNAPPROVED ADULT - Crohn's disease: 75-100 mg PO daily. Myasthenia gravis: 2-3 mg/kg/day PO. Behcet's syndrome, SLE: 2.5 mg/kg/day PO. Vasculitis: 2 mg/kg/day PO.

UNAPPROVED PEDS - JRA: Initial: 1 mg/kg/day PO. Increase by 0.5 mg/kg/day every 4 weeks until response or max dose of 2.5-3 mg/kg/day.

FORMS - Generic/Trade: Tabs 50 mg, scored. Trade only (Azasan): 75, 100 mg, scored.

NOTES - Monitor CBC q 1-2 weeks with dose changes, then q 1-3 months. ACE inhibitors, allopurinol, & methotrexate may increase activity & toxicity. Azathioprine may decrease the activity of anticoagulants, cyclosporine, & neuromuscular blockers.

hydroxychloroquine (Plaquenil) ▶K ♀C ▶+ $$$

ADULT - RA: 400-600 mg PO daily to start, taken with food or milk. After clinical response, decrease to 200-400 mg PO daily. Discontinue if no objective improvement within 6 months. SLE: 400 mg PO daily-bid to start. Decrease to 200-400 PO daily for prolonged maintenance.

PEDS - Not approved in children.

UNAPPROVED PEDS - JRA or SLE: 3-5 mg/kg/day, up to a max of 400 mg/day PO daily or divided bid. Max dose 7 mg/kg/day. Take with food or milk.

FORMS - Generic/Trade: Tabs 200 mg, scored.

NOTES - May exacerbate psoriasis or porphyria. Irreversible retinal damage possible with long-term or high dosage (>6.5 mg/kg/day). Baseline & periodic eye exams recommended. Anorexia, nausea & vomiting may occur. May increase digoxin and metoprolol levels.

methotrexate (Rheumatrex, Trexall) ▶LK

♀X ▶- $$

WARNING - Deaths have occurred from hepatotoxicity, pulmonary disease, intestinal perforation and marrow suppression. According to the manufacturer, use is restricted to severe, recalcitrant, disabling rheumatic disease unresponsive to other therapy. Use with extreme caution in renal insufficiency. May see diarrhea. Folate deficiency states may increase toxicity. The American College of Rheumatology recommends supplementation with 1 mg/day of folic acid.

ADULT - Severe RA, psoriasis: 7.5 mg/week PO single dose or 2.5 mg PO q12h x 3 doses given as a course once weekly. May be increased gradually to a max weekly dose of 20 mg. After clinical response, reduce to lowest effective dose. Psoriasis: 10-25 mg weekly IV/IM until response, then decrease to lowest effective dose. Supplement with 1 mg/day of folic acid. Chemotherapy doses vary by indication. Gestational trophoblastic tumors. ALL, treatment & prophylaxis of meningeal leukemia. Burkitt's lymphoma. Breast cancer. Head & neck cancer. Advanced mycosis fungoides. Squamous cell & small cell lung cancer. Advanced-stage non-Hodgkin's lymphomas, in combination regimens. Non-metastatic osteosarcoma w/leucovorin rescue.

PEDS - Chemotherapy doses vary by indication. ALL, treatment & prophylaxis of meningeal leukemia. Severe JRA: 10 mg/m² PO q week.

UNAPPROVED ADULT - Severe RA, psoriasis: 25 mg PO q week. After clinical response, reduce to lowest effective dose. Supplement with 1 mg/day of folic acid. Non-metastatic osteosarcoma with leucovorin rescue.

FORMS - Trade only (Trexall): Tabs 5, 7.5, 10, 15 mg. Dose Pak (Rheumatrex) 2.5mg (#8,12, 16,20,24's). Generic/Trade: Tabs 2.5 mg, scored.

NOTES - Contraindicated in pregnant & lactating women, alcoholism, liver disease, immunodeficiency, blood dyscrasias. Avoid ethanol. Monitor CBC q month, liver & renal function q 1-3 months.

ANALGESICS: Muscle Relaxants

NOTE: May cause drowsiness and/or sedation, which may be enhanced by alcohol and other CNS depressants.

baclofen (Lioresal, Kemstro) ▶K ♀C ▶+ $$

WARNING - Abrupt discontinuation of intrathecal baclofen has been associated with life-threatening sequelae and/or death.

ADULT - Spasticity related to MS or spinal cord

disease/injury: 5 mg PO tid x 3 days, 10 mg PO tid x 3 days, 15 mg PO tid x 3 days, then 20 mg PO tid x 3 days. Max dose: 20 mg PO qid. Spasticity related to spinal cord disease/injury, unresponsive to oral therapy: Specialized dosing via implantable intrathecal pump.

PEDS - Spasticity related to spinal cord disease/injury: Specialized dosing via implantable intrathecal pump.

UNAPPROVED ADULT - Trigeminal neuralgia: 30-80 mg/day PO divided tid-qid. Tardive dyskinesia: 40-60 mg/day PO divided tid-qid. Intractable hiccoughs: 15-45 mg PO divided tid.

UNAPPROVED PEDS - Spasticity: ≥2 yo: 10-15 mg/day PO divided q8h. Max dose 40 mg/day for 2-7 yo, 60 mg/day for ≥8 yo.

FORMS - Generic: Tabs 10, 20 mg. Trade only: (Kemstro) Tabs-orally disintegrating 10, 20 mg.

NOTES - Hallucinations & seizures with abrupt withdrawal. Administer with caution if impaired renal function. Efficacy not established for rheumatic disorders, stroke, cerebral palsy, or Parkinson's disease.

carisoprodol (Soma) ▶LK ♀? ▶- $

ADULT - Acute musculoskeletal pain: 350 mg PO tid-qid with meals and qhs.

PEDS - Not approved in children.

FORMS - Generic/Trade: Tabs 350 mg.

NOTES - Contraindicated in porphyria, caution in renal or hepatic insufficiency. Abuse potential; caution if addiction-prone. Withdrawal and possible seizures with abrupt discontinuation.

chlorzoxazone (Parafon Forte DSC) ▶LK ♀C ▶? $

WARNING - If signs/symptoms of liver dysfunction are observed, discontinue use.

ADULT - Musculoskeletal pain: Start 500 mg PO tid-qid, increase prn to 750 mg tid-qid. After improvement, decrease to 250 mg PO tid-qid.

PEDS - Not approved in children.

UNAPPROVED PEDS - Musculoskeletal pain: 125-500 mg PO tid-qid or 20 mg/kg/day divided tid-qid depending on age & weight.

FORMS - Generic/Trade: Tabs & caplets 250 & 500 mg (Parafon Forte DSC 500 mg tablets scored).

NOTES - Caution with history of drug allergies. Discontinue if allergic drug reactions occur or for signs/symptoms of liver dysfunction. May turn urine orange or purple-red.

cyclobenzaprine (Amrix, Flexeril) ▶LK ♀B ▶? $

ADULT - Musculoskeletal pain: 5-10 mg PO tid up to max dose of 60 mg/day or 15-30 mg (extended release) PO daily. Not recommended in elderly or for use >2-3 weeks.

PEDS - Not approved in children.

FORMS - Generic/Trade: Tab 5, 10 mg. Generic only: Tab 7.5 mg. Trade only: (Amrix) Extended-release caps 15, 30 mg.

NOTES - Contraindicated with recent or concomitant MAO inhibitor use, immediately post-MI, in patients with arrhythmias, conduction disturbances, heart failure, & hyperthyroidism. Not effective for cerebral or spinal cord disease or in children with cerebral palsy. May have similar adverse effects & drug interactions as TCAs. Caution with urinary retention, angle-closure glaucoma, increased ocular pressure.

dantrolene (Dantrium) ▶LK ♀C ▶- $$$$

WARNING - Hepatotoxicity, monitor LFTs. Use the lowest possible effective dose.

ADULT - Chronic spasticity related to spinal cord injury, stroke, cerebral palsy, MS: 25 mg PO daily to start, increase to 25 mg bid-qid, then by 25 mg up to max of 100 mg bid-qid if necessary. Maintain each dosage level for 4-7 days to determine response. Use the lowest effective dose. Malignant hyperthermia: 2.5 mg/kg rapid IV push q 5-10 minutes continuing until symptoms subside or to a maximum 10 mg/kg/dose. Doses of up to 40 mg/kg have been used. Follow with 4-8 mg/kg/day PO divided tid-qid x 1-3 days to prevent recurrence.

PEDS - Chronic spasticity: 0.5 mg/kg PO bid to start; increase to 0.5 mg/kg tid-qid, then by increments of 0.5 mg/kg up to 3 mg/kg bid-qid. Max dose 100 mg PO qid. Malignant hyperthermia: use adult dose.

UNAPPROVED ADULT - Neuroleptic malignant syndrome, heat stroke: 1-3 mg/kg/day PO/IV divided qid.

FORMS - Generic/Trade: Caps 25, 50, 100 mg.

NOTES - Photosensitization may occur. Warfarin may decrease protein binding of dantrolene & increase dantrolene's effect. The following website may be useful for malignant hyperthermia: www.mhaus.org

metaxalone (Skelaxin) ▶LK ♀? ▶? $$$

ADULT - Musculoskeletal pain: 800 mg PO tid-qid.

PEDS - >12 yo: use adult dose.

FORMS - Trade only: Tabs 800 mg, scored.

NOTES - Contraindicated in serious renal or hepatic insufficiency or history of drug-induced hemolytic or other anemia. Beware of hypersensitivity reactions, leukopenia, hemolytic anemia, & jaundice. Monitor LFTs. Coadministration with food, especially a high fat meal, enhances absorption significantly and may increase CNS depression.

methocarbamol (*Robaxin, Robaxin-750*) ▶LK ♀C ▶? $$
ADULT - Musculoskeletal pain, acute relief: 1500 mg PO qid or 1000 mg IM/IV tid x 48-72h. Maintenance: 1000 mg PO qid, 750 mg PO q4h, or 1500 mg PO tid. Tetanus: specialized dosing.
PEDS - Tetanus: Specialized dosing.
FORMS - Generic/Trade: Tabs 500 & 750 mg. OTC in Canada.
NOTES - Max IV rate 3 mL/min to avoid syncope, hypotension, & bradycardia. Total parenteral dosage should not exceed 3 g/day for >3 consecutive days, except in the treatment of tetanus. Urine may turn brown, black or green.

orphenadrine (*Norflex*) ▶LK ♀C ▶? $$
ADULT - Musculoskeletal pain: 100 mg PO bid. 60 mg IV/IM bid.
PEDS - Not approved in children.
UNAPPROVED ADULT - Leg cramps: 100 mg PO qhs.
FORMS - Generic only: 100 mg extended release. OTC in Canada.
NOTES - Contraindicated in glaucoma, pyloric or duodenal obstruction, BPH, & myasthenia gravis. Some products contain sulfites, which may cause allergic reactions. May increase anticholinergic effects of amantadine & decrease therapeutic effects of phenothiazines. Side effects include dry mouth, urinary retention and hesitancy, constipation, headache & GI upset.

tizanidine (*Zanaflex*) ▶LK ♀C ▶? $$$$
ADULT - Muscle spasticity due to MS or spinal cord injury: 4-8 mg PO q6-8h prn, max dose 36 mg/day.
PEDS - Not approved in children.
FORMS - Generic/Trade: Tabs 2, 4 mg, scored. Trade only: Caps 2, 4, 6 mg.
NOTES - Monitor LFTs. Avoid with hepatic or renal insufficiency. Alcohol, oral contraceptives, fluvoxamine & ciprofloxacin increase tizanidine levels; may cause significant decreases in blood pressure & increased drowsiness and psychomotor impairment. Concurrent antihypertensives may exacerbate hypotension. Dry mouth, somnolence, sedation, asthenia & dizziness most common side effects.

ANALGESICS: Non-Opioid Analgesic Combinations

NOTE: Refer to individual components for further information. Carisoprodol and butalbital may be habit-forming; butalbital contraindicated with porphyria. May cause drowsiness and/or sedation, which may be enhanced by alcohol & other CNS depressants. Avoid exceeding 4 g/day of acetaminophen in combo products. Caution those who drink ≥3 alcoholic drinks/day to limit acetaminophen to 2.5 g/day due to additive liver toxicity.

Ascriptin **(aspirin + aluminum hydroxide + magnesium hydroxide + calcium carbonate, Aspir-Mox)** ▶K ♀D ▶? $
WARNING - Multiple strengths; see FORMS.
ADULT - Pain: 1-2 tabs PO q4h.
PEDS - Not approved in children.
FORMS - OTC: Trade only: Tabs 325 mg ASA/ 50 mg Mg hydroxide/50 mg Al hydroxide/50 mg Ca carbonate (Ascriptin & Aspir-Mox). 500 mg ASA/33 mg Mg hydroxide/33 mg Al hydroxide/ 237 mg Ca carb (Ascriptin Extra Strength).

Bufferin **(aspirin + calcium carbonate + magnesium oxide + magnesium carbonate)** ▶K ♀D ▶? $
ADULT - Pain: 1-2 tabs/caplets PO q4h while symptoms persist. Max 12 in 24 hours.
PEDS - Not approved in children.
FORMS - OTC: Trade only: Tabs/caplets 325 mg ASA/158 mg Ca carbonate/63 mg of Mg oxide/34 mg of Mg carbonate. Bufferin ES: 500 mg ASA/222.3 mg Ca carbonate/88.9 mg of Mg oxide/55.6 mg of Mg carbonate

Esgic **(acetaminophen + butalbital + caffeine)** ▶LK ♀C ▶? $
WARNING - Multiple strengths; see FORMS & write specific product on Rx.
ADULT - Tension or muscle contraction headache: 1-2 tabs/caps PO q4h. Max 6 in 24 hrs.
PEDS - Not approved in children.
FORMS - Generic/Trade: Tabs/caps Esgic is 325/50/40 mg of acetaminophen/butalbital/caffeine. Esgic Plus is 500/50/40 mg.

Excedrin Migraine **(acetaminophen + aspirin + caffeine)** ▶LK ♀D ▶? $
ADULT - Migraine headache: 2 tabs/caps/gel-tabs PO q6h while symptoms persist. Max 8 in 24 hours.
PEDS - ≥12 yo: Use adult dose.
FORMS - OTC/Generic/Trade: Tabs/caplets/gel-tabs acetaminophen 250 mg/ASA 250 mg/caffeine 65 mg.

Fioricet **(acetaminophen + butalbital + caffeine)** ▶LK ♀C ▶? $
ADULT - Tension or muscle contraction headache: 1-2 tabs PO q4h. Max 6 in 24 hours.
PEDS - Not approved in children.
FORMS - Generic/Trade: Tab 325 mg acetaminophen/50 mg butalbital/40 mg caffeine.

Fiorinal **(aspirin + butalbital + caffeine,** ✝*Tecnal, Trianal)* ▶KL ♀D ▶- ©III $
ADULT - Tension or muscle contraction headache: 1-2 tabs PO q4h. Max 6 tabs in 24 hours.
PEDS - Not approved in children.
FORMS - Generic/Trade: Cap 325 mg aspirin/50 mg butalbital/40 mg caffeine.

Goody's Extra Strength Headache Powder **(acetaminophen + aspirin + caffeine)** ▶LK ♀D ▶? $
ADULT - Headache: Place one powder on tongue and follow with liquid, or stir powder into a glass of water or other liquid. Repeat in 4-6 hours prn. Max 4 powders in 24 hours.
PEDS - ≥12 yo: Use adult dose.
FORMS - OTC trade only: 260 mg acetaminophen/520 mg ASA/32.5 mg caffeine per powder paper.

Norgesic **(orphenadrine + aspirin + caffeine)** ▶KL ♀D ▶? $$
WARNING - Multiple strengths; see FORMS & write specific product on Rx.
ADULT - Musculoskeletal pain: Norgesic: 1-2 tabs PO tid-qid. Norgesic Forte: 1 tab tid-qid.
PEDS - Not approved in children.
FORMS - Generic/Trade: Tabs Norgesic 25/385/30 mg of orphenadrine/aspirin/caffeine. Norgesic Forte 50/770/60 mg.

Phrenilin **(acetaminophen + butalbital)** ▶LK ♀C ▶? $
WARNING - Multiple strengths; see FORMS & write specific product on Rx.
ADULT - Tension or muscle contraction headache: Phrenilin: 1-2 tabs PO q4h. Phrenilin Forte: 1 cap PO q4h. Max 6 in 24 hours.
PEDS - Not approved in children.
FORMS - Generic/Trade: Tabs Phrenilin 325/50 mg of acetaminophen/butalbital. Caps Phrenilin Forte 650/50 mg.

Sedapap **(acetaminophen + butalbital)** ▶LK ♀C ▶? $
ADULT - Tension or muscle contraction headache: 1-2 tabs PO q4h. Max 6 tabs in 24 hours.
PEDS - Not approved in children.
FORMS - Generic/Trade: Tab 650 mg acetaminophen/50 mg butalbital.

Soma Compound **(carisoprodol + aspirin)** ▶LK ♀D ▶- $$$
ADULT - Musculoskeletal pain: 1-2 tabs PO qid.
PEDS - Not approved in children.
FORMS - Generic/Trade: Tab 200 mg carisoprodol/325 mg ASA.
NOTES - Carisoprodol may be habit forming. Withdrawal with abrupt discontinuation.

Ultracet **(tramadol + acetaminophen,** ✝*Tramacet)* ▶KL ♀C ▶- $$
ADULT - Acute pain: 2 tabs PO q4-6h prn, max 8 tabs/day for no more than 5 days. If creatinine clearance <30ml/min, increase the dosing interval to 12 hours. Consider a similar adjustment in elderly patients and in cirrhosis.
PEDS - Not approved in children.
FORMS - Generic/Trade: Tab 37.5 mg tramadol/325 mg acetaminophen.
NOTES - Do not use with other acetaminophen-containing drugs due to potential for hepatotoxicity. Contraindicated in acute intoxication with alcohol, hypnotics, centrally-acting analgesics, opioids or psychotropic drugs. Seizures may occur with concurrent antidepressants or with seizure disorder. Use with great caution with MAO inhibitors or in combination with SSRIs due to potential for serotonin syndrome; dose adjustment may be needed. Withdrawal symptoms may occur in patients dependent on opioids or with abrupt discontinuation. Overdose treated with naloxone may increase seizure risk. The most frequent side effects are somnolence & constipation.

ANALGESICS: Nonsteroidal Anti-Inflammatories – COX-2 Inhibitor

celecoxib (*Celebrex*) ▶L ♀C (D in 3rd trimester) ▶? $$$$$
WARNING - The risk of serious cardiovascular events and gastrointestinal bleeding may be increased in patients taking long-term, high-dose NSAIDs, both COX-2 inhibitors as well as non-selective agents. All NSAIDs and COX-2 inhibitors are contraindicated immediately post-CABG surgery. The FDA advises evaluating alternative therapy or using the lowest effective dose. Fewer GI side effects than 1st generation NSAIDs & no effect on platelets, but other NSAID-related side effects (renal dysfunction, fluid retention, CNS) are possible. May cause

fluid retention or exacerbate heart failure. May elevate BP or blunt effects of antihypertensives & loop diuretics. Not substitutes for aspirin for cardiovascular prophylaxis due to lack of anti-platelet effects. Monitor INR with warfarin. May increase lithium levels. Caution in aspirin-sensitive asthma. Use around the time of conception appears to increase the risk of miscarriage (use acetaminophen instead).

ADULT - OA, ankylosing spondilitis: 200 mg PO daily or 100 mg PO bid. RA: 100-200 mg PO bid. Familial adenomatous polyposis (FAP), as an adjunct to usual care: 400 mg PO bid with food. Acute pain, dysmenorrhea: 400 mg x 1, then 200 mg PO bid. May take an additional 200 mg on day 1.

PEDS - JRA: 2-17 yo: 10-25 kg: 50 mg PO bid. >25 kg: 100 mg PO bid.

FORMS - Trade: Caps 50, 100, 200, 400 mg.

NOTES - Contraindicated in sulfonamide allergy. Decrease dose by 50% with hepatic dysfunction. Capsules may be opened and sprinkled into one teaspoon of apple sauce & taken immediately with water.

ANALGESICS: Nonsteroidal Anti-Inflammatories – Salicylic Acid Derivatives

NOTE: The risk of serious cardiovascular events and gastrointestinal bleeding may be increased in patients taking long-term, high-dose NSAIDs, both COX-2 inhibitors as well as non-selective agents (excluding aspirin). All NSAIDs and COX-2 inhibitors are contraindicated immediately post-CABG surgery. The FDA advises evaluating alternative therapy or using the lowest effective dose of these drugs. Avoid in ASA allergy, and in children and teenagers <17 yo with chickenpox or flu due to association with Reye's syndrome. May potentiate warfarin, heparin, valproic acid, methotrexate. Unlike aspirin, derivatives may have less GI toxicity & negligible effects on platelet aggregation & renal prostaglandins. Caution in aspirin-sensitive asthma. Ibuprofen and possibly other NSAIDs may antagonize antiplatelet effects of aspirin if given simultaneously. Use around the time of conception appears to increase the risk of miscarriage (use acetaminophen instead).

aspirin *(Ecotrin, Empirin, Halfprin, Bayer, Anacin, Zorprin, ASA, ♥Asaphen, Entrophen, Novasen)* ▶K ♀D ▶? $

ADULT - Mild to moderate pain, fever: 325-650 mg PO/PR q4h prn. Acute rheumatic fever: 5-8 g/day, initially. RA/OA: 3.2-6 g/day in divided doses. Platelet aggregation inhibition: 81-325 mg PO daily.

PEDS - Mild to moderate pain, fever: 10-15 mg/kg/dose PO q4-6h not to exceed 60-80 mg/kg/day. JRA: 60-100 mg/kg/day PO divided q6-8h. Acute rheumatic fever: 100 mg/kg/day PO/PR x 2 weeks, then 75 mg/kg/day x 4-6 weeks. Kawasaki disease: 80-100 mg/kg/day PO/PR until fever resolves, then 3-5 mg/kg/day PO qam x 7 weeks or longer if there is ECG evidence of coronary artery abnormalities.

UNAPPROVED ADULT - Primary prevention of cardiovascular events (10-year CHD risk >6-10% based on Framingham risk scoring): 75-325 mg PO daily. Post ST-elevation MI: 162-325 mg PO on day 1, continue indefinitely at 75-162 mg/day. Post Non-ST-elevation MI: 160-325 mg PO on day 1, continue indefinitely at 75-160 mg/day. Long-term antithrombotic therapy for chronic atrial fib/flutter in patients with low-moderate risk of stroke (<75 years without risk factors): 325 mg PO daily. Percutaneous coronary intervention pretreatment: Already taking daily ASA therapy: 75-325 mg PO before procedure. Not already taking daily ASA therapy: 300-325 mg PO at least 2-24 hrs before procedure. Post percutaneous coronary intervention: 325 mg daily in combination with clopidogrel for ≥1 month after bare metal stent placement, ≥3 months after sirolimus-eluting stent placement, ≥6 months after paclitaxel-stent placement; then 75-162 mg PO daily indefinitely. Post percutaneous coronary brachytherapy: 75-325 mg daily in combination with clopidogrel indefinitely.

FORMS - Generic/Trade (OTC): tabs, 325,500 mg; chewable 81 mg; enteric-coated 81,162 mg (Halfprin), 81,325,500 mg (Ecotrin), 650, 975 mg. Trade only: tabs, controlled-release 650,800 mg (ZORprin, Rx). Generic only (OTC): suppository 120,200,300,600 mg.

NOTES - Consider discontinuing 1 week prior to surgery (except coronary bypass or in 1st year post-coronary stent) because of the possibility of postoperative bleeding. Aspirin intolerance occurs in 4%-19% of asthmatics. Use caution in liver damage, renal insufficiency, peptic ulcer or bleeding tendencies. Crush or chew tabs (including enteric-coated products) in first dose with acute MI. Higher doses of aspirin (1.3

g/day) have not been shown to be superior to low doses in preventing TIAs and strokes.

choline magnesium trisalicylate (*Trilisate*) ▶K ♀C (D in 3rd trimester) ▶? $$

ADULT - RA/OA: 1500 mg PO bid. Mild to moderate pain, fever: 1000-1500 mg PO bid.

PEDS - RA, mild to moderate pain: 50 mg/kg/day (up to 37 kg) PO divided bid.

FORMS - Generic/Trade: Tabs 750. Generic: Tabs 500, 1000 mg. Solution 500 mg/5mL.

diflunisal (*Dolobid*) ▶K ♀C (D in 3rd trimester) ▶- $$$

ADULT - Mild to moderate pain: Initially: 500 mg-1g PO, then 250-500 mg PO q8-12h. RA/OA: 500 mg-1g PO divided bid. Max dose 1.5g/day.

PEDS - Not approved in children.

FORMS - Generic/Trade: Tabs 250 & 500 mg.

NOTES - Do not crush or chew tablets. Increases acetaminophen levels.

salsalate (*Salflex, Disalcid, Amigesic*) ▶K ♀C (D in 3rd trimester) ▶? $$

ADULT - RA/OA: 3000 mg/day PO divided q8-12h.

PEDS - Not approved in children.

FORMS - Generic/Trade: Tabs 500 & 750 mg, scored.

NSAIDSs – If one class fails, consider another. *Salicylic acid derivatives:* aspirin, diflunisal, salsalate, Trilisate. *Propionic acids:* flurbiprofen, ibuprofen, ketoprofen, naproxen, oxaprozin. *Acetic acids:* diclofenac, etodolac, indomethacin, ketorolac, nabumetone, sulindac, tolmetin. *Fenamates:* meclofenamate. *Oxicams:* meloxicam, piroxicam. *COX-2 inhibitors:* celecoxib.

ANALGESICS: Nonsteroidal Anti-Inflammatories – Other

NOTE: The risk of serious cardiovascular events & gastrointestinal bleeding may be increased when taking long-term, high-dose NSAIDs, both COX-2 inhibitors as well as non-selective agents. All NSAIDs and COX-2 inhibitors are contraindicated immediately post-CABG surgery. The FDA advises evaluating alternative therapy or using the lowest effective dose of these drugs. Chronic use associated with renal insufficiency, gastritis, peptic ulcer disease, GI bleeds. Caution in liver disease. May cause fluid retention or exacerbate heart failure. May elevate BP or blunt effects of antihypertensives & loop diuretics. May increase levels of methotrexate, lithium, phenytoin, digoxin & cyclosporine. May potentiate warfarin. Caution in aspirin-sensitive asthma. Ibuprofen or other NSAIDs may antagonize antiplatelet effects of aspirin if given simultaneously. Use around the time of conception appears to increase the risk of miscarriage (use acetaminophen instead).

Arthrotec (diclofenac + misoprostol) ▶LK ♀X ▶- $$$$$

WARNING - Because of the abortifacient property of the misoprostol component, it is contraindicated in women who are pregnant. Caution in women with childbearing potential; effective contraception is essential.

ADULT - OA: one 50/200 PO tid. RA: one 50/200 PO tid-qid. If intolerant, may use 50/200 or 75/200 PO bid.

PEDS - Not approved in children.

FORMS - Trade only: Tabs 50/200, 75/200 mg

diclofenac/mcg misoprostol.

NOTES - Refer to individual components. Abdominal pain & diarrhea may occur. Check LFTs at baseline then periodically. Do not crush or chew tablets.

diclofenac (*Voltaren, Voltaren XR, Cataflam, Flector*, ♥*Voltaren Rapide*) ▶L ♀B (D in 3rd trimester) ▶- $$$

WARNING - Multiple strengths; see FORMS & write specific product on Rx.

ADULT - OA: immediate or delayed release 50 mg PO bid-tid or 75 mg bid. Extended release 100 mg PO daily. RA: immediate or delayed release 50 mg PO tid-qid or 75 mg bid. Extended release 100 mg PO daily-bid. Ankylosing spondylitis: immediate or delayed release 25 mg PO qid & hs. Analgesia & primary dysmenorrhea: immediate or delayed release 50 mg PO tid. Acute pain of strains, sprains or contusions: Apply one patch to painful area bid.

PEDS - Not approved in children.

UNAPPROVED PEDS - JRA: 2-3 mg/kg/d PO.

FORMS - Generic/Trade: Tabs, immediate-release (Cataflam) 50 mg, extended-release (Voltaren XR) 100 mg. Generic only: Tabs, delayed-release 25, 50, 75 mg. Trade: Patch, 1.3% diclofenac epolamine.

NOTES - Check LFTs at baseline then periodically. Do not apply patch to damaged or non-intact skin. Wash hands and avoid eye contact when handling the patch. Do not wear patch while bathing or showering.

etodolac (Lodine, ✤Ultradol) ▶L ♀C (D in 3rd trimester) ▶- $$$
WARNING - Multiple strengths; write specific product on Rx.
ADULT - OA: 400 mg PO bid-tid. 300 mg PO bid-qid. 200 mg tid-qid. Extended release 400-1200 mg PO daily. Mild to moderate pain: 200-400 mg q6-8h. Max dose 1200 mg/day or if ≤60 kg, 20 mg/kg/day.
PEDS - Not approved in children.
UNAPPROVED ADULT - RA, ankylosing spondylitis: 300-400 mg PO bid. Tendinitis, bursitis & acute gout: 300-400 mg bid-qid then taper.
FORMS - Generic/Trade: Caps, immediate-release 300 mg. Generic only: Tabs, immediate-release 400 & 500 mg. Caps, immediate-release 200 mg. Tabs, extended-release 400, 500, 600 mg.

flurbiprofen (Ansaid, ✤Froben, Froben SR) ▶L ♀B (D in 3rd trimester) ▶+ $$$
ADULT - RA/OA: 200-300 mg/day PO divided bid-qid. Max single dose 100 mg.
PEDS - Not approved in children.
UNAPPROVED ADULT - Ankylosing spondylitis: 150-300 mg/day PO divided bid-qid. Mild to moderate pain: 50 mg PO q6h. Primary dysmenorrhea: 50 mg PO daily at onset, d/c when pain subsides. Tendinitis, bursitis, acute gout, acute migraine: 100 mg PO at onset, then 50 mg PO qid, then taper.
UNAPPROVED PEDS - JRA: 4 mg/kg/day PO.
FORMS - Generic/Trade: Tabs immediate-release 50 & 100 mg.

ibuprofen (Motrin, Advil, Nuprin, Rufen, Neoprofen) ▶L ♀B (D in 3rd trimester) ▶+ $
ADULT - RA/OA: 200-800 mg PO tid-qid. Mild to moderate pain: 400 mg PO q4-6h. Primary dysmenorrhea: 400 mg PO q4h prn. Fever: 200 mg PO q4-6h prn. Migraine pain: 200-400 mg PO not to exceed 400 mg in 24 hours unless directed by a physician (OTC dosing). Max dose 3.2 g/day.
PEDS - JRA: 30-50 mg/kg/day PO divided q6h. Max dose 2400 mg/24h. 20 mg/kg/day may be adequate for milder disease. Analgesic/antipyretic >6 mo: 5-10 mg/kg PO q6-8h, prn. Max dose 40 mg/kg/day. Patent ductus arteriosus in neonates ≤ 32 weeks gestational age weighing 500-1500 g (NeoProfen): Specialized dosing.
FORMS - OTC: Cap/Liqui-Gel Cap 200 mg. Tabs 100, 200 mg. Chewable tabs 50, 100 mg. Liquid & suspension 50 mg/1.25ml, 100 mg/5 mL, suspension 100 mg/2.5 mL. Infant drops 50 mg/1.25 mL (calibrated dropper). Rx only:

Tabs 300, 400, 600, 800 mg.
NOTES - May antagonize antiplatelet effects of aspirin if given simultaneously. Take aspirin 2 hours prior to ibuprofen.

indomethacin (Indocin, Indocin SR, Indocin IV, ✤Indocid-P.D.A.) ▶L ♀B (D in 3rd trimester) ▶+ $
WARNING - Multiple strengths; see FORMS & write specific product on Rx. Use during labor increases risk of fetal/maternal complications: premature closure of the ductus arteriosus, fetal pulmonary hypertension, oligohydramnios, higher rate of postpartum hemorrhage.
ADULT - RA/OA, ankylosing spondylitis: 25 mg PO bid-tid to start. Increase incrementally to a total daily dose of 150-200 mg. Bursitis/tendinitis: 75-150 mg/day PO divided tid-qid. Acute gout: 50 mg PO tid until pain tolerable, rapidly taper dose to D/C. Sustained release: 75 mg PO daily-bid.
PEDS - Closure of patent ductus arteriosus in neonates: Initial dose 0.2 mg/kg IV, if additional doses necessary, dose and frequency (q12h or q24h) based on age and urine output.
UNAPPROVED ADULT - Primary dysmenorrhea: 25 mg PO tid-qid. Cluster headache: 75-150 mg SR PO daily. Polyhydramnios: 2.2-3.0 mg/kg/day PO based on maternal weight; premature closure of the ductus arteriosus has been reported. Preterm labor: initial 50-100 mg PO followed by 25 mg PO q6-12h up to 48 hrs.
UNAPPROVED PEDS - JRA: 1-3 mg/kg/day tid-qid to start. Increase prn to max dose of 4 mg/kg/d or 200 mg/d, whichever is less.
FORMS - Generic/Trade: Caps, immediate-release 25 & 50 mg. Oral suspension 25 mg/5 mL. Cap, sustained-release 75 mg.
NOTES - May aggravate depression or other psychiatric disturbances. Do not crush sustained release capsule.

ketoprofen (Orudis, Orudis KT, Actron, Oruvail, ✤Orudis SR) ▶L ♀B (D in 3rd trimester) ▶- $$$
ADULT - RA/OA: 75 mg PO tid or 50 mg PO qid. Extended release 200 mg PO daily. Mild to moderate pain, primary dysmenorrhea: 25-50 mg PO q6-8h prn.
PEDS - Not approved in children.
UNAPPROVED PEDS - JRA: 100-200 mg/m²/day PO. Max dose 320 mg/day.
FORMS - OTC: Tab immediate-release 12.5mg. Rx: Generic/Trade: Caps ext'd-release 200 mg. Generic only: Caps, immediate-release 25, 50 & 75 mg. Caps, extended-release 100,150 mg.

ketorolac (*Toradol*) ▶L ♀C (D in 3rd trimester) ▶+ $

WARNING - Indicated for short-term (up to 5 days) therapy only. Ketorolac is a potent NSAID and can cause serious GI and renal adverse effects. It may also increase the risk of bleeding by inhibiting platelet function. Contraindicated in patients with active peptic ulcer disease, recent GI bleeding or perforation, a history of peptic ulcer disease or GI bleeding, and advanced renal impairment.

ADULT - Moderately severe, acute pain, single-dose treatment: 30-60 mg IM or 15-30 mg IV. Multiple-dose treatment: 15-30 mg IV/IM q6h. IV/IM doses are not to exceed 60 mg/day in patients ≥65 yo, <50 kg, & for patients with moderately elevated serum creatinine. Oral continuation therapy: 10 mg PO q4-6h prn, max dose 40 mg/day. Combined duration IV/IM and PO is not to exceed 5 days.

PEDS - Not approved in children.

UNAPPROVED PEDS - Pain: 0.5 mg/kg/dose IM/IV q6h not to exceed 30 mg q6h or 120 mg/day. >50 kg: 10 mg PO q6h prn not to exceed 40 mg/day.

FORMS - Generic/Trade: Tab 10 mg.

meclofenamate ▶L ♀B (D in 3rd trimester) ▶- $$$

ADULT - Mild to moderate pain: 50 mg PO q4-6h prn. Max dose 400 mg/day. Menorrhagia & primary dysmenorrhea: 100 mg PO tid for up to 6 days. RA/OA: 200-400 mg/day PO divided tid-qid.

PEDS - Not approved in children.

UNAPPROVED PEDS - JRA: 3-7.5 mg/kg/day PO. Max dose 300 mg/day.

FORMS - Generic only: Caps 50 & 100 mg.

NOTES - Reversible autoimmune hemolytic anemia with use for >12 months.

mefenamic acid (*Ponstel*, ✚*Ponstan*) ▶L ♀D ▶- $$$

ADULT - Mild to moderate pain, primary dysmenorrhea: 500 mg PO initially, then 250 mg PO q6h prn for ≤1 week.

PEDS - >14 yo: use adult dose.

FORMS - Trade only: Cap 250 mg.

meloxicam (*Mobic*, ✚*Mobicox*) ▶L ♀C (D in 3rd trimester) ▶? $$$

ADULT - RA/OA: 7.5 mg PO daily. Max dose 15 mg/day.

PEDS - JRA, ≥2 yo: 0.125 mg/kg PO daily to max of 7.5 mg.

FORMS - Generic/Trade: Tabs 7.5, 15 mg. Trade: Suspension 7.5 mg/5 mL (1.5 mg/mL).

NOTES - Shake suspension gently before using. This is not a selective COX-2 inhibitor.

nabumetone (*Relafen*) ▶L ♀C (D in 3rd trimester) ▶- $$$

ADULT - RA/OA: Initial: two 500 mg tabs (1000 mg) PO daily. May increase to 1500-2000 mg PO daily or divided bid. Dosages >2000 mg/day have not been studied.

PEDS - Not approved in children.

FORMS - Generic/Trade: Tabs 500 & 750 mg.

naproxen (*Naprosyn, Aleve, Anaprox, EC-Naprosyn, Naprelan*) ▶L ♀B (D in 3rd trimester) ▶+ $$$

WARNING - Multiple strengths; see FORMS & write specific product on Rx.

ADULT - RA/OA, ankylosing spondylitis, pain, dysmenorrhea, acute tendinitis & bursitis, fever: 250-500 mg PO bid. Delayed release: 375-500 mg PO bid (do not crush or chew). Controlled release: 750-1000 mg PO daily. Acute gout: 750 mg PO x 1, then 250 mg PO q8h until the attack subsides. Controlled release: 1000-1500 mg PO x 1, then 1000 mg PO daily until the attack subsides.

PEDS - JRA: 10-20 mg/kg/day PO divided bid. Max dose 1250 mg/24h. Pain >2 yo: 5-7 mg/kg/dose PO q8-12h.

UNAPPROVED ADULT - Acute migraine: 750 mg PO x 1, then 250-500 mg PO prn. Migraine prophylaxis, menstrual migraine: 500 mg PO bid beginning one day prior to onset of menses and ending on last day of period.

FORMS - OTC: Generic/Trade: Tab immediate-release 200 mg. OTC Trade: Capsules & Gelcaps immediate-release 200 mg. Rx: Generic/Trade: Tabs immediate-release 250, 375, 500 mg. Delayed-release 375, 500 mg. Tabs delayed-release enteric coated (EC-Naprosyn) 375, 500 mg. Tabs, controlled-release (Naprelan) 375, 500 mg. Generic/Trade: Suspension 125 mg/5 mL.

NOTES - All dosing is based on naproxen; 500 mg naproxen = 550 mg naproxen sodium.

oxaprozin (*Daypro*) ▶L ♀C (D in 3rd trimester) ▶- $$$

ADULT - RA/OA: 1200 mg PO daily. Max dose 1800 mg/day or 26 mg/kg/day, whichever is lower.

PEDS - Not approved in children.

FORMS - Generic/Trade: Caplets, tabs 600 mg, trade scored.

piroxicam (*Feldene, Fexicam*) ▶L ♀B (in 3rd trimester) ▶+ $$$

ADULT - RA/OA: 20 mg PO daily or divided bid.

PEDS - Not approved in children.
UNAPPROVED ADULT - Primary dysmenorrhea: 20-40 mg PO daily x 3 days.
FORMS - Generic/Trade: Caps 10 & 20 mg.

sulindac (*Clinoril*) ▸L ♀B (D in 3rd trimester) ▸- $$$
ADULT - RA/OA, ankylosing spondylitis: 150 mg PO bid. Bursitis, tendinitis, acute gout: 200 mg PO bid, decrease after response. Max dose: 400 mg/day.
PEDS - Not approved in children.
UNAPPROVED PEDS - JRA: 4 mg/kg/day PO divided bid.
FORMS - Generic/Trade: Tabs 150 & 200 mg.
NOTES - Sulindac-associated pancreatitis & a potentially fatal hypersensitivity syndrome have occurred.

tiaprofenic acid (♣*Surgam, Surgam SR*) ▸K ♀C (D in 3rd trimester) ▸- $$
ADULT - Canada only. RA or OA: 600 mg PO daily of sustained release, or 300 mg PO bid of regular release. Some OA patients may be maintained on 300 mg/day.
PEDS - Not approved in children.
FORMS - Generic/Trade: Tab 300 mg. Trade only: Cap, sustained-release 300 mg. Generic only: Tab 200 mg.
NOTES - Caution in renal insufficiency. Cystitis has been reported more frequently than with other NSAIDs.

tolmetin (*Tolectin*) ▸L ♀C (D in 3rd trimester) ▸+ $$$
ADULT - RA/OA: 400 mg PO tid to start. Range 600-1800 mg/day PO divided tid.
PEDS - JRA ≥2 yo: 20 mg/kg/day PO divided tid-qid to start. Range 15-30 mg/kg/day divided tid-qid. Max dose 2g/24h.
UNAPPROVED PEDS - Pain ≥2 yo: 5-7 mg/kg/dose PO q6-8h. Max dose 2g/24h.
FORMS - Generic/Trade: Tabs 200 (trade scored) & 600 mg. Cap 400 mg.
NOTES - Rare anaphylaxis.

ANALGESICS: Opioid Agonist -Antagonists

NOTE: May cause drowsiness and/or sedation, which may be enhanced by alcohol & other CNS depressants. Opioid agonist-antagonists may result in inadequate pain control and/or withdrawal effects in the opioid-dependent. Reserve IM for when alternative routes are not feasible.

buprenorphine (*Buprenex, Subutex*) ▸L ♀C ▸- ©III $ IV, $$$$$ SL
ADULT - Moderate to severe pain: 0.3-0.6 mg IM or slow IV, q6h prn. Max single dose 0.6 mg. Treatment of opioid dependence: Induction 8 mg SL on day 1, 16 mg SL on day 2. Maintenance: 16 mg SL daily. Can individualize to range of 4-24 mg SL daily.
PEDS - Moderate to severe pain: 2-12 yo: 2-6 mcg/kg/dose IM or slow IV q4-6h. Max single dose 6 mcg/kg.
FORMS - Trade only (Subutex): SL tabs 2, 8 mg
NOTES - May cause bradycardia, hypotension, respiratory depression. Concurrent diazepam has resulted in respiratory & cardiovascular collapse. For opioid dependence Subutex is preferred over Suboxone for induction. Suboxone preferred for maintenance. Prescribers must complete training and apply for special DEA number. See www.suboxone.com.

butorphanol (*Stadol, Stadol NS*) ▸LK ♀C ▸+ ©IV $$$
WARNING - Approved as a nasal spray in 1991 and has been promoted as a safe treatment for migraine headaches. There have been numerous reports of dependence-addiction & major psychological disturbances. Stadol NS should be used for patients with infrequent but severe migraine attacks for whom all other common abortive treatments have failed. Experts recommend restriction to ≤2 bottles (30 sprays) per month in patients who are appropriate candidates for this medication.
ADULT - Pain, including post-operative pain: 0.5-2 mg IV q3-4h prn. 1-4 mg IM q3-4h prn. Obstetric pain during labor: 1-2 mg IV/IM at full term in early labor, repeat after 4h. Last resort for migraine pain: 1 mg nasal spray (1 spray in one nostril). If no pain relief in 60-90 min, may give a 2nd spray in the other nostril. Additional doses q3-4h prn.
PEDS - Not approved in children.
FORMS - Generic only: Nasal spray 1 mg/spray, 2.5 mL bottle (14-15 doses/bottle).
NOTES - May increase cardiac workload.

nalbuphine (*Nubain*) ▸LK ♀? ▸? $
ADULT - Moderate to severe pain: 10-20 mg SC/IM/IV q3-6h prn. Max dose 160 mg/day.
PEDS - Not approved in children.

pentazocine (*Talwin NX*) ▸LK ♀C ▸? ©IV $$$
WARNING - The oral form (Talwin NX) may cause fatal reactions if injected.

ADULT - Moderate to severe pain: Talwin: 30 mg IM/IV q3-4h prn, max dose 360 mg/day. Talwin NX: 1 tab PO q3-4h, max 12 tabs/day.
PEDS - Not approved in children.
FORMS - Generic/Trade: Tab 50 mg with 0.5 mg naloxone, trade scored.
NOTES - Rotate injection sites. Can cause hallucinations, disorientation, and seizures. Concomitant sibutramine may precipitate serotonin syndrome.

OPIOID EQUIVALENCY*

Opioid	PO	IV/SC/IM	Opioid	PO	IV/SC/IM
buprenorphine	n/a	0.3-0.4 mg	meperidine	300 mg	75 mg
butorphanol	n/a	2 mg	methadone	5-15 mg	2.5-10 mg
codeine	130 mg	75 mg	morphine	30 mg	10 mg
fentanyl	?	0.1 mg	nalbuphine	n/a	10 mg
hydrocodone	20 mg	n/a	oxycodone	20 mg	n/a
hydromorphone	7.5 mg	1.5 mg	oxymorphone	10 mg	1 mg
levorphanol	4 mg	2 mg	pentazocine	50 mg	30 mg

*Approximate equianalgesic doses as adapted from the 2003 American Pain Society (www.ampainsoc.org) guidelines and the 1992 AHCPR guidelines. Not available = "n/a". See drug entries themselves for starting doses. Many recommend initially using lower than equivalent doses when switching between different opioids. IV doses should be titrated slowly with appropriate monitoring. All PO dosing is with immediate-release preparations. Individualize all dosing, especially in the elderly, children, and in those with chronic pain, opioid naïve, or hepatic/renal insufficiency.

ANALGESICS: Opioid Agonists

NOTE: May cause life-threatening respiratory depression. May cause drowsiness and/or sedation, which may be enhanced by alcohol & other CNS depressants. Patients with chronic pain may require more frequent & higher dosing. Opioids commonly create constipation. All opioids are pregnancy class D if used for prolonged periods or in high doses at term.

codeine ▶LK ♀C ▶- ©II $$
WARNING - Do not use IV in children due to large histamine release, cardiovascular effects. Use in nursing mothers has led to infant death.
ADULT - Mild to moderate pain: 15-60 mg PO/IM/IV/SC q4-6h. Max dose 360 mg in 24 hours. Antitussive: 10-20 mg PO q4-6h prn. Max dose 120 mg in 24 hours.
PEDS - Mild to moderate pain in ≥1yo: 0.5-1 mg/kg PO/SC/IM q4-6h, max dose 60 mg/dose. Antitussive: 2-5 yo: 2.5-5 mg PO q4-6h prn, max dose: 30 mg/day. 6-12 yo: 5-10 mg PO q4-6h prn, max dose 60 mg/day.
FORMS - Generic only: Tabs 15, 30, & 60 mg. Oral soln: 15 mg/5 mL.

fentanyl (*Duragesic, Actiq, Fentora, Sublimaze, IONSYS*) ▶L ♀C ▶+ ©II $$$$$
WARNING - Duragesic Patches, Actiq, & Fentora are contraindicated in the management of acute or postoperative pain due to potentially life-threatening respiratory depression in opioid non-tolerant patients. Instruct patients and their caregivers that even used patches/lozenges on a stick can be fatal to a child or pet. Dispose via toilet. IONSYS: For hospital use only; remove prior to discharge. Can cause life-threatening respiratory depression.
ADULT - Duragesic Patches: Chronic pain: 12.5-100 mcg/hr patch q72 hours. Titrate dose to the needs of the patient. Some patients require q48 hr dosing. May wear more than one patch to achieve the correct analgesic effect. Actiq: Breakthrough cancer pain: 200-1600 mcg sucked over 15 min, if 200 mcg ineffective x 6 units use higher strength. Goal is 4 lozenges on a stick/day in conjunction with long-acting opioid. Buccal tablet (Fentora) for breakthrough cancer pain: 100-800 mcg, titrated to pain relief; may repeat 1x after 30 minutes during single episode of breakthrough pain. See PI for dose conversion from transmucosal lozenges. Post-operative analgesia: 50-100 mcg IM; repeat in 1-2 hours prn. IONSYS: Acute postoperative pain: Specialized dosing.
PEDS - Transdermal (Duragesic): not approved in children <2 yo or in opioid naive. >2 yo: Use adult dosing. Children converting to a 25 mcg patch should be receiving ≥ 45 mg oral morphine equivalents/day. Actiq: not approved <16 yo. IONSYS not approved in children.

UNAPPROVED ADULT - Analgesia/procedural sedation: 50-100 mcg slow IV over 1-2 minutes; carefully titrate to effect. Analgesia: 50-100 mcg IM q1-2h prn.

UNAPPROVED PEDS - Analgesia: 1-2 mcg/kg/dose IV/IM q30-60 minutes prn or continuous IV infusion 1-3 mcg/kg/hr (not to exceed adult dosing). Procedural sedation: 1 to 3 yo: 2 to 3 mcg/kg/dose; 3 to 12 yo: 1 to 2 mcg/kg/dose; > 12 yo: 0.5 to 1 mcg/kg/dose (not to exceed adult dosing); these doses may repeated q30-60 minutes prn.

FORMS - Generic/Trade: Transdermal patches 12.5, 25, 50, 75, 100 mcg/h. Actiq lozenges on a stick, berry flavored 200, 400, 600, 800, 1,200, 1,600 mcg. Trade only: IONSYS: Iontophoretic transdermal system: 40 mcg fentanyl per activation; max 6 doses per hour. Max per system is eighty 40 mcg doses over 24 hours. Trade only: (Fentora) buccal tablet 100, 200, 300, 400, 600, 800 mcg.

NOTES - Do not use patches for acute pain. Oral transmucosal fentanyl doses of 5 mcg/kg provide effects similar to 0.75-1.25 mcg/kg of fentanyl IM. Lozenges on a stick should be sucked, not chewed. Flush lozenge remnants (without stick) down the toilet. For transdermal systems: apply patch to non-hairy skin. Clip (not shave) hair if you have to apply to hairy area. Fever or external heat sources may increase fentanyl released from patch. Dispose of a used patch by folding with the adhesive side of the patch adhering to itself, then flush it down the toilet immediately upon removal. Do not cut the patch in half. For Duragesic patches and Actiq lozenges on a stick: Titrate dose as high as necessary to relieve cancer pain or other types of non-malignant pain when chronic opioids are necessary. Do not suck, chew or swallow buccal tablet. IONSYS: Apply to intact skin on the chest or upper arm. Each dose, activated by the patient, is delivered over a 10-minute period. Remove prior to hospital discharge. Do not allow gel to touch mucous membranes. Dispose of using gloves. Keep all forms of fentanyl out of the reach of children or pets. Concomitant use with potent cytochrome P450 3A4 inhibitors such as ritonavir, ketoconazole, itraconazole, troleandomycin, clarithromycin, nelfinavir, and nefazodone may result in an increase in fentanyl plasma concentrations, which could increase or prolong adverse drug effects and may cause potentially fatal respiratory depression.

FENTANYL TRANSDERMAL DOSE (based on ongoing morphine requirement)*

morphine (IV/IM)	morphine (PO)	Transdermal fentanyl
8-22 mg/day	45-134 mg/day	25 mcg/hr
23-37 mg/day	135-224 mg/d	50 mcg/hr
38-52 mg/day	225-314 mg/d	75 mcg/hr
53-67 mg/day	315-404 mg/d	100 mcg/hr

* *For higher morphine doses see product insert for transdermal fentanyl equivalencies.*

hydromorphone   (***Dilaudid, Dilaudid-5, ♥Hydromorph Contin***) ▶L ♀C ▶? ©II $$

ADULT - Moderate to severe pain: 2-4 mg PO q4-6h. Initial dose (opioid-naive) 0.5-2 mg SC/IM or slow IV q4-6h prn. 3 mg PR q6-8h.

PEDS - Not approved in children.

UNAPPROVED PEDS - Pain ≤12 yo: 0.03-0.08 mg/kg PO q4-6h prn. 0.015 mg/kg/dose IV q4-6h prn. Pain >12 yo: use adult dose.

FORMS - Generic only: Tabs 2, 4. Generic/Trade: Tabs 8 mg (8mg trade scored). Liquid 5 mg/5 mL.

NOTES - In opioid-naive patients, consider an initial dose of 0.5 mg or less IM/SC/IV. SC/IM/IV doses after initial dose may be individualized. May be given by slow IV injection over 2-5 minutes. Titrate dose as high as necessary to relieve cancer pain or other types of non-malignant pain where chronic opioids are necessary. 1.5 mg IV = 7.5 mg PO.

levorphanol (***Levo-Dromoran***) ▶L ♀C ▶? ©II $$$

ADULT - Moderate to severe pain: 2 mg PO q6-8h prn. Increase to 4 mg if necessary.

PEDS - Not approved in children.

FORMS - Generic only: Tabs 2 mg, scored.

meperidine (***Demerol, pethidine***) ▶LK ♀C but + ▶+ ©II $$$

ADULT - Moderate to severe pain: 50-150 mg IM/SC/PO q3-4h prn. OB analgesia: when pains become regular, 50-100 mg IM/SC q1-3h. May also be given slow IV diluted to 10 mg/mL, or by IV infusion diluted to 1 mg/mL.

PEDS - Moderate to severe pain: 1-1.8 mg/kg IM/SC/PO or slow IV (see adult dosing) up to adult dose, q3-4h prn.

FORMS - Generic/Trade: Tabs 50 (trade scored) & 100 mg. Syrup 50 mg/5 mL (trade banana flavored).

NOTES - Avoid in renal insufficiency and in elderly due to risk of metabolite accumulation and increased risk of CNS disturbance and seizures. Multiple drug interactions including MAOIs & SSRIs. Poor oral absorption/efficacy. 75 mg meperidine IV,IM,SC = 300 mg meperidine PO. Take syrup with ½ glass (4 oz) water. Due to the risk of seizures at high doses, meperidine is not a good choice for treatment of chronic pain. Not recommended in children.

methadone (Diskets, Dolophine, Methadose, ♥Metadol) ▶L ♀C ▶+ ©II $

WARNING - High doses (mean ~400 mg/day) have been inconclusively associated with arrhythmia (torsade de pointes), particularly in those with pre-existing risk factors. Caution in opioid-naive patients. Elimination half life (8-59 hours) far longer than its duration of action (4-8 hours); monitor accordingly. Use caution with escalating doses.

ADULT - Severe pain in opioid-tolerant patients: 2.5-10 mg IM/SC/PO q3-4h prn. Opioid dependence: 20-100 mg PO daily.

PEDS - Not approved in children.

UNAPPROVED PEDS - Pain ≤12 yo: 0.7 mg/kg/24h divided q4-6h PO/SC/IM/IV prn. Max 10 mg/dose.

FORMS - Generic/Trade: Tabs 5, 10 mg, Dispersible tabs 40 mg. Oral concentrate: 10 mg/mL. Generic only: Oral soln 5&10 mg/5 mL.

NOTES - Titrate dose as high as necessary to relieve cancer pain or other types of non-malignant pain where chronic opioids are necessary. Every 8-12 hour dosing may decrease the risk of drug accumulation and overdose. Treatment for opioid dependence >3 wks is maintenance and only permitted in approved treatment programs. Drug interactions leading to decreased methadone levels with enzyme-inducing HIV drugs (eg, efavirenz, nevirapine) and other potent inducers such as rifampin. Monitor for opiate withdrawal symptoms and increase dose if necessary. Rapid metabolizers may require more frequent daily dosing.

morphine (MS Contin, Kadian, Avinza, Roxanol, Oramorph SR, MSIR, DepoDur, ♥Statex, M.O.S., Doloral) ▶LK ♀C ▶+ ©II $$$$

WARNING - Multiple strengths; see FORMS & write specific product on Rx. Drinking alcohol while taking Avinza or Kadian may result in a release of a potentially fatal dose of morphine.

ADULT - Moderate to severe pain: 10-30 mg PO q4h (immediate-release tabs, caps, oral soln). Controlled-release (MS Contin, Oramorph SR): 30 mg PO q8-12h. (Kadian): 20 mg PO q12-24h. Extended-release caps (Avinza): 30 mg

PO daily. 10 mg q4h IM/SC. 2.5-15 mg/70kg IV over 4-5 min. 10-20 mg PR q4h. Pain with major surgery (DepoDur): 10-15 mg x 1 epidurally at the lumbar level prior to surgery (max dose 20 mg), or 10 mg epidurally after clamping of the umbilical cord with cesarian section.

PEDS - Moderate to severe pain: 0.1-0.2 mg/kg up to 15 mg IM/SC/IV q2-4h.

UNAPPROVED PEDS - Moderate to severe pain: 0.2-0.5 mg/kg/dose PO (immediate release) q4-6h. 0.3-0.6 mg/kg/dose PO q12h (controlled release).

FORMS - Generic/Trade: Tabs, immediate-release: 15 & 30 mg. Trade only: Caps 15 & 30 mg. Generic/Trade: Oral soln: 10 mg/5 mL, 10 mg/2.5 mL, 20 mg/5 mL, 20 mg/mL (concentrate) & 100 mg/5 mL (concentrate). Rectal suppositories 5, 10, 20 & 30 mg. Controlled-release tabs (MS Contin, Oramorph SR) 15, 30, 60, 100; 200 mg MS Contin only. Controlled-release caps (Kadian) 10, 20, 30, 50, 60, 80, 100, 200 mg. Extended release caps (Avinza) 30, 60, 90 & 120 mg.

NOTES - Titrate dose as high as necessary to relieve cancer pain or other types of non-malignant pain where chronic opioids are necessary. The active metabolites may accumulate in hepatic/renal insufficiency & the elderly leading to increased analgesic & sedative effects. Do not break, chew, or crush MS Contin or Oramorph SR. Kadian & Avinza caps may be opened & sprinkled in applesauce for easier administration, however the pellets should not be crushed or chewed. Doses >1600 mg/day of Avinza contain a potentially nephrotoxic quantity of fumaric acid. Do not mix DepoDur with other medications; do not administer any other medications into epidural space for ≥48 hours.

oxycodone (Roxicodone, OxyContin, Percolone, OxyIR, OxyFAST, ♥Endocodone, Supeudol) ▶L ♀C ▶- ©II $$$$

WARNING - Do not Rx Oxycontin tabs on a prn basis. 80 mg tabs for use in opioid-tolerant patients only. Multiple strengths; see FORMS & write specific product on Rx. Do not break, chew, or crush controlled release preparations.

ADULT - Moderate to severe pain: 5 mg PO q4-6h prn. Controlled-release tabs: 10-40 mg PO q12h. (No supporting data for shorter dosing intervals for controlled release tabs.)

PEDS - Not approved in children.

UNAPPROVED PEDS - Pain ≤12 yo: 0.05-0.3 mg/kg/dose q4-6h PO prn to max 10 mg/dose.

FORMS - Generic/Trade: Immediate-release:

Tabs (scored) & caps 5 mg. Tabs 15, 30 mg. Oral soln 5 mg/5 mL. Oral concentrate 20 mg/mL. Generic only: Immediate release tabs 10, 20 mg. Trade only: Controlled-release tabs: 10, 20, 40, 80 mg.

NOTES - Titrate dose as high as necessary to relieve cancer pain or other types of non-malignant pain where chronic opioids are necessary.

oxymorphone (*Opana*) ▶L ♀C ▶? ©II $$$$
WARNING - Do not break, chew, dissolve or crush extended release tablets due to a rapid release and absorption of a potentially fatal dose of oxymorphone.

ADULT - Moderate to severe pain: 10-20 mg PO q4-6h (immediate release) or 5 mg q12h (extended release) 1 hour pre- or 2 hours post meals. Titrate q3-7 days until adequate pain relief. 5 mg PR q4-6h, prn. 1-1.5 mg IM/SC q4-6h prn. 0.5 mg IV initial dose in healthy patients then q4-6h prn, increase dose until pain adequately controlled.

PEDS - Not approved in children.

FORMS - Trade only: Extended release tabs (Opana ER) 5, 10, 20, 40 mg, Immediate release tabs (Opana IR) 5, 10 mg.

NOTES - Contraindicated in moderate to severe hepatic dysfunction. Decrease dose in elderly and with CrCl <50 ml/min. Avoid alcohol.

propoxyphene (*Darvon-N, Darvon Pulvules*) ▶L ♀C ▶+ ©IV $
ADULT - Mild to moderate pain: 65 mg (Darvon) to 100 mg (Darvon-N) PO q4h prn. Max dose 6 caps/day.

PEDS - Not approved in children.

FORMS - Generic/Trade: Caps 65 mg. Trade only: Tabs 100 mg (Darvon-N).

NOTES - Caution in renal & hepatic dysfunction. Avoid in renal insufficiency and in elderly due to risk of metabolite accumulation, and increased risk of CNS disturbance, seizures, and QRS prolongation.

ANALGESICS: Opioid Analgesic Combinations

NOTE: Refer to individual components for further information. May cause drowsiness and/or sedation, which may be enhanced by alcohol & other CNS depressants. Opioids, carisoprodol, and butalbital may be habit-forming. Avoid exceeding 4 g/day of acetaminophen in combination products. Caution those with ≥3 alcoholic drinks/day to limit acetaminophen use to 2.5 g/day due to additive liver toxicity. Opioids commonly cause constipation -- concurrent laxatives are recommended. All opioids are pregnancy class D if used for prolonged periods or in high doses at term.

Anexsia (hydrocodone + acetaminophen) ▶LK ♀C ▶- ©III $
WARNING - Multiple strengths; see FORMS & write specific product on Rx.
ADULT - Moderate pain: 1 tab PO q4-6h prn.
PEDS - Not approved in children.
FORMS - Generic/Trade: Tabs 5/325, 5/500, 7.5/325, 7.5/650 mg hydrocodone/mg acetaminophen, scored.

Capital with Codeine suspension (acetaminophen + codeine) ▶LK ♀C ▶? ©V $
ADULT - Moderate pain: 15 mL PO q4h prn.
PEDS - Moderate pain 3-6 yo: 5 mL PO q4-6h prn. 7-12 yo: 10 mL PO q4-6h prn. >12 yo use adult dose.
FORMS - Generic = oral soln. Trade = suspension. Both codeine 12 mg and acetaminophen

120 mg per 5 mL (trade, fruit punch flavor).

Combunox (oxycodone + ibuprofen) ▶L ♀C (D in 3rd trimester) ▶? ©II $$$
ADULT - Moderate to severe pain: 1 tab PO q6h prn for ≤7 days. Max dose 4 tabs/24 hours.
PEDS - Moderate to severe pain: ≥14 yo: Use adult dose.
FORMS - Trade only: Tab 5 mg oxycodone/400 mg ibuprofen.
NOTES - For short-term (≤ 7 days) management of pain. See NSAIDs-Other subclass warning & individual components.

Darvocet (propoxyphene + acetaminophen) ▶L ♀C ▶+ ©IV $
WARNING - Multiple strengths; see Forms below & write specific product on Rx.
ADULT - Moderate to severe pain: 1 tab (100/650 or 100/500) or 2 tabs (50/325) PO q4h prn.
PEDS - Not approved in children.
FORMS - Generic/Trade: Tabs 50/325 (Darvocet N-50), 100/650 (Darvocet N-100), & 100/500 (Darvocet A500), mg propoxyphene/mg acetaminophen.
NOTES - Avoid in renal insufficiency and in elderly due to risk of metabolite accumulation, and increased risk of CNS disturbance, seizures, and QRS prolongation.

Darvon Compound Pulvules (propoxyphene + aspirin + caffeine, ✦692 tablet)

▶LK **9**D **▶**- ©IV $

WARNING - Multiple strengths; see FORMS & write specific product on Rx.

ADULT - Moderate pain: 1 cap PO q4h prn.

PEDS - Not approved in children.

FORMS - Generic/Trade: Cap 65 mg propoxyphene/389 mg ASA/32.4 mg caffeine.

NOTES - Avoid in renal insufficiency and in elderly due to risk of metabolite accumulation, and increased risk of CNS disturbance, seizures, and QRS prolongation.

Empirin with Codeine (aspirin + codeine, ❤ *292 tablet*) ▶LK **9**D **▶**- ©III $

WARNING - Multiple strengths; see FORMS & write specific product on Rx.

ADULT - Moderate pain: 1-2 tabs PO q4h prn.

PEDS - Not approved in children.

FORMS - Generic only: Tab 325/30 & 325/60 mg ASA/mg codeine. Empirin brand no longer made.

Fioricet with Codeine (acetaminophen + butalbital + caffeine + codeine) ▶LK **9**C **▶**- ©III $$$

ADULT - Moderate pain: 1-2 caps PO q4h prn, max dose 6 caps/day.

PEDS - Not approved in children.

FORMS - Generic/Trade: Cap 325 mg acetaminophen/50 mg butalbital/40 mg caffeine/30 mg codeine.

Fiorinal with Codeine (aspirin + butalbital + caffeine + codeine, ❤ *Fiorinal C-1/4, Fiorinal C-1/2, Tecnal C-1/4, Tecnal C-1/2*) ▶LK **9**D **▶**- ©III $$$

ADULT - Moderate pain: 1-2 caps PO q4h prn, max dose 6 caps/day.

PEDS - Not approved in children.

FORMS - Generic/Trade: Cap 325 mg ASA/50 mg butalbital /40 mg caffeine/30 mg codeine.

Lorcet (hydrocodone + acetaminophen) ▶LK **9**C **▶**- ©III $

WARNING - Multiple strengths; see FORMS & write specific product on Rx.

ADULT - Moderate pain: 1-2 caps (5/500) PO q4-6h prn, max dose 8 caps/day. 1 tab PO q4-6h prn (7.5/650 & 10/650), max dose 6 tabs/day.

PEDS - Not approved in children.

FORMS - Generic/Trade: Caps 5/500 mg, tabs 7.5/650, 10/650 hydrocodone/acetaminophen.

Lortab (hydrocodone + acetaminophen) ▶LK **9**C **▶**- ©III $$

WARNING - Multiple strengths; see FORMS & write specific product on Rx.

ADULT - Moderate pain: 1-2 tabs 2.5/500 & 5/

500 PO q4-6h prn, max dose 8 tabs/day. 1 tab 7.5/500 & 10/500 PO q4-6h prn, max dose 5 tabs/day. Elixir 15 mL PO q4-6h prn, max 6 doses/day.

PEDS - Not approved in children.

FORMS - Generic/Trade: Lortab 5/500 (scored), Lortab 7.5/500 (trade scored) & Lortab 10/500 mg hydrocodone/mg acetaminophen. Elixir: 7.5/500 mg hydrocodone/mg acetaminophen/15 mL. Trade only: Tabs Lortab 2.5/500.

Magnacet (oxycodone + acetaminophen) ▶L **9**C **▶**- ©II $$$$

WARNING - Multiple strengths; see FORMS & write specific product on Rx.

ADULT - Moderate-severe pain: 1-2 tabs PO q6h prn (2.5/400). 1 tab PO q6h prn (5/400, 7.5/400, 10/400).

PEDS - Not approved in children.

FORMS - Trade only: Tabs 2.5/400, 5/400, 7.5/400, 10/400 oxycodone/acetaminophen.

Maxidone (hydrocodone + acetaminophen) ▶LK **9**C **▶**- ©III $$$

ADULT - Moderate pain: 1 tab PO q4-6h prn, max dose 5 tabs/day.

PEDS - Not approved in children.

FORMS - Trade only: Tab 10/750 mg hydrocodone/mg acetaminophen.

Mersyndol with Codeine (acetaminophen + codeine + doxylamine) ▶LK **9**C **▶**? $

ADULT - Canada only. Headaches, cold symptoms, muscle aches, neuralgia: 1-2 tabs PO q4-6h prn. Maximum 12 tabs/24 hours.

PEDS - Not approved in children.

FORMS - Trade only: OTC tab acetaminophen 325 mg + codeine 8 mg + doxylamine 5 mg.

NOTES - May be habit-forming. Hepatotoxicity may be increased with acetaminophen overdose and may be enhanced with concomitant chronic alcohol ingestion.

Norco (hydrocodone + acetaminophen) ▶L **9**C **▶**? ©III $$$

WARNING - Multiple strengths; see FORMS & write specific product on Rx.

ADULT - Moderate to severe pain: 1-2 tabs PO q4-6h prn (5/325), max dose 12 tabs/day. 1 tab (7.5/325 & 10/325) PO q4-6h prn, max dose 8 & 6 tabs/day, respectively.

PEDS - Not approved in children.

FORMS - Trade: Tabs 5/325, 7.5/325 & 10/325 mg hydrocodone/acetaminophen, scored.

Percocet (oxycodone + acetaminophen, ❤ *Percocet-demi, Oxycocet, Endocet*) ▶L **9**C **▶**- ©II $

WARNING - Multiple strengths; see FORMS &

write specific product on Rx.

ADULT - Moderate-severe pain: 1-2 tabs PO q4-6h prn (2.5/325 & 5/325). 1 tab PO q4-6 prn (7.5/325, 7.5/500, 10/325 & 10/650).

PEDS - Not approved in children.

FORMS - Trade only: Tabs 2.5/325 oxycodone/ acetaminophen. Generic/Trade: Tabs 5/325, 7.5/325, 7.5/500, 10/325, 10/650 mg. Generic only: 2.5/300, 5/300, 7.5/300, 10/300, 2.5/400, 5/400, 7.5/400, 10/400, 10/500 mg.

Percodan (oxycodone + aspirin, ✚Oxycodan, Endodan) ▶LK ♀D ▶- ©II $$

ADULT - Moderate to severe pain: Percodan: 1 tab PO q6h prn. Percodan Demi: 1-2 tabs q6h prn.

PEDS - Not approved in children.

UNAPPROVED PEDS - Moderate to severe pain in 6-12 yo: ¼ Demi tab PO q6h prn. >12 yo ½ Demi tab PO q6h prn.

FORMS - Generic/Trade: Tab Percodan 4.88/ 325 mg oxycodone/ASA (trade scored). Trade only: Percodan Demi 2.44/325 mg scored.

Roxicet (oxycodone + acetaminophen) ▶L ♀C ▶- ©II $

WARNING - Multiple strengths; see FORMS & write specific product on Rx.

ADULT - Moderate to severe pain: 1 tab PO q6h prn. Oral soln: 5 mL PO q6h prn.

PEDS - Not approved in children.

FORMS - Generic/Trade: Tab 5/325 mg, scored. Cap/Caplet 5/500 mg. Trade only: Soln 5/325 per 5 mL, mg oxycodone/acetaminophen.

Soma Compound with Codeine (carisoprodol + aspirin + codeine) ▶L ♀D ▶- ©III $$$

ADULT - Moderate to severe musculoskeletal pain: 1-2 tabs PO qid prn.

PEDS - Not approved in children.

FORMS - Generic/Trade: Tab 200 mg carisoprodol/325 mg ASA/16 mg codeine.

NOTES - Refer to individual components. Withdrawal with abrupt discontinuation.

Synalgos-DC (dihydrocodeine + aspirin + caffeine) ▶L ♀C ▶- ©III $

WARNING - Case reports of prolonged erections when taken concomitantly with sildenafil.

ADULT - Moderate-severe pain: 2 caps PO q4h prn.

PEDS - Not approved in children.

FORMS - Trade only: Cap 16 mg dihydrocodeine/356.4 mg ASA/30 mg caffeine. "Painpack"=12 caps.

NOTES - Most common use is dental pain. Refer to individual components.

Talacen (pentazocine + acetaminophen) ▶L ♀C ▶? ©IV $$$

ADULT - Moderate pain: 1 tab PO q4h prn.

PEDS - Not approved in children.

FORMS - Generic/Trade: Tab 25 mg pentazocine/650 mg acetaminophen, trade scored.

NOTES - Serious skin reactions, including erythema multiforme & Stevens-Johnson syndrome have been reported.

Tylenol with Codeine (codeine + acetaminophen, ✚Lenoltec, Emtec, Triatec) ▶LK ♀C ▶? ©III (Tabs), V(elixir) $

WARNING - Multiple strengths; see FORMS & write specific product on Rx.

ADULT - Moderate pain: 1-2 tabs PO q4h prn.

PEDS - Moderate pain 3-6 yo: 5 mL PO q4-6h prn. 7-12 yo 10 mL PO q4-6h prn. >12 yo: Use adult dose.

FORMS - Generic: Tabs Tylenol #2 (15/ 300), Tylenol #4 (60/300). Tylenol with Codeine Elixir 12/120 per 5 mL, mg codeine/mg acetaminophen. Generic/Trade: Tabs Tylenol #3 (30/ 300). Canadian forms come with (Lenoltec, Tylenol) or without (Empracet, Emtec) caffeine.

Tylox (oxycodone + acetaminophen) ▶L ♀C ▶- ©II $

ADULT - Moderate-severe pain: 1 cap PO q6h prn.

PEDS - Not approved in children.

FORMS - Generic/Trade: Cap 5 mg oxycodone/ 500 mg acetaminophen.

Vicodin (hydrocodone + acetaminophen) ▶LK ♀C ▶? ©III $

WARNING - Multiple strengths; see FORMS & write specific product on Rx.

ADULT - Moderate to severe pain: 5/500 (max dose 8 tabs/day) & 7.5/750 (max dose of 5 tabs/day): 1-2 tabs PO q4-6h prn. 10/660: 1 tab PO q4-6h prn (max of 6 tabs/day).

PEDS - Not approved in children.

FORMS - Generic/Trade: Tabs Vicodin (5/500), Vicodin ES (7.5/750), Vicodin HP (10/660), scored, mg hydrocodone/mg acetaminophen.

Vicoprofen (hydrocodone + ibuprofen) ▶LK ♀- ▶? ©III $$$

ADULT - Moderate pain: 1 tab PO q4-6h prn, max dose 5 tabs/day.

PEDS - Not approved in children.

FORMS - Generic/Trade: Tab 7.5/200 mg hydrocodone/ibuprofen. Generic: Tab 5/200 mg.

NOTES - See NSAIDs-Other subclass warning.

Wygesic (propoxyphene + acetaminophen) ▶L ♀C ▶? ©IV $

ADULT - Moderate pain: 1 tab PO q4h prn.

PEDS - Not approved in children.

FORMS - Generic/Trade: Tab 65 mg propoxyphene/650 mg acetaminophen.

NOTES - Avoid in renal insufficiency and in elderly due to risk of metabolite accumulation, and increased risk of CNS disturbance, seizures, and QRS prolongation.

Xodol (hydrocodone + acetaminophen)
▶LK ♀C ▶- ©III $$

ADULT - Moderate pain: 1 tab PO q4-6 prn, max 6 doses/day.

PEDS - Not approved in children.

FORMS - Trade only: Tabs 5/300, 7.5/300, 10/300 mg hydrocodone/acetaminophen.

Zydone (hydrocodone + acetaminophen)
▶LK ♀C ▶? ©III $$

WARNING - Multiple strengths; see FORMS & write specific product on Rx.

ADULT - Moderate pain: 1-2 tabs (5/400) PO q4-6h prn, max dose 8 tabs/day. 1 tab (7.5/400, 10/400) q4-6h prn, max dose 6 tabs/day.

PEDS - Not approved in children.

FORMS - Trade only: Tabs 5/400, 7.5/400, & 10/400 mg hydrocodone/mg acetaminophen.

ANALGESICS: Opioid Antagonists

NOTE: May result in withdrawal in the opioid dependent, including life-threatening withdrawal if administered to neonates born to opioid-dependent mothers. Rare pulmonary edema, cardiovascular instability, hypotension, hypertension, ventricular tachycardia & ventricular fibrillation have been reported in connection with opioid reversal.

nalmefene (Revex) ▶L ♀B ▶? $$$

ADULT - Opioid overdosage: 0.5 mg/70 kg IV. If needed, this may be followed by a 2nd dose of 1 mg/70 kg, 2-5 minutes later. Max cumulative dose 1.5 mg/70kg. If suspicion of opioid dependency, initially administer a challenge dose of 0.1 mg/70 kg. Post-operative opioid reversal: 0.25 mcg/kg IV followed by 0.25 mcg/kg incremental doses at 2-5 minute intervals, stopping as soon as the desired degree of opioid reversal is obtained. Max cumulative dose 1 mcg/kg.

PEDS - Not approved in children.

FORMS - Trade only: Injection 100 mcg/mL nalmefene for postoperative reversal (blue label). 1 mg/mL nalmefene for opioid overdose (green label).

NOTES - Recurrence of respiratory depression is possible, even after an apparently adequate initial response to nalmefene treatment.

naloxone (Narcan) ▶LK ♀B ▶? $

ADULT - Management of opioid overdose: 0.4-2 mg IV. May repeat IV at 2-3 minute intervals up to 10 mg. Use IM/SC/ET if IV not available. Intravenous infusion: 2 mg in 500 mL D5W or NS (0.004 mg/mL); titrate according to response. Partial post-operative opioid reversal: 0.1-0.2 mg IV at 2-3 minute intervals; repeat IM doses may be required at 1-2 hr intervals.

PEDS - Management of opioid overdose: 0.01 mg/kg IV. Give a subsequent dose of 0.1 mg/kg if inadequate response. Use IM/SC/ET if IV not available. Partial post-operative opioid reversal: 0.005-0.01 mg IV at 2-3 minute intervals.

NOTES - Watch patients for re-emergence of opioid effects.

ANALGESICS: Other

acetaminophen (Tylenol, Panadol, Tempra, paracetamol, ✚Abenol, Atasol, Pediatrix) ▶LK ♀B ▶+ $

ADULT - Analgesic/antipyretic: 325-1000 mg PO q4-6h prn. 650 mg PR q4-6h prn. Max 4 g/day. OA: extended-release: 2 caplets PO q8h around the clock. Max dose 6 caplets/day.

PEDS - Analgesic/antipyretic: 10-15 mg/kg q4-6h PO/PR prn. Max 5 doses/day.

UNAPPROVED ADULT - OA: 1,000 mg PO qid.

FORMS - OTC: Tabs 160, 325, 500, 650 mg. Chewable Tabs 80 mg. Gelcaps 500 mg. Caps 325, 500 mg. Sprinkle caps 80, 160 mg. Extended-release caplets 650 mg. Liquid 160 mg/5 mL & 500 mg/15 mL. Drops 80 mg/0.8 mL. Suppositories 80, 120, 125, 300, 325, 650 mg.

NOTES - Risk of hepatotoxicity with chronic use, especially in alcoholics. Caution in those who drink ≥3 drinks/day. Rectal administration may produce lower/less reliable plasma levels.

cannibis sativa L. extract (✚Sativex) ▶LK ♀X ▶- $$$$

ADULT - Canada only. Adjunctive treatment for the symptomatic relief of neuropathic pain in multiple sclerosis: Start: 1 spray q4h (max 4 times daily), and titrated upwards as tolerated. Limited experience with >12 sprays/day.

PEDS - Not approved in children.

FORMS - Trade only: Buccal spray, 27 mg/ml delta-9-tetrahydrocannabinol & 25 mg/ml cannabidiol, delivers 100 microliters/actuation, 5.5 ml vials containing up to 51 actuations per vial.

NOTES - Contraindicated in pregnancy, child-bearing potential without birth control, history of psychosis, serious heart disease. Contains ethanol. Caution if history of substance abuse.

hyaluronate (*Hyalgan, Supartz, ♥Neo-visc, Orthovisc*) ▶KL ♀? ▶? $$$$$

WARNING - Do not inject extra-articularly; avoid the synovial tissues & capsule. Do not use disinfectants containing benzalkonium chloride for skin preparation.

ADULT - OA (knee): Hyalgan: 2 mL intra-articular injection q week x 3-5 weeks. Supartz: 2.5 mL intra-articular injection q week x 5 weeks. Orthovisc & Neovisc (Canada): 2 mL intra-articular injection q week x 3 weeks. Inject a local anesthetic SC prior to injections.

PEDS - Not approved in children.

FORMS - Trade only: Hyalgan, Neovisc, Orthovisc: 2 mL vials & prefilled syringes. Supartz: 2.5 mL prefilled syringes.

NOTES - For those who have failed conservative therapy. Caution in allergy to eggs, avian proteins or feathers (except Neovisc - synthetic). Remove synovial fluid or effusion before each injection. Knee pain & swelling most common side effects.

hylan GF-20 (*Synvisc*) ▶KL ♀? ▶? $$$$$

WARNING - Do not inject extra-articularly; avoid the synovial tissues & capsule. Do not use disinfectants containing benzalkonium chloride for skin preparation.

ADULT - OA (knee): 2 mL intra-articular injection q week x 3 weeks.

PEDS - Not approved in children.

FORMS - Trade only: 2.25 mL glass syringe w/ 2 mL drug; 3/pack.

NOTES - For those who have failed conservative therapy. Caution in allergy to eggs, avian proteins or feathers. Remove synovial fluid or effusion before each injection. Knee pain & swelling most common side effects.

tramadol (*Ultram, Ultram ER*) ▶KL♀C ▶- $$$

ADULT - Moderate to moderately severe pain: 50-100 mg PO q4-6h prn. Max dose 400 mg/day. If >75 yo, use <300 mg/day PO in divided doses. If CrCl <30 mL/min, increase the dosing interval to 12 hours. If cirrhosis, decrease dose to 50 mg PO q12h. Chronic pain, extended release: 100-300 mg PO daily. Do not use if CrCl <30 mL/min or with severe hepatic dysfunction.

PEDS - Not approved in children <16 yo.

FORMS - Generic/Trade: Tab, immediate-release 50 mg. Trade only: Extended release tabs 100, 200, 300 mg.

NOTES - Contraindicated in acute intoxication with alcohol, hypnotics, centrally acting analgesics, opioids, or psychotropics. Seizures may occur with concurrent antidepressants or in seizure disorder. Great caution with MAO inhibitors or with SSRIs due to potential for serotonin syndrome; dose adjustment may be needed. Withdrawal symptoms may occur in opioid dependent or with abrupt discontinuation. Overdose treated with naloxone may lead to seizures. Carbamazepine decreases levels. The most frequent side effects are nausea & constipation. ER tablets cannot be crushed, chewed or split.

Women's Tylenol Menstrual Relief (acetaminophen + pamabrom) ▶LK ♀B ▶+ $

ADULT - Menstrual cramps: 2 caplets PO q4-6h.

PEDS - >12 yo: use adult dose.

FORMS - OTC: Caplet 500 mg acetaminophen/25 mg pamabrom (diuretic).

NOTES - Hepatotoxicity with chronic use, especially in alcoholics.

ANESTHESIA: Anesthetics & Sedatives

NOTE: Some of these agents are known triggers of malignant hyperthermia, see mahaus.org. 24-hour hotline: 1-800-644-9737.

alfentanil (*Alfenta*) ▶L ♀C ▶? ©II $

ADULT - IV general anesthesia adjunct; specialized dosing. PEDS - Not approved in children.

dexmedetomidine (*Precedex*) ▶LK ♀C ▶?

$$$$

ADULT - ICU sedation <24h: Load 1 mcg/kg over 10 min followed by infusion 0.2-0.7 mcg/kg/h titrated to desired sedation endpoint.

PEDS - Not recommended <18 yo.

NOTES - Alpha 2 adrenergic agonist with sedative properties. Beware of bradycardia and hypotension. Avoid in advanced heart block.

etomidate (*Amidate*) ▶L ♀C ▶? $
ADULT - Anesthesia induction / rapid sequence intubation: 0.3 mg/kg IV.
PEDS - Age ≥10 yo: Adult dosing. Age <10 yo: Not approved.
UNAPPROVED PEDS - Anesthesia induction / rapid sequence intubation: 0.3 mg/kg IV.
NOTES - Adrenocortical suppression, but rarely of clinical significance.

ketamine (*Ketalar*) ▶L ♀? ▶? ©III $
WARNING - Emergence delirium limits value in adults; such reactions are rare in children.
ADULT - Dissociative sedation: 1-2 mg/kg IV over 1-2 min or 4-5 mg/kg IM.
PEDS - Dissociative sedation: 1-2 mg/kg IV over 1-2 min or 4-5 mg/kg IM.
NOTES - Raises BP and intracranial pressure; avoid if coronary artery disease, HTN, head or eye injury. Concurrent atropine minimizes hypersalivation; can be combined in same syringe with ketamine for IM use.

methohexital (*Brevital*) ▶L ♀B ▶? ©IV $
ADULT - Anesthesia induction: 1-1.5 mg/kg IV.
PEDS - Safety in children not established.
UNAPPROVED PEDS - Sedation for diagnostic imaging: 25 mg/kg PR

midazolam (*Versed*) ▶LK ♀D ▶- ©IV $
WARNING - Beware of respiratory depression/apnea. Administer with appropriate monitoring.
ADULT - Sedation/anxiolysis: 0.07-0.08 mg/kg IM (5 mg in average adult); or 1 mg IV slowly q2-3 min up to 5 mg. Anesthesia induction: 0.3-0.35 mg/kg IV over 20-30 seconds.
PEDS - Sedation/anxiolysis: 0.25-1.0 mg/kg to maximum of 20 mg PO, or 0.1-0.15 mg/kg IM. IV route (6 mo to 5 yo): Initial dose 0.05-0.1 mg/kg IV, then titrated to max 0.6 mg/kg. IV route (6-12 yo): Initial dose 0.025-0.05 mg/kg IV, then titrated to max 0.4 mg/kg.
UNAPPROVED PEDS - Sedation/anxiolysis: Intranasal 0.2-0.4 mg/kg. Rectal: 0.25-0.5 mg/kg PR. Higher oral dosing: 0.5-0.75 mg/kg PO, max 20 mg/kg. Status epilepticus: Load 0.15 mg/kg IV followed by infusion 1 mcg/kg/min and titrate dose upward q5 min prn.
FORMS - Oral liquid 2 mg/mL
NOTES - Use lower doses in the elderly, chronically ill, and those receiving concurrent CNS depressants.

pentobarbital (*Nembutal*) ▶LK ♀D ▶? ©II $$
ADULT - Rarely used; other drugs preferred. Hypnotic: 150-200 mg IM or 100 mg IV at a rate of 50 mg/min, maximum dose is 500 mg.
PEDS - FDA approved for active seizing, but other agents preferred.
UNAPPROVED PEDS - Procedural sedation: 1-6 mg/kg IV, adjusted in increments of 1-2 mg/kg to desired effect, or 2-6 mg/kg IM, max 100 mg. Do not exceed 50 mg/min.

propofol (*Diprivan*) ▶L ♀B ▶- $$$
WARNING - Beware of respiratory depression/apnea. Administer with appropriate monitoring.
ADULT - Anesthesia (<55 yo): 40 mg IV q10 sec until induction onset (typical 2-2.5 mg/kg). Follow with maintenance infusion generally 100-200 mcg/kg/min. Lower doses in elderly or for sedation. ICU ventilator sedation: infusion 5-50 mcg/kg/min.
PEDS - Anesthesia (≥3 yo): 2.5-3.5 mg/kg IV over 20-30 seconds, followed with infusion 125-300 mcg/kg/min. Not recommended if <3 yo or for prolonged ICU use.
UNAPPROVED ADULT - Deep sedation: 1 mg/kg IV over 20-30 seconds. Repeat 0.5 mg/kg IV prn. Intubation adjunct: 2.0 to 2.5 mg/kg IV.
UNAPPROVED PEDS - Deep sedation: 1 mg/kg IV (max 40 mg) over 20-30 seconds. Repeat 0.5 mg/kg (max 20 mg) IV prn.
NOTES - Avoid with egg or soy allergies. Prolonged infusions may lead to hypertriglyceridemia. Injection pain can be treated or pre-treated with lidocaine 40-50 mg IV.

remifentanil (*Ultiva*) ▶L ♀C ▶? ©II $$
ADULT, PEDS - IV general anesthesia adjunct; specialized dosing.

sufentanil (*Sufenta*) ▶L ♀C ▶? ©II $$
ADULT, PEDS - IV anesthesia adjunct: specialized dosing.

thiopental (*Pentothal*) ▶L ♀C ▶? ©III $
ADULT - Anesthesia induction: 3-5 mg/kg IV.
PEDS - Anesthesia induction: 3-5 mg/kg IV.
UNAPPROVED PEDS - Sedation for diagnostic imaging: 25 mg/kg PR
NOTES - Duration 5 minutes. Hypotension, histamine release, extravasation tissue necrosis.

ANALGESICS: Local Anesthetics

articaine (*Septocaine, Zorcaine*) ▶LK♀C▶?$
ADULT - Dental local anesthesia: 4% injection.

PEDS - Dental local anesthesia and ≥4 yo: 4% injection.

FORMS - 4% (includes epinephrine 1:100,000)

NOTES - Do not exceed 7 mg/kg total dose

bupivacaine (*Marcaine, Sensorcaine*) ▶LK ♀C ▶? $

ADULT - Local anesthesia, nerve block: 0.25% injection.

PEDS - Not recommended in children <12 yo.

FORMS - 0.25%, 0.5%, 0.75%, all with or without epinephrine.

NOTES - Onset 5 mins, duration 2-4h (longer with epi). Amide group. Max dose 2.5 mg/kg alone, or 3.0 mg/kg with epinephrine.

Duocaine (bupivacaine + lidocaine - local anesthetic) ▶LK ♀C ▶? $

ADULT - Local anesthesia, nerve block for eye surgery.

PEDS - Not recommended in children <12 yo.

FORMS - Vials bupivacaine 0.375% + lido 1%.

NOTES – Do not exceed maximum dosing for both bupivacaine and lidocaine.

lidocaine (*Xylocaine*) ▶LK ♀B ▶? $

ADULT - Local anesthesia: 0.5-1% injection.

PEDS - Local anesthesia: 0.5-1% injection.

FORMS - 0.5,1,1.5,2%. With epi: 0.5,1,1.5,2%.

NOTES - Onset <2 mins, duration 30-60 mins (longer with epi). Amide group. Potentially toxic dose 3-5 mg/kg without epinephrine, and 5-7 mg/kg with epinephrine. Use "cardiac lidocaine" (ie, IV formulation) for Bier blocks at maximum dose of 3 mg/kg so that neither epinephrine nor methylparaben are injected IV.

mepivacaine (*Carbocaine, Polocaine*) ▶LK ♀C ▶? $

ADULT - Nerve block: 1%-2% injection.

PEDS - Nerve block: 1%-2% injection. Use <2% concentration if <3 yo or <30 pounds.

FORMS - 1,1.5,2,3%.

NOTES - Onset 3-5 mins, duration 45-90 mins. Amide group. Max local dose 5 to 6 mg/kg.

Oraquix (prilocaine + lidocaine - local anesthetic) ▶LK ♀B ▶? $$

ADULT - Local anesthetic gel applied to periodontal pockets using blunt-tipped applicator: 4% injection.

PEDS - Not approved in children.

FORMS - Gel 2.5% + 2.5% with applicator.

NOTES - Do not exceed maximum dose for lidocaine or prilocaine.

ANALGESICS: Neuromuscular Blockers

NOTE: Should be administered only by those skilled in airway management and respiratory support.

atracurium (*Tracrium*) ▶Plasma ♀C ▶? $

ADULT - Paralysis: 0.4-0.5 mg/kg IV.

PEDS - Paralysis ≥2yo: 0.4-0.5 mg/kg IV.

NOTES - Duration 15-30 minutes. Hoffman degradation.

cisatracurium (*Nimbex*) ▶Plasma ♀B ▶? $$

ADULT - Paralysis: 0.15-0.2 mg/kg IV.

PEDS - Paralysis: 0.1 mg/kg IV over 5-10 seconds.

NOTES - Duration 30-60 minutes. Hoffman degradation.

pancuronium (*Pavulon*) ▶LK ♀C ▶? $

ADULT - Paralysis: 0.04 to 0.1 mg/kg IV.

PEDS - Paralysis (beyond neonatal age): 0.04 to 0.1 mg/kg IV.

NOTES - Duration 45 minutes. Decrease dose if renal disease.

rocuronium (*Zemuron*) ▶L ♀B ▶? $$

ADULT - Paralysis: 0.6 mg/kg IV bolus. Rapid sequence intubation: 0.6 to 1.2 mg/kg IV. Continuous infusion: 10 to 12 mcg/kg/min; first verify spontaneous recovery from bolus dose.

PEDS - Paralysis (age >3 mo): 0.6 mg/kg IV.

Continuous infusion: 12 mcg/kg/min; first verify spontaneous recovery from bolus dose.

NOTES - Duration 30 minutes. Decrease dose if severe liver disease.

succinylcholine (*Anectine, Quelicin*) ▶Plasma ♀C ▶? $

ADULT - Paralysis: 0.6-1.1 mg/kg IV.

PEDS - Paralysis (≥5 yo): 1 mg/kg IV. Paralysis (<5 yo): 2 mg/kg IV.

NOTES - Avoid in hyperkalemia, myopathies, eye injuries, rhabdomyolysis, subacute burn, syndromes of denervated or disused musculature (eg, paralysis from spinal cord injury or major stroke). If immediate cardiac arrest and ET tube is in correct place & no tension pneumo evident, strongly consider empiric treatment for hyperkalemia. Succinylcholine can trigger malignant hyperthermia: mahaus.org. 24-hour hotline: 1-800-644-9737.

vecuronium (*Norcuron*) ▶LK ♀C ▶? $

ADULT - Paralysis: 0.08-0.1 mg/kg IV bolus. Continuous infusion: 0.8 to 1.2 mcg/kg/min; first verify spontaneous recovery from bolus dose.

PEDS - Paralysis (age ≥10 yrs): 0.08-0.1 mg/kg IV bolus. Continuous infusion: 0.8 to 1.2 mcg/

kg/min; first verify spontaneous recovery from bolus dose. Age 1-10 years: may require a slightly higher initial dose and may also require supplementation slightly more often than older patients. Age 7 weeks to 1 year: moderately more sensitive on a mg/kg dose compared to adults and take 1.5 x longer to recover. Age <7 weeks: Safety has not been established.
NOTES - Duration 15-30 minutes. Decrease dose in severe liver disease.

ANTIMICROBIALS: Aminoglycosides

| NOTE: See also dermatology and ophthalmology |

amikacin (*Amikin*) ▶K ♀D ▶? $$$
WARNING - Nephrotoxicity, ototoxicity.
ADULT - Gram negative infections: 15 mg/kg/day up to 1500 mg/day IM/IV divided q8-12h. Peak 20-35 mcg/mL, trough <5 mcg/mL.
PEDS - Gram neg infections: 15 mg/kg/day up to 1500 mg/day IM/IV divided q8-12h. Neonates: 10 mg/kg load, then 7.5 mg/kg IM/IV q12h.
UNAPPROVED ADULT - Once daily dosing: 15 mg/kg IV q24h. TB (2nd-line treatment): 15 mg/kg up to 1 g IM/IV daily. 10 mg/kg up to 750 mg IM/IV daily if >59 yo.
UNAPPROVED PEDS - Severe infections: 15-22.5 mg/kg/day IV divided q8h. Some experts recommend 30 mg/kg/day. Once daily dosing: 15 mg/kg IV q24h. Some experts consider once-daily dosing of aminoglycosides investigational in children. TB (2nd-line treatment): 15-30 mg/kg up to 1 g IM/IV daily.
NOTES - May enhance effects of neuromuscular blockers. Avoid other ototoxic/nephrotoxic drugs. Individualize dose in renal dysfunction, burn patients. Base dose on average of actual and ideal body weight in obesity.

gentamicin (*Garamycin*) ▶K ♀D ▶+ $$
WARNING - Nephrotoxicity, ototoxicity.
ADULT - Gram negative infections: 3-5 mg/kg/day IM/IV divided q8h. Peak 5-10 mcg/ml, trough <2 mcg/ml. See table for prophylaxis of bacterial endocarditis.
PEDS - Gram neg infections: 2-2.5 mg/kg IM/IV q8h. Infants ≥1 week old, >2 kg: 2.5 mg/ kg IM/IV q8h. Infants <1 week old, >2 kg: 2.5 mg/kg IM/IV q12h. Cystic fibrosis: 9 mg/kg/day IV in divided doses with target peak of 8-12 mcg/mL.
UNAPPROVED ADULT - Once daily dosing for gram negative infections: 5-7 mg/kg IV q24h. Endocarditis: 3 mg/kg/day for synergy with another agent. Give once daily for viridans streptococci, 2-3 divided doses for staphylococci, 3 divided doses for enterococci.
UNAPPROVED PEDS - Once daily dosing: 5-7 mg/kg IV q24h. Age <1 week and full-term: 4 mg/kg IV q24h. Some experts consider once-daily dosing of aminoglycosides investigational in children.
NOTES - May enhance effects of neuromuscular blockers. Avoid other ototoxic/nephrotoxic drugs. Individualize dose in renal dysfunction, burn patients. Base dose on average of actual and ideal body weight in obesity.

streptomycin ▶K ♀D ▶+ $$$$$
WARNING - Nephrotoxicity, ototoxicity. Monitor audiometry, renal function, and electrolytes.
ADULT - Combined therapy for TB: 15 mg/kg up to 1 g IM/IV daily. 10 mg/kg up to 750 mg IM/IV daily if >59 yo.
PEDS - Combined therapy for TB: 20-40 mg/kg up to 1 g IM daily.
UNAPPROVED ADULT - Same IM dosing can be given IV. Streptococcal endocarditis: 7.5 mg /kg IV/IM bid. More info: americanheart.org.
NOTES - Contraindicated in pregnancy. Obtain baseline audiogram, vestibular and Romberg testing, and renal function. Monitor renal function and vestibular and auditory symptoms monthly. May enhance effects of neuromuscular blockers. Avoid other ototoxic/nephrotoxic drugs. Individualize dose in renal dysfunction.

tobramycin (*Nebcin, TOBI*) ▶K ♀D ▶? $$$$
WARNING - Nephrotoxicity, ototoxicity.
ADULT - Gram negative infections: 3-5 mg/kg/day IM/IV divided q8h. Peak 5-10 mcg/mL, trough <2 mcg/mL. Parenteral for cystic fibrosis: 10 mg/kg/day IV divided q6h with target peak of 8-12 mcg/mL. Nebulized for cystic fibrosis (TOBI): 300 mg neb bid 28 days on, then 28 days off.
PEDS - Gram negative infections: 2-2.5 mg/kg IV q8h or 1.5-1.9 mg/kg IV q6h. Premature/full-term neonates ≤1 week old: Up to 4 mg/kg/day divided q12h. Parenteral for cystic fibrosis: 10 mg/kg/day IV divided q6h with target peak of 8-12 mcg/mL. Nebulized for cystic fibrosis (TOBI) ≥6 yo: 300 mg neb bid 28 days on, then 28 days off.
UNAPPROVED ADULT - Once daily dosing: 5-7 mg/kg IV q24h.
UNAPPROVED PEDS - Once daily dosing: 5-7

mg/kg IV q24h. Some experts consider once-daily dosing of aminoglycosides investigational in children.

FORMS - Trade only: TOBI 300 mg ampules for nebulizer.

NOTES - May enhance effects of neuromuscu-lar blockers. Avoid other ototoxic/nephrotoxic drugs. Individualize dose in renal dysfunction, burn patients. Base dose on average of actual and ideal body weight in obesity. Routine monitoring of tobramycin levels not required with nebulized TOBI.

ANTIMICROBIALS: Antifungal Agents

amphotericin B deoxycholate (*Fungizone*)
▶Tissues ♀B ▶? $$$$

WARNING - Do not use IV route for noninvasive fungal infections (oral thrush, vaginal or esophageal candidiasis) in patients with normal neutrophil counts.

ADULT - Life-threatening systemic fungal infections: Test dose 1 mg slow IV. Wait 2-4 h, and if tolerated start 0.25 mg/kg IV daily. Advance to 0.5-1.5 mg/kg/day depending on fungal type. Maximum dose 1.5 mg/kg/day. Infuse over 2-6 h. Hydrate with 500 mL NS before and after infusion to decrease risk of nephrotoxicity.

PEDS - No FDA approved indications.

UNAPPROVED ADULT - Alternative regimen, life-threatening systemic fungal infections: 1 mg test dose as part of 1st infusion (don't need separate IV bag); if tolerated continue infusion, giving target dose of 0.5-1.5 mg/kg on 1st day. Candidemia, non-neutropenic pts: 0.6-1.0 mg/kg IV daily; or 0.7 mg/kg IV daily + fluconazole 800 mg/day for 4-7 days, then fluconazole 800 mg/day. Treat until 14 days past last positive blood culture and signs/sx resolved. Candidemia, neutropenic pts: 0.7-1.0 mg/kg IV daily until 14 days past last positive blood culture, signs/symptoms, and neutropenia resolved. Cryptococcal meningitis in HIV infection: 0.7-1 mg/kg/day IV preferably in combo with flucytosine 25 mg/kg PO q6h x 2 wks. Follow with fluconazole consolidation, then fluconazole chronic suppression until immune reconstitution. Candidal cystitis: Irrigate bladder with 50 mcg/mL soln periodically/ continuously x 5-10 days.

UNAPPROVED PEDS - Systemic life-threatening fungal infections: Test dose 0.1 mg/kg slow IV. Wait 2-4 h, and if tolerated start 0.25 mg/kg IV once daily. Advance to 0.5-1.5 mg/kg/day depending on fungal type. Maximum dose 1.5 mg/kg/day. Infuse over 2-6 h. Hydrate with 10-15 ml/kg NS before infusion to decrease risk of nephrotoxicity. Alternative dosing regimen: Give 1 mg test dose as part of first infusion (separate IV bag not needed); if tolerated continue infusion, giving target dose of 0.5 to 1.5 mg/kg on first day. Candidemia, non-neutropenic pts: 0.6-1.0 mg/kg IV daily until 14-21 days past signs/sx resolved & neg repeat blood culture. Cryptococcal infection in HIV-infected: 0.7-1.5 mg/kg IV once daily preferably in combo with flucytosine depending on site and severity of infection. Tx for ≥2 weeks, followed by fluconazole consolidation, and then fluconazole chronic suppression. Severe histoplasmosis: 1 mg/kg IV once daily until stable for ≥2-3 weeks (treat x 12-16 weeks for meningitis), then consolidation & suppressive therapy.

NOTES - Acute infusion reactions, anaphylaxis, nephrotoxicity, hypokalemia, hypomagnesemia, acidosis, anemia. Monitor renal and hepatic function, CBC, serum electrolytes. Lipid formulations better tolerated, preferred in renal dysfunction.

amphotericin B lipid formulations (*Amphotec, Abelcet, AmBisome*) ▶? ♀B ▶? $$$$$

ADULT - Lipid formulations used primarily in patients refractory/intolerant to amphotericin deoxycholate. Abelcet: Invasive fungal infections: 5 mg/kg/day IV at 2.5 mg/kg/h. Shake infusion bag every 2 h. AmBisome: Infuse IV over 2 h. Empiric therapy of fungal infections in febrile neutropenia: 3 mg/kg/day. Aspergillus, candidal, cryptococcal infections: 3-5 mg/kg/day. Cryptococcal meningitis in HIV infection: 6 mg/kg/day. Amphotec: Test dose of 10 mL over 15-30 minutes, observe for 30 minutes, then 3-4 mg/kg/day IV at 1 mg/kg/h.

PEDS - Lipid formulations used primarily in patients refractory/intolerant to amphotericin deoxycholate. Abelcet: Invasive fungal infections: 5 mg/kg/day IV at 2.5 mg/kg/h. Shake infusion bag every 2 h. AmBisome: Infuse IV over 2 h. Empiric therapy of fungal infections in febrile neutropenia: 3 mg/kg/day. Aspergillus, candidal, cryptococcal infections: 3-5 mg/kg/day. Cryptococcal meningitis in HIV infection: 6 mg/kg/day. Amphotec: Aspergillosis: Test dose of 10 mL over 15-30 minutes, observe for 30 minutes, then 3-4 mg/kg/day IV at 1 mg/kg/h.

NOTES - Acute infusion reactions, anaphylaxis, nephrotoxicity, hypokalemia, hypomagnesemia, acidosis. Lipid formulations better tolerated than amphotericin deoxycholate, preferred in renal dysfunction. Monitor renal and hepatic function, CBC, electrolytes.

anidulafungin (*Eraxis*) ▶Degraded chemically ♀C ▶? $$$$$

ADULT - Candidemia, other systemic candidal infections: 200 mg IV load on day 1, then 100 mg IV once daily until ≥14 days after last positive culture. Esophageal candidiasis: 100 mg IV load on day 1, then 50 mg IV once daily for ≥14 days & continuing for ≥7 days after symptoms resolved. Max infusion rate 1.1 mg/min.

PEDS - Not approved in children.

NOTES - Max infusion rate of 1.1 mg/min to prevent histamine reactions. Diluent contains dehydrated alcohol.

caspofungin (*Cancidas*) ▶KL ♀C ▶? $$$$$

ADULT - Infuse IV over 1 h. Usual dose: 70 mg loading dose on day 1, then 50 mg daily. Patients taking rifampin: 70 mg daily. Consider this dose with other enzyme inducers (such as carbamazepine, dexamethasone, efavirenz, nevirapine, phenytoin) or if inadequate response to lower dose in febrile neutropenia or aspergillosis. Esophageal candidiasis: 50 mg daily. Duration of therapy in invasive aspergillosis is based on severity, treatment response, and resolution of immunosuppression. Treat Candidal infections for ≥14 days after last positive culture. Empiric therapy of febrile neutropenia: Treat until neutropenia resolved. If fungal infection confirmed, treat for ≥14 days and continue tx for ≥7 days after sx and neutropenia resolved.

PEDS - Not approved in children.

NOTES - Administration with cyclosporine increases caspofungin levels & hepatic transaminases; risk of concomitant use unclear. Caspofungin decreases tacrolimus levels. Dosage adjustment in moderate liver dysfunction (Child-Pugh score 7-9): 35 mg IV daily (after 70 mg loading dose in invasive aspergillosis).

clotrimazole (*Mycelex*, ✚*Canesten, Clotrimaderm*) ▶L ♀C ▶? $$$$

ADULT - Oropharyngeal candidiasis: 1 troche dissolved slowly in mouth 5x/day x 14 days. Prevention of oropharyngeal candidiasis in immunocompromised patients: 1 troche dissolved slowly in mouth tid until end of chemotherapy/high-dose corticosteroids.

PEDS - Oropharyngeal candidiasis ≥3 yo: Use adult dose.

FORMS - Generic/Trade: Oral troches 10 mg.

fluconazole (*Diflucan*) ▶K ♀C ▶+ $$$

ADULT - Vaginal candidiasis: 150 mg PO single dose ($). All other dosing regimens IV/PO. Oropharyngeal/ esophageal candidiasis: 200 mg first day, then 100 mg daily for ≥14 days for oropharyngeal, ≥3 weeks & continuing for 2 weeks past symptom resolution for esophageal. Systemic candidiasis: 400 mg daily. Candidal UTI, peritonitis: 50-200 mg daily. Cryptococcal meningitis: 400 mg daily until 10-12 weeks after cerebrospinal fluid is culture negative (see UNAPPROVED ADULT for first-line regimen). Suppression of cryptococcal meningitis relapse in AIDS: 200 mg daily until immune system reconstitution. Prevention of candidiasis after bone marrow transplant: 400 mg daily starting several days before neutropenia and continuing until ANC >1000 cells/mm3 x 7 days.

PEDS - All dosing regimens IV/PO. Oropharyngeal/esophageal candidiasis: 6 mg/kg first day, then 3 mg/kg daily for ≥14 days for oropharyngeal, ≥3 weeks & continuing for 2 weeks past symptom resolution for esophageal. Systemic candidiasis: 6-12 mg/kg daily. Cryptococcal meningitis: 12 mg/kg on first day, then 6 mg/kg daily until 10-12 weeks after cerebrospinal fluid is culture negative. Suppression of cryptococcal meningitis relapse in AIDS: 6 mg/kg daily.

UNAPPROVED ADULT - Onychomycosis, fingernail (2nd line to itraconazole or terbinafine): 150-300 mg PO q week x 3-6 mo. Onychomycosis, toenail (2nd line to itraconazole or terbinafine): 150-300 mg PO q week x 6-12 mo. Recurrent vaginal candidiasis: 150 mg PO every third day x 3 doses, then 100-150 mg PO q week x 6 months. Non-neutropenic candidemia: 400-800 mg/day IV/PO or 800 mg/day + amphotericin B 0.7 mg/kg/day IV for first 4-7 days. Treat until 14 days past last + blood culture and signs/sx resolved. Neutropenic candidemia: 6-12 mg/kg/day IV/PO until 14 days past last + blood culture, signs/sx, and neutropenia resolved. Prevention of candidal infections in high-risk neutropenic pts: 400 mg/day during period of risk for neutropenia. Cryptococcal meningitis: Amphotericin B preferably in combo with flucytosine x ≥2 weeks (induction), followed by fluconazole 400 mg PO once daily x 8 weeks (consolidation), then chronic suppression with fluconazole 200 mg PO once daily until immune system reconstitution.

UNAPPROVED PEDS - Cryptococcal meningitis: Amphotericin B preferably in combo with flucytosine x 2 weeks (induction), followed by fluconazole 5-6 mg/kg IV/PO bid x ≥8 weeks (consolidation), then chronic suppression with lower dose of fluconazole.

FORMS - Generic/Trade: Tabs 50, 100, 200 mg. 150 mg tab in single-dose blister pack. Susp 10 & 40 mg/mL (35 mL).

NOTES - Hepatotoxicity. Many drug interactions, including increased levels of cyclosporine, phenytoin, theophylline, and increased INR with warfarin. Do not use with cisapride. May inhibit metabolism of fluvastatin, and possibly simvastatin/lovastatin at higher doses. Dosing in renal dysfunction: Reduce maintenance dose by 50% for CrCl 11-50 ml/min. Hemodialysis: Give recommended dose after each dialysis. Single dose during 1st trimester of pregnancy does not appear to increase risk of congenital birth defects.

flucytosine (Ancobon) ▶K ♀C ▶- $$$$$

WARNING - Extreme caution in renal or bone marrow impairment. Monitor hematologic, hepatic, renal function in all patients.

ADULT - Candidal/cryptococcal infections: 50-150 mg/kg/day PO divided qid. Initial dose for cryptococcal meningitis: 100 mg/kg/day PO divided qid.

PEDS - Not approved in children.

UNAPPROVED PEDS - Candidal/cryptococcal infections: 50-150 mg/kg/day PO divided qid.

FORMS - Trade only: Caps 250, 500 mg.

NOTES - Flucytosine is given with other antifungal agents. Myelosuppression. Reduce nausea by taking caps a few at a time over 15 mins. Monitor levels. Peak 70-80 mg/L, trough 30-40 mg/L. Reduce dose in renal dysfunction. Avoid in children with severe renal dysfunction.

griseofulvin (Grisactin 500, Grifulvin V, ♥Fulvicin) ▶Skin ♀C ▶? $$$

ADULT - Tinea: 500 mg PO daily x 4-6 weeks for capitis, 2-4 weeks for corporis, 4-8 weeks for pedis, 4 months for fingernails, 6 months for toenails. Can use 1 g/day for pedis and unguium.

PEDS - Tinea: 11 mg/kg PO daily x 4-6 weeks for capitis, 2-4 weeks for corporis, 4-8 weeks for pedis, 4 months for fingernails, 6 months for toenails.

UNAPPROVED PEDS - Tinea capitis: AAP recommends 15-20 mg/kg (max 1 g) PO daily x 4-

6 weeks, continuing for 2 weeks past symptom resolution. Some infections may require 20-25 mg/kg/day or ultramicrosize griseofulvin 5-10 mg/kg (max 750 mg) PO daily.

FORMS - Generic/Trade: Susp 125 mg/5 mL (120 mL), Trade only: Tabs 500 mg.

NOTES - Do not use in liver failure, porphyria. May cause photosensitivity, lupus-like syndrome/ exacerbation of lupus. Decreased INR with warfarin, decreased efficacy of oral contraceptives. Ultramicrosize formulations have greater GI absorption, and are available with different strengths and dosing.

griseofulvin ultramicrosize (Gris-PEG) ▶Skin ♀C ▶? $$

ADULT - Tinea: 375 mg PO daily x 4-6 weeks for capitis, 2-4 weeks for corporis, 4-8 weeks for pedis, 4 months for fingernails, 6 months for toenails. Can use 750 mg/day for pedis and unguium. Best absorption when given after meal containing fat.

PEDS - Tinea, >2 yo: 7.3 mg/kg PO daily x 4-6 weeks for capitis, 2-4 weeks for corporis, 4-8 weeks for pedis, 4 months for fingernails, 6 months for toenails. Give 82.5-165 mg PO daily for 13.6-22.6 kg. Give 165-330 mg for >22.6 kg. Tinea capitis: AAP recommends 5-10 mg/kg (up to 750 mg) PO daily x 4-6 weeks, continuing for 2 weeks past symptom resolution. Best absorption when given after meal containing fat.

FORMS - Generic/Trade: Tabs 125, 250 mg.

NOTES - Do not use in liver failure, porphyria. May cause photosensitivity, lupus-like syndrome/ exacerbation of lupus. Decreased INR with warfarin, decreased efficacy of oral contraceptives. Microsize formulations, which have lower GI absorption, are available with different strengths and dosing.

itraconazole (Sporanox) ▶L ♀C ▶- $$$$$

WARNING - Inhibition of CYP 3A4 metabolism by itraconazole can lead to dangerously high levels of some drugs. High levels of some can prolong QT interval (see QT drugs table). Contraindicated with cisapride, dofetilide, ergot alkaloids, lovastatin, PO midazolam, pimozide, quinidine, simvastatin, triazolam. Negative inotrope; stop treatment if signs/sx of heart failure. Not for onychomycosis if heart failure; use for other indications in heart failure only if benefit exceeds risk.

ADULT - Caps - Take caps with full meal. Onychomycosis, toenails: 200 mg PO daily x 12 weeks. Onychomycosis "pulse dosing", fingernails: 200 mg PO bid for 1st wk of month x 2 months. Test nail specimen to confirm diagnosis before prescribing. IV/PO - Aspergillosis in patients intolerant/ refractory to amphotericin, blastomycosis, histoplasmosis: 200 mg IV bid x 4 doses, each IV dose over 1 h, then 200 mg IV daily. Can also give 200 mg PO bid or daily. Treat for ≥3 months. For life-threatening infections, load with 200 mg IV bid x 4 doses or 200 mg PO tid x 3 days. Empiric therapy of suspected fungal infection in febrile neutropenia: 200 mg IV bid x 4 doses, then 200 mg IV daily for ≤14 days. Continue oral sol'n 200 mg (20 ml) PO bid until significant neutropenia resolved. Oral soln - Swish & swallow in 10 ml increments on empty stomach. Oropharyngeal candidiasis: 200 mg daily x 1-2 weeks. Oropharyngeal candidiasis unresponsive to fluconazole: 100 mg bid. Esophageal candidiasis: 100-200 mg daily x ≥3 weeks & continuing for 2 weeks past symptom resolution.

PEDS - Not approved in children.

UNAPPROVED ADULT - Caps - Onychomycosis "pulse dosing", toenails: 200 mg PO bid for 1st wk of month x 3-4 months. Confirm diagnosis with nail specimen lab testing before prescribing.

UNAPPROVED PEDS - Caps for systemic fungal infections, 3-16 yo: 100 mg PO daily. Oropharyngeal candidiasis: Oral solution 2.5 mg/kg PO bid (max 200-400 mg/day) x 7-14 days. Esophageal candidiasis: Oral solution 2.5 mg/kg PO bid or 5 mg/kg PO once daily for minimum of 14-21 days. Caps usually ineffective for esophageal candidiasis.

FORMS - Generic/Trade: Cap 100 mg. Trade only: Oral soln 10 mg/mL (150 mL).

NOTES - Hepatotoxicity, even during 1st week of therapy. Monitor LFTs if hepatic history; consider monitoring in all. Decreased absorption with antacids, H2 blockers, proton pump inhibitors, or achlorhydria. Itraconazole levels reduced by carbamazepine, isoniazid, nevirapine, phenobarbital, phenytoin, rifabutin & rifampin, and potentially efavirenz. Itraconazole inhibits cytochrome P450 3A4 metabolism of many drugs. Not more than 200 mg bid of itraconazole with unboosted indinavir. May increase adverse effects with trazodone; consider reducing trazodone dose. May increase QT interval with disopyramide or halofantrine. Caps and oral soln not interchangeable. Oral sol'n may be preferred in serious infections due to greater absorption. Oral soln

may not achieve adequate levels in cystic fibrosis patients; consider alternative if no response. Start therapy for onychomycosis on day 1-2 of menses in women of childbearing potential & advise against pregnancy until 2 months after therapy ends. Do not use IV itraconazole if CrCl <30 ml/min. See package insert for instructions before making/ giving IV soln.

ketoconazole (*Nizoral*) ▶L ♀C ▶?+ $$$
WARNING - Hepatotoxicity: inform patients of risk & monitor. Do not use with cisapride, midazolam, pimozide, triazolam.

ADULT - Systemic fungal infections: 200-400 mg PO daily.

PEDS - Systemic fungal infections, ≥2 yo: 3.3-6.6 mg/kg PO daily.

UNAPPROVED ADULT - Tinea versicolor: 400 mg PO single dose or 200 mg PO daily x 7 days. Prevention of recurrent mucocutaneous candidiasis in HIV infection: 200 mg PO daily.

UNAPPROVED PEDS - Prevention of recurrent mucocutaneous candidiasis in HIV infection: 5-10 mg/kg/day PO daily or bid; maximum 400 mg bid.

FORMS - Generic/Trade: Tabs 200 mg.

NOTES - Antacids, H2 blockers, proton pump inhibitors, buffered didanosine, achlorhydria decrease absorption. Ketoconazole levels reduced by isoniazid, rifampin, and potentially efavirenz. Avoid >200 mg/day of ketoconazole with ritonavir or Kaletra. Ketoconazole inhibits cytochrome P450 3A4 metabolism of many drugs. May increase adverse effects with trazodone; consider reducing trazodone dose.

micafungin (*Mycamine*) ▶L, feces ♀C ▶? $$$$$
ADULT - Esophageal candidiasis: 150 mg IV once daily. Prevention of candidal infections in bone marrow transplant patients: 50 mg IV once daily. Infuse over 1 hour. Histamine-mediated reactions possible with more rapid infusion. Flush existing IV lines with normal saline before micafungin infusion.

PEDS - Not approved in children.

NOTES - Increases levels of sirolimus and nifedipine. Not dialyzed. Protect diluted solution from light. Do not mix with other meds; it may precipitate.

nystatin (*Mycostatin*, ✦*Nilstat, Nyaderm, Candistatin*) ▶Not absorbed ♀B ▶? $$$
ADULT - Thrush: 4-6 mL PO swish & swallow qid or suck on 1-2 troches 4-5 x daily.

PEDS - Thrush, infants: 2 mL/dose PO with 1

mL in each cheek qid. Premature and low weight infants: 0.5 mL PO in each cheek qid. Thrush, older children: 4-6 mL PO swish & swallow qid or suck on 1-2 troches 4-5 x daily.

FORMS - Generic/Trade: Susp 100,000 units/ mL (60,480 mL). Trade: Troches 200,000 units.

posaconazole (Noxafil) ▶Glucuronidation ♀C ▶- $$$$$

ADULT - Prevention of invasive Aspergillus or candida infection: 200 mg (5 mL) PO tid. Take with full meal or liquid nutritional supplement.

PEDS - Prevention of invasive Aspergillus or Candida infection, ≥13 yo: 200 mg (5 mL) PO tid. Take with full meal or liquid nutritional supplement.

FORMS - Trade only: Oral susp 40 mg/mL, 105 mL bottle.

NOTES - Consider alternative or monitor for breakthrough fungal infection if patient cannot take with a full meal or liquid nutritional supplement. Monitor for breakthrough fungal infection if severe vomiting/diarrhea. CYP 3A4 inhibitor. Contraindicated with ergot alkaloids and CYP 3A4 substrates that increase the QT interval, including cisapride, pimozide, halofantrine, and quinidine. Consider dosage reduction of vinca alkaloids, calcium channel blockers, lovastatin, simvastatin. Levels reduced by rifabutin, phenytoin, and cimetidine; phenytoin and rifabutin levels increased by posaconazole. Do not coadminister unless benefit exceeds risk. Monitor for rifabutin adverse effects. Reduce cyclosporine dose by 25% and tacrolimus dose by 66% when posaconazole started. Monitor levels of cyclosporine, tacrolimus, sirolimus. Monitor for benzodiazepine adverse effects and consider dosage reduction. Increased LFTs and possible hepatotoxicity.

terbinafine (Lamisil) ▶LK ♀B ▶- $$$$$

ADULT - Onychomycosis: 250 mg PO daily x 6 weeks for fingernails, x 12 weeks for toenails.

PEDS - Not approved in children.

UNAPPROVED ADULT - Onychomycosis "pulse dosing": 500 mg PO daily for 1st week of month x 2 months for fingernails, 4 months for toenails.

UNAPPROVED PEDS - Onychomycosis: 67.5 mg PO daily for <20 kg, 125 mg PO daily for 20-40 kg, 250 mg PO daily for >40 kg x 6 weeks for fingernails, x 12 weeks for toenails.

FORMS - Generic/Trade: Tabs 250 mg.

NOTES - Hepatotoxicity; monitor AST & ALT at baseline. Neutropenia. May rarely cause or exacerbate lupus. Do not use in liver disease or CrCl ≤50 mL/min. Test nail specimen to confirm diagnosis before prescribing. Inhibitor of CYP 2D6.

voriconazole (Vfend) ▶L ♀D ▶? $$$$$

ADULT - Invasive aspergillosis, or Scedosporium, Fusarium infections: 6 mg/kg IV q12h x 2 doses, then 4 mg/kg q12h. Candidemia in nonneutropenic, deep tissue Candida infections: 6 mg/kg IV q12h x 2 doses, then 3-4 mg/kg IV q12h. Treat for ≥2 weeks past symptom resolution or last positive culture, whichever is longer. Dilute IV to ≤5 mg/mL and infuse at ≤3 mg/kg/h over 1-2 h. When PO tolerated, give 200 mg PO q12h if >40 kg or 100 mg PO q12h if <40 kg. Coadministration with efavirenz: voriconazole 400 mg PO bid & efavirenz 300 mg (use caps) PO once daily. See package insert for dosage adjustments due to poor response/ adverse effects. Esophageal candidiasis: 200 mg PO q12h if ≥40 kg; 100 mg PO q12h if <40 kg for ≥2 weeks and continuing for >1 week past symptom resolution. Take tabs/ susp 1 h before/after meals.

PEDS - Safety & efficacy not established in children <12 yo. Use adult dose if ≥12 yo.

FORMS - Trade only: Tabs 50,200 mg (contains lactose), susp 40 mg/mL (75mL).

NOTES - Anaphylactoid reactions (IV only), severe skin reactions & photosensitivity, hepatotoxicity rarely. Transient visual disturbances common; advise against hazardous tasks (if vision impaired), night driving & strong, direct sunlight. Monitor visual (if treated >28 days), liver, and renal function. Many drug interactions. Substrate & inhibitor of CYP 2C9, 2C19, & 3A4. Do not use with carbamazepine, cisapride, ergot alkaloids, lopinavir-ritonavir, phenobarbital, pimozide, quinidine, rifabutin, rifampin, ritonavir 400 mg bid, or sirolimus. Ritonavir decreases voriconazole levels; avoid together unless benefit exceeds risk. Dosage adjustments with cyclosporine, omeprazole, phenytoin, tacrolimus in package insert. Increased INR with warfarin. Could inhibit metabolism of benzodiazepines, calcium channel blockers, statins, and methadone. When combining with oral contraceptives monitor for adverse effects based on increased levels of voriconazole, estrogen, and progestin. Vehicle in IV form may accumulate in renal impairment; oral preferred if CrCl <50 mL/minute. Mild/ moderate cirrhosis (Child-Pugh class A/B): Same loading dose & reduce maintenance dose by 50%. Oral susp stable for 14 days at room temperature.

ANTIMICROBIALS: Antimalarials

NOTE: For help treating malaria or getting anti-malarials, see www.cdc.gov/malaria or call the CDC "malaria hotline" (770) 488-7788 Monday-Friday 8 am to 4:30 pm EST; after hours / week-end (770) 488-7100. Pediatric doses of antima-larials should never exceed adult doses.

chloroquine (*Aralen*) ▶KL ♀C but + ▶+ $$

WARNING - Review product labeling for precau-tions and adverse effects before prescribing.

ADULT - Doses as chloroquine phosphate. Ma-laria prophylaxis, chloroquine-sensitive areas: 500 mg PO q wk from 1-2 weeks before expo-sure to 4 weeks after. Malaria: 1 g PO x 1, then 500 mg PO daily x 3 starting 6 h after 1st dose. Total dose is 2.5 g. Extraintestinal amebiasis: 1 g PO daily x 2, then 500 mg daily x 2-3 weeks.

PEDS - Doses as chloroquine phosphate. Ma-laria prophylaxis, chloroquine-sensitive areas: 8.3 mg/kg (up to 500 mg) PO q wk from 1-2 weeks before exposure to 4 weeks after. Ma-laria: 16.7 mg/kg PO x 1, then 8.3 mg/kg daily x 3 days starting 6 h after 1st dose. Do not ex-ceed adult dose. Chloroquine phosphate 8.3 mg/kg = chloroquine base 5 mg/kg.

FORMS - Generic only: Tabs 250 mg. Ge-neric/Trade: Tabs 500 mg (500 mg phosphate equivalent to 300 mg base).

NOTES - Retinopathy with chronic/high doses; eye exams required. May cause seizures (cau-tion if epilepsy); ototoxicity (caution if hearing loss); myopathy (discontinue if muscle weak-ness develops); bone marrow toxicity (monitor CBC if long-term use); exacerbation of psoria-sis; torsades. Concentrates in liver; caution ad-vised if hepatic disease, alcoholism, or hepato-toxic drugs. Antacids reduce absorption; give at least 4 h apart. Chloroquine reduces ampicil-lin absorption; give at least 2 h apart. May in-crease cyclosporine levels. As little as 1 g can cause fatal overdose in a child. Fatal malaria reported after chloroquine used as malaria prophylaxis in areas with chloroquine resis-tance; use only in areas without resistance. Maternal antimalarial prophylaxis doesn't harm breast-fed infant or protect infant from malaria.

Fansidar (sulfadoxine + pyrimethamine) ▶KL ♀C ▶- $

WARNING - Can cause life-threatening Stevens-Johnson syndrome and toxic epidermal necro-lysis. Stop treatment at first sign of rash, bacte-rial/fungal infection, or change in CBC.

ADULT, PEDS - CDC does not recommend Fansidar for treatment of malaria due to drug resistance and adverse effects.

FORMS - Trade only: Tabs sulfadoxine 500 mg + pyrimethamine 25 mg.

NOTES - Do not use in sulfonamide allergy; megaloblastic anemia due to folate deficiency; or for prolonged period in hepatic/renal failure or blood dyscrasia. Can cause hemolytic ane-mia in G6PD deficiency. Fansidar resistance is common in many malarious regions. Avoid ex-cessive sun exposure.

Malarone (atovaquone + proguanil) ▶Fecal excretion; LK ♀C ▶? $$$$

ADULT - Malaria prophylaxis: 1 adult tab PO daily from 1-2 days before exposure until 7 days after. Malaria treatment: 4 adult tabs PO daily x 3 days. Take with food/milk at same time each day. Repeat dose if vomiting ≤1 h. CDC recommends presumptive self-treatment of malaria (same dose as for treatment, but not for patients taking it for prophylaxis).

PEDS - Safety & efficacy established in children ≥11 kg for prevention, ≥5 kg for treatment. Prevention of malaria: Give PO daily from 1-2 days before exposure until 7 days after: 1 ped tab for 11-20 kg; 2 ped tabs for 21-30 kg; 3 ped tabs for 31-40 kg; 1 adult tab for >40 kg. Treatment of malaria: Give PO daily x 3 days: 2 ped tabs for 5-8 kg; 3 ped tabs for 9-10 kg; 1 adult tab for 11-20 kg; 2 adult tabs for 21-30 kg; 3 adult tabs for 31-40 kg; 4 adult tabs for >40 kg. Take with food or milk at same time each day. Repeat dose if vomiting occurs within 1 h after dose.

FORMS - Trade only: Adult tabs atovaquone 250 mg + proguanil 100 mg; pediatric tabs 62.5 mg + 25 mg.

NOTES - Vomiting common with malaria treat-ment doses (consider antiemetic). Monitor par-asitemia. Atovaquone levels may be decreased by tetracycline, metoclopramide (use another antiemetic if possible), and rifampin (avoid). If CrCl <30 mL/min avoid for malaria prophylaxis and use cautiously for treatment.

mefloquine (*Lariam*) ▶L ♀C ▶? $$

ADULT - Malaria prophylaxis, chloroquine-resis-tant areas: 250 mg PO q week from 1 week be-fore exposure to 4 weeks after. Malaria treat-ment: 1250 mg PO single dose. Take on full stomach with at least 8 oz water.

PEDS - Malaria treatment: 20-25 mg/kg PO; can divide into 2 doses given 6-8 h apart to reduce risk of vomiting. Repeat full dose if vomiting after <30 min; repeat ½ dose if vomiting after <30-60 minutes. Experience limited in infants <3 mo or <5 kg. Malaria prophylaxis: Give PO once weekly starting 1 week before exposure to 4 weeks after: 5-10 kg, 5 mg/kg (prepared by pharmacist); 10-20 kg, ¼ tab; 20-30 kg, ½ tab; 30-45 kg, ¾ tab. Take on full stomach.

UNAPPROVED ADULT - CDC regimen for malaria: 750 mg PO followed by 500 mg PO 6-12 h later, for total of 1250 mg. Quinine + doxycycline/tetracycline/clindamycin or atovaquone-proguanil preferred over mefloquine because of high rate of neuropsychiatric adverse effects with malaria treatment doses of mefloquine.

UNAPPROVED PEDS - Malaria prophylaxis, chloroquine-resistant areas: CDC recommends these PO doses q week starting 1 week before exposure to 4 weeks after: ≤15 kg, 5 mg/kg; 15-19 kg, ¼ tab; 20-30 kg, ½ tab; 31-45 kg, ¾ tab; >45 kg, 1 tab. Malaria treatment, <45 kg: 15 mg/kg PO, then 10 mg/kg PO given 8-12 h after first dose. Take on full stomach with at least 8 oz water.

FORMS - Generic/Trade: Tabs 250 mg.

NOTES - Cardiac conduction disturbances. Do not use with ziprasidone. Do not give until 12 h after the last dose of quinidine, quinine, chloroquine; may cause ECG changes and seizures. Contraindicated for prophylaxis if depression (active/recent), generalized anxiety disorder, psychosis, schizophrenia, other major psychiatric disorder, history of seizures. Tell patients to discontinue if psychiatric symptoms occur during prophylaxis. May cause drowsiness (warn about hazardous tasks). Can crush tabs and mix with a little water, milk, or other liquid. Pharmacists can put small doses into caps to mask bitter taste. Decreases valproate levels. Rifampin decreases mefloquine levels. Maternal use of antimalarial prophylaxis doesn't harm or protect breastfed infant from malaria.

primaquine ▶L ♀- ▶- $

WARNING - Review product labeling for precautions and adverse effects and document normal G6PD level before prescribing.

ADULT - Prevention of relapse, P vivax/ovale malaria: 30 mg base PO daily x 14 days.

PEDS - Not approved in children.

UNAPPROVED ADULT - Pneumocystis in those intolerant to trimethoprim/sulfamethoxazole: 30 mg primaquine base (2 tabs) PO daily plus clindamycin 600-900 mg IV q8h or 300-450 mg PO q8h x 21 days. Primary prevention of malaria in special circumstances: 30 mg base PO once daily beginning 1-2 days before exposure until 7 days after (consult with malaria expert; contact CDC at 770-488-7788 for info).

UNAPPROVED PEDS - Prevention of relapse, P vivax/ovale malaria: 0.5 mg/kg up to 30 mg base PO once daily x 14 d. Primary prevention of malaria in special circumstances: 0.5 mg/kg up to 30 mg base PO once daily beginning 1-2 days before exposure until 7 days after (consult with malaria expert; contact CDC at 770-488-7788 for info).

FORMS - Generic only: Tabs 26.3 mg (equiv to 15 mg base).

NOTES - Hemolytic anemia in G6PD deficiency, methemoglobinemia in NADH methemoglobin reductase deficiency. Contraindicated in pregnancy and G6PD deficiency; screen for deficiency before prescribing. Stop if dark urine or anemia. Avoid in patients with rheumatoid arthritis or SLE, recent quinacrine use, or use of other bone marrow suppressants.

quinine (Qualaquin) ▶L ♀C ▶+? $

ADULT - Malaria: 648 mg PO tid x 3 days (Africa/South America) or 7 days (Southeast Asia). Also give 7-day course of doxycycline, tetracycline or clindamycin.

PEDS - Not approved in children.

UNAPPROVED ADULT - Nocturnal leg cramps: 260-325 mg PO qhs. FDA believes risks outweigh benefits for this indication.

UNAPPROVED PEDS - Malaria: 25-30 mg/kg/day up to 2 g/day PO divided q8h x 3 days (Africa/South America) or 7 days (Southeast Asia). Also give doxycycline, tetracycline or clindamycin.

FORMS - Trade only: Caps 324 mg. Unapproved quinine products removed from US market in February 2007.

NOTES - Thrombocytopenia, thrombotic thrombocytopenic purpura, hemolytic uremic syndrome, cinchonism, hemolytic anemia with G6PD deficiency, cardiac conduction disturbances, hearing impairment. Contraindicated if prolonged QT interval, optic neuritis, myasthenia gravis, or hypersensitivity to quinine, quinidine, mefloquine. Many drug interactions. Do not use with erythromycin, rifampin, neuromuscular blockers. May increase digoxin levels. Monitor INR with warfarin. Antacids decrease absorption. Rule out G6PD deficiency in breastfed at-risk infant before giving to mother.

ANTIMICROBIALS: Antimycobacterial Agents

NOTE: Two or more drugs are needed for the treatment of active mycobacterial infections. See guidelines at http://www.thoracic.org/sections/publications/statements/. Get baseline LFTs, creatinine, and platelet count before treating TB. Evaluate at least monthly for adverse drug reactions. Routine liver and renal function tests not needed unless baseline dysfunction or increased risk of hepatotoxicity.

clofazimine (*Lamprene*) ▶Fecal ♀C ▶?- $
ADULT - Approved for leprosy therapy.
PEDS - Not approved in children.
UNAPPROVED ADULT - Mycobacterium avium complex in immunocompetent patients: 100-200 mg PO daily until "tan", then 50 mg PO daily or 100 mg PO three times weekly. Use in combination with other antimycobacterial agents. Not for general use in AIDS patients due to increased mortality.
FORMS - Trade only: Caps 50 mg. Distributed through investigational new drug application by National Hansen's Disease Program (phone 225-578-9861).
NOTES - Abdominal pain common; rare reports of splenic infarction, bowel obstruction, and GI bleeding. Pink to brownish-black skin pigmentation that may persist for months to years after drug is discontinued. Discoloration of urine, body secretions.

dapsone ▶LK ♀C ▶+ $
ADULT - Leprosy: 100 mg PO daily with rifampin +/- clofazimine or ethionamide.
PEDS - Leprosy: 1 mg/kg (up to 100 mg) PO daily with other antimycobacterial agents.
UNAPPROVED ADULT - Pneumocystis prophylaxis: 100 mg PO daily. Pneumocystis treatment: 100 mg PO daily with trimethoprim 5 mg/kg PO tid x 21 days.
UNAPPROVED PEDS - Pneumocystis prophylaxis, age ≥1 mo: 2 mg/kg (up to 100 mg) PO daily or 4 mg/kg (up to 200 mg) PO q week.
FORMS - Generic only: Tabs 25,100 mg.
NOTES - Blood dyscrasias, severe allergic skin reactions, sulfone syndrome, hemolysis in G6PD deficiency, hepatotoxicity, neuropathy, photosensitivity, leprosy reactional states. Monitor CBC q wk x 4, then monthly x 6, then twice yearly. Monitor LFTs.

ethambutol (*Myambutol*, ✦*Etibi*) ▶LK ♀C but + ▶+ $$$$
ADULT - TB: ATS and CDC recommend 15-20 mg/kg PO daily. Dose with whole tabs: 800 mg PO daily if 40-55 kg, 1200 mg PO daily if 56-75 kg, 1600 mg PO daily if 76-90 kg. Base dose on estimated lean body weight. Max dose regardless of weight is 1600 mg/day.
PEDS - TB: ATS and CDC recommend 15-20 mg/kg up to 1 g PO daily. Use cautiously if visual acuity cannot be monitored. Manufacturer recommends against use in children <13 yo.
UNAPPROVED ADULT - Treatment or prevention of recurrent Mycobacterium avium complex disease in HIV infection: 15-25 mg/kg up to 1600 mg PO daily with clarithromycin/azithromycin +/- rifabutin.
UNAPPROVED PEDS - Treatment or prevention of recurrent Mycobacterium avium complex disease in HIV infection: 15 mg/kg up to 900 mg PO daily with clarithromycin/azithromycin +/- rifabutin.
FORMS - Generic/Trade: Tabs 100,400 mg.
NOTES - Can cause retrobulbar neuritis. Avoid, if possible, in patients with optic neuritis. Test visual acuity and color discrimination at baseline. Ask about visual disturbances monthly. Monitor visual acuity and color discrimination monthly if dose >15-20 mg/kg, duration >2 months, or renal dysfunction. Advise patients to report any change in vision immediately; do not use in those who cannot report visual sx (eg, children, unconscious). Do not give aluminum hydroxide antacid until >4h after ethambutol dose. Reduce dose in renal impairment.

isoniazid (*INH*, ✦*Isotamine*) ▶LK ♀C but + ▶+ $
WARNING – Hepatotoxic; obtain LFT baseline. Monitor LFTs monthly if high-risk (HIV, signs/hx of liver disease, abnormal baseline LFTs, pregnancy/postpartum, alcoholism/regular alcohol use, some patients >35 yo). Stop isoniazid and seek care at once if hepatotoxicity sx. Discontinue if AST >3 x upper limit of normal with hepatotoxicity sx or AST >5 x upper limit of normal without hepatotoxicity sx.
ADULT - TB treatment: 5 mg/kg up to 300 mg PO daily or 15 mg/kg up to 900 mg twice weekly. Latent TB: 300 mg PO daily.
PEDS - TB treatment: 10-15 mg/kg up to 300 mg PO daily. Latent TB: 10 mg/kg up to 300 mg PO daily.
UNAPPROVED ADULT - American Thoracic Society regimen, latent tuberculosis: 5 mg/kg

up to 300 mg PO daily x 9 months (6 months OK if HIV-negative, but less effective than 9 months).

UNAPPROVED PEDS - American Thoracic Society regimen for latent tuberculosis: 10-20 mg/kg up to 300 mg PO daily for 9 months.

FORMS - Generic only: Tabs 100,300 mg, syrup 50 mg/5 mL.

NOTES - To reduce risk of peripheral neuropathy, give pyridoxine 25 mg PO daily if alcoholism, diabetes, HIV, uremia, malnutrition, seizure disorder, pregnant/ breastfeeding woman, breast-fed infant of INH-treated mother. Many drug interactions.

pyrazinamide (PZA, ♣Tebrazid) ▶LK ♀C ▶? $$$

WARNING - The ATS and CDC recommend against general use of 2 mo regimen of rifampin + pyrazinamide for latent TB due to reports of fatal hepatotoxicity.

ADULT - TB: ATS and CDC recommend 20-25 mg/kg PO daily. Dose with whole tabs: 1000 mg PO daily if 40-55 kg, 1500 mg daily if 56-75 kg, 2000 mg if 76-90 kg. Base dose on estimated lean body weight. Max dose regardless of weight is 2000 mg PO daily.

PEDS - TB: 15-30 mg/kg up to 2000 mg PO daily.

FORMS - Generic only: Tabs 500 mg.

NOTES - Hepatotoxicity, hyperuricemia (avoid in acute gout). Obtain LFTs at baseline. Monitor periodically in high-risk patients (HIV infection, alcoholism, pregnancy, signs/history of liver disease, abnormal LFTs at baseline). Discontinue if AST >3 x upper limit of normal with hepatotoxicity sx or AST >5 x upper limit of normal without hepatotoxicity sx. The ATS and CDC recommend against general use of 2 mo regimen of rifampin + pyrazinamide for latent TB due to reports of fatal hepatotoxicity. Consider reduced dose in renal dysfunction.

rifabutin (Mycobutin) ▶L ♀B ▶? $$$$$

ADULT - Prevention of disseminated Mycobacterium avium complex disease in AIDS: 300 mg PO daily or 150 mg PO bid. See www.aidsinfo.nih.gov for dosage adjustments of rifabutin with antiretroviral regimens.

PEDS - Not approved in children.

UNAPPROVED ADULT - TB or Mycobacterium avium complex disease treatment in AIDS: 300 mg PO daily. See www.aidsinfo.nih.gov for dosage adjustments of rifabutin with antiretroviral regimens.

UNAPPROVED PEDS - Mycobacterium avium

complex disease. Prophylaxis: ≥6 yo, 300 mg PO daily. <6 yo, 5 mg/kg (up to 300 mg) PO daily. Treatment: 10-20 mg/kg (max 300 mg/ day) PO once daily. TB: 10-20 mg/kg (up to 300 mg) PO once daily. See www.aidsinfo.nih. gov for dosage adjustment of rifabutin with antiretroviral regimens.

FORMS - Trade only: Caps 150 mg.

NOTES - Uveitis (with high doses or if metabolism inhibited by other drugs), hepatotoxicity, thrombocytopenia, neutropenia. Obtain CBC & LFTs at baseline. Monitor periodically in high-risk patients (HIV infection, alcoholism, pregnancy, signs/ history of liver disease, abnormal LFTs at baseline). Do not use alone in patients with active TB. May induce liver metabolism of other drugs including oral contraceptives, protease inhibitors, and azole antifungals. Substrate of CYP 3A4; fluconazole, clarithromycin, and protease inhibitors increase rifabutin levels (see www.aidsinfo.nih.gov for dosage adjustments). Urine, body secretion, soft contact lenses may turn orange-brown. Consider dosage reduction for hepatic dysfunction.

Rifamate (isoniazid + rifampin) ▶LK ♀C but + ▶+ $$$$

WARNING - Hepatotoxicity.

ADULT - Tuberculosis: 2 caps PO daily on empty stomach.

PEDS - Not approved in children.

FORMS - Trade only: Caps isoniazid 150 mg + rifampin 300 mg.

NOTES - See components. Monitor LFTs at baseline and periodically during therapy.

rifampin (Rimactane, Rifadin, ♣Rofact) ▶L ♀C but + ▶+ $$$$

WARNING - The ATS and CDC recommend against general use of 2 mo regimen of rifampin + pyrazinamide for latent TB due to reports of fatal hepatotoxicity.

ADULT - Tuberculosis: 10 mg/kg up to 600 mg PO/IV daily. Neisseria meningitidis carriers: 600 mg PO bid x 2 days. Take oral doses on empty stomach. IV and PO doses are the same. Neisseria meningitidis carriers: 600 mg PO bid x 2 days. Take on empty stomach. IV & PO doses are the same.

PEDS - Tuberculosis: 10-20 mg/kg up to 600 mg PO/IV daily. Neisseria meningitidis carriers: ≥1 mo, 10 mg/kg up to 600 mg PO bid x 2 days. <1 mo, 5 mg/kg PO bid x 2 days. Take on empty stomach. IV and PO doses are the same. Neisseria meningitidis carriers: age ≥1 mo, 10 mg/kg up to 600 mg PO bid x 2 days.

Age <1 mo, 5 mg/kg PO bid x 2 days. Take on empty stomach.

UNAPPROVED ADULT - Prophylaxis of H influenza type b infection: 20 mg/kg up to 600 mg PO daily x 4 days. Leprosy: 600 mg PO q month with dapsone. American Thoracic Society regimen for latent TB: 10 mg/kg up to 600 mg PO daily x 4 months. Staphylococcal prosthetic valve endocarditis: 300 mg PO q8 hr in combo with gentamicin plus nafcillin, oxacillin, or vancomycin. Take on empty stomach.

UNAPPROVED PEDS - Prophylaxis of H influenza type b infection: ≥1 mo, 20 mg/kg up to 600 mg PO daily x 4 days. <1 mo, 10 mg/kg PO daily x 4 days. Prophylaxis of invasive meningococcal disease: ≥1 mo, 10 mg/kg up to 600 mg PO bid x 2 days. <1 mo, 5 mg/kg PO bid x 2 days. American Thoracic Society regimen for latent TB: 10-20 mg/kg up to 600 mg PO daily x 4 months. Take on empty stomach.

FORMS - Generic/Trade: Caps 150,300 mg. Pharmacists can make oral suspension.

NOTES - Hepatotoxicity, thrombocytopenia. When treating TB, obtain baseline CBC, LFTs. Monitor periodically in high-risk patients (HIV infection, alcoholism, pregnancy, signs/history of liver disease, abnormal LFTs at baseline). Discontinue if AST >3 x upper limit of normal with hepatotoxicity sx or AST >5 x upper limit of normal without hepatotoxicity sx. The ATS and CDC recommend against general use of 2 mo regimen of rifampin + pyrazinamide for latent TB due to reports of fatal hepatotoxicity. Induces hepatic metabolism of many drugs; check other sources for dosage adjustments before prescribing. See www.aidsinfo.nih.gov for dosage adjustments of antiretroviral regimens with rifampin. If used with rifampin, consider increasing efavirenz to 800 mg qhs if weight ≥50 kg. Do not use rifampin with protease inhibitors. Decreased efficacy of oral con-traceptives; use non-hormonal method. Decreased INR with warfarin; monitor daily or as needed. Adjust dose for hepatic impairment. Colors urine, body secretions, soft contact lenses red-orange. IV rifampin is stable for 4h after dilution in dextrose 5%.

rifapentine (*Priftin*) ▶Esterases, fecal ♀C ▶? $$$$

ADULT - TB: 600 mg PO twice weekly x 2 months, then once weekly x 4 months. ATS and CDC recommend use only for continuation therapy in selected HIV-negative patients.

PEDS - Not approved in children <12 yo.

FORMS - Trade only: Tabs 150 mg.

NOTES - Hepatotoxicity, thrombocytopenia, exacerbation of porphyria. Obtain CBC and LFTs at baseline. Monitor LFTs periodically in high-risk patients (HIV infection, alcoholism, pregnancy, signs/ history of liver disease, abnormal LFTs at baseline). Do not use in porphyria. Urine, body secretions, contact lenses, and dentures may turn red-orange. May induce liver metabolism of other drugs including oral contraceptives. Avoid with protease inhibitors or NNRTIs.

Rifater (isoniazid + rifampin + pyrazinamide) ▶LK ♀C ▶? $$$$$

WARNING - Hepatotoxicity.

ADULT - TB, initial 2 mo of treatment: 6 tabs PO daily if ≥55 kg, 5 tabs daily if 45-54 kg, 4 tabs daily if ≤44 kg. Additional pyrazinamide tablets required to provide adequate dose in patient >90 kg. Take on empty stomach. Can finish treatment with Rifamate.

PEDS - Ratio of formulation may not be appropriate for children <15 yo.

FORMS - Trade only: Tab Isoniazid 50 mg + rifampin 120 mg + pyrazinamide 300 mg.

NOTES - See components. Monitor LFTs at baseline and during therapy. Do not use in patients with renal dysfunction.

ANTIMICROBIALS: Antiparasitics

albendazole (*Albenza*) ▶L ♀C ▶? $$$

ADULT - Hydatid disease, neurocysticercosis: ≥60 kg - 400 mg PO bid. <60 kg - 15 mg/kg/day (up to 800 mg/day) PO divided bid. Treatment duration varies. Take with food.

PEDS - Hydatid disease, neurocysticercosis: ≥60 kg - 400 mg PO bid. <60 kg: 15 mg/kg/day (up to 800 mg/day) PO divided bid. Treatment duration varies. Take with food.

UNAPPROVED ADULT - Hookworm, whipworm, pinworm, roundworm: 400 mg PO single dose. Repeat in 2 weeks for pinworm. Cutaneous larva migrans: 200 mg PO bid x 3 days. Giardia: 400 mg PO daily x 5 days.

UNAPPROVED PEDS - Roundworm, hookworm, pinworm, whipworm: 400 mg PO single dose. Repeat in 2 weeks for pinworm. Cutaneous larva migrans: 200 mg PO bid x 3 days.

Giardia: 400 mg PO daily x 5 days.

FORMS - Trade only: Tabs 200 mg.

NOTES - Monitor LFTs, WBC. Consider corticosteroids & anticonvulsants in neurocysticercosis. Get negative pregnancy test before treatment & warn against getting pregnant until a month after treatment. Treat close contacts for pinworms.

atovaquone (*Mepron*) ▶Fecal ♀C ▶? $$$$$

ADULT - Pneumocystis in patients intolerant to trimethoprim/sulfamethoxazole: Treatment 750 mg PO bid x 21 days. Prevention 1500 mg PO daily. Take with meals.

PEDS - Pneumocystis in patients intolerant to trimethoprim/sulfamethoxazole, 13-16 yo: Treatment, 750 mg PO bid x 21 days. Prevention, 1500 mg PO daily. Take with meals. Efficacy & safety not established for <13 yo.

UNAPPROVED PEDS - Prevention of recurrent Pneumocystis in HIV infection: 1-3 mo, 30 mg/kg PO daily. 4-24 mo, 45 mg/kg PO daily. >24 mo, 30 mg/kg PO daily. Take with meals.

FORMS - Trade only: Susp 750 mg/5 mL, foil pouch 750 mg/5 mL.

NOTES - Efficacy of atovaquone may be decreased by lopinavir/ ritonavir (Kaletra), rifampin (consider using alternative), rifabutin, rifapentine, and ritonavir.

ivermectin (*Stromectol*) ▶L ♀C ▶+ $

ADULT - Strongyloidiasis: 200 mcg/kg PO single dose. Onchocerciasis: 150 mcg/kg PO q3-12 months. Take on empty stomach with water.

PEDS - For children ≥15 kg. Strongyloidiasis: 200 mcg/kg PO single dose. Onchocerciasis: 150 mcg/kg PO single dose q 3-12 months. Take on empty stomach with water.

UNAPPROVED ADULT - Scabies: 200 mcg/kg PO repeated in 2 weeks. Pubic lice: 250 mcg/kg PO repeated in 2 weeks. Cutaneous larva migrans: 150-200 mcg/kg PO single dose. Take on empty stomach with water.

UNAPPROVED PEDS - Scabies: 200 mcg/kg PO single dose. Cutaneous larva migrans: 150-200 mcg/kg PO single dose. Take on empty stomach with water. Safety and efficacy not established in children <15 kg.

FORMS - Trade only: Tab 3, 6 mg.

NOTES - Mazzotti & ophthalmic reactions with treatment for onchocerciasis. May need repeat/monthly treatment for strongyloidiasis in immunocompromised/HIV-infected patients.

mebendazole (*Vermox*) ▶L ♀C ▶? $$

ADULT - Pinworm: 100 mg PO x 1; repeat in 2 weeks. Roundworm, whipworm, hookworm:

100 mg PO bid x 3 days.

PEDS - Pinworm: 100 mg PO x 1; repeat dose in 2 weeks. Roundworm, whipworm, hookworm: 100 mg PO bid x 3 days.

UNAPPROVED ADULT, PEDS - Roundworm, whipworm, hookworm: 500 mg PO single dose.

FORMS - Generic/Trade: Chew tab 100 mg.

NOTES - Treat close contacts for pinworms.

nitazoxanide (*Alinia*) ▶L ♀B ▶? $$$

ADULT - Cryptosporidial or Giardial diarrhea: 500 mg PO bid with food x 3 days.

PEDS - Cryptosporidial or Giardial diarrhea: 100 mg bid for 1-3 yo, 200 mg bid for 4-11 yo, 500 mg bid for ≥12 yo. Give PO with food x 3 days. Use suspension for <12 yo.

UNAPPROVED ADULT - C difficile colitis: 500 mg PO bid x 10 days.

FORMS - Trade only: Oral susp 100 mg/5 mL 60 mL bottle, tab 500 mg.

NOTES - Contains 1.5 g sucrose/5 mL. Turns urine bright yellow. Store at room temperature for up to 7 days.

paromomycin (*Humatin*) ▶Not absorbed ♀C ▶- $$$

ADULT, PEDS - Intestinal amebiasis: 25-35 mg/kg/day PO divided tid with/after meals x 5-10 d.

UNAPPROVED ADULT - Giardiasis: 500 mg PO tid x 7 days.

UNAPPROVED PEDS - Giardiasis: 25-35 mg/kg/day PO divided tid with/after meals x 7 days.

FORMS - Generic/Trade: Caps 250 mg.

NOTES - Nephrotoxicity possible with systemic absorption in inflammatory bowel disease. Not effective for extra-intestinal amebiasis.

pentamidine (*Pentam, NebuPent, ✦Pentacarinat*) ▶K ♀C ▶- $$$

ADULT - Pneumocystis treatment: 4 mg/kg IM/IV daily x 21 days. IV infused over 60-90 minutes. NebuPent for Pneumocystis prevention: 300 mg nebulized q 4 weeks.

PEDS - Pneumocystis treatment: 4 mg/kg IM/IV daily x 21 days. NebuPent not approved in children.

UNAPPROVED PEDS - Pneumocystis prevention, ≥5 yo: 300 mg NebuPent nebulized q 4 weeks.

FORMS - Trade only: Aerosol 300 mg.

NOTES - Contraindicated with ziprasidone. Fatalities due to severe hypotension, hypoglycemia, cardiac arrhythmias with IM/IV. Have patient lie down, check BP, and keep resuscitation equipment handy during IM/IV injection. May cause torsades, hyperglycemia, neutropenia, nephrotoxicity, pancreatitis, hypocalcemia. Monitor BUN, serum creatinine, blood glucose, CBC, LFTs, serum calcium, and ECG. Bronchospasm with inhalation (consider bronchodilator). Reduce IM/IV dose in renal dysfunction.

praziquantel (*Biltricide*) ▶LK ♀B ▶- $$$

ADULT, PEDS - Schistosomiasis: 20 mg/kg PO q4-6h x 3 doses. Liver flukes: 25 mg/kg PO q4-6h x 3 doses.

UNAPPROVED ADULT - Neurocysticercosis: 50 mg/kg/day PO divided tid x 15 days. Fish, dog, beef, pork intestinal tapeworms: 10 mg/kg PO single dose.

UNAPPROVED PEDS - Neurocysticercosis: 50-100 mg/kg/day PO divided tid x 15 days. Fish, dog, beef, pork intestinal tapeworms: 10 mg/kg PO single dose.

FORMS - Trade only: Tabs 600 mg.

NOTES - Contraindicated in ocular cysticercosis. May cause drowsiness; do not drive or operate machinery for 48 h. Phenytoin, carbamazepine, rifampin (avoid using together), and dexamethasone may lower praziquantel levels enough to cause treatment failure. Take with liquids during a meal. Do not chew tabs. Manufacturer advises against breast feeding until 72 h after treatment.

pyrantel (*Antiminth, Pin-X, Pinworm, ✤Combantrin*) ▶Not absorbed ♀- ▶? $

ADULT, PEDS - Pinworm, roundworm: 11 mg/kg up to 1 g PO single dose. Repeat in 2 weeks for pinworm.

UNAPPROVED ADULT, PEDS - Hookworm: 11 mg/kg up to 1 g PO daily x 3 days.

FORMS - OTC: Caps 62.5 mg, liquid 50 mg/mL.

NOTES - Purging not necessary. Treat close contacts for pinworms.

pyrimethamine (*Daraprim*) ▶L ♀C ▶+ $$

ADULT - Toxoplasmosis, immunocompetent patients: 50-75 mg PO daily x 1-3 weeks, then reduce by 50% for 4-5 more weeks. Give with leucovorin (10-15 mg daily) and sulfadiazine. Reduce initial dose in seizure disorders.

PEDS - Toxoplasmosis: 1 mg/kg/day PO divided bid x 2-4 days, then reduce by 50% x 1 month. Give with sulfadiazine & leucovorin. Reduce initial dose in seizure disorders.

UNAPPROVED ADULT - CNS toxoplasmosis in AIDS. Acute therapy: 200 mg PO x 1, then 50 mg (<60 kg) to 75 mg (≥60 kg) PO once daily + sulfadiazine 1000 mg (<60 kg) to 1500 mg (≥60 kg) PO q6h + leucovorin 10-20 mg PO once daily (can increase to ≥50 mg/day). Treat for ≥6 weeks. Secondary prevention: 25-50 mg

PO once daily + sulfadiazine 500-1000 mg PO qid +.leucovorin 10-25 mg PO once daily. Reduce initial dose in seizure disorders.

UNAPPROVED PEDS - Congenital toxoplasmosis: 2 mg/kg PO once daily x 2 days, then 1 mg/kg once daily x 2-6 months, then 1 mg/kg three times weekly + sulfadiazine 50 mg/kg PO bid. Give leucovorin 10 mg PO/IM with each dose of pyrimethamine. Treat x 1 year. Acquired toxoplasmosis: 2 mg/kg (up to 50 mg) PO once daily x 3 days, then 1 mg/kg (up to 25 mg) PO once daily + sulfadiazine 25-50 mg/kg PO (up to 1-1.5 g/dose) qid. Give leucovorin 10-25 mg/day PO. Treat ≥6 weeks followed by chronic suppressive therapy.

FORMS - Trade only: Tabs 25 mg.

NOTES - Hemolytic anemia in G6PD deficiency, dose-related folate deficiency, hypersensitivity. Monitor CBC.

thiabendazole (*Mintezol*) ▶LK ♀C ▶? $

ADULT - Helminths: 22 mg/kg/dose up to 1500 mg PO bid. Treat x 2 days for strongyloidiasis, cutaneous larva migrans. Take after meals.

PEDS - Helminths: 22 mg/kg/dose up to 1500 mg PO bid. Treat x 2 days for strongyloidiasis, cutaneous larva migrans. Limited use in children <13.5 kg. Take after meals.

FORMS - Trade only: Chew tab 500 mg, susp 500 mg/5 mL (120 mL).

NOTES - May cause drowsiness.

tinidazole (*Tindamax*) ▶KL ♀C ▶?- $

ADULT - Trichomoniasis or giardiasis: 2 g PO single dose. Amebiasis: 2 g PO daily x 3 days. Bacterial vaginosis: 2 g PO once daily x 2 days or 1 g PO once daily x 5 days. Take with food.

PEDS - Giardiasis, >3 yo: 50 mg/kg (up to 2 g) PO single dose. Amebiasis, >3 yo: 50 mg/kg (up to 2 g) PO daily x 3 days. Take with food.

UNAPPROVED ADULT - Recurrent/persistent urethritis: 2 g PO single dose.

FORMS - Trade only: Tabs 250,500 mg. Pharmacists can compound oral suspension.

NOTES - Give iodoquinol/ paromomycin after treatment for amebic dysentery or liver abscess. Disulfiram reaction; avoid alcohol until ≥3 days after treatment. Can minimize infant exposure by withholding breastfeeding for 3 days after maternal single dose. May increase levels of cyclosporine, fluorouracil, lithium, phenytoin, tacrolimus. May increase INR with warfarin. Do not give at same time as cholestyramine. CYP 450 3A4 substrate. For patients undergoing hemodialysis: Give supplemental ½ dose after dialysis session.

ANTIMICROBIALS: Antiviral Agents – Anti-CMV

cidofovir (*Vistide*) ▶K ♀C ▶- $$$$$
WARNING - Severe nephrotoxicity. Granulocytopenia - monitor neutrophil counts.
ADULT - CMV retinitis: 5 mg/kg IV q wk x 2 wks, then 5 mg/kg every other week. Give probenecid 2 g PO 3h before and 1 g 2h and 8h after infusion. Give normal saline with each infusion.
PEDS - Not approved in children.
NOTES - Fanconi-like syndrome. Stop nephrotoxic drugs ≥1 week before cidofovir. Get serum creatinine, urine protein before each dose. See package insert for dosage adjustments based on renal function. Do not use if creatinine >1.5 mg/dl, CrCl ≤55 mL/min, or urine protein ≥100 mg/dl (≥2+). Hold/ decrease zidovudine dose by 50% on days cidofovir is given. Tell women not to get pregnant until 1 month after and men to use barrier contraceptive until 3 months after cidofovir. Ocular hypotony - monitor intraocular pressure.

foscarnet (*Foscavir*) ▶K ♀C ▶? $$$$$
WARNING - Nephrotoxicity; seizures due to mineral/electrolyte imbalance.
ADULT - Hydrate before infusion. CMV retinitis: 60 mg/kg IV (over 1 h) q8h or 90 mg/kg IV (over 1.5-2 h) q12h x 2-3 weeks, then 90-120 mg/kg IV daily over 2h. Acyclovir-resistant HSV infection: 40 mg/kg IV (over 1 h) q8-12h x 2-3 weeks or until healed.
PEDS - Not approved in children. Deposits into teeth & bone of young animals.
UNAPPROVED PEDS - Hydrate before infusion. CMV retinitis: 60 mg/kg IV (over 1 h) q8h or 90 mg/kg IV (over 1.5-2 h) q12h x 2-3 weeks, then 90-120 mg/kg IV daily over 2h. Acyclovir-resistant HSV infection: 40 mg/kg IV (over 1 h) q8h x 2-3 weeks or until healed. Acyclovir-resistant varicella zoster infection: 40-60 mg/kg IV q8h x 7-10 days.
NOTES - Granulocytopenia, anemia, vein irritation, penile ulcers. Decreased ionized serum calcium, especially with IV pentamidine. Must use IV pump to avoid rapid administration. Monitor renal function, serum calcium, magnesium, phosphate, potassium. Reduce dose in renal impairment. Stop foscarnet if CrCl decreases to <0.4 mL/min/kg.

ganciclovir (*DHPG*) ▶K ♀C ▶- $$$$$
WARNING - Neutropenia, anemia, thrombocytopenia. Do not use if ANC <500/mm3 or platelets <25,000/mm3.

ADULT - CMV retinitis. Induction: 5 mg/kg IV q12h x 14-21 days. Maintenance: 6 mg/kg daily x 5 days/week; 5 mg/kg IV daily; 1000 mg PO tid; or 500 mg PO 6 times/day (q3h while awake) with food. Prevention of CMV disease in advanced AIDS: 1000 mg PO tid with food. Prevention of CMV disease after organ transplant: 5 mg/kg IV q12h x 7-14 days, then 6 mg/kg IV daily x 5 days/week or 1000 mg PO tid with food. Give IV infusion over 1 h.
PEDS - Safety and efficacy not established in children; potential carcinogenic or reproductive adverse effects.
UNAPPROVED PEDS - CMV retinitis in immunocompromised patient: Induction 5 mg/kg IV q12h x 14-21 days. Maintenance 5 mg/kg IV daily or 6 mg/kg IV daily x 5 days/week. Symptomatic congenital CMV infection: 6 mg/kg IV q12 h x 6 weeks.
FORMS - Generic only: Caps 250, 500 mg.
NOTES - Neutropenia (worsened by zidovudine), phlebitis/pain at infusion site, increased seizure risk with imipenem. Monitor CBC, creatinine. Reduce dose if CrCl <70 mL/min. Adequate hydration required. Potential teratogen, carcinogen. Tell women not to get pregnant during & men to use barrier contraceptive until ≥3 months after treatment. Follow guidelines for handling/ disposal of cytotoxic agents.

valganciclovir (*Valcyte*) ▶K ♀C ▶- $$$$$
WARNING - Myelosuppression may occur at any time. Monitor CBC frequently. Do not use if ANC <500/mm3, platelets <25,000/mm3, hemoglobin <8 g/dL.
ADULT - CMV retinitis: 900 mg PO bid x 21 days, then 900 mg PO daily. Prevention of CMV disease in high-risk kidney, kidney-pancreas, and heart transplant patients: 900 mg PO daily from within 10 days after transplant until 100 days post-transplant. Give with food. Valganciclovir tabs and ganciclovir caps not interchangeable on mg per mg basis.
PEDS - Safety and efficacy not established in children; potential carcinogenic or reproductive adverse effects.
FORMS - Trade only: Tabs 450 mg.
NOTES - Contraindicated in ganciclovir allergy. Greater bioavailability than oral ganciclovir. Potential teratogen. Tell women not to get pregnant during and men to use barrier contraceptive until ≥3 months after treatment. CNS toxic-

ity; warn against hazardous tasks. May increase creatinine; monitor renal function. Reduce dose if CrCl <60 ml/min. Use ganciclovir instead in hemodialysis patients. Potential drug interactions with didanosine, mycophenolate.

Potential carcinogen. Avoid direct contact with broken/crushed tabs; do not intentionally break/crush tabs. Follow guidelines for handling/ disposal of cytotoxic agents.

ANTIMICROBIALS: Antiviral Agents – Anti-Herpetic

acyclovir (*Zovirax*) ▶K ♀B ▶+ $
ADULT - Genital herpes: 200 mg PO q4h (5x/day) x 10 days for first episode, x 5 days for recurrent episodes. Chronic suppression: 400 mg PO bid. Zoster: 800 mg PO q4h (5x/day) x 7-10 days. Chickenpox: 800 mg PO qid x 5 days. IV: 5-10 mg/kg IV q8h, each dose over 1 h. Zoster in immunocompromised patients: 10 mg/kg IV q8h x 7 days. Herpes simplex encephalitis: 10 mg/kg IV q8h x 10 days. Mucosal/cutaneous herpes simplex in immunocompromised patients: 5 mg/kg IV q8h x 7 days. Treat ASAP after symptom onset.
PEDS – Safety/efficacy of PO acyclovir not established for <2 yo. Chickenpox: 20 mg/kg PO qid x 5 days. Use adult dose if >40 kg. AAP does not recommend routine treatment of chickenpox with acyclovir. Consider use if >12 yo, chronic cutaneous or pulmonary disease, or corticosteroid or chronic salicylate use. IV: 250-500 mg/m² q8h, each dose over 1h. Zoster in immunocompromised patients <12 yo: 20 mg/kg IV q8h x 7 days. Herpes simplex encephalitis: 20 mg/kg IV q8h x 10 days for 3 mo-12 yo, adult dose for ≥12 yo. Neonatal herpes simplex (birth to 3 mo): 10 mg/kg IV q8 h x 10 days; CDC regimen is 20 mg/kg IV q8h x 21 days for disseminated/CNS disease, x 14 days for skin/mucous membranes. Mucosal/cutaneous herpes simplex in immunocompromised: 10 mg/kg IV q8h x 7 days for <12 yo, adult dose for ≥12 yo. Treat ASAP after symptoms.
UNAPPROVED ADULT - Genital herpes: 400 mg PO tid x 7-10 days for first episode, x 5 days for recurrent episodes, x 5-10 days for recurrent episodes in HIV+ patients. Alternative regimens for recurrent episodes in HIV negative patients: 800 mg PO bid x 5 days or 800 mg PO tid x 2 days. Chronic suppression of genital herpes in HIV+ patients: 400-800 mg PO bid-tid. Orolabial herpes (controversial indication): 400 mg PO 5x/day. Bell's palsy: 400 mg PO 5x/day x 10 days. Treat ASAP after symptom onset.
UNAPPROVED PEDS - Primary herpes gingivostomatitis: 15 mg/kg PO 5x/day x 7 days. First-episode genital herpes: 80 mg/kg/day PO divided tid (max 1.2 g/day) x 7-10 days. Use dose in unapproved adult for adolescents. Zoster (mild) in mild immunosuppression: 20 mg/kg (max 800 mg/dose) PO qid x 7-10 days. Treat ASAP after symptom onset.
FORMS - Generic/Trade: Caps 200 mg, tabs 400,800 mg. Susp 200 mg/5 mL.
NOTES - Maintain adequate hydration. Severe drowsiness with acyclovir plus zidovudine. Reduce dose in renal dysfunction and in elderly. Base IV dose on ideal body weight in obese adults.

famciclovir (*Famvir*) ▶K ♀B ▶? $$
ADULT - Recurrent genital herpes: 1000 mg PO bid x 2 doses. Chronic suppression of genital herpes: 250 mg PO bid. Recurrent herpes labialis: 1500 mg PO single dose. Recurrent orolabial/ genital herpes in HIV patients: 500 mg PO bid x 7 days. Zoster: 500 mg PO tid x 7 days. Treat ASAP after symptom onset.
PEDS - Not approved in children.
UNAPPROVED ADULT - First-episode genital herpes: 250 mg PO tid x 7-10 days. Chronic suppression of genital herpes in HIV+ patients: 500 mg PO bid. Chickenpox in young adults: 500 mg PO tid x 5 days. Bell's palsy: 750 mg PO tid plus prednisone 1 mg/kg PO daily x 7 days. Treat ASAP after symptom onset.
UNAPPROVED PEDS - Chickenpox in adolescents: 500 mg PO tid x 5 days. First-episode genital herpes in adolescents: Use dose in unapproved adult.
FORMS - Trade only: Tabs 125, 250, 500 mg. All tabs contain lactose.
NOTES - Reduce dose for CrCl <60 mL/min.

valacyclovir (*Valtrex*) ▶K ♀B ▶+ $$$$$
ADULT - First-episode genital herpes: 1 g PO bid x 10 days. Recurrent genital herpes: 500 mg PO bid x 3 days. Chronic suppression of genital herpes in immunocompetent patients: 1 g PO daily. Can use 500 mg PO daily if ≤9 recurrences/year; transmission of genital herpes reduced with use of this regimen by source

partner, in conjunction with safer sex practices. Chronic suppression of genital herpes in HIV-infected patients: 500 mg PO bid. Herpes labialis: 2 g PO q12h x 2 doses. Zoster: 1 g PO tid x 7 days. Treat ASAP after symptom onset.
PEDS - Herpes labialis, ≥12 yo: 2 g PO q12h x 2 doses. Treat ASAP after symptom onset.
UNAPPROVED ADULT - Recurrent genital herpes: 1 g PO daily x 5 days. Recurrent genital herpes in HIV+ patients: 1 g PO bid x 5-10 days. Bell's palsy: 1 g PO bid plus prednisone 1 mg/kg PO daily x 7 days. Orolabial herpes in immunocompromised patients, including HIV infection: 1 g PO tid x 7 days. Chickenpox in young adults: 1 g PO tid x 5 days. Treat ASAP after symptom onset.
UNAPPROVED PEDS - Chickenpox in adolescents: 1 g PO tid x 5 days. Treat ASAP after symptom onset. First-episode genital herpes in adolescents: Use adult dose.
FORMS - Generic/Trade: Tabs 500,1000 mg.
NOTES - Maintain adequate hydration. CNS and renal adverse effects more common if elderly or renal impairment; avoid inappropriately high doses in these patients. Thrombotic thrombocytopenic purpura/hemolytic uremic syndrome at dose of 8 g/day. Reduce dose for CrCl <50 mL/min. Metabolized to acyclovir.

ANTIMICROBIALS: Antiviral Agents – Anti-HIV – CCR5 Antagonists

NOTE: AIDS treatment guidelines available online at www.aidsinfo.nih.gov. Consider monitoring LFTs in patients receiving highly active anti-retroviral therapy (HAART).

maraviroc (*Selzentry*) ▶LK ♀B ▶- $$$$$
WARNING - Hepatotoxicity with features of allergy; consider discontinuing if signs/symptoms of hepatitis, or increased LFTs with rash/systemic symptoms. Caution if baseline liver dysfunction or coinfection with hepatitis B/C.
ADULT - Combination therapy for HIV infection, treatment-experienced patients: 150 mg PO bid with strong CYP 3A4 inhibitors (delavirdine, most protease inhibitors, ketoconazole, itraconazole, clarithromycin); 300 mg PO bid with drugs that are not strong CYP 3A4 inducers/inhibitors (NRTIs, tipranavir-ritonavir, nevirapine, enfuvirtide); 600 mg PO bid with strong CYP 3A4 inducers (efavirenz, rifampin, carbamazepine, phenobarbital, phenytoin). Tropism test before treatment; not for dual/mixed or CXCR4-tropic HIV infection.
PEDS - Not recommended for <16 yo based on lack of data.
FORMS - Trade only: Tabs 150,300 mg.
NOTES - Caution for patients with liver dysfunction or coinfection with hepatitis B/C. May increase risk of myocardial ischemia or MI. Theoretical risk of infection/malignancy due to effects on immune system. Metabolized by CYP 3A4; do not use with St John's wort. Co-administration of CYP 3A4 inhibitor in patients with CrCl <50 mL/min may increase maraviroc levels and risk of adverse drug reactions.

ANTIMICROBIALS: Antiviral Agents – Anti-HIV - Combinations

NOTE: AIDS treatment guidelines available online at www.aidsinfo.nih.gov. Consider monitoring LFTs in patients receiving highly active anti-retroviral therapy (HAART). WARNING: Nucleoside reverse transcriptase inhibitors can cause lactic acidosis and hepatic steatosis. Fatalities reported in pregnant women receiving didanosine + stavudine.

Atripla (efavirenz + emtricitabine + tenofovir) ▶KL ♀D ▶- $$$$$
WARNING - Emtricitabine and tenofovir: Potentially fatal lactic acidosis and hepatosteatosis; severe acute exacerbation of hepatitis B after discontinuation in patients coinfected with HIV and hepatitis B; not indicated for treatment of hepatitis B.
ADULT - Combination therapy for HIV infection: 1 tab PO once daily on empty stomach, preferably at bedtime. Atripla can be used alone or in combo with other anti-retrovirals that are not already in the tab.
PEDS - Safety and efficacy not established.
FORMS - Trade only: Tabs efavirenz 600 mg + emtricitabine 200 mg + tenofovir 300 mg.
NOTES - See components. Do not give Atripla with lamivudine. Not for CrCl ≤50 mL/min. Efavirenz induces cytochrome P450 3A4, causing many drug interactions.
Epzicom (abacavir + lamivudine) ▶LK ♀C ▶- $$$$$

WARNING - Abacavir: Potentially fatal hypersensitivity reactions. Abacavir and lamivudine: Lactic acidosis and hepatosteatosis. Lamivudine: Exacerbation of hepatitis B after discontinuation in patients co-infected with HIV and hepatitis B.

ADULT - Combination therapy for HIV infection: 1 tab PO daily.

PEDS - Safety and efficacy not established.

FORMS - Trade only: Tabs abacavir 600 mg + lamivudine 300 mg.

NOTES - See components. Contraindicated if previous hypersensitivity reaction to abacavir due to risk of fatal rechallenge reaction. Not for patients with CrCl ≤50 mL/min, hepatic dysfunction, or if dosage adjustment required.

Trizivir (abacavir + lamivudine + zidovudine) ▶LK ♀C ▶- $$$$$

WARNING - Abacavir: Life-threatening hypersensitivity (see abacavir entry for details). Never restart after a reaction. Zidovudine: Bone marrow suppression, myopathy.

ADULT - HIV infection, alone (not preferred) or in combo with other agents: 1 tab PO bid.

PEDS - HIV infection in adolescents ≥40 kg, alone (not a preferred regimen) or in combo with other agents: 1 tab PO bid.

FORMS - Trade only: Tabs abacavir 300 mg + lamivudine 150 mg + zidovudine 300 mg.

NOTES - See components. Monitor CBC. Not for weight <40 kg, CrCl ≤50 mL/min or if dosage adjustment required.

Truvada (emtricitabine + tenofovir) ▶K ♀B ▶- $$$$$

WARNING - Emtricitabine and tenofovir: Potentially fatal lactic acidosis and hepatosteatosis; severe acute exacerbation of hepatitis B after discontinuation in patients coinfected with HIV and hepatitis B.

ADULT - Combination therapy for HIV infection: 1 tab PO daily.

PEDS - Safety and efficacy not established.

UNAPPROVED ADULT - Antiviral-resistant chronic hepatitis B in HIV-coinfected patients: 1 tab PO daily.

FORMS - Trade only: Tabs emtricitabine 200 mg + tenofovir 300 mg.

NOTES - See components. Do not use in a triple nucleoside regimen. Not for patients with CrCl ≤30 mL/min or hemodialysis; hepatic dysfunction; or if dosage adjustment required. Increase dosing interval to q48h if CrCl 30-49 mL/min. Coadminister didanosine and Truvada cautiously; monitor for didanosine adverse effects, and discontinue didanosine if they occur. Reduce didanosine dose to 250 mg in adults >60 kg; dosage adjustment of didanosine unclear if <60 kg. Give Videx EC + Truvada on empty stomach or with light meal. Give buffered didanosine + Truvada on empty stomach. Atazanavir and lopinavir/ ritonavir increase tenofovir levels; monitor and discontinue Truvada if tenofovir adverse effects. Tenofovir decreases atazanavir levels. If atazanavir is used with Truvada, use 300 mg atazanavir + 100 mg ritonavir. Do not use Truvada with lamivudine.

ANTIMICROBIALS: Antiviral Agents – Anti-HIV – Fusion Inhibitors

NOTE: AIDS treatment guidelines available online at www.aidsinfo.nih.gov.

enfuvirtide (Fuzeon, T-20) ▶Serum ♀B ▶- $$$$$

WARNING - Not for monotherapy.

ADULT - Combination therapy for HIV infection: 90 mg SC bid. Give each injection at new site in upper arm, anterior thigh, or abdomen, avoiding areas with current injection site reaction.

PEDS - Combination therapy for HIV infection, 6-16 yo: 2 mg/kg up to 90 mg SC bid. Give each injection at new site in upper arm, anterior thigh, or abdomen, avoiding areas with current injection site reaction.

FORMS - 30-day kit with vials, diluent, syringes, alcohol wipes. Single-dose vials contain 108 mg to provide 90 mg enfuvirtide.

NOTES - Increased risk of bacterial pneumonia; monitor for signs and sx. Biojector 2000 can cause persistent nerve pain if used near large nerves, bruising, hematomas. Anticoagulants, hemophilia, or other coagulation disorder may increase risk of post-injection bleeding. Reconstitute with 1.1 mL sterile water for injection. This provides 1.2 mL of solution, of which only 1 mL (90 mg) is injected. Allow vial to stand until powder dissolves completely (up to 45 minutes). Do not shake. Second daily dose can be reconstituted ahead of time if stored in refrigerator in original vial and used within 24 h. Return to room temp before injecting. Discard unused solution. Patient education on administration available 1-877-438-9366 or fuzeon.com.

ANTIMICROBIALS: Antiviral Agents – Anti-HIV – Non-Nucleoside Reverse Transcriptase Inhibitors

NOTE: AIDS guidelines at aidsinfo.nih.gov. Many serious drug interactions - always check before prescribing! See aidsinfo.nih.gov for use of rifamycins with NNRTIs. Consider monitoring LFTs with highly active anti-retroviral therapy (HAART).

efavirenz (*Sustiva, EFV*) ▶L ♀D ▶- $$$$$
WARNING - Not for monotherapy.
ADULT - Combination therapy for HIV infection: 600 mg PO qhs. Coadministration with voriconazole: Use voriconazole maintenance dose of 400 mg PO bid & reduce efavirenz to 300 mg (use caps) PO once daily. Avoid with high-fat meal. Take on empty stomach, bedtime best.
PEDS - Consider antihistamine rash prophylaxis before starting. Combination therapy for HIV infection, ≥3 yo: 10-15 kg: 200 mg PO qhs. 15-20 kg: 250 mg qhs. 20 to <25 kg: 300 mg qhs. 25 to <32.5 kg: 350 mg qhs. 32.5 to <40 kg: 400 mg qhs. ≥40 kg: 600 mg qhs. Do not give with high-fat meal.
FORMS - Trade only: Caps 50,100,200 mg, tabs 600 mg.
NOTES - Psychiatric/CNS reactions (warn about hazardous tasks), rash (consider antihistamines and/or corticosteroids; stop treatment if severe), increased cholesterol (monitor). To avoid "hangover", give 1st dose at 6-8 pm & start drug over weekend. False-positive with Microgenics cannabinoid screening test. Monitor LFTs if given with ritonavir, hepatotoxic drugs, or to patients with hepatitis B/C. Induces cytochrome P450 3A4. Many drug interactions including decreased levels of anticonvulsants, atorvastatin, diltiazem, itraconazole, methadone, pravastatin, simvastatin, and probably ketoconazole. Do not give with cisapride, pimozide, triazolam, ergot alkaloids, or St John's wort. Midazolam contraindicated in labeling; but can use single dose IV cautiously with monitoring for procedural sedation. See www.aidsinfo.nih.gov for use of rifamycins with NNRTIs. If used with rifampin, consider increasing efavirenz to 800 mg qhs if weight ≥50 kg. High risk of rash when taken with clarithromycin; consider alternative antimicrobial. Potentially teratogenic; get negative pregnancy test before use by women of child-bearing potential and recommend barrier contraceptive.

nevirapine (*Viramune, NVP*) ▶LK ♀C ▶- $$$$$

WARNING - Life-threatening skin reactions, hypersensitivity, hepatotoxicity. Monitor clinical & lab status intensively during first 18 weeks of therapy (risk of rash and/or hepatotoxicity greatest during first 6 weeks) and frequently thereafter. Consider LFTs at baseline, before and 2 weeks after dose increase, and at least once monthly. Rapidly progressive liver failure can occur after only a few weeks of therapy. Stop nevirapine and never rechallenge if clinical hepatitis, severe rash, or rash with constitutional sx. Obtain LFTs if rash occurs. Risk of hepatotoxicity with rash high in women or high CD4 count (women with CD4 count >250 especially high risk, including pregnant women). Do not use if CD4 count >250 in women or >400 in men unless benefit clearly outweighs risk. Elevated LFTs or hepatitis B/C infection at baseline increases risk of hepatotoxicity. Hepatotoxicity not reported after single doses of nevirapine or in children. Not for monotherapy.
ADULT - Combination therapy for HIV infection: 200 mg PO daily x 14 days, then 200 mg PO bid. Dose titration reduces risk of rash. If rash develops, do not increase dose until resolution. If stopped for >7 days, restart with initial dose.
PEDS - Combination therapy for HIV infection, 2 mo - 8 yo: 4 mg/kg PO daily x 14 days, then 7 mg/kg PO bid. ≥8 yo: 4 mg/kg PO daily x 14 days, then 4 mg/kg PO bid. Max dose 400 mg/day. Dose titration reduces rash risk. If rash develops, do not increase dose until resolution. If stopped for >7 days, restart with initial dose.
UNAPPROVED ADULT - Combination therapy for HIV infection: 200 mg PO daily x 14 days, then 400 mg PO daily. Prevention of maternal-fetal HIV transmission, maternal dosing: 200 mg PO single dose at onset of labor.
UNAPPROVED PEDS - Prevention of maternal-fetal HIV transmission, neonatal dosing: 2 mg/kg PO single dose within 3 days of birth.
FORMS - Trade only: Tabs 200 mg, susp 50 mg/5 mL (240 mL).
NOTES - Cytochrome P450 3A inducer. May require increased methadone dose. Do not give with ketoconazole, hormonal contraceptives, St John's wort. See www.aidsinfo.nih.gov for use of rifamycins with NNRTIs. Granulocytopenia more common in children receiving zidovudine and nevirapine.

ANTIMICROBIALS: Antiviral Agents – Anti-HIV – Nucleoside/Nucleotide Reverse Transcriptase Inhibitors

NOTE: AIDS treatment guidelines available online at www.aidsinfo.nih.gov. Consider monitoring LFTs in patients receiving highly active anti-retroviral therapy (HAART). WARNING: Nucleoside reverse transcriptase inhibitors can cause lactic acidosis and hepatic steatosis. Fatalities reported in pregnant women receiving didanosine + stavudine.

abacavir (*Ziagen, ABC*) ▶L ♀C ▶- $$$$$
WARNING - Potentially fatal hypersensitivity (look for fever, rash, GI symptoms, cough, dyspnea, pharyngitis, or other respiratory symptoms). Stop at once & never rechallenge after suspected reaction. Fatal reactions can recur within hours of rechallenge in patients with previously unrecognized reaction.
ADULT - Combination therapy for HIV infection: 300 mg PO bid or 600 mg PO daily. Severe hypersensitivity may be more common with once-daily dose.
PEDS - Combination therapy for HIV, 3 mo - 16 yo: 8 mg/kg up to 300 mg PO bid.
FORMS - Trade only: Tabs 300 mg, oral soln 20 mg/mL (240 mL).
NOTES - Dosage reduction for mild hepatic dysfunction (Child-Pugh score 5-6): 200 mg (10 mL of oral soln) PO bid.

Combivir (lamivudine + zidovudine) ▶LK ♀C ▶- $$$$$
WARNING - Zidovudine: bone marrow suppression, myopathy. Lamivudine: Severe acute exacerbation of hepatitis B can occur after discontinuation of lamivudine in patients coinfected with HIV + hepatitis B. Monitor closely for ≥2 mo after discontinuing lamivudine in such patients; consider treating hepatitis B.
ADULT - Combination therapy for HIV infection: 1 tab PO bid.
PEDS - Combination therapy for HIV infection, ≥12 yo: 1 tab PO bid.
FORMS - Trade only: Tabs lamivudine 150 mg + zidovudine 300 mg.
NOTES - See components. Monitor CBC. Not for weight <50 kg, CrCl ≤50 mL/min, hepatic dysfunction, or if dosage adjustment required.

didanosine (*Videx, Videx EC, ddI*) ▶LK ♀B ▶- $$$$$
WARNING - Potentially fatal pancreatitis; avoid use with other drugs that can cause pancreatitis. Avoid didanosine + stavudine in pregnancy due to reports of fatal lactic acidosis with pancreatitis or hepatic steatosis.
ADULT - Combination therapy for HIV infection: Buffered powder: 250 mg PO bid for ≥60 kg, 167 mg PO bid for <60 kg. Videx EC: 400 mg PO daily for ≥60 kg, 250 mg PO daily for <60 kg. All formulations usually taken on empty stomach. Dosage reduction of Videx EC with tenofovir: 250 mg if ≥60 kg, 200 mg if <60 kg. Dosage reduction unclear with tenofovir if CrCl <60 mL/min. Give tenofovir + Videx EC on empty stomach or with light meal; give tenofovir + buffered didanosine on empty stomach.
PEDS - Combination therapy for HIV infection: 100 mg/m^2 PO bid for age 2 weeks-8 mo. 120 mg/m^2 PO bid for age >8 mo. Give on empty stomach. Videx EC not approved for children.
FORMS - Generic/Trade: Pediatric powder for oral solution 10 mg/mL (buffered with antacid), delayed-release caps 200, 250, 400 mg. Trade only: (Videx EC) delayed-release caps 125 mg, chewable tabs 25, 50, 100, 150, 200 mg.
NOTES - Peripheral neuropathy (use cautiously with other neurotoxic drugs), retinal changes, optic neuritis, retinal depigmentation in children, hyperuricemia. Risk of lactic acidosis, pancreatitis, and peripheral neuropathy increased by concomitant stavudine. Diarrhea with buffered powder. See package insert for reduced dose if CrCl <60 mL/min. Do not use with allopurinol. Give some medications at least 1 h (amprenavir, delavirdine, indinavir), 2 h (atazanavir, ciprofloxacin, levofloxacin, norfloxacin, ofloxacin, itraconazole, ketoconazole, ritonavir, dapsone, tetracyclines), or 4 h (moxifloxacin, gatifloxacin) before buffered didanosine. Contraindicated with ribavirin due to risk of didanosine toxicity.

emtricitabine (*Emtriva, FTC*) ▶K ♀B ▶- $$$$$
WARNING - Severe acute exacerbation of hepatitis B can occur after discontinuation in patients coinfected with HIV + hepatitis B. Monitor closely for ≥2 mo; consider treating hepatitis B.
ADULT - Combination therapy for HIV infection: 200 mg cap PO daily. Oral soln: 240 mg (24 mL) PO daily.
PEDS - Combination therapy for HIV, ≥3 mo: 6 mg/kg up to 240 mg (24 mL) of oral soln PO once daily. Can give 200 mg cap PO once

daily if >33 kg.

UNAPPROVED PEDS - Combination therapy for HIV infection. Oral soln: 3 mg/kg PO once daily for ≤3 mo, 6 mg/kg up to 240 mg for 3 mo-17 yo. Caps, >33 kg: 200 mg PO once daily.

FORMS - Trade only: Caps 200 mg, oral soln 10 mg/mL (170 mL).

NOTES - Lactic acidosis/hepatic steatosis. Exacerbation of hepatitis B after discontinuation. Dosage reduction in adults with renal dysfunction. Caps: 200 mg PO q48h if CrCl 30-49 mL/min; 200 mg PO q72h if CrCl 15-29 mL/min; 200 mg PO q96h if CrCl <15 mL/min or hemodialysis. Oral soln: 120 mg q24h if CrCl 30-49 mL/min; 80 mg q24h if CrCl 15-29 mL/min, 60 mg q24h if CrCl <15 mL/min or hemodialysis. Refrigerate oral soln if possible; stable for 3 months stored at room temp.

lamivudine (Epivir, Epivir-HBV, 3TC, ♥Heptovir) ▶K ♀C ▶- $$$$$

WARNING - Lower dose of lamivudine in Epivir-HBV can cause HIV resistance - test for HIV before prescribing Epivir-HBV. Severe acute exacerbation of hepatitis B can occur after discontinuation of lamivudine in patients coinfected with HIV + hepatitis B. Monitor closely for ≥2 mo after discontinuing lamivudine in such patients; consider treating hepatitis B.

ADULT - Epivir for combination therapy for HIV infection: 300 mg PO daily or 150 mg PO bid. Epivir-HBV for chronic hepatitis B: 100 mg PO daily.

PEDS - Epivir for HIV infection: 3 mo-16 yo, 4 mg/kg (up to 150 mg) PO bid. Epivir-HBV for chronic hepatitis B, 2-17 yo: 3 mg/kg up to 100 mg PO daily.

UNAPPROVED PEDS - Epivir for HIV infection in adolescents ≥50 kg: 300 mg PO daily.

FORMS - Trade only: Epivir, 3TC: Tabs 150, 300 mg, oral soln 10 mg/mL. Epivir-HBV, Heptovir: Tabs 100 mg, oral soln 5 mg/mL.

NOTES - Lamivudine-resistant hepatitis B reported. Epivir: Pancreatitis in children. Monitor for hepatic decompensation (potentially fatal), neutropenia, and anemia if also receiving interferon for hepatitis C. If hepatic decompensation occurs, consider discontinuing lamivudine, and reducing or discontinuing interferon, and/or ribavirin. Dosage reduction for CrCl <50 mL/min in package insert.

stavudine (Zerit, d4T) ▶LK ♀C ▶- $$$$$

WARNING - Warn patients to report early signs of lactic acidosis (eg, abdominal pain, N/V, fa-

tigue, dyspnea, weakness). Symptoms can mimic Guillain-Barre syndrome. Stop stavudine if weakness or lactic acidosis. Potentially fatal pancreatitis & hepatotoxicity with didanosine + stavudine +/- hydroxyurea. Avoid this combo in pregnancy.

ADULT - Combination therapy for HIV infection: 40 mg PO q12h; 30 mg PO q12h if <60 kg. Hold for peripheral neuropathy. If symptoms resolve completely, can restart at 20 mg PO q12h or 15 mg q12h if <60 kg. If symptoms recur, consider stopping permanently.

PEDS - Combination therapy for HIV infection: <30 kg and ≥2 weeks old: 1 mg/kg PO bid. 30-59.9 kg: 30 mg bid. ≥60 kg: 40 mg bid.

FORMS - Trade only: Caps 15,20,30,40 mg; oral soln 1 mg/mL (200 mL).

NOTES - Peripheral neuropathy, lactic acidosis, pancreatitis; risk of these adverse reactions increased by concomitant didanosine. Do not use with zidovudine. Dosage reduction for CrCl <50 mL/min in package insert. Oral soln stable in refrigerator for 30 days.

tenofovir (Viread, TDF) ▶K ♀B ▶- $$$$$

WARNING - Stop tenofovir if hepatomegaly or steatosis occur, even if LFTs normal. Severe acute exacerbation of hepatitis B can occur after discontinuation of tenofovir in patients coinfected with HIV + hepatitis B. Monitor closely for ≥2 mo after discontinuing tenofovir in such patients; consider treating hepatitis B.

ADULT - Combination therapy for HIV infection: 300 mg PO daily with a meal. High rate of virologic failure with tenofovir + didanosine + lamivudine; avoid this regimen.

PEDS - Not approved in children. Decreased bone mineral density reported. Insufficient data to recommend as initial HIV therapy in children.

UNAPPROVED ADULT - Coinfection with HIV + hepatitis B: 300 mg PO daily with a meal.

FORMS - Trade only: Tab 300 mg.

NOTES - Decreased bone mineral density; consider bone monitoring if hx of pathologic fracture or high risk of osteopenia. Consider calcium + vitamin D supplement. Tenofovir increases didanosine levels and possibly serious didanosine adverse effects (eg pancreatitis, lactic acidosis, hyperlactatemia, neuropathy). Reduce Videx EC to 250 mg in patients ≥60 kg or 200 mg if <60 kg. Dosage adjustment of Videx EC unclear if CrCl <60 mL/min. Give tenofovir + Videx EC on empty stomach or with light meal; give tenofovir + buffered didanosine on empty stomach. If atazanavir is used with tenofovir, use 300 mg atazanavir + 100 mg ritonavir. Atazanavir and lopinavir/ritonavir increase tenofovir levels; monitor and discontinue tenofovir if adverse effects. Tenofovir can cause renal impairment including acute renal failure & Fanconi syndrome. Avoid tenofovir if current / recent nephrotoxic drug use. Drugs that reduce renal function or undergo renal elimination (eg acyclovir, adefovir, ganciclovir) may increase tenofovir levels. Monitor creatinine & phosphate if risk/ history of renal insufficiency or nephrotoxic drug. Dosage reduction if CrCl <50 ml/min: 300 mg q48h if CrCl 30-49 ml/min; 300 mg twice weekly if CrCl 10-29 ml/min; 300 mg once weekly for dialysis patients (given after dialysis).

zidovudine (*Retrovir, AZT, ZDV*) ▶LK ♀C ▶-
$$$$$
WARNING - Bone marrow suppression, myopathy.
ADULT – HIV combination therapy: 600 mg/day PO divided bid or tid. IV dosing: 1 mg/ kg IV over 1 h 5-6 x/day. Prevention of maternal-fetal HIV transmission, maternal dosing (>14 weeks of pregnancy): 200 mg PO tid or 300 mg PO bid until start of labor. During labor, 2 mg/kg IV over 1 h, then 1 mg/kg/h until delivery.
PEDS - Combination therapy for HIV infection. 6 wk -12 yo: 160 mg/m^2 up to 200 mg PO q8h. Adolescents: Use adult dose. Prevention of maternal-fetal HIV transmission, infant dosing: 2 mg/kg PO q6h from within 12 h of birth until 6 weeks old. Can also give infants 1.5 mg/kg IV over 30 min q6h.
FORMS - Generic/Trade: Tab 300 mg, syrup 50 mg/5 mL (240 mL). Trade only: Cap 100 mg.
NOTES - Do not use with stavudine. Hematologic toxicity; monitor CBC. Increased bone marrow suppression with ganciclovir or valganciclovir. Granulocytopenia more common in children receiving zidovudine and nevirapine. Monitor for hepatic decompensation, neutropenia, and anemia if also receiving interferon regimen for hepatitis C. If hepatic decompensation occurs, consider discontinuing zidovudine, interferon, and/or ribavirin. See package insert for dosage adjustments based on renal function or hematologic toxicity.

ANTIMICROBIALS: Antiviral Agents – Anti-HIV – Protease Inhibitors

NOTE: Many serious drug interactions - always check before prescribing! Protease inhibitors inhibit CYP 3A4. Contraindicated with most antiarrhythmics, cisapride, ergot alkaloids, lovastatin, pimozide, simvastatin, St. John's wort, triazolam; caution with atorvastatin. Midazolam contraindicated in labeling; but can use single dose IV cautiously with monitoring for procedural sedation. See www.aidsinfo.nih.gov for use of rifamycins with protease inhibitors. Do not use rifampin with protease inhibitors. Monitor INR with warfarin. Avoid inhaled/nasal fluticasone with ritonavir if possible; increased fluticasone levels can cause Cushing's syndrome/adrenal suppression. Other protease inhibitors may increase fluticasone levels; find alternatives for long-term use. Trazodone levels and adverse effects increased by ritonavir and possibly other protease inhibitors; may need to reduce trazodone dose. Not more than a single 25 mg dose of sildenafil in 48 hours with protease inhibitors. Vardenafil initial dose is 2.5 mg; not more than a single 2.5 mg dose in 72 hours. Sildenafil preferred over vardenafil with unboosted indinavir. Tadalafil initial dose is 5 mg; not more than 10 mg single dose in 72 hours. Adverse effects include spontaneous bleeding in hemophiliacs, hyperglycemia, hyperlipidemia, immune reconstitution syndrome, and fat redistribution. Coinfection with hepatitis C or other liver disease increases the risk of hepatotoxicity with protease inhibitors; monitor LFTs at least twice in 1st month of therapy, then every 3 months.

amprenavir (*Agenerase, APV*) ▶L ♀C ▶-
$$$$$
WARNING - Oral solution contraindicated in children <4 yo, pregnancy, hepatic/renal failure, therapy with metronidazole/ disulfiram due to potential propylene glycol toxicity.
ADULT - Combination therapy for HIV infection: 1200 mg PO bid. In combination with ritonavir: Give amprenavir 1200 mg PO daily with ritonavir 200 mg PO daily. Or amprenavir 600 mg bid with ritonavir 100 mg bid. Do not take with high-fat meal.
PEDS – HIV combination therapy. Do not take with high-fat meal. Caps: 1200 mg PO bid if 13-16 yo; 20 mg/kg bid or 15 mg/kg tid if 4-12 yo or 13-16 yo and <50 kg. Max for caps is 2400 mg/day. Oral soln: 22.5 mg/kg PO bid or 17 mg/kg tid if 4-12 yo or 13-16 yo and <50 kg.

Max for oral soln is 2800 mg/day. Switch from oral soln to caps as soon as possible.

FORMS - Trade only: Caps 50 mg, oral soln 15 mg/mL (240 mL).

NOTES - Life-threatening skin reactions; cross-sensitivity with sulfonamides possible. Monitor lipids. Contains vitamin E; tell patients not to take more. Multivitamin containing minimal vitamin E probably OK. Inhibits cytochrome P450 3A4. Do not give amprenavir plus ritonavir with flecainide or propafenone. Monitor levels of antiarrhythmics, immunosuppressants, tricyclic antidepressants. Avoid delavirdine. Using amprenavir with methadone can decrease levels of both drugs. See www.aidsinfo.nih.gov for dosage adjustment of rifamycins. Take ≥1 h before/after buffered didanosine/ antacids. Hormonal contraceptives may reduce levels; do not use. Oral sol'n and caps not interchangeable on mg per mg basis. Dosage reduction of caps for moderate/ severe hepatic dysfunction: 450 mg bid for Child-Pugh score of 5-8; 300 mg bid for Child-Pugh score of 9-12. Oral solution contraindicated in hepatic/renal failure.

atazanavir (*Reyataz, ATV*) ▶L ♀B ▶- $$$$$
ADULT - Combination therapy for HIV infection. Therapy-naive patients: 400 mg PO daily. Efavirenz regimen, therapy-naive patients: atazanavir 300 mg + ritonavir 100 mg + efavirenz 600 mg all PO daily. Therapy-experienced patients: atazanavir 300 mg PO daily + ritonavir 100 mg PO daily. Tenofovir regimen (must include ritonavir): atazanavir 300 mg + ritonavir 100 mg + tenofovir 300 mg all PO daily with food. Give atazanavir with food; give 2 h before or 1 h after buffered didanosine.
PEDS - Not approved in children. Use adult dose if ≥16 yo. Do not use in infants; may cause kernicterus.
FORMS - Trade: Caps 100, 150, 200, 300 mg.
NOTES - Does not appear to increase cholesterol or triglycerides. Asymptomatic increases in indirect bilirubin due to inhibition of UDP-glucuronosyl transferase (UGT); may cause jaundice/ scleral icterus. Do not use with indinavir; both may increase bilirubin. Consider other etiology for associated increases in transaminases. May inhibit UGT1A1 metabolism of irinotecan. Prolongs PR interval and rare cases of second degree AV block reported; caution advised for patients with AV block or on drugs that prolong PR interval. Monitor ECG with calcium channel blockers; consider reducing diltiazem dose by 50%. Reduce clarithromycin dose by 50%; consider alternative therapy for indications other than Mycobacterium avium complex. Acid required for atazanavir absorption; acid-suppressing drugs can cause treatment failure. Give atazanavir with food. Do not use proton pump inhibitors. Regimens for H2 blockers in treatment-naive patients: atazanavir 400 mg once daily ≥2 h before and ≥10 h after H2 blocker OR atazanavir 300 mg + ritonavir 100 mg once daily and H2 blocker at any time. Treatment-experienced patients: atazanavir 300 mg + ritonavir 100 mg once daily ≥2 h before and ≥10 h after H2 blocker. Give atazanavir 2 h before or 1 h after antacids or buffered didanosine. Give atazanavir and EC didanosine at different times. Inhibits cytochrome P450 1A2, 2C9, and 3A4. See aidsinfo.nih.gov for rifamycin dosage adjustment. Monitor antiarrhythmics, immunosuppressants, tricyclic antidepressant levels. Increases levels of ethinyl estradiol and norethindrone; use lowest dose of both in oral contraceptives. In mild to moderate hepatic impairment (Child-Pugh class B), consider dosage reduction to 300 mg daily with food. Do not use in Child-Pugh Class C.

darunavir (*Prezista*) ▶L ♀B ▶- $$$$$
ADULT - Combination therapy for HIV infection in therapy-experienced patients: 600 mg boosted by ritonavir 100 mg PO bid with food. Darunavir should always be boosted with ritonavir.
PEDS - Not approved in children.
FORMS - Trade only: Tab 300 mg.
NOTES - Cross-sensitivity with sulfas possible; caution if allergy. CYP 3A4 inhibitor and substrate. Do not give with lopinavir/ritonavir or saquinavir. Monitor levels of antiarrhythmics. Clarithromycin dosage reduction if CrCl <60 mL/min (see clarithromycin entry for details). Not >200 mg/day ketoconazole or itraconazole. Ritonavir decreases voriconazole levels; do not use darunavir/ritonavir unless benefit exceeds risk. Reduce rifabutin to 150 mg PO every other day. May decrease oral contraceptive efficacy; consider additional or alternative method. Give didanosine 1 h before/2 h after darunavir/ritonavir. Increases pravastatin levels up to 5-fold; consider alternatives.

fosamprenavir (*Lexiva, 908,* ✦*Telzir*) ▶L ♀C ▶- $$$$$
ADULT - Combination therapy for HIV infection. Therapy-naives: 1400 mg PO bid (without ritonavir). OR fosamprenavir 1400 mg + ritonavir 200 mg both PO daily. OR 700 mg fosamprenavir + 100 mg ritonavir both PO bid.

Protease inhibitor-experienced patients: 700 mg fosamprenavir + 100 mg ritonavir both PO bid. Do not use once-daily regimen. If once-daily ritonavir-boosted regimen given with efavirenz, increase ritonavir to 300 mg/day; no increase of ritonavir dose needed for bid regimen with efavirenz. Can give nevirapine with fosamprenavir only if bid ritonavir-boosted regimen used. No meal restrictions for tabs; advise adults to take suspension with food. Re-dose if vomiting occurs within 30 minutes of giving oral suspension.

PEDS - Combination therapy for HIV infection. Therapy-naïve, 2-5 yo: 30 mg/kg susp PO bid (max 1400 mg bid). Therapy naïve, >6 yo: 30 mg/kg susp PO bid (max 1400 mg bid) or 18 mg/kg susp PO bid + ritonavir 3 mg/kg PO bid (max fosamprenavir 700 mg + ritonavir 100 mg PO bid). Protease inhibitor-experienced, ≥6 yo: 18 mg/kg susp PO bid + ritonavir 3 mg/kg PO bid (max fosamprenavir 700 mg + ritonavir 100 mg PO bid). For fosamprenavir without ritonavir, can use tabs if ≥47 kg (fosamprenavir 1400 mg PO bid). For fosamprenavir + ritonavir, can use tabs if ≥39 kg (fosamprenavir 700 mg + ritonavir 100 mg PO bid). Use adult dose if ≥16 yo. Do not use in infants; may cause kernicterus. Advise children to take susp with food. Re-dose if vomiting occurs within 30 minutes of giving oral suspension.

FORMS - Trade only: Tabs 700 mg (equivalent to amprenavir 600 mg), Susp 50 mg/mL (equivalent to amprenavir 43 mg/mL).

NOTES - Lower pill burden than amprenavir. Life-threatening skin reactions possible (reported with amprenavir). Cross-sensitivity with sulfonamides possible; use caution in sulfonamide-allergic patients. Hypertriglyceridemia; monitor lipids. Fosamprenavir is inhibitor & substrate of cytochrome P450 3A4. Do not use fosamprenavir + ritonavir with flecainide or propafenone. Do not use fosamprenavir with delavirdine. Use lowest possible dose of atorvastatin or rosuvastatin with monitoring for myopathy or consider fluvastatin/pravastatin. See aidsinfo.nih.gov for dosage adjustment of rifamycins. Monitor CBC at least weekly if taking rifabutin. Monitor levels of antiarrhythmics, immunosuppressants, tricyclic antidepressants. May need to increase dose of methadone. Monitor INR with warfarin. Not >200 mg/day ketoconazole/ itraconazole with fosamprenavir + ritonavir; may need to reduce antifungal dose if >400 mg/day itraconazole/ ketoconazole with

unboosted fosamprenavir. Contraindicated with lovastatin or simvastatin; not >20 mg/day of atorvastatin. Not >2.5 mg vardenafil q24h with unboosted fosamprenavir or q72h for fosamprenavir + ritonavir. Do not use hormonal contraceptives. More adverse reactions when fosamprenavir given with Kaletra; appropriate dose for combination therapy unclear. Mild to moderate hepatic dysfunction (Child-Pugh score 5-8): 700 mg PO bid for unboosted fosamprenavir; no data for ritonavir-boosted regimen. Refrigeration not required, but may improve taste of oral suspension.

indinavir (*Crixivan, IDV*) ▶LK ♀C ▶- $$$$$

ADULT - Combination therapy for HIV infection: 800 mg PO q8h between meals with water (at least 48 oz/day).

PEDS - Not approved in children. Do not use in infants; may cause kernicterus.

UNAPPROVED ADULT - Combination therapy for HIV infection: 800 mg PO bid with ritonavir 100-200 mg PO bid. Or 400 mg bid with ritonavir 400 mg bid. 600 mg PO bid with Kaletra 400/100 mg PO bid. Can be given without regard to meals when given with ritonavir.

UNAPPROVED PEDS - Combination therapy for HIV infection, adolescents: 800 mg PO q8h between meals with water (at least 48 oz/day). Children: 350-500 mg/m2/dose (max of 800 mg/dose) PO q8h.

FORMS - Trade: Caps 100, 200, 333, 400 mg.

NOTES - Nephrolithiasis (may be more common in children), hemolytic anemia, indirect hyperbilirubinemia, possible hepatitis, interstitial nephritis with asymptomatic pyuria. Do not use with atazanavir; both may increase bilirubin. Inhibits cytochrome P450 3A4. Avoid using with carbamazepine if possible. Give indinavir and buffered didanosine 1 h apart on empty stomach. See www.aidsinfo.nih.gov for dosage adjustment of rifamycins and indinavir. Reduce indinavir dose to 600 mg PO q8h when given with ketoconazole, itraconazole 200 mg bid, or delavirdine 400 mg tid. Increase indinavir dose to 1000 mg PO q8h when given with efavirenz, nevirapine. For mild to moderate hepatic cirrhosis, give 600 mg PO q8h. Indinavir not recommended in pregnancy because of dramatic reduction in blood levels.

lopinavir-ritonavir (*Kaletra, LPV/r*) ▶L ♀C ▶- $$$$$

ADULT - Combination therapy for HIV infection: Give tabs without regard to meals; give oral soln with food. Therapy-naive patients: 2 tabs

(400/100 mg) PO bid or 4 tabs (800/200 mg) once daily. 5 mL PO bid or 10 mL once daily of oral soln. Increase oral soln to 6.5 mL PO bid (not once daily) with efavirenz, nevirapine, fosamprenavir, or nelfinavir (dosage increase not needed with tabs). Therapy-experienced patients: No once-daily regimen. 2 tabs (400/100 mg) PO bid or 5 mL oral soln bid. Increase oral soln to 6.5 mL PO bid with efavirenz, nevirapine, amprenavir, or nelfinavir. Consider 3 tabs (600/150 mg) bid with efavirenz, nevirapine, fosamprenavir without ritonavir, or nelfinavir if reduced lopinavir susceptibility suspected.

PEDS - Combination therapy for HIV infection, 6 mo-12 yo: lopinavir 12 mg/kg PO bid for 7 to <15 kg, 10 mg/kg PO bid for 15-40 kg. Do not exceed adult dose. Use adult dose for >12 yo or >40 kg. With efavirenz, nevirapine, or amprenavir increase to 13 mg/kg PO bid for 7 to <15 kg, 11 mg/kg PO bid for 15-45 kg. Do not exceed adult dose. Use adult dose for >12 yo or >45 kg. Give tabs without regard to meals; give oral soln with food. Beware of medication errors with highly concentrated Kaletra oral soln; fatal overdose reported in infant given excessive volume of Kaletra oral soln.

FORMS - Trade only: Tabs 200/50 mg lopinavir-ritonavir. Oral soln 80/20 mg/ml (160 mL).

NOTES - Errors can occur if Keppra (levetiracetam) confused with Kaletra. May cause pancreatitis. Ritonavir (inhibits cytochrome P450 3A4 & 2D6) included in formulation to inhibit metabolism and boost levels of lopinavir. Increases tenofovir levels; monitor for adverse drug reaction. Many other drug interactions including decreased efficacy of oral contraceptives. Ritonavir decreases voriconazole levels; do not give with voriconazole unless benefit exceeds risk. See www.aidsinfo.nih.gov for dosage adjustment of rifamycins. May require higher methadone dose. Avoid inhaled/nasal fluticasone if possible; concomitant use may cause Cushing's syndrome and adrenal suppression. Ritonavir increases trazodone levels and adverse effects; consider reducing trazodone dose. Clarithromycin dosage reduction if CrCl <60 mL/min (see clarithromycin entry for details). Give buffered didanosine 1 h before/ 2 h after Kaletra oral soln. Kaletra tabs can be given at same time as didanosine without food. Do not give Kaletra with tipranavir 500 mg + ritonavir 100 mg both bid. Monitor INR with warfarin. Oral soln contains alcohol. Use oral soln within 2 months if patient stores at room temperature. Tabs do not require refrigeration. Do not crush, cut, or chew tabs.

nelfinavir (*Viracept, NFV*) ▶L ♀B ▶- $$$$$

ADULT - Combination therapy for HIV infection: 750 mg PO tid or 1250 mg PO bid with meals. Absorption improved when meal contains ≥500 calories with 11-28 g of fat.

PEDS - Combination therapy for HIV infection, ≥2 yo: 45-55 mg/kg PO bid or 25-35 mg/kg PO tid to max of 2500 mg/day. Take with meals. Use powder or 250 mg tabs.

UNAPPROVED PEDS - Combination therapy for HIV infection: Up to 45 mg/kg/dose PO tid with meals. Absorption improved when meal contains ≥500 calories with 11-28 g of fat.

FORMS - Trade only: Tab 250, 625 mg, powder 50 mg/g (114 g).

NOTES - Diarrhea common. Inhibits cytochrome P450 3A4. Decreases efficacy of oral contraceptives. May require higher methadone dose. See aidsinfo.nih.gov for dosage adjustment of rifamycins and nelfinavir. Give nelfinavir 2 h before/1 h after buffered didanosine. Oral powder stable for 6 h after mixing if refrigerated. No dosage adjustment for mild hepatic impairment (Child-Pugh Class A); not recommended for more severe hepatic failure (Child-Pugh B/C).

ritonavir (*Norvir, RTV*) ▶L ♀B ▶- $$$$$

WARNING - Contraindicated with many drugs due to risk of drug interactions.

ADULT - Full-dose regimen (600 mg PO bid) poorly tolerated. Lower doses of 100 mg PO daily to 400 mg PO bid used to boost levels of other protease inhibitors. Best tolerated regimen with saquinavir may be ritonavir 400 mg bid with Invirase 400 mg bid. Saquinavir 1000 mg bid (Invirase) with ritonavir 100 mg bid also used. In combination with amprenavir: Give amprenavir 1200 mg PO daily with ritonavir 200 mg daily. Or amprenavir 600 mg bid with ritonavir 100 mg bid.

PEDS - Combination therapy for HIV infection, ≥1 month old: 250 mg/m^2 PO q12h, increasing by 50 mg/m^2/dose every 2-3 days to 400 mg/m^2 PO q12h. Max dose 600 mg PO bid. Give with meals.

UNAPPROVED ADULT - Combination therapy for HIV infection: 100-200 mg PO bid with indinavir 800 mg PO bid.

UNAPPROVED PEDS - Used at lower than labeled doses to boost levels of other protease inhibitors.

FORMS - Trade only: Cap 100 mg, oral soln 80 mg/mL (240 mL).

NOTES - Nausea & vomiting, pancreatitis, alterations in AST, ALT, GGT, CPK, uric acid. Inhibits hepatic cytochrome P450 3A & 2D6. Contraindicated with alfuzosin. Ritonavir decreases voriconazole levels. Do not use ritonavir 400 mg bid with voriconazole; use ritonavir 100 mg bid with voriconazole only if benefit exceeds risk. Not >200 mg/day of ketoconazole with ritonavir. See aidsinfo.nih.gov for dosage adjustment of rifamycins. Do not use with rifampin; it decreases ritonavir levels and may increase hepatotoxicity risk. Not more than a single dose of vardenafil 2.5 mg or tadalafil 10 mg in 72 h with ritonavir. Decreases efficacy of combined oral or patch contraceptives; consider alternative. Increases methadone dosage requirements. May cause serotonin syndrome with fluoxetine. Increases trazodone levels and adverse effects; consider reducing trazodone dose. Clarithromycin dosage reduction if CrCl <60 mL/min (see clarithromycin entry for details). Avoid inhaled/nasal fluticasone if possible; concomitant use may cause Cushing's syndrome and adrenal suppression. Give ritonavir 2.5h before/after buffered didanosine. Monitor digoxin; may increase levels. Caps and oral soln contain alcohol. Do not refrigerate oral soln. Try to refrigerate caps, but stable for 30 days at <77 degrees F.

saquinavir (*Invirase, SQV*) ▶L ♀B ▶? $$$$$

ADULT - Combination therapy for HIV infection. Regimen must contain ritonavir. Invirase 1000 mg + ritonavir 100 mg both PO bid taken within 2 h after meals. Invirase 1000 mg + lopinavir-ritonavir (Kaletra) 400/100 mg both PO bid. If serious toxicity occurs, do not reduce Invirase dose; efficacy unclear for lower doses.

PEDS - ≥16 yo: Use adult dose.

FORMS - Trade only: Invirase (hard gel) caps 200 mg, tabs 500 mg.

NOTES - Do not use saquinavir with garlic supplements or tipranavir/ritonavir. Delavirdine, omeprazole, or ketoconazole increase saquinavir levels. Monitor LFTs if given with delavirdine. Rifampin contraindicated with ritonavir-boosted saquinavir due to risk of hepatotoxicity. See www.aidsinfo.nih.gov for dosage adjustment of rifamycins. Monitor for increased digoxin levels. May reduce methadone levels. Clarithromycin dosage reduction if CrCl <60 mL/min (see clarithromycin entry for details).

tipranavir (*Aptivus*) ▶Feces ♀C ▶- $$$$$

WARNING - Potentially fatal hepatotoxicity. Monitor clinical status and LFTs frequently. Risk increased by coinfection with hepatitis B/C. Contraindicated in moderate to severe hepatic failure (Child Pugh B /C). Intracranial hemorrhage can occur with tipranavir + ritonavir; caution if at risk of bleeding from trauma, surgery, other medical conditions, or receiving antiplatelet agents or anticoagulants.

ADULT - HIV infection, boosted by ritonavir in treatment-experienced patients or for strain resistant to multiple protease inhibitors: 500 mg + ritonavir 200 mg PO bid with food.

PEDS - Safety and efficacy not established.

FORMS - Trade only: Caps 250 mg.

NOTES - Contains sulfonamide moiety; potential for cross-sensitivity unknown. Al/Mg antacids may decrease absorption; separate doses. Ritonavir-boosted tipranavir inhibits CYP 3A4 and 2D6. Contraindicated with CYP 3A4 substrates that can cause life-threatening toxicity at high concentrations. May increase immunosuppressant, tricyclic antidepressant levels. May need higher methadone dose. Ritonavir decreases voriconazole levels; do not give together unless benefit exceeds risk. Do not use tipranavir/ritonavir with amprenavir, Kaletra, or saquinavir. Decreases ethinyl estradiol levels; consider non-hormonal contraception. Reduce rifabutin to 150 mg PO every other day. Clarithromycin dosage reduction if CrCl <60 mL/min (see clarithromycin entry for details). Caps contain alcohol. Refrigerate bottle of caps before opening. Stable at room temp for 60 days.

ANTIMICROBIALS: Antiviral Agents – Anti-Influenza

NOTE: Whenever possible, immunization is the preferred method of prophylaxis. Consider chemoprophylaxis in high-risk patients vaccinated after influenza activity has begun, care-givers for high-risk patients, patients with immunodeficiency (including HIV infection), and those who request it. Provide chemoprophylaxis to all residents during institutional outbreaks of influenza, continuing for ≥2 weeks or until 1 week after end of outbreak. Avoid anti-influenza antivirals from 48 hours before until 2 weeks after a dose of live influenza vaccine unless medically necessary. Patients with suspected influenza may have primary/ concomitant bacterial pneumonia; antibiotics may be indicated.

amantadine (*Symmetrel*, ✦*Endantadine*) ▶K ♀C ▶? $

WARNING - The CDC does not recommend for treatment/prevention of influenza A in the US due to high levels of resistance.

ADULT - Influenza A: 100 mg PO bid. ≥65 yo: 100 mg PO daily. Parkinsonism: 100 mg PO bid. Max 400 mg/day divided tid-qid. Drug-induced extrapyramidal disorders: 100 mg PO bid. Max 300 mg/day divided tid-qid.

PEDS - Safety and efficacy not established in infants <1 yo. Influenza A, treatment or prophylaxis, ≥10 yo: 100 mg PO bid. 1-9 yo and any child <40 kg: 5 mg/kg/day up to 150 mg/day PO divided bid.

FORMS - Generic: Cap 100 mg. Generic/Trade: Tab 100 mg, syrup 50 mg/5 mL (120 mL).

NOTES - CNS toxicity, suicide attempts, neuroleptic malignant syndrome with dosage reduction/withdrawal, anticholinergic effects, orthostatic hypotension. Do not stop abruptly in Parkinson's disease. Dosage reduction in adults with renal dysfunction: 200 mg PO 1st day, then 100 mg PO daily for CrCl 30-50 mL/min. 200 mg PO 1st day, then 100 mg PO qod for CrCl 15-29 mL/min. 200 mg PO q week for CrCl <15 mL/min or hemodialysis.

oseltamivir (*Tamiflu*) ▶LK ♀C ▶? $$$

ADULT - Influenza A/B, treatment: 75 mg PO bid x 5 days starting within 2 days of symptom onset. Prophylaxis: 75 mg PO daily. Start within 2 days of exposure and continue for ≥7 days. Take with food to improve tolerability.

PEDS - Influenza A/B, ≥1 yo: Each dose is 30 mg if ≤15 kg, 45 mg if 16-23 kg, 60 mg if 24-40 kg, 75 mg if >40 kg or ≥13 yo. For treatment, give twice daily x 5 days starting within 2 days of sx onset. For prophylaxis, give once daily x 10 days starting within 2 days of exposure. Take with food to improve tolerability. Suspension comes with graduated syringe calibrated to 30, 45, and 60 mg; use 30 mg plus 45 mg to measure 75 mg dose.

FORMS - Trade only: Caps 30, 45, 75 mg, susp 12 mg/mL (25 mL).

NOTES - Not for infants <1 yo; immature blood brain barrier could lead to high oseltamivir levels in CNS. Increased INR with warfarin. Postmarketing reports (mostly from Japan) of self-injury and delirium, primarily among children and adolescents; monitor for abnormal behavior. Dosage adjustment for CrCl 10-30 mL/min: 75 mg PO daily x 5 days for treatment, 75 mg PO qod for prophylaxis. Susp stable for 10 days at room temperature.

rimantadine (*Flumadine*) ▶LK ♀C ▶- $$

WARNING - The CDC does not recommend for treatment/prevention of influenza A in the US due to high levels of resistance.

ADULT - Prophylaxis/treatment of influenza A: 100 mg PO bid. Start treatment ≤48 h of symptom onset and continue x 7 days. Reduce to 100 mg/day if side effects in patients ≥65 yo, severe hepatic dysfunction, CrCl ≤10 mL/min, elderly nursing home patient.

PEDS - Prophylaxis of influenza A, ≥10 yo: 100 mg PO bid. 1-9 yo or any child <40 kg: 5 mg/kg/day up to 150 mg/day divided daily or bid.

FORMS - Trade only: Tabs 100 mg, syrup 50 mg/5 mL (240 mL).

zanamivir (*Relenza*) ▶K ♀C ▶? $$

ADULT - Influenza A/B, treatment: 2 puffs bid x 5 days. Take 2 doses on day 1 at least 2 h apart. Start within 2 days of symptom onset. Influenza A/B, prevention: 2 puffs once daily x 10 days.

PEDS - Influenza A/B, treatment, ≥7 yo: 2 puffs bid x 5 days. Take 2 doses on day 1 at least 2 h apart. Start within 2 days of symptom onset. Influenza A/B, prevention, ≥5 yo: 2 puffs once daily x 10 days.

FORMS - Trade only: Rotadisk inhaler 5 mg/puff (20 puffs).

NOTES - May cause bronchospasm & worsen pulmonary function in asthma or COPD; avoid if underlying airways disease. Stop if bronchospasm/ decline in respiratory function. Show patient how to use inhaler.

ANTIMICROBIALS: Antiviral Agents – Other

adefovir (*Hepsera*) ▶K ♀C ▶- $$$$$

WARNING - Nephrotoxic; monitor renal function. HIV resistance in untreated HIV infection; test for HIV before prescribing. Lactic acidosis with hepatic steatosis. Severe acute exacerbation of hepatitis B can occur after discontinuation of adefovir in patients with HIV + hepatitis B coinfection. Monitor closely for ≥2 mo after discontinuing adefovir in such patients; consider retreating hepatitis B.

ADULT - Chronic hepatitis B: 10 mg PO daily.

PEDS - Not approved in children.

FORMS - Trade only: Tabs 10 mg.
NOTES - Monitor renal function. See package insert for dosage reduction if CrCl <50 mL/minute. Other nephrotoxic drugs may increase risk of nephrotoxicity.

entecavir (*Baraclude*) ▶K ♀C ▶- $$$$$
WARNING - Nucleoside analogues can cause lactic acidosis with hepatic steatosis. Severe acute exacerbation of hepatitis B can occur after discontinuation. Monitor closely for ≥2 mo after discontinuation. Patients coinfected with HIV + hepatitis B should not receive entecavir for hepatitis B unless they also receive HAART for HIV; failure to treat HIV in such patients could lead to HIV resistance to NRTIs.
ADULT - Chronic hepatitis B: 0.5 mg PO once daily if treatment naive; 1 mg if lamivudine-resistant or history of viremia despite lamivudine treatment. Give on empty stomach (2 h after last meal and 2 h before next meal).
PEDS - Chronic hepatitis B, ≥16 yo: 0.5 mg PO once daily if treatment naive; 1 mg if lamivudine-resistant or history of viremia despite lamivudine treatment.
FORMS - Trade only: 0.5, 1 mg tabs, solution 0.05 mg/mL (210 mL).
NOTES - Entecavir treatment of co-infected patients not receiving HIV treatment may increase the risk of lamivudine/emtricitabine resistance. Do not mix oral solution with water or other liquid. Reduce dose if CrCl <50 mL/min or dialysis. Give dose after dialysis sessions.

interferon alfa-2b (*Intron A*) ▶K ♀C ▶?+ $$$$$
WARNING - May cause or worsen serious neuropsychiatric, autoimmune, ischemic, & infectious diseases. Frequent clinical & lab monitoring required. Stop interferon if signs/sx of these conditions are persistently severe or worsen.
ADULT - Chronic hepatitis B: 5 million units/day or 10 million units 3 times/week SC/IM x 16 weeks if HBeAg +, x 48 weeks if HBeAg. Chronic hepatitis C: 3 million units SC/IM 3 times/wk x 16 weeks. Continue for 18-24 mo if ALT normalized. Other indications: condylomata acuminata, AIDS-related Kaposi's sarcoma, hairy-cell leukemia, melanoma, follicular lymphoma.
PEDS - Chronic hepatitis C, ≥3 yo: Interferon alfa-2b 3 million units/m² SC 3 times/week and PO ribavirin according to weight. Ribavirin: 200 mg bid for 25-36 kg; 200 mg q am and 400 mg q pm for 37-49 kg; 400 mg bid for 50-61 kg. Use adult dose for >61 kg. If ribavirin contraindicated use interferon 3-5 million units/m² (max

3 million units/dose) SC/IM three times/week. Chronic hepatitis B, ≥1 yo: 3 million units/m² three times/week for first week, then 6 million units/m² (max 10 million units/dose) SC three times/week.
UNAPPROVED ADULT - Prevention of chronic hepatitis C in acute hepatitis C: 5 million units SC daily x 4 weeks then 5 million units SC 3 times/week x 20 weeks. Superficial bladder tumors. Chronic myelogenous leukemia. Cutaneous T-cell lymphoma. Essential thrombocythemia. Non-Hodgkin's lymphoma. Chronic granulocytic leukemia.
FORMS - Trade only: Powder/soln for injection 3,5,10 million units/vial. Soln for injection 18,25 million units/multidose vial. Multidose injection pens 3,5,10 million units/dose (6 doses/pen).
NOTES - Monitor for depression, suicidal behavior (esp. in adolescents), other severe neuropsychiatric effects. Thyroid abnormalities, hepatotoxicity, flu-like sx, pulmonary & cardiovascular reactions, retinal damage, neutropenia, thrombocytopenia, hypertriglyceridemia (consider monitoring). Increases theophylline levels. Monitor CBC, TSH, LFTs, electrolytes. Dosage adjustments for hematologic toxicity in package insert.

interferon alfacon-1 (*Infergen*) ▶Plasma ♀C ▶? $$$$$
WARNING - May cause or worsen serious neuropsychiatric, autoimmune, ischemic, & infectious diseases. Frequent clinical & lab monitoring required. Stop interferon if signs/sx of these conditions are persistently severe or worsen.
ADULT - Chronic hepatitis C: 9 mcg SC 3 times/week x 24 weeks. Increase to 15 mcg SC 3 times/week x 24 weeks if relapse/no response. Reduce to 7.5 mcg SC 3 times/week if intolerable adverse effects.
PEDS - Not approved in children.
FORMS - Trade: Vials injectable soln 9,15 mcg.
NOTES - Monitor for depression, suicidal behavior, other severe neuropsychiatric effects. Thyroid dysfunction, cardiovascular reactions, retinal damage, flu-like symptoms, thrombocytopenia, neutropenia, exacerbation of autoimmune disorders, hypertriglyceridemia (consider monitoring). Monitor CBC, thyroid function. Refrigerate injectable soln.

interferon alfa-n3 (*Alferon N*) ▶K ♀C ▶- $$$$$
WARNING - Flu-like syndrome, myalgias, alopecia. Contraindicated in egg protein allergy.
ADULT - Doses vary by indication. Condylomata

acuminata, intralesional.

PEDS - Not approved in children.

palivizumab (Synagis) ▶L ♀C ▶? $$$$$

PEDS - Prevention of respiratory syncytial virus pulmonary disease in high-risk patients: 15 mg/kg IM q month during RSV season with first injection before season starts (November to April in northern hemisphere). Consider for children <2 yo treated for chronic lung disease in last 6 mo or with hemodynamically significant congenital heart disease; infants born <28 wk gestation who are now <12 mo; infants born 29-32 wk gestation who are now <6 mo. Give a dose ASAP after cardiopulmonary bypass (due to decreased palivizumab levels) even if <1 month after last dose.

NOTES - Preservative-free - use within 6 h of reconstitution. Not >1 mL per injection site.

peginterferon alfa-2a (Pegasys) ▶LK ♀C ▶- $$$$$

WARNING - May cause or worsen serious neuropsychiatric, autoimmune, ischemic, infectious diseases. Frequent clinical & lab monitoring recommended. Discontinue if signs/sx of these conditions are persistently severe or worsen.

ADULT - Chronic hepatitis C not previously treated with alfa interferon: 180 mcg SC in abdomen or thigh once weekly for 48 weeks +/- PO ribavirin 800-1200 mg/day. Ribavirin dose and duration depends on genotype and body weight (see PO ribavirin entry). Chronic hepatitis C in patients coinfected with HIV: 180 mcg SC once weekly plus ribavirin 800 mg/day PO for 48 weeks regardless of genotype. Hepatitis B: 180 mcg SC in abdomen or thigh once weekly for 48 weeks.

PEDS - Not approved in children.

FORMS - Trade: 180 mcg/1 mL solution in single-use vial, 180 mcg/0.5 mL prefilled syringe.

NOTES - Contraindicated in autoimmune hepatitis; hepatic decompensation in cirrhotic patients (Child-Pugh score >6 if HCV only; score ≥6 if HIV co-infected). Monitor for depression, suicidal behavior, relapse of drug addiction, other severe neuropsychiatric effects. Interferons can cause thrombocytopenia, neutropenia, thyroid dysfunction, hyperglycemia, hypoglycemia, cardiovascular events, colitis, pancreatitis, hypersensitivity, flu-like sx, pulmonary & ophthalmologic disorders. Risk of severe neutropenia/ thrombocytopenia greater in HIV infected patients. Monitor CBC, blood chemistry. Interferons increase risk of hepatic decompensation in hep C/HIV coinfected patients receiving HAART with NRTI. Monitor LFTs and clinical status; discontinue peginterferon if Child-Pugh score ≥6. Exacerbation of hepatitis during tx of hepatitis B: Monitor LFTs more often and consider dosage reduction if ALT flares. Discontinue tx if ALT increase is progressive despite dosage reduction or if flares accompanied by hepatic decompensation or bilirubin increase. Cytochrome P450 1A2 inhibitor; may increase theophylline levels (monitor). May increase methadone levels. Use cautiously if CrCl <50 ml/min. Dosage adjustments for adverse effects, hepatic dysfunction, or hemodialysis in package insert. Store in refrigerator.

peginterferon alfa-2b (PEG-Intron) ▶K? ♀C ▶- $$$$$

WARNING - May cause or worsen serious neuropsychiatric, autoimmune, ischemic, infectious diseases. Frequent clinical & lab monitoring recommended. Discontinue if signs/sx of these conditions are persistently severe or worsen.

ADULT - Chronic hepatitis C not previously treated with alfa interferon. Give SC once weekly for 1 year. Dose and vial strength based on weight. Monotherapy: 1 mcg/kg/week. ≤45 kg: 40 mcg (0.4 ml, 50 mcg/0.5 ml vial). 46-56 kg: 50 mcg (0.5 ml, 50 mcg/0.5 ml vial). 57-72 kg: 64 mcg (0.4 ml, 80 mcg/0.5 ml vial). 73-88 kg: 80 mcg (0.5 ml, 80 mcg/0.5 ml vial). 89-106 kg: 96 mcg (0.4 ml, 120 mcg/0.5 ml vial). 107-136 kg: 120 mcg (0.5 ml, 120 mcg/0.5 ml vial). 137-160 kg: 150 mcg (0.5 ml, 150 mcg/0.5 ml vial). In combo with oral ribavirin (see Rebetol entry): 1.5 mcg/kg/week. <40 kg: 50 mcg (0.5 ml, 50 mcg/0.5 ml vial). 40-50 kg: 64 mcg (0.4 ml, 80 mcg/0.5 ml vial). 51-60 kg: 80 mcg (0.5 ml, 80 mcg/0.5 ml vial). 61-75 kg: 96 mcg (0.4 ml, 120 mcg/0.5 ml vial). 76-85 kg: 120 mcg (0.5 ml, 120 mcg/0.5 ml vial). >95 kg: 150 mcg (0.5 ml, 150 mcg/0.5 ml vial). Give at bedtime or with antipyretic to minimize flu-like sx. Consider stopping if HCV RNA is not below limit of detection after 24 weeks of therapy.

PEDS - Not approved in children.

FORMS - Trade only: 50,80,120,150 mcg/0.5 mL single-use vials with diluent, 2 syringes, and alcohol swabs. Disposable single-dose Redipen 50,80,120,150 mcg.

NOTES - Monitor for depression, suicidality, other severe neuropsychiatric effects. Thrombocytopenia, neutropenia, thyroid dysfunction, hyperglycemia, cardiovascular events, colitis, pancreatitis, hypersensitivity, flu-like sx, pulmonary damage. Caution if CrCl <50 mL/min.

Monitor CBC, blood chemistry. May increase methadone levels. Dosage adjustments for adverse effects in package insert. Peginterferon should be used immediately after reconstitution, but can be refrigerated for up to 24 h.

ribavirin - inhaled (*Virazole*) ▶Lung ♀X ▶- $$$$$

WARNING - Beware of sudden pulmonary deterioration with ribavirin. Drug precipitation may cause ventilator dysfunction.

PEDS - Severe respiratory syncytial virus infection: Aerosol 12-18 hours/day x 3-7 days.

NOTES - Minimize exposure to health care workers, especially pregnant women.

ribavirin - oral (*Rebetol, Copegus, Ribasphere*) ▶Cellular, K ♀X ▶- $$$$$

WARNING - Teratogen with extremely long half-life; contraindicated if pregnancy possible in patient/ partner. Female patients and female partners of male patients must avoid pregnancy by using 2 forms of birth control during and for 6 months after stopping ribavirin. Obtain pregnancy test at baseline and monthly. Hemolytic anemia that may worsen cardiac disease. Assess for underlying heart disease before tx with ribavirin. Do not use in significant/ unstable heart disease. Baseline ECG if pre-existing cardiac dysfunction.

ADULT - Chronic hepatitis C. Rebetol in combo with interferon alfa-2b (Intron A): 600 mg PO bid if >75 kg; 400 mg q am and 600 mg q pm if ≤75 kg. Take without regard to meals, but consistently the same. Rebetol in combo with peginterferon alfa 2b (PEG-Intron): 400 mg PO bid with food. Copegus in combo with peginterferon alfa 2a (Pegasys): For genotype 1 or 4, treat x 48 wks with 1200 mg/day if ≥75 kg; 1000 mg/day if <75 kg. For genotype 2 or 3, treat x 24 wks with 800 mg/day PO. For patients coinfected with HIV: 800 mg/day PO for 48 weeks regardless of genotype. Take bid with food. See package inserts for dosage reductions if Hb declines.

PEDS - Rebetol in combo with interferon alfa-2b: For patients ≤25 kg or who cannot swallow caps: 15 mg/kg/day of soln PO divided bid. Caps: 200 mg PO bid for 25-36 kg; 200 mg qam and 400 mg q pm for 37-49 kg; 400 mg bid for 50-61 kg. Use adult dose for >61 kg. Take without regard to meals, but consistently the same.

UNAPPROVED PEDS - Combination therapy with interferon alfa for chronic hepatitis C. 200 mg bid for 25-36 kg; 200 mg qam and 400 mg q pm for 37-49 kg; 400 mg bid for 50-61 kg. Use adult dosing for >61 kg.

FORMS - Generic/Trade: Caps 200 mg, tabs 200,400 mg. Generic only: tabs 600mg. Trade only (Rebetol): oral soln 40mg/mL (100ml).

NOTES - Contraindicated in hemoglobinopathies; autoimmune hepatitis; hepatic decompensation in cirrhosis (Child-Pugh score >6 if HCV only; score ≥6 if HIV co-infected). Get CBC at baseline, weeks 2 & 4, and prn. Risk of anemia increased if >50 yo or if renal dysfunction. Do not use if CrCl <50 mL/min. Decreased INR with warfarin; monitor INR weekly for 4 weeks after ribavirin started/stopped. May increase risk of lactic acidosis with nucleoside reverse transcriptase inhibitors. Avoid didanosine, stavudine, zidovudine.

telbivudine (*Tyzeka*) ▶K ♀B ▶- $$$$$

WARNING - Nucleoside analogues can cause lactic acidosis with hepatic steatosis. Severe acute exacerbation of hepatitis B can occur after discontinuation. Monitor closely for ≥2 months after discontinuation.

ADULT - Chronic hepatitis B: 600 mg PO once daily.

PEDS - Not approved in children.

FORMS - Trade only: 600 mg tabs.

NOTES - No dosage adjustment needed for hepatic dysfunction. Renal dysfunction: 600 mg PO q48h for CrCl 30-49 mL/min; q72h for CrCl <30 mL/min but not hemodialysis; q96h for ESRD. Give dose after hemodialysis session.

ANTIMICROBIALS: Carbapenems

ertapenem (*Invanz*) ▶K ♀B ▶? $$$$$

ADULT - Community-acquired pneumonia, diabetic foot, complicated intra-abdominal, skin, urinary tract, acute pelvic infections: 1g IM/IV over 30 minutes q24h x ≤14 days for IV, x ≤7 days for IM. Prophylaxis, elective colorectal surgery: 1 g IV 1 h before incision.

PEDS - Community-acquired pneumonia, complicated intra-abdominal, skin, urinary tract, acute pelvic infections (3 mo-12 yo): 15 mg/kg IV/IM q12h (max 1 g/day). Use adult dose for ≥13 yo. Infuse IV over 30 minutes. Can give IV for ≤14 days, IM for ≤7 days.

NOTES - Possible cross-sensitivity with other

beta-lactams; pseudomembranous colitis; superinfection; seizures (especially if renal dysfunction or CNS disorder). Not active against Pseudomonas or Acinetobacter species. IM diluted with lidocaine; contraindicated if amide-type local anesthetic allergy. Renal dysfunction (adults): 500 mg q24h for CrCl ≤30 mL/min or hemodialysis. Give 150 mg supplemental dose if daily dose given within 6 h before hemodialysis session. Do not dilute in dextrose.

imipenem-cilastatin (Primaxin) ▶K ♀C ▶? $$$$$

ADULT - Pneumonia, sepsis, endocarditis, polymicrobic, intra-abdominal, gynecologic, bone & joint, skin infections. Normal renal function, ≥70 kg - Mild infection: 250-500 mg IV q6h. Moderate infection: 500 mg IV q6-8h or 1 g IV q8h. Severe infection: 500 mg IV q6h to 1 g IV q6-8h. Complicated UTI: 500 mg IV q6h. See product labeling for doses in adults <70 kg. Can give up to 1.5 g/day IM for mild/moderate infections.

PEDS - Pneumonia, sepsis, endocarditis, polymicrobic, intra-abdominal, bone & joint, skin infections. Age >3 mo: 15-25 mg/kg IV q6h. 1-3 mo: 25 mg/kg IV q6h. 1-4 weeks old: 25 mg/kg IV q8h. <1 week old: 25 mg/kg IV q12h. Not for children with CNS infections, or <30 kg with renal dysfunction.

UNAPPROVED ADULT - Malignant otitis externa, empiric therapy for neutropenic fever: 500 mg IV q6h.

NOTES - Possible cross-sensitivity with other beta-lactams, pseudomembranous colitis, superinfection, seizures (especially with ganciclovir or in elderly with renal dysfunction, cerebrovascular/seizure disorder). See product labeling for dose if CrCl <70 mL/min. Not for CrCl <5 mL/min unless dialysis started within 48 h.

meropenem (Merrem IV) ▶K ♀B ▶? $$$$$

ADULT - Intra-abdominal infections: 1 g IV q8h. Complicated skin infections: 500 mg IV q8h.

PEDS - Meningitis: 40 mg/kg IV q8h for age ≥3 mo; 2 g IV q8h if >50 kg. Intra-abdominal infection: 20 mg/kg IV q8h for age ≥3 mo; 1 g IV q8h for weight >50 kg. Complicated skin infections: 10 mg/kg IV q8h for age ≥3 mo; 500 mg IV q8h for weight >50 kg.

UNAPPROVED ADULT - Meningitis: 40 mg/kg (max 2 g) IV q 8h. Hospital-acquired pneumonia, complicated UTI, malignant otitis externa: 1 g IV q8h.

UNAPPROVED PEDS - Infant >2 kg: 20 mg/kg IV q12h for ≤1 week old, q8h for 1-4 wks old.

NOTES - Possible cross-sensitivity with other beta-lactams; pseudomembranous colitis; superinfection; seizures; thrombocytopenia in renal dysfunction. Reduces valproic acid levels. For adults with renal dysfunction: Give normal dose q12h for CrCl 26-50 mL/min, 50% of normal dose q12h for CrCl 10-25 mL/min, 50% of normal dose q24h for CrCl <10 mL/min.

OVERVIEW OF BACTERIAL PATHOGENS (selected)

Gram Positive Aerobic Cocci: *Staph epidermidis* (coagulase negative), *Staph aureus* (coagulase positive), Streptococci: *S pneumoniae* (pneumococcus), *S pyogenes* (Group A), *S agalactiae* (Group B), enterococcus

Gram Positive Aerobic / Facultatively Anaerobic Bacilli: *Bacillus, Corynebacterium diphtheriae, Erysipelothrix rhusiopathiae, Listeria monocytogenes, Nocardia*

Gram Negative Aerobic Diplococci: *Moraxella catarrhalis, Neisseria gonorrhoeae, Neisseria meningitidis*

Gram Negative Aerobic Coccobacilli: *Haemophilus ducreyi, Haemoph. influenzae*

Gram Negative Aerobic Bacilli: *Acinetobacter, Bartonella* species, *Bordetella pertussis, Brucella, Burkholderia cepacia, Campylobacter, Francisella tularensis, Helicobacter pylori, Legionella pneumophila, Pseudomonas aeruginosa, Stenotrophomonas maltophilia, Vibrio cholerae, Yersinia*

Gram Neg Facultatively Anaerobic Bacilli: *Aeromonas hydrophila, Eikenella corrodens, Pasteurella multocida,* Enterobacteriaceae: *E coli, Citrobacter, Shigella, Salmonella, Klebsiella, Enterobacter, Hafnia, Serratia, Proteus, Providencia*

Anaerobes: *Actinomyces, Bacteroides fragilis, Clostridium botulinum, Clostridium difficile, Clostridium perfringens, Clostridium tetani, Fusobacterium, Lactobacillus, Peptostreptococcus*

Defective Cell Wall Bacteria: *Chlamydia pneumoniae, Chlamydia psittaci, Chlamydia trachomatis, Coxiella burnetii, Mycoplasma pneumoniae, Rickettsia prowazekii, Rickettsia rickettsii, Rickettsia typhi, Ureaplasma urealyticum*

Spirochetes: *Borrelia burgdorferi, Leptospira, Treponema pallidum*

Mycobacteria: *M avium complex, M kansasii, M leprae, M tuberculosis*

CEPHALOSPORINS – GENERAL ANTIMICROBIAL SPECTRUM

1st generation: gram positive (including Staph aureus); basic gram neg. coverage

2nd generation: diminished Staph aureus, improved gram negative coverage compared to 1st generation; some with anaerobic coverage

3rd generation: further diminished Staph aureus, further improved gram negative coverage compared to 1st & 2nd generation; some with Pseudomonal coverage & diminished gram positive coverage

4th generation: same as 3rd generation plus coverage against Pseudomonas

ANTIMICROBIALS: Cephalosporins – 1st Generation

NOTE: Cephalosporins are 2nd-line to penicillin for group A strep pharyngitis, can be cross-sensitive with penicillin, and can cause pseudomembranous colitis.

cefadroxil (*Duricef*) ▶K ♀B ▶+ $$$
ADULT - Simple UTI: 1-2 g/day PO divided once daily-bid. Other UTIs: 1 g PO bid. Skin infections: 1 g/day PO divided once daily-bid. Group A strep pharyngitis: 1 g/day PO divided once daily-bid x 10 days. See table for prophylaxis of bacterial endocarditis.
PEDS - UTIs, skin infections: 30 mg/kg/day PO divided bid. Group A streptococcal pharyngitis/tonsillitis, impetigo: 30 mg/kg/day PO divided once daily-bid. Treat pharyngitis for 10 days.
FORMS - Generic/Trade: Tabs 1 g, caps 500 mg, susp 125, 250, & 500 mg/5 mL.
NOTES - Renal dysfunction in adults: 1 g load, then 500 mg PO q12h for CrCl 25-50 mL/min, 500 mg PO q24h for CrCl 10-25 mL/min, 500 mg PO q36h for CrCl <10 mL/min.

cefazolin (*Ancef*) ▶K ♀B ▶+ $$$
ADULT - Pneumonia, sepsis, endocarditis, skin, bone & joint, genital infections. Mild infections due to gram-positive cocci: 250-500 mg IM/IV q8h. Moderate/severe infections: 0.5-1 g IM/IV q6-8h. Life-threatening infections: 1-1.5 g IV q6h. Simple UTI: 1 g IM/IV q12h. Pneumococcal pneumonia: 500 mg IM/IV q12h. Surgical prophylaxis: 1 g IM/IV 30-60 min preop, additional 0.5-1 g during surgery >2h, and 0.5-1 g q6-8h x 24h postop. See table for prophylaxis of bacterial endocarditis.
PEDS - Pneumonia, sepsis, endocarditis, skin, bone & joint infections. Mild/moderate infections, age ≥1 mo: 25-50 mg/kg/day IM/IV divided q6-8h. Severe infections, age ≥1 mo:

100 mg/kg/day IV divided q6-8h. See table for prophylaxis of bacterial endocarditis.
NOTES - Renal dysfunction in adults: Usual 1st dose, then usual dose q8h for CrCl 35-54 mL/min, 50% of usual dose q12h for CrCl 11-34 mL/min, 50% of usual dose q18-24h for CrCl <10 mL/min. Renal dysfunction in children: Usual 1st dose, then 60% of usual dose q12h for CrCl 40-70 mL/min, 25% of usual dose q12h for 20-40 mL/min, 10% of usual dose q24h for CrCl 5-20 mL/min.

cephalexin (*Keflex, Panixine DisperDose*) ▶K ♀B ▶? $$$
ADULT - Pneumonia, bone, GU infections. Usual dose: 250-500 mg PO qid. Max: 4 g/day. Group A strep pharyngitis, skin infections, simple UTI: 500 mg PO bid. Treat pharyngitis x 10 days. See table for prophylaxis of bacterial endocarditis.
PEDS - Pneumonia, GU, bone, skin infections, group A strep pharyngitis. Usual dose: 25-50 mg/kg/day PO divided doses. Max dose: 100 mg/kg/day. Can give bid for strep pharyngitis in children >1 yo, skin infections. Group A strep pharyngitis, skin infections, simple UTI in patients >15 yo: 500 mg PO bid. Treat pharyngitis x 10 days. Not for otitis media, sinusitis.
FORMS - Generic/Trade: Caps 250, 500 mg. Generic only: Tabs 250, 500 mg, susp 100,125 & 250 mg/5 mL. Panixine DisperDose 125, 250 mg scored tabs for oral susp. Trade only: Caps 333, 750 mg.
NOTES - Mix Panixine tab with 2 tsp water and drink mixture, then rinse container with a little water and drink that. Do not chew or swallow tab whole. Use only for doses that can be delivered by half or whole tabs.

ANTIMICROBIALS: Cephalosporins – 2nd Generation

NOTE: Cephalosporins are 2nd-line to penicillin for group A strep pharyngitis, can be cross-sensitive with penicillin, and can cause pseudomembranous colitis.

cefaclor (Ceclor, Raniclor) ▶K ♀B ▶? $$$

ADULT - Otitis media, pneumonia, group A strep pharyngitis, UTI, skin infections: 250-500 mg PO tid. Extended release tabs: Acute exacerbation of chronic bronchitis, secondary bacterial infection of acute bronchitis: 500 mg PO bid with food. Group A streptococcal pharyngitis, skin infections: 375 mg PO bid with food. Treat pharyngitis x 10 days.

PEDS - Pneumonia, group A strep pharyngitis, UTI, skin infections: 20-40 mg/kg/day up to 1 g/day PO divided bid for pharyngitis, tid for other infections. Treat pharyngitis x 10d. Otitis media: 40 mg/kg/day PO divided bid.

FORMS - Generic/Trade: Caps 250,500 mg, susp 125,187,250,375 mg/5 mL. Generic only: Chew tabs 125,187,250,375 mg. Extended release tabs 375, 500 mg.

cefoxitin (Mefoxin) ▶K ♀B ▶+ $$$$$

ADULT - Pneumonia, UTI, sepsis, intra-abdominal, gynecologic, skin, bone & joint infections: Uncomplicated, 1 g IV q6-8h. Moderate to severe, 1 g IV q4h or 2 g IV q6-8h. Infections requiring high doses, 2 g IV q4h or 3 g IV q6h. Uncontaminated gastrointestinal surgery, vaginal/abdominal hysterectomy: 2 g IV 30-60 min preop, then 2 g IV q6h x 24h. C-section: 2 g IV after cord clamped or 2 g IV q4h x 3 doses with 1st dose given after cord clamped.

PEDS - Pneumonia, UTI, sepsis, intra-abdominal, skin, bone/joint infections, age ≥3 mo: 80-160 mg/kg/day IV divided into 4-6 doses, not to exceed 12 g/day. Mild-moderate infections: 80-100 mg/kg/day IV divided into 3-4 doses. Surgical prophylaxis: 30-40 mg/kg IV 30-60 min preop and for not more than 24h postop.

NOTES - Eosinophilia & increased AST with high doses in children. Reduced adult dosing in renal dysfunction: Load with 1-2 g IV; then 1-2 g IV q8-12h for CrCl 30-50 mL/min, 1-2 g IV q12-24h for CrCl 10-29 mL/min, 0.5-1 g IV q12-24h for CrCl 5-9 mL/min, 0.5 g IV q24-48h for CrCl <5 mL/min. Give 1-2 g loading dose after each hemodialysis.

cefprozil (Cefzil) ▶K ♀B ▶+ $$$$

ADULT - Group A strep pharyngitis: 500 mg PO daily x 10 days. Sinusitis: 250-500 mg PO bid. Acute exacerbation of chronic/secondary infection of acute bronchitis: 500 mg bid. Skin infections: 250-500 mg bid or 500 mg once daily.

PEDS - Otitis media: 15 mg/kg/dose PO bid. Group A strep pharyngitis: 7.5 mg/kg/dose PO bid x 10 days. Sinusitis: 7.5-15 mg/kg/dose PO bid. Skin infections: 20 mg/kg PO daily. Use adult dose for ≥13 yo.

FORMS - Generic/Trade: Tabs 250,500 mg. Susp 125 & 250 mg/5 mL.

NOTES - Give 50% of usual dose at usual interval for CrCl <30 mL/min.

cefuroxime (Zinacef, Ceftin, Kefurox) ▶K ♀B ▶? $$$

ADULT - IM/IV cefuroxime. Uncomplicated simple UTI, pneumonia, skin infections, disseminated gonorrhea: 750 mg IM/IV q8h. Bone & joint, or severe/complicated infections: 1.5 g IV q8h. Sepsis: 1.5 g IV q6h to 3 g IV q8h. Gonorrhea: 1.5g IM single dose split into 2 injections, given with probenecid 1 g PO. Surgical prophylaxis: 1.5 g IV 30-60 min preop, then 750 mg IM/IV q8h for prolonged procedures. Open heart surgery: 1.5 g IV q12h x 4 with 1st dose at anesthesia induction. Cefuroxime axetil tabs: Group A strep pharyngitis, acute sinusitis: 250 mg PO bid x 10 days. Acute exacerbation of chronic/secondary infection of acute bronchitis, skin infections: 250-500 mg PO bid. Lyme disease: 500 mg PO bid x 14 days for early disease, x 28 days for Lyme arthritis. Simple UTI: 125-250 mg PO bid. Gonorrhea: 1 g PO single dose.

PEDS - IM/IV cefuroxime. Most infections: 50-100 mg/kg/day IM/IV divided q6-8h. Bone & joint infections: 150 mg/kg/day IM/IV divided q8h not to exceed max adult dose. Cefuroxime axetil tabs: Group A strep pharyngitis: 125 mg PO bid x 10 days. Otitis media, sinusitis: 250 mg PO bid x 10 days. Cefuroxime axetil oral susp: Group A strep pharyngitis: 20 mg/kg/day (up to 500 mg/day) PO divided bid x 10 days. Otitis media, sinusitis, impetigo: 30 mg/kg/day (up to 1 g/day) PO divided bid x 10 days. Use adult dose for ≥13 yo.

UNAPPROVED PEDS - Lyme disease: 30 mg/kg/day PO divided bid (max 500 mg/dose) x 14 days for early disease, x 28 days for Lyme arthritis. Community-acquired pneumonia: 150 mg/kg/day IV divided q8h.

FORMS - Generic/Trade: Tabs 250,500 mg. Generic only: 125 mg tab. Trade only: Susp 125 & 250 mg/5 mL.

NOTES - AAP recommends 5-7 days of therapy for older (≥6 yo) children with non-severe otitis media, and 10 days for younger children and those with severe disease. Dosage adjustment for renal dysfunction in adults: 750 mg IM/IV q12h for CrCl 10-20 mL/min, 750 mg IM/IV q24h for CrCl <10 mL/min. Give supplemental dose after hemodialysis. Tabs & susp not bioequivalent on mg/mg basis. Do not crush tabs.

ANTIMICROBIALS: Cephalosporins – 3rd Generation

NOTE: Cephalosporins are 2nd-line to penicillin for group A strep pharyngitis, can be cross-sensitive with penicillin, and can cause pseudomembranous colitis.

cefdinir (*Omnicef*) ▶K ♀B ▶? $$$$

ADULT - Community-acquired pneumonia, skin infections: 300 mg PO bid x 10 days. Sinusitis: 600 mg PO once daily or 300 mg PO bid x 10 days. Group A strep pharyngitis, acute exacerbation of chronic bronchitis: 600 mg PO once daily x 10 days or 300 mg PO bid x 5-10 days.

PEDS - Group A strep pharyngitis, otitis media: 14 mg/kg/day PO divided bid x 5-10 days or once daily x 10 days. Sinusitis: 14 mg/kg/day PO divided once daily-bid x 10 days. Skin infections: 14 mg/kg/day PO divided bid x 10 days. Use adult dose for ≥13 yo.

FORMS - Generic/Trade: Cap 300 mg. Susp 125 & 250 mg/5 mL.

NOTES - AAP recommends 5-7 days of therapy for older (≥6 yo) children with non-severe otitis media, and 10 days for younger children and those with severe disease. Give iron, multivitamins with iron, or antacids ≥2 h before/after. Cefdinir complex with iron may turn stools red. Dosage reduction for renal dysfunction: 300 mg PO daily for adults with CrCl <30 mL/min. 7 mg/kg/day PO once daily up to 300 mg/day for children with CrCl <30 mL/min. Hemodialysis: 300 mg or 7 mg/kg PO after hemodialysis, then 300 mg or 7 mg/kg PO q48h.

cefditoren (*Spectracef*) ▶K ♀B ▶? $$$

ADULT - Skin infections, group A strep pharynxgitis: 200 mg PO bid x 10 days. Give 400 mg bid x 10 days for acute exacerbation of chronic bronchitis, x 14 days for community-acquired pneumonia. Take with food.

PEDS - Not approved for <12 yo. Skin infections, group A strep pharyngitis, adolescents ≥12 yo: 200 mg PO bid with food x 10 days.

FORMS - Trade only: Tabs 200 mg.

NOTES - Contraindicated if milk protein allergy or carnitine deficiency. Not for long-term use due to potential risk of carnitine deficiency. Do not take with drugs that reduce gastric acid (antacids, H2 blockers, etc). Dosage adjustment for renal dysfunction: Max 200 mg bid if CrCl 30-49 mL/min; max 200 mg once daily if CrCl <30 mL/min.

cefixime (*Suprax*) ▶K/Bile ♀B ▶? $

ADULT - Simple UTI, pharyngitis, acute bacterial bronchitis, acute exacerbation of chronic bronchitis: 400 mg PO once daily. Gonorrhea: 400 mg PO single dose.

PEDS - Otitis media: 8 mg/kg/day susp PO divided once daily-bid. Pharyngitis: 8 mg/kg/day PO divided once daily-bid x 10 days. Use adult dose for >50 kg or ≥13 yo.

UNAPPROVED ADULT - Disseminated gonorrhea, CDC regimen: 500 mg PO bid of suspension or 400 mg PO bid of tabs.

UNAPPROVED PEDS - Febrile UTI (3-24 mo): 16 mg/kg PO on first day, then 8 mg/kg PO daily to complete 14 days. Gonorrhea: 8 mg/kg (max 400 mg) PO single dose for <45 kg, 400 mg PO single dose for ≥45 kg.

FORMS - Trade only: Susp 100 & 200 mg/5 mL, tab 400 mg (Canada only).

NOTES - Cross-sensitivity with penicillins possible, pseudomembranous colitis. Poor activity against S aureus. Increased INR with warfarin. May increase carbamazepine levels. Susp stable at room temp or refrigerated x 14 days. Dosing in renal dysfunction: 75% of usual dose at usual interval for CrCl 21-60 mL/min or hemodialysis. 50% of usual dose at usual interval for CrCl <20 mL/min or continuous peritoneal dialysis.

cefoperazone (*Cefobid*) ▶Bile/K ♀B ▶? $$$$$

ADULT - Peritonitis, sepsis, respiratory, intra-abdominal, skin infections, endometritis, pelvic inflammatory disease & other gynecologic infections: Usual dose 2-4 g/day IV divided q12h. Infections with less serious organisms/severe infections: 6-12 g/day IV divided q6-12h. Use q6h for Pseudomonas infections. 1-2 g doses can be given IM.

PEDS - Not approved in children.

UNAPPROVED PEDS - Mild to moderate infections, age ≥1 mo: 100-150 mg/kg/day IM/IV divided q8-12h.

NOTES - Possible clotting impairment. Disulfiram-like reaction with alcohol. Not for meningitis.

cefotaxime (*Claforan*) ▶KL ♀B ▶+ $$$$$

ADULT - Pneumonia, sepsis, GU & gynecologic, skin, intra-abdominal, bone & joint infections: Uncomplicated, 1 g IM/IV q12h. Moderate/severe, 1-2 g IM/IV q8h. Infections usually requiring high doses, 2 g IV q6-8h. Life-threatening, 2 g IV q4h. Meningitis: 2g IV q4-6h. Gonorrhea: 0.5-1 g IM single dose.

SEXUALLY TRANSMITTED DISEASES & VAGINITIS*

Bacterial vaginosis: 1) metronidazole 5 g of 0.75% gel intravaginally daily x 5 days OR 500 mg PO bid x 7 days. 2) clindamycin 5 g of 2% cream intravaginally qhs x 7 days. In pregnancy: 1) metronidazole 500 mg PO bid x 7 days OR 250 mg PO tid x 7 days. 2) clindamycin 300 mg PO bid x 7 days.

Candidal vaginitis: 1) intravaginal clotrimazole, miconazole, terconazole, nystatin, tioconazole, or butoconazole. 2) fluconazole 150 mg PO single dose.

Chancroid: Single dose of: 1) azithromycin 1 g PO or 2) ceftriaxone 250 mg IM.

Chlamydia: First line either azithromycin 1 g PO single dose or doxycycline 100 mg PO bid x 7 days. Second line fluoroquinolones or erythromycin. In pregnancy: 1) azithromycin 1 g PO single dose. 2) amoxicillin 500 mg PO tid x 7 days. Repeat NAAT‡ 3 weeks after treatment.

Epididymitis: 1) ceftriaxone 250 mg IM single dose + doxycycline 100 mg PO bid x 10 days. 2) ofloxacin 300 mg PO bid or levofloxacin 500 mg PO daily x 10 days if enteric organisms suspected, or negative gonococcal culture or NAAT.†.

Gonorrhea: Single dose of: 1) ceftriaxone 125 mg IM 2) cefixime 400 mg PO (not for pharynx).† Treat chlamydia empirically. Cephalosporin desensitization advised for cephalosporin-allergic patients (e.g. pregnant women). Consider azithromycin 2 g PO single dose for uncomplicated gonorrhea, but no efficacy/safety data for this regimen in pregnant women.

Gonorrhea, disseminated: Initially treat with ceftriaxone 1 g IM/IV q24h until 24-48 h after improvement. Second-line alternatives: 1) cefotaxime 1 g IV q8h. 2) ceftizoxime 1 g IV q8h. Complete 1 week of treatment with: 1) cefixime tabs 400 mg PO bid (not available in US). 2) cefixime susp 500 mg PO bid. 3) cefpodoxime 400 mg PO bid.† Cephalosporin desensitization advised for cephalosporin-allergic patients (e.g. pregnant women).

Gonorrhea, meningitis: ceftriaxone 1-2 g IV q12h for 10-14 days.

Gonorrhea, endocarditis: ceftriaxone 1-2 g IV q12h for at least 4 weeks.

Granuloma inguinale: doxycycline 100 mg PO bid x >= 3 weeks and until lesions completely healed. Alternative azithromycin 1 g PO once weekly x 3 weeks.

Herpes simplex (genital, first episode): 1) acyclovir 400 mg PO tid x 7-10 days. 2) famciclovir 250 mg PO tid x 7-10 days. 3) valacyclovir 1 g PO bid x 7-10 days.

Herpes simplex (genital, recurrent): 1) acyclovir 400 mg PO tid x 5 days. 2) acyclovir 800 mg PO tid x 2 days or bid x 5 days. 3) famciclovir 125 mg PO bid x 5 days. 4) famciclovir 1 g PO bid x 1 day. 5) valacyclovir 500 mg PO bid x 3 days. 6) valacyclovir 1 g PO daily x 5 days.

Herpes simplex (suppressive therapy): 1) acyclovir 400mg PO bid. 2) famciclovir 250 mg PO bid. 3) valacyclovir 500-1000 mg PO daily.

Herpes simplex (genital, recurrent in HIV infection): 1) Acyclovir 400 mg PO tid x 5-10 days. 2) famciclovir 500 mg PO bid x 5-10 days. 3) Valacyclovir 1 g PO bid x 5-10 days.

Herpes simplex (suppressive therapy in HIV infection): 1) Acyclovir 400-800 mg PO bid-tid. 2) Famciclovir 500 mg PO bid. 3) Valacyclovir 500 mg PO bid.

Herpes simplex (prevention of transmission in immunocompetent patients with ≤9 recurrences/year): Valacyclovir 500 mg PO daily by source partner, in conjunction with safer sex practices.

Lymphogranuloma venereum: 1) doxycycline 100 mg PO bid x 21 days. Alternative: erythromycin base 500 mg PO qid x 21 days.

Pelvic inflammatory disease (PID), inpatient regimens: 1) cefoxitin 2 g IV q6h + doxycycline 100 mg IV/PO q12h. 2) clindamycin 900 mg IV q8h + gentamicin 2 mg/kg IM/IV loading dose, then 1.5 mg/kg IM/IV q8h (See gentamicin entry for alternative daily dosing). Can switch to PO therapy within 24 h of improvement.

Pelvic inflammatory disease (PID), outpatient treatment: 1) ceftriaxone 250 mg IM single dose + doxycycline 100 mg PO bid +/- metronidazole 500 mg PO bid x 14 days.

Proctitis, proctocolitis, enteritis: ceftriaxone 125 mg IM single dose + doxycycline 100 mg PO bid x7d.

Sexual assault prophylaxis: ceftriaxone 125 mg IM single dose + metronidazole 2 g PO single dose + azithromycin 1 g PO single dose/doxycycline 100 mg PO bid x 7 days. Consider giving antiemetic.

Syphilis (primary and secondary): 1) benzathine penicillin 2.4 million units IM single dose. 2) doxycycline 100 mg PO bid x 2 weeks if penicillin allergic.

Syphilis (early latent, i.e. duration <1 y): 1) benzathine penicillin 2.4 million units IM single dose. 2) doxycycline 100 mg PO bid x 2 weeks if penicillin allergic.

SEXUALLY TRANSMITTED DISEASES & VAGINITIS, continued

Syphilis (late latent or unknown duration): 1) benzathine penicillin 2.4 million units IM q week x 3 doses. 2) doxycycline 100 mg PO bid x 4 weeks if penicillin allergic.

Syphilis (tertiary): 1) benzathine penicillin 2.4 million units IM q week x 3 doses. 2) doxycycline 100 mg PO bid x 4 weeks if penicillin allergic.

Syphilis (neuro): 1) penicillin G 18-24 million units/day continuous IV infusion or 3-4 million units IV q4h x 10-14 days. 2) procaine penicillin 2.4 million units IM daily + probenecid 500 mg PO qid, both x 10-14 days.

Syphilis in pregnancy: Treat only with penicillin regimen for stage of syphilis as noted above. Use penicillin desensitization protocol if penicillin-allergic.

Trichomoniasis: metronidazole (can use in pregnancy) or tinidazole, each 2 g PO single dose.

Urethritis, Cervicitis: Test for Chlamydia and gonorrhea with NAAT‡. Treat based on test results or treat presumptively if high-risk of infection (Chlamydia: age ≤25 y, new/ multiple sex partners, or unprotected sex; gonorrhea: population prevalence >5%), esp. if NAAT‡ unavailable or patient unlikely to return for follow-up.

Urethritis (persistent/recurrent): 1) metronidazole/ tinidazole 2 g PO single dose + azithromycin 2 g PO single dose (if not used in first episode).

* *MMWR 2006;55:RR-11 or http://www.cdc.gov/STD/treatment/. Treat sexual partners for all except herpes, candida, and bacterial vaginosis.*

† *As of April 2007, the CDC no longer recommends fluoroquinolones for gonorrhea because of high resistance rates. Do not consider fluoroquinolone unless antimicrobial susceptibility can be documented by culture. If parenteral cephalosporin not feasible for PID (and NAAT is negative or culture documents fluoroquinolone susceptibility), can consider levofloxacin 500 mg PO once daily or ofloxacin 400 mg PO bid +/- metronidazole 500 mg PO bid x 14 days.*

‡ *NAAT = nucleic acid amplification test.*

PEDS - Neonates, ≤1 week old: 50 mg/kg/dose IV q12h. 1-4 weeks old: 50 mg/kg/dose IV q8h. Labeled dose for pneumonia, sepsis, GU, skin, intra-abdominal, bone/joint, CNS infections, 1 mo-12 yo: 50-180 mg/kg/day IM/IV divided q4-6h. AAP recommendations: 225-300 mg/kg/day IV divided q6-8h for S pneumoniae meningitis. Mild to moderate infections: 75-100 mg/kg/day IV/IM divided q6-8h. Severe infections: 150-200 mg/kg/day IV/IM divided q6-8h.

UNAPPROVED ADULT - Disseminated gonorrhea, CDC regimen: 1 g IV q8h.

NOTES - Bolus injection through central venous catheter can cause arrhythmias. Decrease dose by 50% for CrCl <20 mL/min.

cefpodoxime (*Vantin*) ▶K ♀B ▶? $$$$

ADULT - Acute exacerbation of chronic bronchitis, acute sinusitis: 200 mg PO bid x 10 days. Community-acquired pneumonia: 200 mg PO bid x 14 days. Group A strep pharyngitis: 100 mg PO bid x 5-10 days. Skin infections: 400 mg PO bid x 7-14 days. Simple UTI: 100 mg PO bid x 7 days. Gonorrhea: 200 mg PO single dose. Give tabs with food.

PEDS - 5 mg/kg PO bid x 5 days for otitis media, x 5-10 days for group A strep pharyngitis, x 10 days for sinusitis. Adult dose if ≥12 yo.

FORMS - Generic/Trade: Tabs 100, 200 mg. Susp 50 & 100 mg/5 mL.

NOTES - AAP recommends 5-7 days of therapy for older (≥6 yo) children with non-severe otitis media, and 10 days for younger children and those with severe disease. Do not give antacids within 2 h before/after cefpodoxime. Dosing in renal dysfunction: Increase dosing interval to q24h for CrCl <30 mL/min. Give 3 times/week after dialysis session for hemodialysis patients. Susp stable for 14 days refrigerated.

ceftazidime (*Ceptaz, Fortaz, Tazicef*) ▶K ♀B ▶+ $$$$$

ADULT - Simple UTI: 250 mg IM/IV q12h. Complicated UTI: 500 mg IM/IV q8-12h. Uncomplicated pneumonia, mild skin infections: 500 mg - 1g IM/IV q8h. Serious gynecologic, intra-abdominal, bone & joint, life-threatening infections, meningitis, empiric therapy of neutropenic fever: 2 g IV q8h. Pseudomonas lung infections in cystic fibrosis: 30-50 mg/kg IV q8h to max of 6 g/day.

PEDS - Use sodium formulations in children (Fortaz, Tazicef). UTIs, pneumonia, skin, intra-abdominal, bone & joint infections, 1 mo-12 yo: 100-150 mg/kg/day IV divided q8h to max of 6 g/day. Meningitis, 1 mo-12 yo: 150 mg/kg/day

IV divided q8h to max of 6 g/day. Infants up to 4 weeks old: 30 mg/kg IV q12h. Use adult dose & formulations if ≥12 yo.

UNAPPROVED ADULT - P aeruginosa foot osteomyelitis from nail puncture: 2 g IV q8h.

UNAPPROVED PEDS - AAP dosing for infants >2 kg: 50 mg/kg IV q8-12h for <1 week old, q8h for ≥1 week old.

NOTES - High levels in renal dysfunction can cause CNS toxicity. Adult renal dysfunction dosing: 1 g IV q12h for CrCl 31-50 mL/min; 1 g q24h for CrCl 16-30 mL/min; load with 1 g, then 500 mg q24h for CrCl 6-15 mL/min; load with 1 g, then 500 mg q48h for CrCl <5 mL/min. 1 g IV load in hemodialysis patients, then 1 g IV after hemodialysis sessions.

ceftibuten (*Cedax*) ▶K ♀B ▶? $$$$

ADULT - Group A strep pharyngitis, acute exacerbation of chronic bronchitis, otitis media not due to S pneumoniae: 400 mg PO once daily x 10 days.

PEDS - Group A strep pharyngitis, otitis media not due to S pneumoniae, age >6 mo: 9 mg/kg up to 400 mg PO once daily. Give susp on empty stomach.

FORMS - Trade only: Cap 400 mg, susp 90 mg/5 mL.

NOTES - Poor activity against S aureus and S pneumoniae. Dosing in adults with renal dysfunction: 200 mg PO once daily for CrCl 30-49 mL/min, 100 mg PO daily for CrCl 5-29 mL/min. Dosing in children with renal dysfunction: 4.5 mg/kg PO once daily for CrCl 30-49 mL/min, 2.25 mg/kg PO daily for CrCl 5-29 mL/min. Hemodialysis: adults 400 mg PO and children 9 mg/kg PO after each dialysis session. Susp stable for 14 days refrigerated.

ceftizoxime (*Cefizox*) ▶K ♀B ▶? $$$$$

ADULT - Simple UTI: 500 mg IM/IV q12h. Pneumonia, sepsis, intra-abdominal, skin, bone & joint infections: 1-2 g IM/IV q8-12h. Pelvic inflammatory disease: 2g IV q8h. Life-threatening infections: 3-4 g IV q8h. Gonorrhea: 1 g IM single dose. Split 2 g IM dose into 2 injections.

PEDS - Pneumonia, sepsis, intra-abdominal, skin, bone/joint infections, age ≥6 mo: 50 mg/kg/dose IV q6-8h. Up to 200 mg/kg/day for serious infections, not to exceed max adult dose.

UNAPPROVED PEDS - Gonorrhea, CDC regimens: 500 mg IM single dose for uncomplicated; 1 g IV q8h for disseminated infection.

NOTES - Can cause transient rise in eosinophils, ALT, AST, CPK in children. Not for meningitis. Dosing in adults with renal dysfunction:

For less severe infection load with 500 mg - 1 g IM/IV, then 500 mg q8h for CrCl 50-79 mL/min, 250-500 mg q12h for CrCl 5-49 mL/min, 500 mg q48h or 250 mg q24h for hemodialysis. For life-threatening infection, give loading dose, then 750 mg - 1.5 g IV q8h for CrCl 50-79 mL/min, 500 mg q12h for CrCl 5-49 mL/min, 500 mg - 1 g q48h or 500 mg q24h for hemodialysis. For hemodialysis patients, give dose at end of dialysis.

ceftriaxone (*Rocephin*) ▶K/Bile ♀B ▶+ $$$$$

ADULT - Pneumonia, UTI, pelvic inflammatory disease (hospitalized), sepsis, meningitis, skin, bone & joint, intra-abdominal infections: Usual dose 1-2 g IM/IV q24h (max 4 g/day divided q12h). Gonorrhea: single dose 125 mg IM (250 mg if ambulatory treatment of PID).

PEDS - Meningitis: 100 mg/kg/day (max 4 g/day) IV divided q12-24h. Skin, pneumonia, other serious infections: 50-75 mg/kg/day (max 2 g/day) IM/IV divided q12-24h. Otitis media: 50 mg/kg (max 1 g) IM single dose.

UNAPPROVED ADULT - Lyme disease carditis, meningitis: 2 g IV daily x 14 days. Chancroid: 250 mg IM single dose. Disseminated gonorrhea: 1 g IV q24h. Prophylaxis, invasive meningococcal disease: 250 mg IM single dose.

UNAPPROVED PEDS - Refractory otitis media (no response after 3 days of antibiotics): 50 mg/kg IM q24h x 3 doses. Lyme disease carditis, meningitis: 50-75 mg/kg IM/IV daily (max 2 g/day) x 14 days. Prophylaxis, invasive meningococcal disease: Single IM dose of 125 mg for ≤15 yo, 250 mg for >15 yo. Gonorrhea: 125 mg IM single dose; use adult regimens in STD table if ≥45 kg. Gonococcal bacteremia/arthritis: 50 mg/kg (max 1 g if ≤45 kg) IM/IV daily x 7 days. Gonococcal ophthalmia neonatorum/ gonorrhea prophylaxis in newborn: 25-50 mg/kg up to 125 mg IM/IV single dose at birth. Disseminated gonorrhea, infants: 25-50 mg/kg/day IM/IV daily x 7 days. Typhoid fever: 50-75 mg/kg IM/IV daily x 14 days.

NOTES - Can cause prolonged prothrombin time (due to vitamin K deficiency), biliary sludging/symptoms of gallbladder disease. Do not give to neonates with hyperbilirubinemia. Risk of life-threatening precipitates when administered to neonates within 48 hours of calcium-containing products or solutions, even if via separate IV lines. Do not dilute with Ringers/ Hartmann's soln. Dilute in 1% lidocaine for IM use. Do not exceed 2 g/day in patients with both hepatic & renal dysfunction.

ANTIMICROBIALS: Cephalosporins – 4th Generation

NOTE: Cross-sensitivity with penicillins possible. May cause pseudomembranous colitis.

cefepime (*Maxipime*) ▶K ♀B ▶? $$$$$
ADULT - Mild, moderate UTI: 0.5-1 g IM/IV q12h. Severe UTI, skin, complicated intra-abdominal infections: 2 g IV q12h. Pneumonia: 1-2 g IV q12h. Empiric therapy of febrile neutropenia: 2 g IV q8h.
PEDS - UTI, skin infections, pneumonia, ≤40 kg: 50 mg/kg IV q12h. Empiric therapy for feb-rile neutropenia, ≤40 kg: 50 mg/kg IV q8h. Do not exceed adult dose.
UNAPPROVED ADULT - P aeruginosa osteomyelitis of the foot from nail puncture: 2 g IV q12h. Meningitis: 2 g IV q8h.
UNAPPROVED PEDS - Meningitis, cystic fibrosis: 50 mg/kg IV q8h (max 6 g/day).
NOTES - High levels in renal dysfunction can cause CNS toxicity; dosing for CrCl <60 mL/min in package insert.

ANTIMICROBIALS: Macrolides

azithromycin (*Zithromax, Zmax*) ▶L♀B▶? $$
ADULT - Community-acquired pneumonia: 500 mg IV over 1 h daily x ≥2 days, then 500 mg PO daily x 7-10 days total. Pelvic inflammatory disease: 500 mg IV daily x 1-2 days, then 250 mg PO daily to complete 7 days. Oral for acute exacerbation of chronic bronchitis, community-acquired pneumonia, group A streptococcal pharyngitis (second-line to penicillin), skin infections: 500 mg PO on 1st day, then 250 mg PO daily to complete 5 days. Acute sinusitis, alternative for acute exacerbation of chronic bronchitis: 500 mg PO daily x 3 days. Chlamydia, chancroid: 1 g PO single dose. Gonorrhea: 2 g PO single dose. Observe patient for ≥30 minutes for poor GI tolerability. Prevention of disseminated Mycobacterium avium complex disease: 1200 mg PO q week. Zmax for acute sinusitis, community-acquired pneumonia: 2 g PO single dose taken on empty stomach.
PEDS - Oral for otitis media, community-acquired pneumonia: 10 mg/kg up to 500 mg PO on 1st day, then 5 mg/kg up to 250 mg PO daily to complete 5 days. Acute sinusitis: 10 mg/kg PO daily x 3 days. Short regimens for otitis media: 30 mg/kg PO single dose or 10 mg/kg PO daily x 3 days. Group A streptococcal pharyngitis (second-line to penicillin): 12 mg/kg up to 500 mg PO daily x 5 days. Take susp on empty stomach.
UNAPPROVED ADULT - See table for prophylaxis of bacterial endocarditis. Nongonococcal urethritis: 1 g PO single dose. See STD table for recurrent/persistent urethritis. Chlamydia in pregnancy: 1 g PO single dose. Campylobacter gastroenteritis: 500 mg PO daily x 3 days. Traveler's diarrhea: 500 mg PO on 1st day, then 250 mg PO daily to complete 5 days; or 1 g PO single dose. Mycobacterium avium complex disease treatment in AIDS: 500 mg PO daily (use ≥2 drugs for active infection). Pertussis treatment/ post-exposure prophylaxis: 500 mg PO on 1st day, then 250 mg PO daily to complete 5 days. Early primary/latent syphilis: 2 g PO single dose (CDC recommends only for penicillin-allergic non-pregnant patients; azithromycin treatment failures reported in US).
UNAPPROVED PEDS - Prevention of disseminated Mycobacterium avium complex disease: 20 mg/kg PO q week not to exceed adult dose. Mycobacterium avium complex disease treatment: 5 mg/kg PO daily (use ≥2 drugs for active infection). Cystic fibrosis & colonized with P aeruginosa (≥6 yo): 250 mg (<40 kg) or 500 mg (≥40 kg) PO three times weekly x 24 weeks. Chlamydia trachomatis (≥8 yo or <8 yo & ≥45 kg): 1 g PO single dose. Pertussis treatment/ post-exposure prophylaxis: Infants <6 mo, 10 mg/kg PO once daily x 5 days. Age ≥6 mo; 10 mg/kg (max 500 mg) PO single dose on day 1, then 5 mg/kg (max 250 mg) PO once daily on days 2–5. See table for bacterial endocarditis prophylaxis. Traveler's diarrhea: 5-10 mg/kg PO single dose. Cholera: 20 mg/kg up to 1 g PO single dose.
FORMS - Generic/Trade: Tab 250, 500, 600 mg, Susp 100 & 200/5 mL. Trade only: Packet 1000 mg. Z-Pak: #6, 250 mg tab. Tri-Pak: #3, 500 mg tab. Zmax extended release oral susp: 2 g in 60 mL single dose bottle.
NOTES - Severe allergic/skin reactions rarely, IV site reactions, hearing loss with prolonged use. Potential for QT interval prolongation and torsades cannot be excluded in patients at risk for prolonged cardiac repolarization. Does not inhibit cytochrome P450 enzymes. Do not take

at the same time as Al/Mg antacids (except Zmax which can be taken with antacids). Contraindicated with pimozide. Single dose and 3-day regimens cause more vomiting than 5-day regimen for otitis media. Mechanism of action in cystic fibrosis is unknown; macrolides may inhibit P aeruginosa virulence factors or reduce inflammation. Zmax: Store at room temperature and use within 12 hours of reconstitution. Additional treatment required for vomiting within 5 minutes of dose; consider for vomiting within 1 hour of dose; unnecessary for vomiting >1 hour after dose.

clarithromycin (Biaxin, Biaxin XL) ▶KL ♀C ▶? $$$

ADULT - Group A streptococcal pharyngitis (second-line to penicillin): 250 mg PO bid x 10 days. Acute sinusitis: 500 mg PO bid x 14 days. Acute exacerbation of chronic bronchitis (S pneumoniae/M catarrhalis), community-acquired pneumonia, skin infections: 250 mg PO bid x 7-14 days. Acute exacerbation of chronic bronchitis (H influenzae): 500 mg PO bid x 7-14 days. H pylori: See table in GI section. Mycobacterium avium complex disease prevention/ treatment: 500 mg PO bid. Two or more drugs are needed for the treatment of active mycobacterial infections. Biaxin XL: Acute sinusitis: 1000 mg PO daily x 14 days. Acute exacerbation of chronic bronchitis, community-acquired pneumonia: 1000 mg PO daily x 7 days. Take Biaxin XL with food.

PEDS - Group A streptococcal pharyngitis (second-line to penicillin), community-acquired pneumonia, sinusitis, otitis media, skin infections: 7.5 mg/kg PO bid x 10 days. Mycobacterium avium complex prevention/treatment: 7.5 mg/kg up to 500 mg PO bid. Two or more drugs are needed for the treatment of active mycobacterial infections.

UNAPPROVED ADULT - See table for prophylaxis of bacterial endocarditis. Pertussis treatment/ post-exposure prophylaxis: 500 mg PO bid x 7 days. Community-acquired pneumonia: 500 mg PO bid.

UNAPPROVED PEDS - See table for prophylaxis of bacterial endocarditis. Pertussis treatment/ post-exposure prophylaxis (≥1 mo): 7.5 mg/kg up to 500 mg PO bid x 7 days.

FORMS - Generic/Trade: Tab 250, 500 mg. Extended release 500 mg. Trade only: susp 125 & 250 mg/5 mL. Biaxin XL-Pak: #14, 500 mg tabs. Generic only: Extended release 1000 mg.

NOTES - Rare arrhythmias in patients with pro-longed QT. Cytochrome P450 3A4 & 1A2 inhibitor. Contraindicated with cisapride, pimozide. Many drug interactions including increased levels of carbamazepine, cyclosporine, digoxin, disopyramide, lovastatin, rifabutin, simvastatin (avoid), tacrolimus, theophylline. Toxicity with ergotamine, dihydroergotamine, or colchicine (esp. if elderly or renal dysfunction). Monitor INR with warfarin. Clarithromycin levels decreased by efavirenz (avoid concomitant use) and nevirapine enough to impair efficacy in Mycobacterium avium complex disease. AAP recommends 5-7 days of therapy for older (≥6 yo) children with non-severe otitis media, and 10 days for younger children and those with severe disease. Dosage reduction for renal insufficiency in patients taking ritonavir, lopinavir/ritonavir (Kaletra), or ritonavir-boosted tipranavir or darunavir: Decrease by 50% for CrCl 30-60 ml/min, decrease by 75% for CrCl <30 ml/min. Reduce clarithromycin dose by 50% if given with atazanavir; consider alternative for indications other than Mycobacterium avium complex. Do not refrigerate susp.

erythromycin base (Eryc, E-mycin, Ery-Tab, ✚Erybid, Erythromid, P.C.E.) ▶L ♀B ▶+ $

ADULT - Respiratory, skin infections: 250-500 mg PO qid or 333 mg PO tid. Pertussis, treatment/post-exposure prophylaxis: 500 mg PO q6h x 14 days. S aureus skin infections: 250 mg PO q6h or 500 mg PO q12h. Secondary prevention of rheumatic fever: 250 mg PO bid. Chlamydia in pregnancy, nongonococcal urethritis: 500 mg PO qid x 7 days. Alternative for chlamydia in pregnancy if high dose not tolerated: 250 mg PO qid x 14 days. Erythrasma: 250 mg PO tid x 21 days. Legionnaires' disease: 2 g/day in divided doses x 14-21 days.

PEDS - Usual dose: 30-50 mg/kg/day PO divided qid x 10 days. Can double dose for severe infections. Pertussis: 40-50 mg/kg/day PO divided qid x 14 days (azithromycin preferred for infants <1 mo due to risk of hypertrophic pyloric stenosis with erythro). Chlamydia, newborn - <45 kg: 50 mg/kg/day divided qid x 14 days.

UNAPPROVED ADULT - Chancroid: 500 mg PO tid x 7 days. Campylobacter gastroenteritis: 500 mg PO bid x 5 days.

FORMS - Generic/Trade: Tab 250, 333, 500 mg, delayed-release cap 250.

NOTES - Rare arrhythmias in patients with pro-longed QT. Incidence of sudden death may be increased when erythromycin is combined with potent CYP 3A4 inhibitors. May aggravate myasthenia gravis. Hypertrophic pyloric stenosis in infants primarily ≤2 weeks of age. Cytochrome P450 3A4 & 1A2 inhibitor. Many drug interactions including increased levels of carbamazepine, cyclosporine, digoxin, disopyramide, tacrolimus, theophylline, some benzodiazepines and statins (avoid simvastatin). Monitor INR with warfarin. Contraindicated with cisapride, pimozide.

erythromycin estolate ▶L ♀B ▶+ $

WARNING - Hepatotoxicity, primarily in adults.

ADULT - Other erythromycin forms preferred in adults.

PEDS - Usual dose: 30-50 mg/kg/day PO divided bid-qid. Can double for severe infections. Group A streptococcal pharyngitis: 20-40 mg/kg/day (up to 1 g/day) PO divided bid to qid x 10d. Secondary prevention of rheumatic fever: 250 mg PO bid. Pertussis: 40-50 mg/kg/day PO divided qid x 14 days.

FORMS - Generic: Susp 125 & 250 mg/5 mL.

NOTES - Contraindicated in liver disease. Rare arrhythmias in patients with prolonged QT. Incidence of sudden death may be increased when erythromycin is combined with potent CYP 3A4 inhibitors. May aggravate myasthenia gravis. Hypertrophic pyloric stenosis in infants primarily ≤2 weeks of age. Cytochrome 450 3A4 & 1A2 inhibitor. Many drug interactions including increased levels of carbamazepine, cyclosporine, digoxin, disopyramide, tacrolimus, theophylline, some benzodiazepines and statins. Monitor INR with warfarin. Contraindicated with cisapride, pimozide.

erythromycin ethyl succinate (*EES, Eryped*) ▶L ♀B ▶+ $

ADULT - Usual dose: 400 mg PO qid. Nongonococcal urethritis: 800 mg PO qid x 7 days. Chlamydia in pregnancy: 800 mg PO qid x 7 days or 400 mg PO qid x 14 days if high dose not tolerated. Secondary prevention of rheumatic fever: 400 mg PO bid. Legionnaires' disease: 3.2 g/day in divided doses x 14-21 days.

PEDS - Usual dose: 30-50 mg/kg/day PO divided qid. Max dose: 100 mg/kg/day. Group A streptococcal pharyngitis: 40 mg/kg/day (up to 1 g/day) PO divided bid to qid x 10 days. Secondary prevention of rheumatic fever: 400 mg PO bid. Pertussis: 40-50 mg/kg/day up to 2 g/day PO divided qid x 14 days.

FORMS - Generic/Trade: Tab 400 tab, susp 200 & 400 mg/5 mL. Trade only (EryPed): Susp 100 mg/2.5mL.

NOTES - Rare arrhythmias in patients with prolonged QT. Incidence of sudden death may be increased when erythromycin is combined with potent CYP 3A4 inhibitors. May aggravate myasthenia gravis. Hypertrophic pyloric stenosis in infants primarily ≤2 weeks of age. Cytochrome P450 3A4 & 1A2 inhibitor. Many drug interactions including increased levels of carbamazepine, cyclosporine, digoxin, disopyramide, tacrolimus, theophylline, some benzodiazepines and statins (avoid simvastatin). Monitor INR with warfarin. Contraindicated with cisapride, pimozide.

erythromycin lactobionate (✤*Erythrocin IV*) ▶L ♀B ▶+ $$$$

ADULT - For severe infections/PO not possible: 15-20 mg/kg/day (max 4g) IV divided q6h. Legionnaires' disease: 4 g/day IV divided q6h.

PEDS - For severe infections/PO not possible: 15-20 mg/kg/day (max 4g) IV divided q6h.

UNAPPROVED PEDS - 20-50 mg/kg/day IV divided q6h.

NOTES - Dilute and give slowly to minimize venous irritation. Reversible hearing loss (risk increased in elderly given ≥4 g/day), allergy, arrhythmias in patients with prolonged QT, exacerbation of myasthenia gravis. Incidence of sudden death may be increased when erythromycin is combined with potent CYP 3A4 inhibitors. Hypertrophic pyloric stenosis in infants primarily ≤2 weeks of age. CYP P450 3A4 & 1A2 inhibitor. Many drug interactions including increased levels of carbamazepine, cyclosporine, digoxin, disopyramide, tacrolimus, theophylline, some benzodiazepines & statins (avoid simvastatin). Monitor INR with warfarin. Contraindicated with cisapride, pimozide.

Pediazole (erythromycin ethyl succinate + sulfisoxazole) ▶KL ♀C ▶- $$

PEDS - Otitis media, age >2 mo: 50 mg/kg/day (based on EES dose) PO divided tid-qid.

FORMS - Generic/Trade: Susp, erythromycin ethyl succinate 200 mg + sulfisoxazole 600 mg/ 5 mL.

NOTES - Sulfisoxazole: Stevens-Johnson syndrome, toxic epidermal necrolysis, hepatotoxicity, blood dyscrasia, hemolysis in G6PD deficiency. Increased INR with warfarin. Erythromycin: Rare arrhythmias in patients with prolonged QT. Incidence of sudden death may be increased when erythromycin is combined with potent CYP 3A4 inhibitors. May aggravate myasthenia gravis. Cytochrome P450 3A4 & 1A2 inhibitor. Many drug interactions including increased levels of carbamazepine, cyclosporine, digoxin, disopyramide, tacrolimus, theophylline, some benzodiazepines/statins. Monitor INR with warfarin. Contraindicated with cisapride, pimozide. AAP recommends 5-7 days of therapy for older (≥6 yo) children with nonsevere otitis media, and 10 days for younger children and those with severe disease.

PENICILLINS - GENERAL ANTIMICROBIAL SPECTRUM

1st generation: Most streptococci; oral anaerobic coverage
2nd generation: Most streptococci; Staph aureus
3rd generation: Most streptococci; basic gram negative coverage
4th generation: Pseudomonas

ANTIMICROBIALS: Penicillins – 1st Generation (Natural)

NOTE: Anaphylaxis occurs rarely with penicillins; cross-sensitivity with cephalosporins is possible.

benzathine penicillin (Bicillin L-A, ✝Megacillin) ▶K ♀B ▶? $$

ADULT - Group A streptococcal pharyngitis: 1.2 million units IM single dose. Secondary prevention of rheumatic fever: 1.2 million units IM q month (q 3 weeks for high-risk patients) or 600,000 units IM q 2 weeks. Primary, secondary, early latent syphilis: 2.4 million units IM single dose. Tertiary, late latent syphilis: 2.4 million units IM q week x 3 doses.

PEDS - Group A streptococcal pharyngitis (AHA regimen): 600,000 units IM for ≤27 kg, 1.2 million units IM for >27 kg. Secondary prevention of rheumatic fever: 1.2 million units IM q month (q 3 weeks for high-risk patients) or 600,000 units IM q 2 weeks. Primary, secondary, early latent syphilis: 50,000 units/kg (up to 2.4 million units) IM single dose. Late latent syphilis: 50,000 units/kg (up to 2.4 million units) IM x 3 weekly doses.

UNAPPROVED ADULT - Prophylaxis of diphtheria/treatment of carriers: 1.2 million units IM single dose.

UNAPPROVED PEDS - Prophylaxis of diphtheria/treatment of carriers: 1.2 million units IM single dose for ≥30 kg or ≥6 yo. 600,000 units IM single dose for <30 kg or <6 yo.

FORMS - Trade only: for IM use, 600,000 units/mL; 1, 2 and 4 mL syringes.

NOTES - Do not give IV. Doses last 2-4 wks. Not for neurosyphilis.

benzylpenicilloyl polylysine (Pre-Pen) ▶K ♀? ▶? $

ADULT - Skin testing for penicillin allergy: 1 drop in needle scratch, then 0.01-0.02 mL intradermally if no reaction.

PEDS - Not approved in children.

NOTES - Systemic allergic reactions; do not test if known to be highly sensitive to penicillin. Pre-Pen has been temporarily unavailable but is expected to return. In unavailable, desensitization in a hospital is indicated for patients with a history of anaphylaxis, angioedema, bronchospasm, or urticaria with penicillin. Consider outpatient oral desensitization or monitored test doses if symptoms do not appear to be IgE mediated. See CDC 2006 STD guideline for penicillin allergy skin testing protocols.

Bicillin C-R (procaine penicillin + benzathine penicillin) ▶K ♀B ▶? $$$

ADULT - Scarlet fever, erysipelas, upper-respiratory, skin and soft-tissue infections due to Group A strep: 2.4 million units IM single dose. Pneumococcal infections other than meningitis: 1.2 million units IM q2-3 days until temperature normal x 48 h. Not for treatment of syphilis.

PEDS - Scarlet fever, erysipelas, upper-respiratory, skin & soft-tissue infections due to Group A strep: 2.4 million units IM for >27 kg, 900,000-1.2 million units IM for 13.6-27 kg, 600,000 units IM for <13.6 kg. Pneumococcal infections other than meningitis: 600,000 units IM q2-3 days until temperature normal x 48 h. Not for treatment of syphilis.

FORMS - Trade only: for IM use 300/300 thousand units procaine/benzathine penicillin; 1, 2, and 4 mL syringes.

NOTES - Contraindicated if allergic to procaine. Do not give IV. Do not substitute Bicillin CR for Bicillin LA in treatment of syphilis.

penicillin G ▶K ♀B ▶? $$$

ADULT - Penicillin-sensitive pneumococcal pneumonia: 8-12 million units/day IV divided q4-6h. Penicillin-sensitive pneumococcal meningitis: 24 million units/day IV divided q2-4h. Empiric therapy, native valve endocarditis: 20 million units/day IV continuous infusion or divided q4h plus nafcillin/oxacillin and gentamicin. Neurosyphilis: 18-24 million units/day continuous IV infusion or 3-4 million units IV q4h x 10-14 days. Bioterrorism anthrax: See idsociety.org/BT/ToC.htm.

PEDS - Mild to moderate infections: 25,000-50,000 units/kg/day IV divided q6h. Severe infections including pneumococcal and meningococcal meningitis: 250,000-400,000 units/kg/day IV divided q4-6h. Neonates <1 week, >2 kg: 25,000-50,000 units/kg IV q8h. Neonates ≥1 week, >2 kg: 25,000-50,000 units/kg IV q6h. Group B streptococcal meningitis: ≤7 days old, 250,000-450,000 units/kg/d IV divided q8h. >7 days old, 450,000-500,000 units/kg/day IV divided q4-6h. Congenital syphilis: 50,000 units/kg/dose IV q12h during first 7 days of life, then q8h thereafter to complete 10 days. Congenital syphilis or neurosyphilis in children >1 month old: 50,000 units/kg IV q4-6 h x 10 days.

UNAPPROVED ADULT - Prevention of perinatal group B streptococcal disease: Give to mother 5 million units IV at onset of labor/after membrane rupture, then 2.5 million units IV q4h until delivery. Diphtheria: 100,000-150,000 units/kg/day IV divided q6h x 14 days.

UNAPPROVED PEDS - Diphtheria: 100,000-150,000 units/kg/day IV divided q6h x 14 days.

NOTES - Decrease dose by 50% if CrCl <10 mL/min.

penicillin V (*Veetids*, ♥*PVF-K, Nadopen-V*) ▶K ♀B ▶? $

ADULT - Usual dose: 250-500 mg PO qid. AHA dosing for group A streptococcal pharyngitis: 500 mg PO bid or tid x 10 days. Secondary prevention of rheumatic fever: 250 mg PO bid. Vincent's infection: 250 mg PO q6-8h.

PEDS - Usual dose: 25-50 mg/kg/day PO divided tid or qid. Use adult dose for ≥12 yo. AHA dosing for group A streptococcal pharyngitis: 250 mg PO bid or tid x 10 days. Secondary prevention of rheumatic fever: 250 mg PO bid.

UNAPPROVED PEDS - Prevention of pneumococcal infections in functional/anatomic asplenia: 125 mg PO bid for <3 yo, 250 mg PO bid for ≥3 yo.

FORMS - Generic/Trade: Tabs 250,500 mg, oral soln 125 & 250 mg/5 mL.

NOTES - Oral soln stable in refrigerator x 14 d.

procaine penicillin (*Wycillin*) ▶K ♀B ▶? $$$$

ADULT - Pneumococcal & streptococcal infections, Vincent's infection, erysipeloid: 0.6-1.0 million units IM daily. Neurosyphilis: 2.4 million units IM daily plus probenecid 500 mg PO q6h, both x 10-14 days.

PEDS - Pneumococcal & streptococcal infections, Vincent's infection, erysipeloid, <27 kg: 300,000 units IM daily. AAP dose for mild-to-moderate infections, >1 mo: 25,000-50,000 units/kg/day IM divided daily-bid. Congenital syphilis: 50,000 units/kg IM daily x 10 days.

NOTES - Peak 4h, lasts 24h. Contraindicated if procaine allergy; skin test if allergy suspected. Transient CNS reactions with high doses.

ANTIMICROBIALS: Penicillins – 2nd Generation (Penicillinase-Resistant)

NOTE: Anaphylaxis occurs rarely with penicillins; cross-sensitivity with cephalosporins is possible.

cloxacillin ▶KL ♀B ▶? $$

ADULT - Staph infections: 250-500 mg PO qid on empty stomach. Severe infections: 1-2 g IV/IM q4h. Staph osteomyelitis: 2 g IV/IM q6h. IV/IM not available in US.

PEDS - Staph infections: 50-100 mg/kg/day PO divided q6h on empty stomach. Use adult dose for ≥20 kg.

FORMS - Generic: Caps 250,500 mg, oral soln 125 mg/5 mL. Parenteral not available in US.

NOTES - Oral soln stable in refrigerator x 14 d.

dicloxacillin (*Dynapen*) ▶KL ♀B ▶? $$

ADULT - Usual dose: 250-500 mg PO qid. Take on empty stomach.

PEDS - Mild to moderate upper respiratory, skin & soft-tissue infections, age >1 mo: 12.5 mg/kg/day PO divided qid. Pneumonia, disseminated infections, age >1 mo: 25 mg/kg/day PO divided qid. Follow-up therapy after IV antibiotics for Staph osteomyelitis: 50-100 mg/kg/day PO divided qid. Use adult dose for ≥40 kg. Give on empty stomach.

FORMS - Generic only: Caps 250,500 mg. Trade only: Susp 62.5 mg/5 mL.

NOTES - Oral susp stable at room temperature for 7d, in refrigerator 14d.

nafcillin ▶L ♀B ▶? $$$$$

ADULT - Staph infections, usual dose: 500 mg IM q4-6h or 500-2000 mg IV q4h. Osteomyelitis: 1-2 g IV q4h. Empiric therapy, native valve endocarditis: 2 g IV q4h plus penicillin/ampicillin and gentamicin.

PEDS - Staph infections, usual dose: Neonates, 10 mg/kg IM q12h. <40 kg, 25 mg/kg IM q12h.

UNAPPROVED PEDS - Mild to moderate infections: 50-100 mg/kg/day IM/IV divided q6h. Severe infections: 100-200 mg/kg/day IM/IV divided q4-6h. Neonates <1 week, >2 kg: 25 mg/kg IM/IV q8h. Neonates ≥1 week, >2 kg: 25-35 mg/kg IM/IV q6h.

NOTES - Reversible neutropenia with prolonged use. Decreased INR with warfarin. Decreased cyclosporine levels.

oxacillin (*Bactocill*) ▶KL ♀B ▶? $$$$$
ADULT - Staph infections: 250 mg-2g IM/IV q4-6h. Osteomyelitis: 1.5-2 g IV q4h. Empiric therapy, native valve endocarditis: 2 g IV q4h with penicillin/ampicillin and gentamicin.

PEDS - Mild to moderate infections: 100-150 mg/kg/day IM/IV divided q6h. Severe infections: 150-200 mg/kg/day IM/IV divided q4-6h. Use adult dose for ≥40 kg. AAP regimens for newborns >2 kg: <1 week, 25-50 mg/kg IM/IV q8h. ≥1 week, 25-50 mg/kg IM/IV q6h.

NOTES - Hepatic dysfunction possible with doses >12 g/day; monitor LFTs. Oral soln stable for 3 days at room temperature, 14 days refrigerated.

PROPHYLAXIS FOR BACTERIAL ENDOCARDITIS*

Limited to dental or respiratory tract procedures in patients at highest risk: prosthetic heart valve, prior infective endocarditis, valvulopathy after cardiac transplantation, or some types of congenital heart disease (unrepaired congenital cyanotic disease, repairs for the first 6 months, repairs with residual defect). All regimens are single doses administered 30-60 minutes prior to procedure.

Standard regimen	amoxicillin[1] 2 g PO
Unable to take oral meds	ampicillin[1] 2 g IV/IM; or cefazolin[1] or ceftriaxone[1] 1 g IM/IV
Allergic to penicillin	clindamycin[2] 600 mg PO; or cephalexin[1†] 2 g PO; or azithromycin[3] or clarithromycin[3] 500 mg PO
Allergic to penicillin and unable to take oral meds	clindamycin[2] 600 mg IV/IM; or cefazolin[1†] or ceftriaxone[1†] 1 g IV/IM

* Footnotes for pediatric doses: 1 = 50 mg/kg; 2 = 20 mg/kg; 3 = 15 mg/kg. Total pediatric dose should not exceed adult dose. For additional details of the 2007 AHA guidelines, see americanheart.org. Prophylaxis is no longer recommended for GU or GI tract procedures, and skin procedure prophylaxis is only recommended if the skin structure or musculoskeletal tissue is infected (use anti-staphylococcal penicillin or cephalosporin, or clindamycin or vancomycin if patient cannot tolerate beta-lactam or MRSA suspected).
†Avoid cephalosporins if prior penicillin-associated anaphylaxis, angioedema, or urticaria.

ANTIMICROBIALS: Penicillins – 3rd Generation (Aminopenicillins)

NOTE: Anaphylaxis occurs rarely with penicillins; cross-sensitivity with cephalosporins is possible.

amoxicillin (*Amoxil, DisperMox, Polymox, Trimox, ✦Novamoxin*) ▶K ♀B ▶+ $
ADULT - ENT, skin, GU infections: 250-500 mg PO tid or 500-875 mg PO bid. Pneumonia: 500 mg PO tid or 875 mg PO bid. H pylori: See table in GI section. See table for prophylaxis of bacterial endocarditis.

PEDS - ENT, skin, GU infections: 20-40 mg/kg/day PO divided tid or 25-45 mg/kg/day PO divided bid. See "unapproved" for AAP acute otitis media dosing. Pneumonia: 40 mg/kg/day PO divided tid or 45 mg/kg/day PO divided bid. Infants <3 mo: 30 mg/kg/day PO divided q12h. See table above for bacterial endocarditis.

UNAPPROVED ADULT - Acute sinusitis with antibiotic use in past month &/or drug-resistant S pneumoniae rate >30%: 3-3.5 g/day PO. High-dose for community-acquired pneumonia: 1 g PO tid. Lyme disease: 500 mg PO tid x 14 days for early disease, x 28 days for Lyme arthritis. Chlamydia in pregnancy: 500 mg PO tid x 7 days. Bioterrorism anthrax: See idsociety.org/BT/ToC.htm.

UNAPPROVED PEDS - Otitis media (AAP high-dose): 80-90 mg/kg/day PO divided bid-tid. Community-acquired pneumonia, 4 mo-4 yo: 80-100 mg/kg/day PO divided tid-qid. Lyme disease: 50 mg/kg/day (up to 1500 mg/day) PO divided tid x 14 days for early disease, x 28 days for Lyme arthritis. Bioterrorism anthrax: See www.idsociety.org/BT/ToC.htm.

FORMS - Generic/Trade: Caps 250,500 mg, tabs 500,875 mg, chews 125, 200,250,400mg, susp 125, 250 mg/5 mL, susp 200 & 400 mg/5 mL. Trade: Infant drops 50 mg/mL (Amoxil). DisperMox 200,400,600 mg tabs for oral susp.

NOTES - Rash with mononucleosis. AAP recommends 5-7 days of therapy for older (≥6 yo) children with non-severe otitis media, and 10 days for younger children and those with severe disease. Dosing in adults with renal dysfunction: Do not use 875 mg tab for CrCl <30 mL/min. Use 250-500 mg PO bid for CrCl 10-30 mL/min, 250-500 mg PO daily for CrCl <10 mL/min or hemodialysis. Give additional dose both during & at end of dialysis. Oral susp & infant drops stable for 14 days at room temperature or in the refrigerator. Mix DisperMox tab with 2 tsp water and drink mixture, then rinse container with a little water and drink that. Do not chew or swallow tab whole. Use only for doses that can be delivered by whole tabs.

amoxicillin-clavulanate (*Augmentin, Augmentin ES-600, Augmentin XR,* ✚*Clavulin*) ▶K ♀B ▶? $$$

ADULT - Pneumonia, otitis media, sinusitis, skin infections, UTIs: Usual dose - 500 mg PO bid or 250 mg PO tid. More severe infections: 875 mg PO bid or 500 mg PO tid. Augmentin XR: 2 tabs PO q12h with meals x 10 days for acute sinusitis, x 7-10 days for community-acquired pneumonia.

PEDS - 200,400 chewables & 200,400/5 mL susp for bid administration: Pneumonia, otitis media, sinusitis: 45 mg/kg/day PO divided bid. (See "unapproved" for AAP high-dose for otitis media.) Less severe infections such as skin, UTIs: 25 mg/kg/day PO divided bid. 125,250 chewables & 125,250/5 mL susp for tid administration: Pneumonia, otitis media, sinusitis: 40 mg/kg/day PO divided tid. Less severe infections such as skin, UTIs: 20 mg/kg/day PO divided tid. Age <3 months: Use 125 mg/5 mL susp and give 30 mg/kg PO q12 hr. Use adult dose for ≥40 kg. Augmentin ES-600 susp for ≥3 mo and <40 kg. Recurrent/ persistent otitis media with risk factors (antibiotics for otitis media in past 3 months and either age ≤2 yo or daycare): 90 mg/kg/day PO divided bid with food x 10 days.

UNAPPROVED ADULT - Prevention of infection after dog/cat bite: 875 mg PO bid or 500 mg PO tid x 3-5 days. Treatment of infected dog/cat bite: 875 mg PO bid or 500 mg PO tid, duration of treatment based on response.

UNAPPROVED PEDS - AAP otitis media, sinusitis: Augmentin ES-600 susp 90 mg/kg/day PO divided bid. Group A streptococcal pharyngitis, repeated culture-positive episodes: 45 mg/kg/day PO divided bid x 10 days.

FORMS - Generic/Trade: (amoxicillin + clavulanate) Tabs 250+125, 500+125, 875+125 mg, chewables and susp 200+28.5, 400+57 mg per tab or 5 mL, (ES) susp 600+42.9 mg/5mL Trade only: Chewables and susp 125+31.25, 250+62.5 mg per tab or 5 mL. Extended-release tabs (Augmentin XR) 1000+62.5 mg.

NOTES - Rash with mononucleosis; diarrhea common (less with bid dosing). AAP recommends 5-7 days of therapy for older (≥6 yo) children with non-severe otitis media, and 10 days for younger children and those with severe disease. Do not interchange Augmentin products with different clavulanate content. 250 mg tab contains too much clavulanate for children <40 kg. Suspensions stable in refrigerator x 10 days. See package insert for dosage reduction if CrCl <30 mL/min. Augmentin XR contraindicated if CrCl <30 mL/min.

ampicillin (*Principen,* ✚*Penbritin*) ▶K ♀B ▶? $ PO $$$$$ IV

ADULT - Usual dose: 1-2 g IV q4-6h or 250-500 mg PO qid. Sepsis, meningitis: 150-200 mg/kg/day IV divided q3-4h. Empiric therapy, native valve endocarditis: 12 g/day IV continuous infusion or divided q4h plus nafcillin/oxacillin and gentamicin. See table for prophylaxis of bacterial endocarditis. Take oral ampicillin on an empty stomach.

PEDS - AAP recommendations: Mild to moderate infections: 100-150 mg/kg/day IM/IV divided q6h or 50-100 mg/kg/day PO divided qid. Severe infections: 200-400 mg/kg/day IM/IV divided q6h. Infants >2 kg: 25-50 mg/kg IV q8h if <1 week old and q6h if ≥1 week old. Use adult doses for ≥40 kg. Give oral ampicillin on an empty stomach. Group B streptococcal meningitis: ≤1 week old, 200-300 mg/kg/day IV divided q8h. ≥1 week old, 300 mg/kg/day IV divided q4-6h. Give with gentamicin initially. See table for prophylaxis of bacterial endocarditis.

UNAPPROVED ADULT - Prevention of neonatal group B strep disease: Give to mother 2 g IV during labor, then 1-2 g IV q4-6h until delivery.

FORMS - Generic/Trade: Caps 250,500 mg, susp 125 & 250 mg/5 mL.

NOTES - Rash in patients with mononucleosis or taking allopurinol; pseudomembranous colitis. Susp stable for 7 days at room temperature, 14 days in the refrigerator. Reduce dosing interval to q12-24h for CrCl <10 mL/min. Give dose after hemodialysis.

ampicillin-sulbactam (*Unasyn*) ▶K ♀B ▶? $$$$$

ADULT - Skin, intra-abdominal, gynecologic infections: 1.5-3 g IM/IV q6h.

PEDS - Skin infections, ≥1 yo: <40 kg, 300 mg/kg/day IV divided q6h. ≥40 kg: adult dose.

UNAPPROVED ADULT - Community-acquired pneumonia. 1.5-3 g IM/IV q6h with a macrolide or doxycycline.

UNAPPROVED PEDS - AAP regimens. Mild to moderate infections: 100-150 mg/kg/day of ampicillin IM/IV divided q6h. Severe infections: 200-400 mg/kg/day IM/IV divided q6h.

NOTES - Rash with mononucleosis or allopurinol; pseudomembranous colitis. Dosing in renal impairment: Give usual dose q6-8h for adults with CrCl ≥30 mL/min, q12h for CrCl 15-29 mL/min, q24 h for CrCl 5-14 mL/min.

pivampicillin (*Pondocillin*) ▶K ♀? ▶? $

ADULT - Canada only. Respiratory tract, ENT, gynecologic, urinary tract infections: Usual dose is 500 mg PO bid; 1000 mg PO bid for severe infections. Treat pharyngitis x 10 d.

PEDS - Canada only. Not recommended for severe infections. Avoid in infants <3 mo. Susp, 3-12 mo: 40-60 mg/kg/day PO divided bid. Susp, ≤10 yo: 25-35 mg/kg/day up to 525 mg PO bid. 5 mL PO bid for 1-3 yo, 7.5 mL PO bid for 4-6 yo, 10 mL PO bid for 7-10 yo. Treat pharyngitis x 10 d.

FORMS - Trade only: Tabs 500 mg (377 mg ampicillin), # 20, oral susp 35 mg/mL (26 mg ampicillin), 100,150,200 mL bottles.

NOTES - Long-term therapy or repeated courses may increase carnitine excretion; avoid with valproate or in carnitine deficiency. Avoid with lymphocytic leukemia or infectious mononucleosis due to high risk of rash; allopurinol can also increase risk of rash. Pseudomembranous colitis. Susp stable for 7 days at room temperature, 14 days in the refrigerator. Reduce dose in severe renal dysfunction.

ANTIMICROBIALS: Penicillins – 4th Generation (Extended Spectrum)

NOTE: Anaphylaxis occurs rarely with penicillins; cross-sensitivity with cephalosporins is possible.

carbenicillin (*Geocillin*) ▶K ♀B ▶? $$$$$

ADULT - UTI: 382-764 mg PO qid. Prostatitis: 764 mg PO qid.

UNAPPROVED PEDS - 30-50 mg/kg/day PO divided q6h.

FORMS - Trade only: Tab 382 mg.

NOTES - Do not use if CrCl <10 mL/minute.

piperacillin ▶K/Bile ♀B ▶? $$$$$

ADULT - Simple UTI, community-acquired pneumonia: 6-8 g/day IM/IV divided q6-12h. Complicated UTI: 8-16 g/day IV divided q6-8h. Serious infections: 12-18 g/day IV divided q4-6h. Max dose: 24 g/day.

PEDS - Safety and efficacy not established in children <12 yo. Use adult dose for ≥12 yo.

UNAPPROVED ADULT - Empiric therapy of neutropenic fever: 3 g IV q4h or 4 g IV q6h with an aminoglycoside.

UNAPPROVED PEDS - Mild to moderate infections: 100-150 mg/kg/day IV divided q6h. Severe infections: 200-300 mg/kg/day IV divided q4-6h.

NOTES - Hypokalemia; bleeding & coagulation abnormalities possible especially with renal impairment. May prolong neuromuscular blockade with non-depolarizing muscle relaxants. May reduce renal excretion of methotrexate; monitor methotrexate levels and toxicity. Adult dosing with renal dysfunction: Serious infections: 4 g IV q8h for CrCl 20-40 mL/min, 4 g IV q12h for CrCl <20 mL/min. Complicated UTI: 3 g IV q8h for CrCl 20-40 mL/min, 3 g IV q12h for CrCl <20 mL/min. Simple UTI: 3 g IV q12h for CrCl <20 mL/min.

piperacillin-tazobactam (*Zosyn*, ♣*Tazocin*) ▶K ♀B ▶? $$$$$

ADULT - Appendicitis, peritonitis, skin infections, postpartum endometritis, pelvic inflammatory disease, moderate community-acquired pneumonia: 3.375 g IV q6h. Nosocomial pneumonia: 4.5 g IV q6h (with aminoglycoside initially and if P. aeruginosa is cultured).

PEDS - Appendicitis/peritonitis: 100 mg/kg of piperacillin IV q8h for ≥9 months old; 80 mg/kg q8h for 2-9 months old; adult dose if >40 kg.

UNAPPROVED ADULT - Serious infections: 4.5 g IV q6h.

UNAPPROVED PEDS - 300-400 mg/kg/day piperacillin IV divided q6-8h for >6 months old; 150-300 mg/kg/day IV divided q6-8h for <6 months old.

NOTES - Hypokalemia; bleeding & coagulation abnormalities possible especially with renal impairment. May prolong neuromuscular blockade with non-depolarizing muscle relaxants. False-positive result possible with Bio-Rad Laboratories Platelia Aspergillus EIA test. May reduce renal excretion of methotrexate; monitor methotrexate levels and toxicity. Dosing in renal impairment: 2.25 g IV q6h for CrCl 20-40 mL/min, 2.25 g IV q8h for CrCl <20 mL/min. Hemodialysis: Maximum dose of 2.25 g IV q8h plus 0.75 g after each dialysis.

ticarcillin (Ticar) ▶K ♀B ▶+ $$$$$
ADULT - Sepsis, pneumonia, skin & soft tissue, intra-abdominal, female GU infections: 3 g IV q4h or 4 g IV q6h. Simple UTI: 1 g IM/IV q6h. Complicated UTI: 3 g IV q6h.
PEDS - Sepsis, pneumonia, skin & soft tissue, intra-abdominal infections, <40 kg: 200-300 mg/kg/day IV divided q4-6h. Simple UTI, <40 kg: 50-100 mg/kg/day IM/IV divided q6-8h. Complicated UTI, <40 kg: 150-200 mg/kg/day IV divided q4-6h. Use adult dose for ≥40 kg. Severe infections, neonates ≥2 kg: <1 week, 75 mg/kg IV q8h. >1 week, 100 mg/kg IV q8h or 75 mg/kg IV q6h.
NOTES - Hypokalemia; bleeding & coagulation abnormalities possible especially with renal impairment. Not more than 2 g/IM injection site. Up to 6.5 mEq sodium/g ticarcillin. Adult dosing with renal dysfunction: 3 g IV load, then 2 g IV q4h for CrCl 30-60 mL/min, 2 g IV q8h for CrCl 10-30 mL/min, 2 g IV q12h or 1 g IM q6h for CrCl <10 mL/min. Liver dysfunction and CrCl <10 mL/min: 2 g IV q24h or 1 g IM q12h. Peri-

toneal dialysis: 3 g IV q12h. Hemodialysis: 2 g IV q12h and 3 g IV after each dialysis session.

ticarcillin-clavulanate (Timentin) ▶K ♀B ▶? $$$$$
ADULT - Systemic infections or UTIs: 3.1 g IV q4-6h. Gynecologic infections: Moderate, 200 mg/kg/day IV divided q6h. Severe, 300 mg/kg/day IV divided q4h. Adults <60 kg: 200-300 mg/kg/day (based on ticarcillin content) IV divided q4-6h. Use q4h dosing interval for Pseudomonas infections.
PEDS - Mild to moderate infections: ≥60 kg, 3.1 g IV q6h. Age ≥3 mo and <60 kg, 200 mg/kg/day (based on ticarcillin content) IV divided q6h. Severe infections: ≥60 kg, 3.1 g IV q4h. Age ≥3 mo and <60 kg, 300 mg/kg/day (based on ticarcillin content) IV divided q4h.
NOTES - Timentin 3.1 g = 3 g ticarcillin + 0.1 g clavulanate. Hypokalemia; bleeding & coagulation abnormalities possible especially in renal impairment. 4.75 mEq sodium/g Timentin. IV dosing in adults with renal dysfunction: Load with 3.1 g, then 2 g q4h for CrCl 30-60 mL/min, 2 g q8h for CrCl 10-30 mL/min, 2 g q12h for CrCl <10 mL/min, 2 g q24h for CrCl <10 mL/min and liver dysfunction. Peritoneal dialysis: 3.1 g q12h. Hemodialysis: 3.1 g load, then 2 g q12h and 3.1 g after each dialysis.

ANTIMICROBIALS: Quinolones – 1st Generation

NOTE: Important quinolone drug interactions with warfarin, antacids, iron, zinc, magnesium, sucralfate, cimetidine, caffeine, cyclosporine, hydantoins, theophylline, etc.

nalidixic acid (NegGram) ▶KL ♀C ▶? $$$$
ADULT - UTI: 1 g PO qid for 1-2 weeks, may reduce to 2 g/day thereafter.
PEDS - UTI, age ≥3 mo: 55 mg/kg/day PO divided qid, may reduce to 33 mg/kg/day thereafter. Use cautiously in children; arthropathy ob-

served in animal studies. Stop therapy if arthralgia develops.
FORMS - Trade only: Tabs 0.25, 0.5, 1 g.
NOTES - CNS toxicity; photosensitivity; hemolytic anemia in G6PD deficiency. Contraindicated if seizure history. Monitor CBC and LFTs if used for >2 weeks. Do not use with alkylating agents such as melphalan. Give at least 2 h before or after Al/Mg antacids, iron, sucralfate, calcium, zinc, buffered didanosine.

ANTIMICROBIALS: Quinolones – 2nd Generation

NOTE: As of April 2007, the CDC no longer recommends fluoroquinolones for gonorrhea because of high resistance rates. Fluoroquinolones can cause tendon rupture (rare; risk increased by corticosteroids, especially in elderly), phototoxicity (risk varies among agents), pseudomembranous colitis (risk may vary among agents), QT interval prolongation (risk varies among agents; see QT drugs table), exacerbation of myasthenia gravis, CNS toxicity, peripheral neuropathy (rare), and hypersensitivity. Important quinolone drug interactions with antacids, iron, zinc, magnesium, sucralfate, buffered didanosine, cimetidine, caffeine, cyclosporine, phenytoin, anticoagulants, theophylline, etc.

ciprofloxacin *(Cipro, Cipro XR, ProQuin XR)* ▶LK ♀C but teratogenicity unlikely ▶?+ $$$$

ADULT - UTI: 250-500 mg PO bid or 200-400 mg IV q12h. Simple UTI: 250 mg PO bid x 3 days or Cipro XR/Proquin XR 500 mg PO daily x 3 days. Give Proquin XR with main meal of day, preferably dinner. Cipro XR for complicated UTI, uncomplicated pyelonephritis: 1000 mg PO daily x 7-14 days. Pneumonia, skin, bone/joint infections: 400 mg IV q8-12h or 500-750 mg PO bid. Treat bone/joint infections x 4-6 weeks. Acute sinusitis: 500 mg PO bid x 10 days. Chronic bacterial prostatitis: 500 mg PO bid x 28 days. Infectious diarrhea: 500 mg PO bid x 5-7 days. Typhoid fever: 500 mg PO bid x 10 days. Nosocomial pneumonia: 400 mg IV q8h. Complicated intra-abdominal infection (with metronidazole): 400 mg IV q12 h, then 500 mg PO bid. Empiric therapy of febrile neutropenia: 400 mg IV q8h with piperacillin. Bioterrorism anthrax. Inhalation or severe cutaneous anthrax treatment: 400 mg IV q12h with ≥1 other drug initially, then monotherapy with 500 mg PO bid to complete 60 days. Monotherapy for post-exposure prophylaxis or treatment of less severe cutaneous anthrax: 500 mg PO bid x 60 days. See www.idsociety.org/BT/ToC.htm for more info.

PEDS - Safety and efficacy not established for most indications in children; arthropathy in juvenile animals. Still limited data, but case series of treated children show no evidence of arthropathy other than transient large-joint arthralgias. Musculoskeletal adverse events reported with ciprofloxacin treatment of complicated UTI in peds patients were mild to moderate in severity and resolved within 1 month after treatment. Complicated UTI, pyelonephritis, 1-17 yo: 6-10 mg/kg IV q8h, then 10-20 mg/kg PO q12h. Max dose is 400 mg IV or 750 mg PO even for peds patients >51 kg. Bioterrorism anthrax. Treatment of inhalation anthrax, severe cutaneous anthrax, or cutaneous anthrax in any case <2 yo: 10-15 mg/kg IV q12h with ≥1 other drug initially, then monotherapy with 10-15 mg/kg up to 500 mg PO bid to complete 60 days. Monotherapy for post-exposure prophylaxis or less severe cutaneous anthrax treatment: 10-15 mg/kg up to 500 mg PO bid x 60 days. See www.idsociety.org/BT/ToC.htm for more info.

UNAPPROVED ADULT - Acute uncomplicated pyelonephritis: 500 mg PO bid x 7 days. Chan-croid: 500 mg PO bid x 3 days. Prophylaxis, high-risk GU surgery: 500 mg PO or 400 mg IV. Prophylaxis, invasive meningococcal disease: 500 mg PO single dose. Traveler's diarrhea (treatment preferred over prophylaxis): Treatment - 500 mg PO bid x 1-3 days or 750 mg PO single dose. Prophylaxis - 500 mg PO daily x ≤3 weeks. Infectious diarrhea: 500 mg PO bid x 1-3 days for shigella, x 5-7 days for non-typhi salmonella (usually not treated). Malignant otitis externa: 400 mg IV or 750 mg PO q12h. TB (2nd-line treatment): 750-1500 mg/day IV/PO.

UNAPPROVED PEDS - Acute pulmonary exacerbation of cystic fibrosis: 10 mg/kg/dose IV q8h x 7 days, then 20 mg/kg/dose PO q12h to complete 10-21 days of treatment. TB (2nd-line treatment): 10-15 mg/kg PO bid (max: 1.5 g/day). Cholera, 2-15 yo: 20 mg/kg up to 750 mg PO single dose.

FORMS - Generic/Trade: Susp 250 & 500 mg/5 mL. Tabs 100, 250, 500, 750 mg. Extended release tabs 500 mg (Cipro XR & ProQuin XR), 1000 mg (Cipro XR only). Trade only: ProQuin XR blister pack 500 mg #3.

NOTES - Crystalluria if alkaline urine. Ciprofloxacin inhibits cytochrome P450 1A2, an enzyme that metabolizes caffeine, clozapine, tacrine, theophylline, and warfarin. Give ciprofloxacin immediate-release or Cipro XR 2 h before or 6 h after antacids, iron, sucralfate, calcium, zinc, buffered didanosine, or other highly buffered drugs (Proquin XR is 2h before or 4 h after these multivalent cations). Can give with meals containing dairy products, but not with yogurt, milk, or calcium-fortified fruit juice alone. Do not give Cipro XR within 2h of calcium doses >800 mg. Watch for hypoglycemia with glyburide. Do not give oral susp in feeding tube. Cipro XR, Proquin XR, and immediate-release tabs are not inter-changeable. Do not split, crush, or chew Cipro XR or Proquin XR. In patients with complicated UTI or acute pyelonephritis and CrCl <30 mL/min, reduce dose of Cipro XR to 500 mg daily. Dosing of immediate-release ciprofloxacin in adults with renal dysfunction: 250-500 mg PO q12h for CrCl 30-50 ml/min; 250-500 mg PO q18h or 200-400 mg IV q18-24h for CrCl 5-29 ml/min; 250-500 mg PO q24h given after dialysis session for hemodialysis/ peritoneal dialysis.

lomefloxacin *(Maxaquin)* ▶LK ♀C ▶? $$$
ADULT - Acute exacerbation of chronic bronchitis not due to S pneumoniae, simple UTI due to

K pneumoniae, P mirabilis, S saprophyticus: 400 mg PO daily x 10 days. Simple E coli UTI: 400 mg PO daily x 3 days. Complicated UTI: 400 mg PO daily x 14 days. Take in the evening to decrease risk of phototoxicity.

PEDS - Safety and efficacy not established in children; arthropathy in juvenile animals.

FORMS - Trade only: Tabs 400 mg.

NOTES - High risk of phototoxicity. Avoid sunlight during and for several days after treatment. Give Al/Mg antacids, sucralfate 4 h before or 2 h after lomefloxacin. Dosing in renal dysfunction: 400 mg PO load, then 200 mg PO daily for CrCl 11-39 mL/min or hemodialysis.

norfloxacin (Noroxin) ►LK ♀C ▶? $$$

ADULT - Simple UTI due to E coli, K pneumoniae, P mirabilis: 400 mg PO bid x 3 days. UTI due to other organisms: 400 mg PO bid x 7-10 days. Complicated UTI: 400 mg PO bid x 10-21 days. Acute/chronic prostatitis: 400 mg PO bid x 28 days. Take on an empty stomach.

PEDS - Safety and efficacy not established in children; arthropathy in juvenile animals.

UNAPPROVED ADULT - Traveler's diarrhea (treatment preferred over prophylaxis): Treatment - 400 mg PO bid x 1-3 days. Prophylaxis - 400 mg PO daily for up to 3 weeks. Infectious diarrhea: 400 mg PO bid x 5-7 days for non-typhi salmonella (usually not treated), x 1-3 days for shigella. Take on an empty stomach.

FORMS - Trade only: Tabs 400 mg.

NOTES - Crystalluria with high doses. Maintain adequate hydration. Norfloxacin inhibits cytochrome P450 1A2, an enzyme that metabolizes caffeine, clozapine, ropinirole, tacrine, theophylline, tizanidine, and warfarin. Increased

INR with warfarin. Do not take with dairy products. Give antacids, zinc, iron, sucralfate, multivitamins, or buffered didanosine 2 h before/after norfloxacin. Dosing for CrCl <30 mL/min: 400 mg PO daily.

ofloxacin (Floxin) ►LK ♀C ▶?+ $$$

ADULT - Acute exacerbation of chronic bronchitis, community-acquired pneumonia, skin infections: 400 mg PO bid x 10 days. Simple UTI due to E coli, K pneumoniae: 200 mg PO bid x 3 days. Simple UTI due to other organisms: 200 mg PO bid x 7 days. Complicated UTI: 200 mg PO bid x 10 days. Chronic bacterial prostatitis: 300 mg PO bid x 6 weeks.

PEDS - Safety and efficacy not established in children; arthropathy in juvenile animals.

UNAPPROVED ADULT - Epididymitis: 300 mg PO bid x 10 days. Traveler's diarrhea, treatment: 300 mg PO bid x 1-3 days. Infectious diarrhea: 300 mg PO bid x 1-3 days for shigella, 5-7 days for non-typhi salmonella (usually not treated). TB (2nd-line): 600-800 mg PO daily.

FORMS - Generic/Trade: Tabs 200,300,400 mg.

NOTES - May prolong QT interval; avoid using in proarrhythmic conditions or with drugs that prolong QT interval, including Class 1A and III antiarrhythmics. Give antacids, iron, sucralfate, multivitamins containing zinc, buffered didanosine 2h before or after ofloxacin. May decrease metabolism of theophylline, increase INR with warfarin. Monitor glucose with antidiabetic agents. Can cause false positive on opiate urine screening immunoassay; may need confirmation test. Dosing in renal dysfunction: Usual dose given q24h for CrCl 20-50 mL/min, 50% of usual dose q24h for CrCl <20 mL/min.

QUINOLONES- GENERAL ANTIMICROBIAL SPECTRUM

1st generation: gram negative (excluding Pseudomonas), urinary tract only, no atypicals. 2nd generation: gram negative (including Pseudomonas); Staph aureus but not pneumococcus; some atypicals. 3rd generation: gram negative (including Pseudomonas); gram positive (including Staph aureus and pneumococcus); expanded atypical coverage. 4th generation: same as 3rd generation plus enhanced coverage of pneumococcus, decreased activity vs. Pseudomonas.

ANTIMICROBIALS: Quinolones – 3rd Generation

NOTE: As of April 2007, the CDC no longer recommends fluoroquinolones for gonorrhea because of high resistance rates. Can cause tendon rupture (rare; risk increased by corticosteroids, especially in elderly), pseudomembranous colitis (risk may vary among agents), phototoxicity (risk varies among agents), CNS toxicity, peripheral neuropathy (rare), hypersensitivity, and QT interval prolongation (risk varies among agents). Avoid using in proarrhythmic conditions or with drugs that prolong QT including Class 1A and Class III antiarrhythmics. Important quinolone drug interactions with antacids, iron, zinc, magnesium, sucralfate, cimetidine, caffeine, cyclosporine, phenytoin, anticoagulants, theophylline, etc.

levofloxacin (Levaquin) ▶KL ♀C ▶? $$$$

ADULT - IV & PO doses are the same. 750 mg once daily x 5 days for community-acquired pneumonia or acute sinusitis, x 7-14 days for nosocomial pneumonia or complicated skin infections, 500 mg once daily x 7 days for acute exacerbation of chronic bronchitis, x 7-10 days for uncomplicated skin infections, x 7-14 days for community-acquired pneumonia, x 10-14 days for acute sinusitis, x 28 days for chronic bacterial prostatitis. 250 mg PO daily x 3 days for simple UTI, x 10 days for complicated UTI or acute pyelonephritis. Post-exposure anthrax prophylaxis: 500 mg PO once daily x 60 days. See www.idsociety.org/BT/ToC.htm for more info. Infuse IV doses over 60 minutes (250-500 mg) to 90 minutes (750 mg). Take oral sol'n on empty stomach.

PEDS - Safety and efficacy not established in children; arthropathy in juvenile animals.

UNAPPROVED ADULT - Legionnaires' disease: 1 g IV/PO on 1st day, then 500 mg IV/PO once daily. Chlamydia, epididymitis: See STD table. TB (2nd-line treatment): 500-1000 mg/day IV/PO. Traveler's diarrhea, treatment: 500 mg PO once daily x 1-3 days. Infectious diarrhea: 500 mg PO once daily x 1-3 days for shigella, x 5-7 days for salmonella.

FORMS - Trade only: Tabs 250,500,750 mg. Trade only: oral soln 25 mg/mL. Leva-Pak: #5, 750 mg tabs.

NOTES - Give Mg/Al antacids, iron, sucralfate, multivitamins containing zinc, buffered didanosine 2 h before/after PO levofloxacin. Increased INR with warfarin. Monitor glucose with antidiabetic agents. Can cause false positive on opiate urine screening immunoassay; may need confirmation test. Dosing in renal dysfunction: For most indications and CrCl <50 mL/min, load with 500 mg, then 250 mg daily for CrCl 20-49 mL/min, 250 mg q48h for CrCl 10-19 mL/min, hemodialysis, peritoneal dialysis. For complicated UTI/ pyelonephritis and CrCl 10-19 mL/min, give 250 mg q48h.

ANTIMICROBIALS: Quinolones – 4th Generation

NOTE: As of April 2007, the CDC no longer recommends fluoroquinolones for gonorrhea because of high resistance rates. Can cause tendon rupture (rare; risk increased by corticosteroids, especially in elderly), pseudomembranous colitis (risk may vary among agents), phototoxicity (risk varies among agents), CNS toxicity, peripheral neuropathy (rare), hypersensitivity, and QT interval prolongation (risk varies among agents; see QT drugs table). Avoid using in proarrhythmic conditions or with drugs that prolong QT interval, including Class 1A and Class III antiarrhythmics. Important quinolone drug interactions with antacids, iron, zinc, magnesium, sucralfate, cimetidine, caffeine, cyclosporine, phenytoin, anticoagulants, theophylline, etc. Monitor INR with warfarin.

gatifloxacin ▶K ♀C ▶- $$$

ADULT - IV & PO doses are the same. Community-acquired pneumonia: 400 mg daily x 7-14 days. Acute exacerbation of chronic bronchitis: 400 mg daily x 5 days. Complicated UTI, acute pyelonephritis, uncomplicated skin infections: 400 mg daily x 7-10 days. Acute sinusitis: 400 mg daily x 10 days. Simple UTI: 400 mg single dose or 200 mg daily x 3 days.

PEDS - Safety and efficacy not established in children; arthropathy in juvenile animals.

UNAPPROVED ADULT - IV & PO doses are the same. Acute uncomplicated pyelonephritis: 400 mg daily x 7 days. TB (2nd-line treatment): 400 mg IV/PO daily.

FORMS - Generic only: Tabs 200, 400 mg. Tequin brand left US market in June 2006; generics are expected.

NOTES - Do not exceed recommended IV dose or infusion rate due to QT prolongation risk. Contraindications: ziprasidone, diabetes. Can cause hyper- or hypoglycemia in non-diabetics. Monitor for hypo/ hyperglycemia if risk factors (renal dysfunction, old age, meds that alter glucose) and stop if either occurs. Give PO gatifloxacin 4 h before Al/Mg antacids, iron, multivitamins with zinc, buffered didanosine. May increase digoxin levels. Dosing for renal dysfunction in adults: 400 mg loading dose on day 1. On day 2, reduce dose to 200 mg PO daily for CrCl <40 mL/min, hemodialysis, continuous peritoneal dialysis. PO susp can be given through GI feeding tube.

gemifloxacin (Factive) ▶Feces, K ♀C ▶- $$$

ADULT - Acute exacerbation of chronic bronchitis: 320 mg PO daily x 5 days. Community-acquired pneumonia: 320 mg PO daily x 5-7 days (x 7 days for multi-drug resistant S pneumoniae).

PEDS - Safety and efficacy not established in children; arthropathy in juvenile animals.

FORMS - Trade only: Tabs 320 mg.

NOTES - Maintain fluid intake to prevent crystalluria. Give 2 h before or 3 h after Al/Mg antacids, iron, multivitamins with zinc, buffered didanosine. Give ≥2 h before sucralfate. May increase INR with warfarin. Discontinue if rash. Dosage reduction for CrCl ≤40 mL/min, hemodialysis, or CAPD: 160 mg PO daily.

moxifloxacin (Avelox) ▶LK ♀C ▶- $$$

ADULT - 400 mg PO/IV daily x 5 days (chronic bronchitis exacerbation), 5-14 days (complicated intra-abdominal infection; usually given IV initially), 7 days (uncomplicated skin infections), 10 days (acute sinusitis), 7-14 days (community acquired pneumonia, including penicillin-resistant S pneumoniae), 7-21 days (complicated skin infections). IV infused over 60 minutes.

PEDS - Safety and efficacy not established in children; arthropathy in juvenile animals.

UNAPPROVED ADULT - TB (2nd-line treatment): 400 mg IV/PO daily.

FORMS - Trade only: Tabs 400 mg.

NOTES - Do not exceed recommended IV dose or infusion rate due to QT prolongation risk. Contraindicated with ziprasidone. Give tabs ≥4 h before or 8 h after Mg/Al antacids, iron, multivitamins with zinc, sucralfate, buffered didanosine. Avoid in moderate or severe hepatic insufficiency.

ANTIMICROBIALS: Sulfonamides

NOTE: Sulfonamides can cause Stevens-Johnson syndrome; toxic epidermal necrolysis; hepatotoxicity; blood dyscrasias; hemolysis in G6PD deficiency. Avoid maternal sulfonamides when the breastfed infant is ill, stressed, premature, has hyperbilirubinemia, or has glucose-6-phosphate dehydrogenase deficiency.

sulfadiazine ▶K ♀C ▶+ $$$$

ADULT - Usual dose: 2-4 g PO initially, then 2-4 g/day divided into 3-6 doses. Secondary prevention of rheumatic fever: 1 g PO daily. Toxoplasmosis treatment: 1-1.5 g PO qid with pyrimethamine and leucovorin.

PEDS - Not for infants <2 mo, except as adjunct to pyrimethamine for congenital toxoplasmosis. Usual dose: Give 75 mg/kg PO initially, then 150 mg/kg/day up to 6 g/day divided in 4-6 doses. Secondary prevention of rheumatic fever, <27 kg: 500 mg PO daily. Use adult dose for >27 kg.

UNAPPROVED ADULT - CNS toxoplasmosis in AIDS. Acute therapy: Pyrimethamine 200 mg PO x 1, then 50 mg (<60 kg) to 75 mg (≥60 kg) PO once daily + sulfadiazine 1000 mg (<60 kg) to 1500 mg (≥60 kg) PO q6h + leucovorin 10-20 mg PO once daily (can increase to ≥50 mg). Secondary prevention: Pyrimethamine 25-50 mg PO once daily + sulfadiazine 500-1000 mg PO qid + leucovorin 10-25 mg PO once daily.

UNAPPROVED PEDS - Not for infants <2 mo, except as adjunct to pyrimethamine for congenital toxoplasmosis. AAP regimen for toxoplasmosis: 100-200 mg/kg/day PO with pyrimethamine and leucovorin (duration varies). Secondary prevention after CNS toxoplasmosis in HIV infection: 85-120 mg/kg/day PO divided in 2-4 doses with pyrimethamine and leucovorin.

FORMS - Generic only: Tab 500 mg.

NOTES - Not effective for streptococcal pharyngitis. Maintain fluid intake to prevent crystalluria & stone formation. Reduce dose in renal insufficiency. May increase INR with warfarin. May increase levels of methotrexate, phenytoin.

sulfisoxazole (Gantrisin Pediatric) ▶KL ♀C ▶+ $

PEDS - Usual dose: 75 mg/kg PO load, then 150 mg/kg/day PO divided q4-6h (max 6 g/day). Not for infants <2 mo, except as adjunct to pyrimethamine for congenital toxoplasmosis.

UNAPPROVED PEDS - Prophylaxis for recurrent otitis media: 50 mg/kg PO qhs.

FORMS - Trade only: susp 500 mg/5 mL. Generic only: Tabs 500 mg.

NOTES - May increase levels of methotrexate, phenytoin. Significantly increased INR with warfarin; avoid concomitant use if possible. Reduce dose in renal failure. Maintain fluid intake to prevent crystalluria/stone formation.

trimethoprim-sulfamethoxazole (Bactrim, Septra, Sulfatrim, cotrimoxazole) ▶K ♀C ▶+ $

ADULT - UTI, shigellosis, acute exacerbation of chronic bronchitis: 1 tab PO bid, double strength (DS, 160 TMP/800 SMX). Travelers' diarrhea: 1 DS tab PO bid x 5 days. Pneumocystis treatment: 15-20 mg/kg/day (based on

TMP) IV divided q6-8h or PO divided tid x 21 days total. Pneumocystis prophylaxis: 1 DS tab PO daily.

PEDS - UTI, shigellosis, otitis media: 5 mL susp/10 kg (up to 20 mL)/dose PO bid. Pneumocystis treatment: 15-20 mg/kg/day (based on TMP) IV divided q6-8h or 5 mL susp/8 kg/dose PO q6h. Pneumocystis prophylaxis: 150 mg/m²/day (based on TMP) PO divided bid on 3 consecutive days each week. Do not use in infants <2 mo; may cause kernicterus.

UNAPPROVED ADULT - Bacterial prostatitis: 1 DS tab PO bid x 10-14 days for acute, x 1-3 months for chronic. Sinusitis: 1 DS tab PO bid x 10 days. Burkholderia cepacia pulmonary infection in cystic fibrosis: 5 mg/kg (based on TMP) IV q6h. Pneumocystis prophylaxis: 1 SS tab PO daily. Primary prevention of toxoplasmosis in AIDS: 1 DS PO daily. Pertussis: 1 DS tab PO bid x 14 days (2nd line to macrolides). High-dose for community-acquired MRSA skin infections: 2 DS tabs PO bid-tid x 7-10 days.

UNAPPROVED PEDS - Head lice unresponsive to usual therapy: 10 mg/kg/day (based on TMP) PO divided bid x 10 days in combo with standard doses of permethrin 1%. Pertussis: 8 mg/kg/day (based on TMP) PO divided bid x 14 days (second-line to macrolides).

FORMS - Generic/Trade: Tabs 80 mg TMP/400 mg SMX (single strength), 160 mg TMP/800 mg SMX (double strength; DS), susp 40 mg TMP/200 mg SMX per 5 mL. 20 mL susp = 2 SS tabs = 1 DS tab.

NOTES - Not effective for streptococcal pharyngitis. No activity against penicillin-nonsusceptible pneumococci. Bone marrow depression with high IV doses. Significantly increased INR with warfarin; avoid concomitant use if possible. Increases levels of methotrexate, phenytoin. Rifampin reduces TMP/SMX levels. AAP recommends 5-7 days of therapy for older (≥6 yo) children with non-severe otitis media, and 10 days for younger children and those with severe disease. Dosing in renal dysfunction: Use 50% of usual dose for CrCl 15-30 mL/min. Don't use for CrCl <15 mL/min.

ANTIMICROBIALS: Tetracyclines

NOTE: Tetracyclines can cause photosensitivity and pseudotumor cerebri (avoid with isotretinoin which is also linked to pseudotumor cerebri). May decrease efficacy of oral contraceptives. Increased INR with warfarin. May increase risk of ergotism with ergot alkaloids.

demeclocycline (Declomycin) ▶K, feces ♀D ▶?+ $$$$$
ADULT - Usual dose: 150 mg PO qid or 300 mg PO bid on empty stomach.

PEDS - Avoid in children <8 yo due to teeth staining. Usual dose: 6.6-13.2 mg/kg/day PO divided bid-qid on empty stomach.

UNAPPROVED ADULT - SIADH: 600-1200 mg/day PO given in 3-4 divided doses.

FORMS - Generic/Trade : Tabs 150,300 mg.

NOTES - Diabetes insipidus, high risk of photosensitivity. Caution in renal dysfunction; doxycycline preferred. Absorption impaired by iron, calcium, Al/ Mg antacids. Take with fluids (not milk) to decrease esophageal irritation. SIADH onset of action occurs within 5-14 days; do not increase dose more frequently than q3-4 days. Increased INR with warfarin. May decrease oral contraceptive effectiveness.

doxycycline (Adoxa, Doryx, Monodox, Oracea, Periostat, Vibramycin, Vibra-Tabs, ✦Doxycin) ▶LK ♀D ▶?+ $
ADULT - Usual dose: 100 mg PO bid on first day, then 100 mg/day PO daily or divided bid. Severe infections: 100 mg PO bid. Chlamydia, nongonococcal urethritis: 100 mg PO bid x 7 days. Acne vulgaris: Up to 100 mg PO bid. Periostat for periodontitis: 20 mg PO bid 1 h before breakfast and dinner. Oracea for inflammatory rosacea (papules & pustules): 40 mg PO once every morning on empty stomach. Cholera: 300 mg PO single dose. Primary, secondary, early latent syphilis if penicillin-allergic: 100 mg PO bid x 14 days. Late latent or tertiary syphilis if penicillin allergic: 100 mg PO bid x 4 weeks. Not for neurosyphilis. Malaria prophylaxis: 100 mg PO daily starting 1-2d before exposure until 4 wks after. Intravenous: 200 mg on first day in 1-2 infusions, then 100-200 mg/day in 1-2 infusions. Bioterrorism anthrax: 100 mg bid x 60 days. Use IV with ≥1 other drug for initial treatment of inhalation or severe cutaneous anthrax. PO monotherapy for less severe cutaneous anthrax or post-exposure prophylaxis. See idsociety.org/BT/ToC.htm for more info.

PEDS - Avoid in children <8 yo due to teeth staining. Usual dose, children ≤45 kg: 4.4

mg/kg/day PO divided bid on first day, then 2.2-4.4 mg/kg/day PO divided daily or bid. Use adult dose for children >45 kg. Malaria prophylaxis: 2 mg/kg/day up to 100 mg PO daily starting 1-2 days before exposure until 4 weeks after. Most PO and IV doses are equivalent. Bioterrorism anthrax: 100 mg bid for >8 yo and >45 kg, 2.2 mg/kg bid for >8 yo and ≤45 kg, or ≤8 yo. Treat x 60 days. Use IV with ≥1 other drug for initial treatment of inhalation anthrax, severe cutaneous anthrax, or cutaneous anthrax in any case <2 yo. PO monotherapy for less severe cutaneous anthrax and post-exposure prophylaxis: idsociety.org/BT/ToC.htm for more info.

UNAPPROVED ADULT - See sexually-transmitted diseases table for granuloma inguinale, lymphogranuloma venereum, pelvic inflammatory disease treatment. Lyme disease: 100 mg PO bid x 14 days for early disease, x 28 days for Lyme arthritis. Prevention of Lyme disease in highly endemic area, with deer tick attachment ≥48h: 200 mg PO single dose with food within 72 h of tick bite. Ehrlichiosis: 100 mg IV/PO bid x 7-14 days. Malaria, co-therapy with quinine/quinidine: 100 mg IV/PO bid x 7 days. Lymphatic filariasis: 100 mg PO bid x 8 weeks.

UNAPPROVED PEDS - Avoid in children <8 yo due to teeth staining. Lyme disease: 4 mg/kg/day PO divided bid (max 200 mg/day) x 14 days for early disease, x 28 days for Lyme arthritis. Malaria, co-therapy with quinine/quinidine: 2.2 mg/kg IV/PO bid (max 100 mg bid) x 7 days.

FORMS - Generic/Trade: Tabs 75,100 mg, caps 20, 50,100 mg. Trade only: (Vibramycin) Susp 25 mg/5 mL (60 mL), Syrup 50 mg/5 mL (480 mL). Delayed Release (Doryx): Tabs 75,100 mg, Caps 40 mg (Oracea). Generic only: Caps 75,150 mg tabs 50,150 mg.

NOTES - Photosensitivity, pseudotumor cerebri, increased BUN, painful IV infusion. Do not use Oracea for treatment of infections. Do not give antacids or calcium supplements within 2 h of doxycycline. Barbiturates, carbamazepine, rifampin, and phenytoin may decrease doxycycline levels. Preferred over tetracycline in renal dysfunction. Take with fluids to decrease esophageal irritation; can take with food/milk. Can break Doryx tabs and give immediately in a spoonful of applesauce. Do not crush or chew delayed-release pellets in tab. Maternal antimalarial prophylaxis doesn't harm breast-fed infant or protect infant from malaria.

minocycline (Minocin, Dynacin, Solodyn, ♣Enca) ▶LK ♀D ▶?+ $$$

ADULT - Usual dose: 200 mg IV/PO 1st dose, then 100 mg q12h. IV and PO doses are the same. Not more than 400 mg/day IV. Solodyn for inflammatory non-nodular moderate to severe acne: 1 mg/kg PO once daily. Dose is 45 mg for 45-<60 kg, 90 mg for 60-90 kg, 135 mg for 91-136 kg.

PEDS - Avoid in children <8 yo due to teeth staining. Usual dose: 4 mg/kg PO 1st dose, then 2 mg/kg bid. IV and PO doses are the same. Solodyn for inflammatory non-nodular moderate to severe acne, ≥12yo: 1 mg/kg PO once daily. Dose is 45-<60 kg, 90 mg for 60-90 kg, 135 mg for 91-136 kg.

UNAPPROVED ADULT - Acne vulgaris (traditional dosing before Solodyn): 50 mg PO bid. Rheumatoid arthritis: 100 mg PO bid.

FORMS - Generic/Trade: Caps, tabs 50,75,100 mg. Trade only (Solodyn): Extended release tabs 45, 90, 145 mg.

NOTES - Dizziness, hepatotoxicity, lupus. Do not use Solodyn for treatment of infections. Do not give antacids or calcium supplements within 2h of minocycline. May cause drowsiness. Take with fluids (not milk) to decrease esophageal irritation. Use with caution in renal dysfunction; doxycycline preferred.

tetracycline (Sumycin) ▶LK ♀D ▶?+ $

ADULT - Usual dose: 250-500 mg PO qid on empty stomach. H pylori: See table in GI section. Primary, secondary, early latent syphilis if penicillin-allergic: 500 mg PO qid x 14 days. Late latent syphilis if penicillin allergic: 500 mg PO qid x 28 days.

PEDS - Avoid in children <8 yo due to teeth staining. Usual dose: 25-50 mg/kg/day PO divided bid-qid on empty stomach.

UNAPPROVED ADULT - Malaria, co-therapy with quinine: 250 mg PO qid x 7 days.

UNAPPROVED PEDS - Malaria, co-therapy with quinine: 25 mg/kg/day PO divided qid x 7 days.

FORMS - Generic/Trade: Caps 250,500 mg. Trade only: Tabs 250, 500 mg, susp 125 mg/5 mL.

NOTES - Increased BUN/hepatotoxicity in patients with renal dysfunction. Increased INR with warfarin. Do not give antacids or calcium supplements within 2 h of tetracycline. Use with caution in renal dysfunction; doxycycline preferred. Take with fluids (not milk) to decrease esophageal irritation.

ANTIMICROBIALS: Other

aztreonam (*Azactam*) ▶K ♀B ▶+ $$$$$
ADULT - UTI: 500 mg-1 g IM/IV q8-12h. Pneumonia, sepsis, skin, intra-abdominal, gynecologic infections: Moderate, 1-2 g IM/IV q8-12h. Severe or P aeruginosa infections, 2 g IV q6-8h. Use IV route for doses >1 g.
PEDS - Serious gram-negative infections, usual dose: 30 mg/kg/dose IV q6-8h.
UNAPPROVED ADULT - Meningitis: 2 g IV q6-8h.
UNAPPROVED PEDS - P aeruginosa pulmonary infection in cystic fibrosis: 50 mg/kg/dose IV q6-8h.
NOTES - Dosing in adults with renal dysfunction: 1-2 g IV load, then 50% of usual dose for CrCl 10-30 mL/min. 0.5-2 g IV load, then 25% of usual dose for CrCl <10 mL/min. For life-threatening infections, also give 12.5% of initial dose after each hemodialysis.

chloramphenicol (*Chloromycetin*) ▶LK ♀C ▶- $$$$$
WARNING - Serious & fatal blood dyscrasias. Dose-dependent bone marrow suppression common.
ADULT - Typhoid fever, rickettsial infections: 50 mg/kg/day IV divided q6h. Up to 75-100 mg/kg/day IV for serious infections untreatable with other agents.
PEDS - Severe infections including meningitis: 50-100 mg/kg/day IV divided q6h. AAP recommends 75-100 mg/kg/day for invasive pneumococcal infections only in patients with life-threatening beta-lactam allergy.
NOTES - Monitor CBC every 2 days. Monitor levels. Therapeutic peak: 10-20 mcg/mL. Trough: 5-10 mcg/mL. Use cautiously in acute intermittent porphyria/G6PD deficiency. Gray baby syndrome in preemies and newborns. Barbiturates, rifampin decrease chloramphenicol levels. Chloramphenicol increases barbiturate, phenytoin levels and may increase INR with warfarin. Dosing in adults with hepatic dysfunction: 1 g IV load, then 500 mg q6h.

clindamycin (*Cleocin*, ✙*Dalacin C*) ▶L ♀B ▶?+ $$$
WARNING - Pseudomembranous colitis.
ADULT - Serious anaerobic, Staph, streptococcal infections: 600-900 mg IV q8h or 150-450 mg PO qid. See tables for bacterial endocarditis and treatment of sexually transmitted diseases (pelvic inflammatory disease).
PEDS - Serious anaerobic, streptococcal, Staph infections: 20-40 mg/kg/day IV divided q6-8h or 8-20 mg/kg/day (as caps) PO divided tid-qid or 8-25 mg/kg/day (as palmitate oral soln) PO divided tid-qid. Do not give <37.5 mg of oral soln PO tid for ≤10 kg. Infants <1 mo: 15-20 mg/kg/day IV divided tid-qid. See table for prophylaxis of bacterial endocarditis.
UNAPPROVED ADULT - Bacterial vaginosis: 300 mg PO bid x 7 days. Oral/dental infection: 300 mg PO qid. Prevention of perinatal group B streptococcal disease: 900 mg IV to mother q8h until delivery. CNS toxoplasmosis, AIDS (with leucovorin, pyrimethamine): Acute treatment 600 mg PO/IV q6h; secondary prevention 300-450 mg PO q6-8h. Group A streptococcal pharyngitis, repeated culture-positive episodes: 600 mg/day PO in 2-4 divided doses x 10 days. Malaria, co-therapy with quinine/quinidine: 10 mg/kg base IV loading dose followed by 5 mg/kg IV q8h or 20 mg/kg/day base PO divided tid to complete 7 days.
UNAPPROVED PEDS - Group A streptococcal pharyngitis, repeated culture-positive episodes: 20-30 mg/kg/day PO divided q8h x 10 days. Otitis media: 30-40 mg/kg/day PO divided tid. Toxoplasmosis, substitute for sulfadiazine in sulfonamide-intolerant children: 5-7.5 mg/kg (up to 600 mg/dose) PO/IV qid + pyrimethamine + leucovorin. Malaria, co-therapy with quinine/quinidine: 10 mg/kg base IV loading dose followed by 5 mg/kg IV q8h or 20 mg/kg/day base PO divided tid to complete 7 days.
FORMS - Generic/Trade: Cap 75,150,300 mg. Trade only: Oral soln 75 mg/5 mL.
NOTES - Not for meningitis. Not more than 600 mg/IM injection site. Avoid if lincomycin hypersensitivity.

daptomycin (*Cubicin*, *Cidecin*) ▶K ♀B ▶? $$$$$
ADULT - Complicated skin infections: 4 mg/kg IV once daily x 7-14 days. S aureus bacteremia, including endocarditis: 6 mg/kg IV once daily x ≥2-6 weeks. Infuse over 30 minutes.
PEDS - Not approved in children.
NOTES - May cause myopathy; monitor CK weekly. Stop if myopathy symptoms and CK >5 x upper limit of normal, or no symptoms and CK ≥10 x upper limit of normal. Consider withholding statins during daptomycin treatment. May cause neuropathy. Can falsely elevate PT

with certain thromboplastin reagents; can minimize effect by drawing PT/INR sample just before daptomycin dose or use another reagent. Not effective for community-acquired pneumonia. Dosage reduction in adults with CrCl <30 mL/min: 4 mg/kg IV q48h. Reconstituted soln stable for up to 12 h at room temp or 48 h in refrigerator (combined time in vial + IV bag).

drotrecogin (*Xigris*) ▸Plasma ♀C ▸? $$$$$

ADULT - To reduce mortality in sepsis: 24 mcg/kg/h IV x 96 h. Reduced mortality only in patients with APACHE II score ≥25.

PEDS - Not approved in children, and was ineffective in a clinical trial of severe sepsis in children with a trend toward increased CNS bleeding.

NOTES - Can cause severe bleeding. Contraindicated with conditions and drugs that increase risk of bleeding; see package insert for details. Xigris may not be indicated in patients with single organ dysfunction and recent surgery; these patients do not have high enough risk of mortality to require treatment and Xigris increased mortality. Criteria for use include systemic inflammatory response plus acute organ dysfunction. Stop infusion 2 h before invasive procedure, or if bleeding occurs. May prolong APTT. Complete IV infusion within 12 h of reconstitution. Do not expose IV solution to heat or direct sunlight.

fosfomycin (*Monurol*) ▸K ♀B ▸? $$

ADULT - Simple UTI in women: One 3 g packet PO single dose. Dissolve granules in 1/2 cup of water.

PEDS - Not approved in children <12 yo.

FORMS - Trade only: 3 g packet of granules.

NOTES - Metoclopramide decreases urinary excretion of fosfomycin. No benefit with multiple dosing. Single dose less effective than ciprofloxacin or TMP/SMX; equivalent to nitrofurantoin.

lincomycin (*Lincocin*) ▸LK ♀C ▸- $$$$$

WARNING - Pseudomembranous colitis.

ADULT - Serious gram-positive infections: 600 mg IM q12-24h. 600-1000 mg IV q8-12h. Max IV daily dose is 8 g. Dilute to 1 g/100 mL or less, and infuse over at least 1 h. Reserve for patients who are allergic or do not respond to penicillins.

PEDS - Serious gram-positive infections, >1 mo: 10-20 mg/kg/day IV divided q8-12h. Dilute to 1 g/100 mL or less, and infuse over at least 1 h. Reserve for patients who are allergic or do not respond to penicillins.

NOTES - Do not use in patients with clindamycin hypersensitivity. Monitor hepatic and renal function and CBC during prolonged therapy. Do not coadminister with erythromycin due to potential antagonism. May enhance effects of neuromuscular blockers. Reduce dose by 25% to 30% in patients with severe renal dysfunction and consider monitoring levels.

linezolid (*Zyvox*, ✱*Zyvoxam*) ▸Oxidation/K ♀C ▸? $$$$$

ADULT - IV & PO doses are the same. Vancomycin-resistant E. faecium infections: 600 mg IV/PO q12h x 14-28 days. Pneumonia, complicated skin infections (including diabetic foot): 600 mg IV/PO q12h x 10-14 days. Uncomplicated skin infections: 400 mg PO q12h x 10-14 days. Infuse over 30-120 minutes.

PEDS - Pneumonia, complicated skin infections, ≤11 yo: 10 mg/kg IV/PO q8h x 10-14 days. Vancomycin-resistant E. faecium infections, ≤11 yo: 10 mg/kg IV/PO q8h x 14-28 days. Uncomplicated skin infections: 10 mg/kg PO q8h if <5 yo, q12h if 5-11 yo x 10-14 days.

FORMS - Trade only: Tabs 600 mg, susp 100 mg/5 mL.

NOTES – Myelosuppression; check CBC weekly, esp. if >2 weeks of therapy, pre-existing myelosuppression, other myelosuppressive drugs, or chronic infection treated with other antibiotics. Consider stopping if myelosuppression occurs or worsens. Peripheral and optic neuropathy, primarily in those treated for >1 month. Ophthalmic exam recommended for visual changes at any time; monitor visual function in all treated for ≥3 months. In a study comparing linezolid with vancomycin, oxacillin, or dicloxacillin for catheter-related bloodstream infections, mortality was increased in linezolid-treated patients infected only with gram-negative bacteria. Inhibits MAO; may interact with adrenergic and serotonergic drugs, high tyramine foods. Limit tyramine to <100 mg/ meal. Reduce initial dose of dopamine/epinephrine. Serotonin syndrome reported with concomitant administration of serotonergic drugs (SSRIs). Store susp at room temperature; stable for 21 days. Gently turn bottle over 3-5 times before giving a dose; do not shake.

metronidazole (*Flagyl*, ✱*Florazole ER*, *Trikacide*, *Nidazol*) ▸KL ♀B ▸?- $

ADULT - Trichomoniasis: Treat patient & sex partners with 2 g PO single dose (may be used in pregnancy per CDC), 250 mg PO tid x 7 days, or 375 mg PO bid x 7 days. Flagyl ER for bacterial vaginosis: 750 mg PO daily x 7 days on empty stomach. H pylori: See table in GI section. Anaerobic bacterial infections: Load 1 g or 15 mg/kg IV, then 500 mg or 7.5 mg/kg IV/PO q6-8h, each IV dose over 1h (not to exceed 4 g/day). Prophylaxis, colorectal surgery: 15 mg/kg IV completed 1 h preop, then 7.5 mg/kg IV q6h x 2 doses. Acute amebic dysentery: 750 mg PO tid x 5-10 days. Amebic liver abscess: 500-750 mg PO tid x 5-10 days.

PEDS - Amebiasis: 35-50 mg/kg/day PO (max of 750 mg/dose) divided tid x 10 days.

UNAPPROVED ADULT - Bacterial vaginosis: 500 mg PO bid x 7 days. Bacterial vaginosis in pregnancy: 500 mg PO bid or 250 mg PO tid x 7 days. Trichomoniasis (CDC alternative to single dose): 500 mg PO bid x 7 days. Pelvic inflammatory disease & recurrent/persistent urethritis: see STD table. Clostridium difficile diarrhea: 250 mg PO qid or 500 mg PO tid x 10 days. Giardia: 250 mg PO tid x 5-7 days.

UNAPPROVED PEDS - Clostridium difficile diarrhea: 30-50 mg/kg/day PO divided tid or qid x 7-10 days (not to exceed adult dose). Trichomoniasis: 5 mg/kg PO tid (max 2 g/day) x 7 days. Giardia: 15 mg/kg/day PO divided tid x 5-7 days. Anaerobic bacterial infections: 30 mg/kg/day IV/PO divided q6h, each IV dose over 1h (not to exceed 4 g/day).

FORMS - Generic/Trade: Tabs 250,500 mg, ER tabs 750 mg, Caps 375 mg.

NOTES - Peripheral neuropathy (chronic use), seizures. Disulfiram reaction; avoid alcohol until ≥1 day after tabs, ≥3 days with caps/ Flagyl ER. Do not give within 2 weeks of disulfiram. Interacts with barbiturates, lithium, phenytoin. Increased INR with warfarin. Darkens urine. Give iodoquinol/paromomycin after treatment for amebic dysentery or liver abscess. Can minimize infant exposure by withholding breastfeeding for 12-24 h after maternal single dose. Decrease dose in liver dysfunction.

nitrofurantoin (*Furadantin, Macrodantin, Macrobid*) ▶KL ♀B ▶+? $$

WARNING - Pulmonary fibrosis with prolonged use.

ADULT - Acute uncomplicated cystitis: 50-100 mg PO qid with food/milk x 7 days or x 3 days after sterile urine. Long-term suppressive therapy: 50-100 mg PO qhs. Sustained release Macrobid: 100 mg bid with food/milk x 7 days.

PEDS - UTI: 5-7 mg/kg/day divided qid x 7 days or x 3 days after sterile urine. Long-term suppressive therapy: Doses as low as 1 mg/kg/

day PO divided daily-bid. Give with food/milk. Macrobid, >12 yo: 100 mg PO bid with food/ milk x 7 days.

FORMS - Macrodantin: Caps 25,50,100 mg. Generic only: Caps 50,100 mg. Furadantin: Susp 25 mg/5 mL. Macrobid: Caps 100 mg.

NOTES - Contraindicated if CrCl <60 mL/min, pregnancy ≥38 weeks, infant <1 mo. Hemolytic anemia in G6PD deficiency (including susceptible infants exposed through breast milk), hepatotoxicity, peripheral neuropathy. May turn urine brown. Do not use for complicated UTI or pyelonephritis.

rifaximin (*Xifaxan*) ▶Feces, no GI absorption ♀C ▶? $$

ADULT - Travelers diarrhea: 200 mg PO tid x 3 days.

PEDS - Not approved in children <12 yo.

FORMS - Trade only: Tab 200 mg.

NOTES - Not effective for diarrhea complicated by fever/blood in stool or caused by pathogens other than E coli. Consider switching to another agent if diarrhea persists (24-48h) or worsens.

Synercid (quinupristin + dalfopristin) ▶Bile ♀B ▶? $$$$$

ADULT - Vancomycin-resistant E faecium infections (Not active against E. faecalis): 7.5 mg/kg IV q8h. Complicated staphylococcal/streptococcal skin infections: 7.5 mg/kg IV q12h. Infuse over 1 h.

PEDS - Safety and efficacy not established.

UNAPPROVED PEDS - Vancomycin-resistant E faecium infections (Not active against E. faecalis): 7.5 mg/kg IV q8h. Complicated staphylococcal/streptococcal skin infections: 7.5 mg/kg IV q12h. Infuse over 1 h.

NOTES - Venous irritation (flush with D5W after peripheral infusion; do not use normal saline/heparin), arthralgias/myalgias, hyperbilirubinemia. Cytochrome P450 3A4 inhibitor. Increases levels of cyclosporine, midazolam, nifedipine, and others.

telithromycin (*Ketek*) ▶LK ♀C ▶? $$$

WARNING - Contraindicated in myasthenia gravis due to reports of exacerbation, including fatal acute respiratory depression. Warn patients about exacerbation of myasthenia gravis, hepatotoxicity, visual disturbances, and loss of consciousness.

ADULT - Community-acquired pneumonia: 800 mg PO daily x 7-10 days. Indications for acute sinusitis & acute exacerbation of chronic bronchitis removed from labeling in Jan 07 because potential benefit no longer justifies risk of adverse effects.

PEDS - Safety and efficacy not established.

FORMS - Trade only: 300,400 mg tabs. Ketek Pak: #10, 400 mg tabs.

NOTES - May prolong QT interval. Avoid in proarrhythmic conditions or with drugs that prolong QT interval. Life-threatening hepatotoxicity. Monitor for signs/sx of hepatitis. Contraindicated if history of hepatitis due to any macrolide or telithromycin. Contraindicated in myasthenia gravis. Cytochrome P450 3A4 substrate and inhibitor. Contraindicated with cisapride, pimozide, rifampin, ergot alkaloids. Withhold simvastatin, lovastatin, or atorvastatin during course of telithromycin. Consider monitoring INR with warfarin. Give telithromycin and theophylline at least 1 h apart. Monitor for increased toxicity of digoxin, midazolam, metoprolol. CYP P450 3A4 inducers (ie phenytoin, carbamazepine) could reduce telithromycin levels. Dosage adjustment for CrCl <30 mL/min (including hemodialysis) is 600 mg once daily. On dialysis days, give after hemodialysis session. Dosage adjustment for CrCl <30 mL/min with hepatic dysfunction is 400 mg once daily.

tigecycline (Tygacil) ▶Bile, K ♀D ▶?+ $$$$$

ADULT - Complicated skin or intra-abdominal infections: 100 mg IV first dose, then 50 mg IV q12h. Infuse over 30-60 minutes.

PEDS - Not approved in children. Avoid in children <8 yo due to teeth staining.

NOTES - May decrease oral contraceptive efficacy. Monitor INR with warfarin. Dose adjustment for severe liver dysfunction (Child Pugh C): 100 mg IV first dose, then 25 mg IV q12h.

trimethoprim (Primsol, ✷Proloprim) ▶K ♀C ▶- $

ADULT - Uncomplicated UTI: 100 mg PO bid or 200 mg PO daily.

PEDS - Safety not established in infants <2 mo; Otitis media, age ≥6 mo (not for M catarrhalis): 10 mg/kg/day PO divided bid x 10 days.

UNAPPROVED ADULT - Prophylaxis of recurrent UTI: 100 mg PO qhs. Pneumocystis treatment: 5 mg/kg PO tid with dapsone 100 mg PO daily x 21 days.

FORMS - Generic only: Tabs 100, 200 mg. Primsol: Oral soln 50 mg/5 mL.

NOTES - Contraindicated in megaloblastic anemia due to folate deficiency. Blood dyscrasias. Trimethoprim alone not first-line for otitis media. Inhibits metabolism of phenytoin and procainamide. Dosing in adults with renal dysfunction: 50 mg PO q12h for CrCl 15-30 mL/min. Do not use if CrCl <15 mL/min.

vancomycin (Vancocin) ▶K ♀C ▶? $$$$$

ADULT - Severe Staph infections, endocarditis: 1g IV q12h, each dose over 1h or 30 mg/kg/day IV divided q12h. Empiric therapy, native valve endocarditis: 15 mg/kg (max 2 g/day unless levels monitored) IV q12h with gentamicin. Clostridium difficile diarrhea: 500-2000 mg/day PO divided tid to qid x 7-10 days. IV administration ineffective for this indication. See table for prophylaxis of bacterial endocarditis.

PEDS - Severe Staph infections, endocarditis: 10 mg/kg IV q6h. Infants <1 week old: 15 mg/kg IV load, then 10 mg/kg q12h. Infants 1 week - 1 mo: 15 mg/kg IV load, then 10 mg/kg q8h. Clostridium difficile diarrhea: 40-50 mg/kg/day up to 500 mg/day PO divided qid x 7-10 days. IV administration ineffective for this indication.

UNAPPROVED ADULT - Clostridium difficile diarrhea: 125 mg PO qid x 7-10 days.

UNAPPROVED PEDS - AAP dosing for infants: 10-15 mg/kg IV q8-12h for infants <1 week. 10-15 mg/kg IV q6-8h for infants ≥1 week. Bacterial meningitis: 60 mg/kg/day IV divided q6h. Nonmeningeal pneumococcal infections: 40-45 mg/kg/day IV divided q6h.

FORMS - Trade only: Caps 125,250 mg

NOTES - "Red Neck" (or "Red Man") syndrome with rapid IV administration, vein irritation with IV extravasation, reversible neutropenia, rare ototoxicity or nephrotoxicity. Enhanced effects of neuromuscular blockers. Use caution with other ototoxic/nephrotoxic drugs. Role of levels is controversial, but one approach is peak 30-40 mcg/mL 1.5-2.5 hours after 1-hour infusion, trough 5-20 mcg/mL. Individualize dose if renal dysfunction. Oral vancomycin poorly absorbed; do not use for extraluminal infections.

CARDIOVASCULAR: ACE Inhibitors

NOTE: See also antihypertensive combinations. Hyperkalemia possible, especially if used concomitantly with other drugs that increase K+ (including K+ containing salt substitutes) and in patients with heart failure, diabetes mellitus, or renal impairment. Monitor closely for hypoglycemia during first month of treatment when combined with insulin or oral antidiabetic agents. An increase in serum creatinine up to 35% above baseline is acceptable and is not reason to withhold therapy unless hyperkalemia occurs. ACE inhibitors are contraindicated during pregnancy. Contraindicated with a history of angioedema. Consider intestinal angioedema if abdominal pain (with or without N/V). African Americans and smokers may be at higher risk for angioedema. Swelling of tongue, glottis, or larynx may result in airway obstruction, especially with history of airway surgery. Rarely associated with syndrome starting with cholestatic jaundice or hepatitis progressing to fulminant hepatic necrosis and sometimes death. Increases risk of hypotension with volume depleted or hyponatremic patients. African Americans may need higher dose to achieve adequate response. Renoprotection and decreased cardiovascular morbidity/mortality seen with some ACE inhibitors are most likely a class effect.

benazepril (*Lotensin*) ▶LK ♀- ▶? $$

ADULT - HTN: Start 10 mg PO daily, usual maintenance dose 20-40 mg PO daily or divided bid, max 80 mg/day, but added effect not apparent above 40 mg/day. Elderly, renal impairment, or concomitant diuretic therapy: Start 5 mg PO daily.

PEDS - HTN: Start 0.2 mg/kg/day (max 10 mg/day) as monotherapy; doses >0.6 mg/kg/day (or >40 mg/day) have not been studied. Do not use if age <6 years or if glomerular filtration rate <30 mL/min.

UNAPPROVED ADULT - Renoprotective dosing: 10 mg PO daily. Heart failure: Start 5 mg PO daily, usual 5-20 mg/day, max 40 mg/day (in 1-2 doses).

FORMS - Generic/Trade: Tabs, non-scored 5, 10,20,40 mg.

NOTES - BID dosing may be required for 24-hour BP control.

captopril (*Capoten*) ▶LK ♀- ▶+ $

ADULT - HTN: Start 25 mg PO bid-tid, usual maintenance dose 25-150 mg PO bid-tid, max 450 mg/day. Elderly, renal impairment, or concomitant diuretic therapy: Start 6.25-12.5 mg PO bid-tid. Heart failure: Start 6.25-12.5 mg PO tid, usual 50-100 mg PO tid, max 450 mg/day. Diabetic nephropathy: 25 mg PO tid.

PEDS - Not approved in children.

UNAPPROVED ADULT - Hypertensive urgency: 12.5-25 mg PO, repeated once or twice if necessary at intervals of ≥30-60 minutes.

UNAPPROVED PEDS - Neonates: 0.1-0.4 mg/kg/day PO divided q6-8h. Infants: initial dose

0.15-0.3 mg/kg/dose, titrate to effective dose, max dose 6 mg/kg/day divided daily-qid. Children: initial dose 0.3-0.5 mg/kg/dose PO q8h, titrate to effective dose, max dose 6 mg/kg/day (not to exceed 450 mg/day) divided bid-qid.

FORMS - Generic/Trade: Tabs, scored 12.5,25, 50,100 mg.

NOTES - A captopril solution or suspension (1 mg/mL) can be made by dissolving Tabs in distilled water or flavored syrup. The solution is stable for 7days at room temperature.

cilazapril (✦*Inhibace*) ▶LK ♀- ▶? $

ADULT - Canada only. HTN: Initial dose 2.5 mg PO daily, usual maintenance dose 2.5-5 mg daily, max 10 mg daily. Elderly or concomitant diuretic therapy: initiate 1.25 mg PO daily. Heart failure adjunct: Initially 0.5 mg PO daily, increase to usual maintenance of 1-2.5 mg daily. Renal Impairment with CrCl 10-40 mL/min, initiate 0.5 mg daily, max 2.5mg/day. CrCl <10 mL/min 0.25-0.5 mg once or twice per week, adjust dose according to BP response.

PEDS - Not approved in children.

FORMS - Generic/Trade: Scored tabs 1, 2.5, 5 mg.

NOTES - Reduce dose in hepatic / renal impairment

enalapril (*enalaprilat, Vasotec*) ▶LK ♀- ▶+ $$

ADULT - HTN: Start 5 mg PO daily, usual maintenance dose 10-40 mg PO daily or divided bid, max 40 mg/day. If oral therapy not possible, can use enalaprilat 1.25 mg IV q6h over 5 minutes, and increase up to 5 mg IV q6h if needed. Renal impairment or concomitant diuretic therapy: Start 2.5 mg PO daily. Heart failure: Start 2.5 mg PO bid, usual 10-20 mg PO bid, max 40 mg/day.

PEDS - Not approved in children.

UNAPPROVED ADULT - Hypertensive crisis: enalaprilat 1.25-5 mg IV q6h. Renoprotective dosing: 10-20 mg PO daily.

UNAPPROVED PEDS - HTN: Start 0.1 mg/kg/day PO daily or divided bid, titrate to effective dose, maximum dose 0.5 mg/kg/day; 0.005-0.01 mg/kg/dose IV q8-24 hours.

FORMS - Generic/Trade: Tabs, scored 2.5,5 mg, non-scored 10, 20 mg.

NOTES - BID dosing may be required for 24-hour BP control. An enalapril oral suspension (0.2 mg/mL) can be made by dissolving one 2.5 mg tab in 12.5 mL sterile water, use immediately. Enalaprilat is the active metabolite of enalapril.

HYPERTENSION THERAPY[1]

Area of concern	BP target	Preferred Therapy[2]	Comments
General coronary artery disease prevention	<140/90 mm Hg	ACEI, ARB, CCB, thiazide, or combination	Start 2 drugs if systolic BP ≥160 or diastolic BP ≥100
High coronary artery disease risk[3]	<130/80 mm Hg		
Stable angina, unstable angina, MI	<130/80 mm Hg	β-blocker[4] + (ACEI or ARB)[5]	May add dihydropyridine CCB or thiazide
Left heart failure[6, 7]	<120/80 mm Hg	β-blocker + (ACEI or ARB) + diuretic[8] + aldosterone antagonist[9]	

1. ACEI = angiotensin converting enzyme inhibitor; ARB = angiotensin-receptor blocker; CCB = calcium-channel blocker; MI = myocardial infarction. Adapted from Circulation 2007;115:2761-2788. **2**. All patients should attempt lifestyle modifications: optimize weight, healthy diet, sodium restriction, exercise, smoking cessation, alcohol moderation. **3**. Diabetes mellitus, chronic kidney disease, known coronary artery disease or risk equivalent (eg, peripheral artery disease, abdominal aortic aneurysm), 10-year Framingham risk score ≥10%. **4**. Use only if hemodynamically stable. If β-blocker contraindications or intolerable side effects (and no bradycardia or heart failure), may substitute verapamil or diltiazem. **5**. Preferred if anterior wall MI, persistent HTN, heart failure, or diabetes mellitus. **6**. Avoid verapamil, diltiazem, clonidine, α-blockers. **7**. For Blacks with New York Heart Association class III or IV HF, consider adding hydralazine/isosorbide dinitrate. **8**. Loop or thiazide. **9**. Use if New York Heart Association class III or IV, or if clinical heart failure + LV ejection fraction < 40%.

ACE INHIBITOR DOSING

ACE INHIBITOR DOSING	Hypertension		Heart Failure		
	Initial	Max/day	Initial	Target	Max
benazepril (*Lotensin*)	10 mg qd*	80 mg	-	-	-
captopril (*Capoten*)	25 mg bid/tid	450 mg	6.25-12.5 mg tid	50 mg tid	150 mg tid
enalapril (*Vasotec*)	5 mg qd*	40 mg	2.5 mg bid	10 mg bid	20 mg bid
fosinopril (*Monopril*)	10 mg qd*	80 mg	10 mg qd	20 mg qd	40 mg qd
lisinopril (*Zestril/Prinivil*)	10 mg qd	80 mg	5 mg qd	20 mg qd	40 mg qd
moexipril (*Univasc*)	7.5 mg qd*	30 mg	-	-	-
perindopril (*Aceon*)	4 mg qd*	16 mg	-	-	-
quinapril (*Accupril*)	10-20 mg qd*	80 mg	5 mg bid	10 mg bid	20 mg bid
ramipril (*Altace*)	2.5 mg qd*	20 mg	2.5 mg bid	5 mg bid	10 mg bid
trandolapril (*Mavik*)	1-2 mg qd*	8 mg	1 mg qd	4 mg qd	4 mg qd

Data taken from prescribing information.   *May require bid dosing for 24-hour BP control.

fosinopril (*Monopril*) ▶LK ♀- ▶? $$
ADULT - HTN: Start 10 mg PO daily, usual maintenance dose 20-40 mg PO daily or divided bid, max 80 mg/day, but added effect not apparent above 40 mg/day. Elderly, renal impairment, or concomitant diuretic therapy: Start 5 mg PO daily. Heart failure: Start 5-10 mg PO daily, usual 20-40 mg daily, max 40 mg/day.
PEDS - HTN: 6-16 years & weight >50 kg: 5-10 mg PO daily.
UNAPPROVED ADULT - Renoprotective dosing: 10-20 mg PO daily.
FORMS - Generic/Trade: Tabs, scored 10, non-scored 20,40 mg.
NOTES - Elimination 50% renal, 50% hepatic. Accumulation of drug negligible with impaired renal function.

lisinopril (*Prinivil, Zestril*) ▶K ♀- ▶? $
ADULT - HTN: Start 10 mg PO daily, usual maintenance dose 20-40 mg PO daily, max 80 mg/day, but added effect not apparent above 40 mg/day. Renal impairment or concomitant diuretic therapy: Start 2.5-5 mg PO daily. Heart failure, acute MI: start 2.5-5 mg PO daily, usual 5-20 mg PO daily, max 40 mg/day.
PEDS - HTN ≥6 yo: 0.07 mg/kg PO daily; 5 mg/day max. Not recommended <6 yo or with glomerular filtration rate <30 mL/min/1.73 meters squared.
UNAPPROVED ADULT - Renoprotective dosing: 10-20 mg PO daily.
FORMS - Generic/Trade: Tabs, non-scored 2.5, 10, 20, 30, 40, scored 5 mg.

moexipril (*Univasc*) ▶LK ♀- ▶? $$

ADULT - HTN: Start 7.5 mg PO daily, usual maintenance dose 7.5-30 mg PO daily or divided bid, max 30 mg/day. Renal impairment or concomitant diuretic therapy: Start 3.75 mg PO daily; max 15 mg/day with renal impairment.
PEDS - Not approved in children.
FORMS - Generic/Trade: Tabs, scored 7.5, 15 mg.
NOTES - BID dosing may be required for 24-hour BP control.

perindopril (*Aceon*, ✚*Coversyl*) ▶K♀-▶? $$
ADULT - HTN: Start 4 mg PO daily, usual maintenance dose 4-8 mg PO daily or divided bid, max 16 mg/day. Renal impairment or concomitant diuretic therapy: Start 2 mg PO daily or divided bid. Reduction of cardiovascular events in stable coronary artery disease: Start 4 mg PO daily x 2 weeks, max 8 mg/day. Elderly (>70 years): 2 mg PO daily x 1 week, 4 mg PO daily x 1 week, max 8 mg/day.
PEDS - Not approved in children.
UNAPPROVED ADULT - Heart failure: Start 2 mg PO daily, usual dose 4 mg daily, max dose 8 mg daily. Recurrent stroke prevention: 4 mg PO daily with indapamide.
FORMS - Trade only: Tabs, scored 2,4,8 mg.
NOTES - BID dosing does not provide clinically significant BP lowering compared to once daily.

quinapril (*Accupril*) ▶LK ♀- ▶? $$
ADULT - HTN: Start 10-20 mg PO daily (start 10 mg/day if elderly), usual maintenance dose 20-80 mg PO daily or divided bid, max 80 mg/day, but added effect not apparent above 40 mg/day. Renal impairment or concomitant diuretic therapy: Start 2.5-5 mg PO daily. Heart failure: Start 5 mg PO bid, usual maintenance dose 20-40 mg/day divided bid.
PEDS - Not approved in children.
FORMS - Generic/Trade: Tabs, scored 5, non-

scored 10, 20, 40 mg.
NOTES - BID dosing may be required for 24-hour BP control.

ramipril (*Altace*) ▶LK ♀- ▶? $$
ADULT - HTN: Start 2.5 mg PO daily, usual maintenance dose 2.5-20 mg PO daily or divided bid, max 20 mg/day. Renal impairment or concomitant diuretic therapy: Start 1.25 mg PO daily. Heart failure post-MI: Start 2.5 mg PO bid, usual maintenance dose 5 mg PO bid. Reduce risk of MI, stroke, death from cardiovascular causes: Start 2.5 mg PO daily for 1 week, then 5 mg daily for 3 weeks, increase as tolerated to maintenance dose 10 mg daily.
PEDS - Not approved in children.
UNAPPROVED ADULT - Renoprotective dosing: Titrate to 10 mg PO daily.
FORMS - Generic/Trade: Caps 1.25, 2.5, 5, 10 mg.
NOTES - BID dosing may be required for 24-hour BP control. cap contents can be sprinkled on applesauce and eaten or mixed with 120 mL of water or apple juice and swallowed. Mixtures are stable for 24 hr at room temperature or 48 hr refrigerated. Hypoglycemia may occur with co-administration with insulin or hypoglycemic agents.

trandolapril (*Mavik*) ▶LK ♀- ▶? $$
ADULT - HTN: Start 1 mg PO daily in non-black patients or 2 mg PO daily in black patients, usual maintenance dose 2-4 mg PO daily or divided bid, max 8 mg/day, but added effect not apparent above 4 mg/day. Renal impairment or concomitant diuretic therapy: Start 0.5 mg PO daily. Heart failure/post-MI: Start 0.5-1 mg PO daily, titrate to target dose 4 mg PO daily.
PEDS - Not approved in children.
FORMS - Generic/Trade: Tabs, 1, 2, 4 mg.

CARDIOVASCULAR: Aldosterone Antagonists

NOTE: Hyperkalemia possible, especially if used concomitantly with other drugs that increase K+ and in patients with renal impairment.

eplerenone (*Inspra*) ▶L ♀B ▶? $$$$
ADULT - HTN: Start 50 mg PO daily, increase after 4 weeks if needed to max dose 50 mg bid. Start 25 mg daily if concomitant drugs that mildly inhibit CYP 3A4 isoenzyme (eg, erythromycin, verapamil, fluconazole, saquinavir). Improve survival of stable patients with left ventricular systolic dysfunction (EF ≤40%) and

heart failure post-MI: Start 25 mg PO daily; titrate to target dose 50 mg PO daily within 4 weeks, if tolerated.
PEDS - Not approved in children.
FORMS - Trade: Tabs non-scored 25, 50 mg
NOTES - Contraindicated if K+ >5.5 mEq/L; CrCl ≤30 mL/min; strong CYP 3A4 inhibitors (ketoconazole, itraconazole, nefazodone, troleandomycin, clarithromycin, ritonavir, nelfinavir). For treatment of HTN, contraindications include Type 2 DM with microalbuminuria; creat >2 mg/

dL in males or >1.8 mg/dL in females; CrCl <50 mL/min; concomitant K+ supplementation, K-sparing diuretics. Hyperkalemia more common with concomitant ACE inhibitors/ARBs. Measure serum K+ before initiating, within 1st week , at 1 month after starting treatment or dose adjustment, then prn. Monitor lithium levels. Monitor BP if used with NSAIDs.

spironolactone (*Aldactone*) ▶LK ♀D ▶+ $

ADULT - Edema (heart failure, cirrhotic ascites, nephrotic syndrome): Start 100 mg PO daily or divided bid, maintain for 5 days, increase as needed to achieve diuretic response, usual dose range 25-200 mg/day. Other diuretics may be needed. HTN: 50-100 mg PO daily or divided bid, generally used in combination with a thiazide diuretic to maintain serum potassium, increase dose as needed based on serum potassium and BP. Diuretic-induced hypokalemia: 25-100 mg PO daily when potassium supplements/sparing regimens inappropriate.

Primary hyperaldosteronism, maintenance therapy: 100-400 mg/day PO until surgery or indefinitely if surgery not an option. Cirrhotic ascites: Start 100 mg once daily or in divided doses. Dose may range from 25-200 mg/day.

PEDS - Edema: 3.3 mg/kg PO daily or divided bid.

UNAPPROVED ADULT - Severe heart failure: Start 12.5-25 mg PO daily, usual maintenance dose 25–50 mg daily. Hirsutism: 50-200 mg PO daily, maximal regression of hirsutism in 6 months. Acne: 50-200 mg PO daily.

UNAPPROVED PEDS - Edema/HTN: 1-3.3 mg/kg/day, PO daily or divided bid, max 200 mg/day.

FORMS - Generic/Trade: Tabs, non-scored 25; scored 50,100 mg.

NOTES - Dosing more frequently than BID not necessary. Hyperkalemia more likely with ≥50 mg/day and with concomitant ACE inhibitors or K+ supplements.

CARDIOVASCULAR: Angiotensin Receptor Blockers (ARBs)

NOTE: See also antihypertensive combinations. An increase in serum creatinine up to 35% above baseline is acceptable and is not reason to withhold therapy unless hyperkalemia occurs. ARB use during pregnancy may cause injury or death to the developing fetus: use reliable form of contraception in women of child bearing age; discontinue as soon as pregnancy is detected. Use with caution in patients with a history of ACE inhibitor-induced angioedema. African Americans may be at higher risk for angioedema. Rare cases of angioedema and rhabdomyolysis have been reported with ARBs. Increased risk of hypotension with volume-depleted, hyponatremic patients, or during anesthesia/major surgery. Coadministration with NSAIDS, including selective COX-2 inhibitors, may further deteriorate renal function (usually reversible) and decrease antihypertensive effects.

candesartan (*Atacand*) ▶K ♀- ▶? $$$

ADULT - HTN: Start 16 mg PO daily, max 32 mg/day. Volume depleted patients: Start 8 mg PO daily. Reduce cardiovascular death and hospitalizations from heart failure (NYHA II-IV & ejection fraction ≤40%): Start 4 mg PO daily, may double dose q2 wk; maximum 32 mg/day; has an added effect with ACE inhibitor.

PEDS - Not approved in children.

UNAPPROVED ADULT - Reduce heart failure hospitalizations in chronic heart failure & ejection fraction >40%: Start 4 mg PO daily, double dose q 2 weeks; target dose 32 mg/day.

FORMS - Trade: Tabs non-scored 4,8,16,32mg.

NOTES - May increase lithium levels. Initiate/titrate cautiously with heart failure; with symptomatic hypotension, may need to reduce dose temporarily and give fluids.

eprosartan (*Teveten*) ▶Fecal excretion ♀- ▶? $$

ADULT - HTN: Start 600 mg PO daily, maximum 800 mg/day given daily or divided bid.

PEDS - Not approved in children.

FORMS - Trade: Tabs non-scored 400, 600 mg.

irbesartan (*Avapro*) ▶L ♀- ▶? $$$

ADULT - HTN: Start 150 mg PO daily, max 300 mg/day. Volume depleted patients: Start 75 mg PO daily. Type 2 diabetic nephropathy: Start 150 mg PO daily, target dose 300 mg daily.

PEDS - Not approved in children.

FORMS – Trade only: Tabs, non-scored 75, 150, 300 mg.

losartan (*Cozaar*) ▶L ♀- ▶? $$$

ADULT - HTN: Start 50 mg PO daily, max 100 mg/day given daily/divided bid. Volume-depleted patients or history of hepatic impairment: Start 25 mg PO daily. Stroke risk reduction in patients with HTN & left ventricular hypertrophy (does not appear to apply to Blacks): Start 50 mg PO daily. If need more BP reduction add HCTZ 12.5 mg PO daily; then increase losartan to 100 mg/day, then increase HCTZ to 25mg/day. Type 2 diabetic nephropathy: Start 50 mg PO daily, target dose 100 mg/day.

PEDS - HTN: Start 0.7 mg/kg/day (up to 50 mg), doses >1.4 mg/kg/day (or >100 mg) have not been studied. Do not use if age <6 years or if glomerular filtration rate <30 mL/min.

UNAPPROVED ADULT - Heart failure: Start 12.5 mg PO daily, target dose 50 mg daily. Renoprotective dosing: Start 50 mg PO daily, increase to 100 mg daily prn BP control.

FORMS - Trade only: Tabs, non-scored 25,50, 100 mg.

NOTES - Black patients with HTN & left ventricular hypertrophy may not have the same stroke risk reduction than non-Blacks. Monitor BP control when adding or discontinuing rifampin, fluconazole, or erythromycin.

olmesartan (*Benicar*) ▶K ♀- ▶? $$$
ADULT - HTN: Start 20 mg PO daily, maximum 40 mg/day.

PEDS - Not approved in children.

FORMS - Trade only: Tabs, non-scored 5,20,40 mg.

telmisartan (*Micardis*) ▶L ♀- ▶? $$$
ADULT - HTN: Start 40 mg PO daily, maximum 80 mg/day.

PEDS - Not approved in children.

FORMS - Trade only: Tabs, non-scored 20,40, 80 mg.

NOTES - Swallow tabs whole, do not break or crush. Caution in hepatic insufficiency. May need to monitor digoxin levels when initiating, adjusting dose, or discontinuing.

valsartan (*Diovan*) ▶L ♀- ▶? $$$
ADULT - HTN: Start 80-160 mg PO daily, max 320 mg/d. Heart failure: Start 40 mg PO bid, target dose 160 mg bid; provides no added effect when used with adequate dose of ACE inhibitor. Reduce mortality/morbidity post-MI with left ventricular systolic dysfunction/failure: Start 20 mg PO bid, increase to 40 mg PO bid within 7 days, target dose 160 mg bid.

PEDS - Not approved in children.

UNAPPROVED ADULT - Renoprotective dosing: 80-160 mg PO daily.

FORMS - Trade only: Tabs, scored 40 mg, non-scored 80, 160, 320 mg.

CARDIOVASCULAR: Antiadrenergic Agents

clonidine (*Catapres, Catapres-TTS,* ❦*Dixarit*) ▶LK ♀C ▶? $$
ADULT - HTN: Start 0.1 mg PO bid, usual maintenance dose 0.2-1.2 mg/day divided bid-tid, max 2.4 mg/day. Transdermal (Catapres-TTS): Start 0.1 mg/24 hour patch q week, titrate to desired effect, max effective dose 0.6 mg/24 hour (two, 0.3 mg/24 hour patches).

PEDS - HTN: Start 5-7 mcg/kg/day PO divided q6-12 hr, titrate at 5-7 intervals to 5-25 mcg/kg/day divided q6h; max 0.9 mg/day. Transdermal not recommended in children.

UNAPPROVED ADULT - HTN urgency: Initially 0.1-0.2 mg PO, followed by 0.1 mg q1h as needed up to a total dose of 0.5-0.7 mg. Menopausal flushing: 0.1-0.4 mg/day PO divided bid-tid; transdermal applied weekly 0.1 mg/day. Tourette's syndrome: 3-5 mcg/kg/day PO divided bid-qid. Opioid withdrawal, adjunct: 0.1-0.3 mg PO tid-qid or 0.1-0.2 mg PO q4h tapering off over days 4-10. Alcohol withdrawal, adjunct: 0.1-0.2 mg PO q4h prn. Smoking cessation: Start 0.1 mg PO bid, increase 0.1 mg/day at weekly intervals to 0.75 mg/day as tolerated; transdermal (Catapres TTS): 0.1-0.2 mg/24 h

patch q week for 2-3 weeks after cessation. ADHD: 5 mcg/kg/day PO x 8 weeks. Post-traumatic stress disorder: Start 0.1 mg PO hs, max 0.6 mg/day in divided doses.

UNAPPROVED PEDS - ADHD: Start 0.05 mg PO qhs, titrate based on response over 8 weeks to max 0.2 mg/day (<45 kg) or 0.4 mg/day (> 45 kg) in 2-4 divided doses. Tourette's syndrome: 3-5 mcg/kg/day PO divided bid-qid.

FORMS - Generic/Trade: Tabs, non-scored 0.1, 0.2, 0.3 mg. Trade only: transdermal weekly patch 0.1 mg/day (TTS-1), 0.2 mg/day (TTS-2), 0.3 mg/day (TTS-3).

NOTES - Sedation. Bradycardia. Rebound HTN with abrupt discontinuation of tabs, especially at doses ≥0.8 mg/day. Taper therapy over 4-7 days to avoid rebound HTN. Dispose of used patches carefully, keep away from children. Remove patch before MRI to avoid skin burns.

doxazosin (*Cardura, Cardura XL*) ▶L ♀C ▶? $$
WARNING - Not 1st line for HTN. Increased risk of heart failure in patients who used doxazosin compared to diuretic in treating HTN.

ADULT - BPH, immediate release: Start 1 mg

PO qhs, titrate by doubling the dose over at least 1-2 week intervals up to a maximum of 8 mg PO qhs. Extended release (not approved for HTN): Start 4 mg PO qam with breakfast, titrate dose in 3-4 weeks to max dose 8 mg PO qam. HTN: Start 1 mg PO qhs, max 16 mg/day. Avoid use of doxazosin alone to treat combined HTN and BPH.

PEDS - Not approved in children.

UNAPPROVED ADULT - Promote spontaneous passage of ureteral calculi: 4 mg (XL formulation only) PO daily usually combined with an NSAID, antiemetic and opioid of choice.

FORMS - Generic/Trade: Tabs, scored 1,2,4,8 mg. Trade only: XL tabs 4,8 mg.

NOTES - Dizziness, drowsiness, lightheadedness, syncope. Bedtime dosing may minimize side effects. Initial 1 mg dose is used to decrease postural hypotension that may occur after the first few doses. If therapy is interrupted for several days, restart at the 1 mg dose. Monitor BP after first dose, after each dose adjustment, and periodically thereafter. Contraindicated with vardenafil or tadalafil; increases risk of hypotension.

guanabenz (*Wytensin*) ▶LK ♀C ▶- $$$

WARNING - Sedation, rebound HTN with abrupt discontinuation especially with high doses.

ADULT - HTN: Start 2-4 mg PO bid, max 32 mg bid.

PEDS - Children >12 years of age: initial dose 0.5-2 mg/day divided bid, usual maintenance dose 4-24 mg/day divided bid.

FORMS - Generic only: Tabs, 4, 8 mg.

NOTES - Sedation. Rebound HTN with abrupt discontinuation, especially at higher doses (32 mg/day). Taper therapy over 4-7 days to avoid rebound HTN.

guanfacine (*Tenex*) ▶K ♀B ▶? $

ADULT - HTN: Start 1 mg PO qhs, increase to 2-3 mg qhs if needed after 3-4 weeks, max 3 mg/day.

PEDS - HTN: ≥12 years of age, same as adult.

UNAPPROVED PEDS - ADHD: Start 0.5 mg PO daily, titrate by 0.5 mg q3-4 days as tolerated to 0.5 mg PO tid.

FORMS - Generic/Trade: Tabs, non-scored 1, 2 mg.

NOTES - Most of the drug's therapeutic effect is seen at 1 mg/day. Rebound HTN with abrupt discontinuation, but generally BP returns to pretreatment measurements slowly without ill effects. Less sedation and hypotension compared to clonidine.

methyldopa (*Aldomet*) ▶LK ♀B ▶+ $

ADULT - HTN: Start 250 mg PO bid-tid, usual maintenance dose 500-3000 mg/day divided bid-qid, max 3000 mg/day. Hypertensive crisis: 250-500 mg IV q6h, maximum 1gm IV q6h, maximum 4000 mg/day.

PEDS - HTN: 10 mg/kg/day PO divided bid-qid, titrate dose to a max dose 65 mg/kg/day or 3000 mg/day, whichever is less.

FORMS - Generic/Trade: Tabs, non-scored 500 mg. Generic: Tabs, non-scored 125, 250 mg.

NOTES - Not 1st or 2nd line for HTN (other agents preferred) except pregnancy-induced HTN. IV form has a slow onset of effect and other agents preferred for rapid reduction of BP. Hemolytic anemia possible.

prazosin (*Minipress*) ▶L ♀C ▶? $

WARNING - Not first line agent for hypertension. Increased risk of heart failure in patients who used doxazosin compared to diuretic in treating HTN.

ADULT - HTN: Start 1 mg PO bid-tid, usual maintenance dose 20 mg/day divided bid-tid, max 40 mg/day, but doses >20 mg/day usually do not increase efficacy.

PEDS - Not approved in children.

UNAPPROVED ADULT - Post-traumatic stress disorder: Start 1 mg PO hs, increase weekly by 1-2 mg/day to max dose of 20 mg/day. Doses >10 mg/day are divided early evening and hs.

UNAPPROVED PEDS - HTN: Start 0.005 mg/kg PO single dose; increase slowly as needed up to maintenance dose 0.025-0.150 mg/kg/day divided q6 hours; max dose 0.4 mg/kg/day.

FORMS - Generic/Trade: Caps 1,2,5 mg.

NOTES - To avoid syncope, start with 1 mg qhs, and increase dose gradually. Contraindicated with vardenafil or tadalafil; increases risk of hypotension.

reserpine (*Serpasil*) ▶LK ♀C ▶- $

ADULT - HTN: Start 0.05-0.1 mg PO daily or 0.1 mg PO qod, max dose 0.25 mg/day.

PEDS - Not approved in children.

FORMS - Generic: Tabs, scored, 0.1,0.25 mg.

NOTES - Should be used in combination with a diuretic to counteract fluid retention and augment BP control. May cause depression at higher doses, avoid use in patients with depression or active peptic ulcer disease.

terazosin (*Hytrin*) ▶LK ♀C ▶? $

WARNING - Not first line agent for HTN. Increased risk of heart failure in patients who used related-drug doxazosin compared to diuretic in treating HTN.

ADULT - HTN: Start 1 mg PO qhs, usual effective dose 1-5 mg PO daily or divided bid, max 20 mg/day. BPH: Start 1 mg PO qhs, titrate dose in a stepwise fashion to 2, 5, or 10 mg PO qhs to desired effect. Treatment with 10 mg PO qhs for 4-6 weeks may be needed to assess benefit. Maximum 20 mg/day.

PEDS - Not approved in children.

FORMS - Generic (Caps, Tabs)/Trade (Caps): 1, 2, 5, 10 mg.

NOTES - Dizziness, drowsiness, lightheadedness, syncope. Bedtime dosing may minimize side effects. Initial 1 mg dose is used to decrease postural hypotension that may occur after the first few doses. If therapy is interrupted for several days, restart at the 1 mg dose. Monitor BP after first dose, after each dose adjustment, and periodically thereafter. Contraindicated with vardenafil or tadalafil; increases risk of hypotension.

SELECTED DRUGS THAT MAY PROLONG THE QT INTERVAL

alfuzosin	dofetilide*	indapamide*	pimozide*†	tamoxifen
amiodarone*†	dolasetron	isradipine	polyethylene glycol	telithromycin*
apomorphine	droperidol*	levofloxacin*	(PEG-salt solution)§	thioridazine‡
arsenic trioxide*	epirubicin	lithium	procainamide*	tizanidine
azithromycin*	erythromycin*†	mefloquine	quetiapine‡	tolterodine
chloroquine*	felbamate	methadone*†	quinidine*†	vardenafil
chlorpromazine*†	flecainide*	moexipril/HCTZ	quinine	venlafaxine
cisapride*†	foscarnet	moxifloxacin	ranolazine	Visicol§
clarithromycin*	fosphenytoin	nicardipine	risperidone‡	voriconazole*
clozapine	gemifloxacin	octreotide	salmeterol	vorinostat
cocaine*	granisetron	ofloxacin	sotalol*†	ziprasidone‡
dasatinib	haloperidol*‡	ondansetron	sunitinib	
disopyramide*†	ibutilide*†	pentamidine*†	tacrolimus	

See www.qtdrugs.com. This table may not include all drugs that prolong the QT interval or cause torsades. Risk of drug-induced QT prolongation may be increased in women, elderly, ↓K, ↓Mg, bradycardia, starvation, CHF, & CNS injuries. Hepatorenal dysfunction & drug interactions can ↑ the concentration of QT interval-prolonging drugs. Coadministration of QT interval-prolonging drugs can have additive effects. Avoid these (and other) drugs in congenital prolonged QT syndrome. *Torsades reported in product labeling/case reports. †↑Risk in women. ‡QT prolongation with PO administration: thioridazine > ziprasidone > haloperidol, quetiapine, risperidone; with IM administration: haloperidol > ziprasidone. §May be due to electrolyte imbalance.

CARDIOVASCULAR: Anti-Dysrhythmics / Cardiac Arrest

adenosine (*Adenocard*) ▶Plasma ♀C ▶? $$$

ADULT - PSVT conversion (not A-fib): 6 mg rapid IV & flush, preferably through a central line. If no response after 1-2 mins then 12 mg. A third dose of 12 mg may be given prn.

PEDS - PSVT conversion <50 kg: initial dose 50-100 mcg/kg IV, give subsequent doses q1-2 min prn by increasing 50-100 mcg/kg each time, up to a max single dose of 300 mcg/kg or 12 mg, whichever less. ≥50 kg: Same as adult.

UNAPPROVED PEDS - PSVT conversion: Initial dose 0.1-0.2 mg/kg IV bolus.

NOTES - Half-life is <10 seconds. Give doses by rapid IV push followed by normal saline flush. Need higher dose if on theophylline or caffeine, lower dose if on dipyridamole or carbamazepine. May cause respiratory collapse in asthma, COPD. Use in setting with cardiac resuscitation readily available. Do not confuse with adenosine phosphate used for the symptomatic relief of varicose vein complications.

amiodarone (*Cordarone, Pacerone*) ▶L ♀D ▶- $$$$

WARNING - Life-threatening pulmonary and hepatoxicity. Proarrhythmic. Contraindicated in cardiogenic shock and with marked sinus bradycardia or 2nd/3rd degree heart block if no pacemaker. Loading doses for inpatients only.

ADULT - Life-threatening ventricular arrhythmia without cardiac arrest: Load 150 mg IV over 10 min, then 1 mg/min x 6 hrs, then 0.5 mg/min x 18h. Mix in D5W. Oral loading dose 800-1600 mg PO daily for 1-3 weeks, reduce dose to 400-800 mg daily for 1 month when arrhythmia is controlled or adverse effects are prominent, then reduce to lowest effective dose, usually 200-400 mg daily.

PEDS - Not approved in children.

UNAPPROVED ADULT - Refractory atrial fibrillation: loading dose 600-800 mg PO daily for 7-14 days, then 200-400 mg daily. Maintain sinus rhythm with A-fib: 100-400 mg PO daily. Shock refractory VF/pulseless VT: 300 mg or 5 mg/kg IV bolus followed by unsynchronized shock, additional 150 mg bolus may be given if serious arrhythmias recur. Stable monomorphic ventricular tachycardia: 150 mg IV over 10 min, repeat q10-15 min prn.

UNAPPROVED PEDS - May cause death or other serious side effects (see NOTES); do not use in infants <30 days old and use only if medically warranted if >30 days old. Ventricular arrhythmia: IV therapy limited data; 5 mg/kg IV over 30 minutes; followed by 5 mcg/kg/min infusion; increase infusion as needed up to max 10 mcg/kg/min or 20 mg/kg/ day. Give loading dose in 1 mg/kg aliquots with each aliquot given over 5-10 min; do not exceed 30 mg/min.

FORMS - Trade only: Tabs, 100 mg (Pacerone). Generic/Trade: Tabs, 200, 400 mg.

NOTES - Consider inpatient rhythm monitoring during initiation of therapy, especially when treating life-threatening arrhythmias. Consult cardiologist before using with other antiarrhythmics. Do not use with iodine allergy. Photosensitivity with oral therapy. Hypo or hyperthyroidism possible. Monitor LFTs, TFTs, and PFTs. Prompt ophthalmic examination needed with changes in visual acuity or decreased peripheral vision. Most manufacturers of laser refractive devices contraindicate eye laser surgery when taking amiodarone. Long elimination half-life, approximately 25-50 days. Drug interactions may persist after discontinuance due to long half-life. May increase levels of substrates of p-glycoprotein and drugs metabolized by CYP450 enzymes (CYP1A2, CYP2C9, CYP 2D6, CYP3A4). Co-administration of fluoroquinolones, macrolides, loratadine, trazodone, or azoles may prolong QTc. May double or triple phenytoin level. May increase cyclosporine levels. May increase digoxin levels; discontinue digoxin or reduce dose by 50%. May increase INR with warfarin therapy up to 100%; reduce warfarin dose by 33-50%. Increased risk of myopathy when used with simvastatin or lovastatin. Caution with simvastatin >20 mg/day or lovastatin >40 mg/day, unless clinical benefit outweighs risk of myopathy. Co-administration with clopidogrel may result in ineffective platelet inhibition. Do not use with grapefruit juice. Use cautiously with beta blockers and calcium channel blockers. Protease inhibitors, cimetidine may increase levels. Give bid if intolerable GI effects occur with once-daily dosing. IV therapy may cause hypotension and bradycardia in adults. Administer IV infusion using a nonevacuated glass bottle and in-line IV filter. Use central line when concentration >2 mg/ml. May cause congenital hypothyroidism and hyperthyroidism if given during pregnancy. Avoid use if <1 month of age: IV form contains benzyl alcohol, which may cause gasping syndrome (gasping respirations, hypotension, bradycardia, and cardiovascular collapse). In those 1 month to 15 yo may cause life-threatening hypotension, bradycardia, AV block. May adversely affect male reproductive tract development in infants & toddlers from plasticizer exposure from IV tubing; use syringes instead of IV tubing to administer doses to infants and toddlers.

atropine (*AtroPen*) ▶K ♀C ▶- $

ADULT - Bradyarrhythmia/CPR: 0.5-1.0 mg IV q3-5 mins, max 0.04 mg/kg (3 mg). Treatment of muscarinic symptoms of insecticide or nerve agent poisonings: Mild symptoms: 1 injection of 2 mg auto-injector pen, 2 additional injections after 10 minutes may be given in rapid succession if severe symptoms develop. Severe symptoms: 3 injections of 2 mg pen in rapid succession. Administer injection in mid-lateral thigh. Max 3 injections.

PEDS - CPR: 0.02 mg/kg/dose IV q5 mins for 2-3 doses prn (max single dose 0.5 mg); minimum single dose, 0.1 mg; max cumulative dose 1 mg. Treatment of muscarinic symptoms of insecticide or nerve agent poisonings: Follow adult dosing instructions, but if <7 kg use 0.25 mg pen, if 7-18 kg use 0.5 mg pen, if 18-41 kg use 1 mg pen, if >41 kg use 2 mg pen.

UNAPPROVED ADULT - ET administration prior to IV access: 2-2.5 x the recommended IV dose in 10 mL of NS or distilled water.

FORMS - Trade only: Prefilled auto-injector pen: 0.25 mg (yellow), 0.5 mg (blue), 1 mg (dark red), 2 mg (green).

NOTES - Injector should be used by someone with adequate training in recognizing & treating nerve agent or insecticide intoxication. Seek immediate medical attention after injection(s).

bicarbonate ▶K ♀C ▶? $

ADULT - Cardiac arrest: 1 mEq/kg/dose IV initially, followed by repeat doses up to 0.5 mEq/kg at 10 minute intervals during continued arrest. Severe acidosis: 2-5 mEq/kg dose IV administered as a 4-8 hour infusion. Repeat dosing based on lab values.

PEDS - Cardiac arrest: Neonates or infants <2 years of age, 1 mEq/kg dose IV slow injection initially, followed by repeat doses up to 1 mEq/kg at 10 minute intervals during continued arrest. To avoid intracranial hemorrhage due to hypertonicity, use a 1:1 dilution of 8.4% (1 mEq/mL) sodium bicarbonate and dextrose 5% or use the 4.2% (0.5 mEq/mL) product.

UNAPPROVED ADULT - Prevention of contrast-induced nephropathy: Administer sodium bicarbonate 154 mEq/L soln at 3 mL/kg/hr IV x 1h before contrast, followed by infusion of 1 mL/kg/hr x 6 hrs post-procedure. If >110 kg dose based on 110 kg weight.

NOTES - Full correction of bicarb deficit should not be attempted during the first 24h. May paradoxically exacerbate intracellular acidosis.

digoxin (Lanoxin, Lanoxicaps, Digitek) ▶KL ♀C ▶+ $

ADULT - Systolic heart failure/rate control of chronic A-fib: <70 years: 0.25 mg PO daily; >70 years: 0.125 mg PO daily; impaired renal function: 0.0625-0.125 mg PO daily; titrate based on response. Rapid A-fib: Load 0.5 mg IV, then 0.25 mg IV q6h x 2 doses, maintenance 0.125-0.375 mg IV/PO daily; titrate to minimum effective dose. Other agents (ie, beta blockers, diltiazem, verapamil) generally are more effective in controlling ventricular rate in A-fib.

PEDS - Arrhythmia: Oral total loading dose with tabs or elixir: premature neonate, 20-30 mcg/kg; full-term neonate, 25-35 mcg/kg; 1-24 months, 35-60 mcg/kg; 2-5 years, 30-40 mcg/kg; 5-10 years, 20-35 mcg/kg; >10 years, 10-15 mcg/kg. Initially, give half of the total loading dose; other half of loading dose may be given in 6-8h after reassessment. Use 25-35% of oral loading dose in divided doses (bid) for <10 years for maintenance dose. Caution - peds doses are in mcg, elixir is labeled in mg/mL.

UNAPPROVED ADULT - Reentrant PSVT (after carotid massage, IV adenosine, IV beta blocker, IV diltiazem): 8-15 mcg/kg IV, give 50% of total dose initially, 25% 4-6 hours later, and then the final 25% 4-6 hours later.

FORMS - Generic/Trade: Tabs, scored (Lanoxin, Digitek) 0.125,0.25 mg; elixir 0.05 mg/mL. Trade: Caps (Lanoxicaps), 0.05,0.1,0.2 mg.

NOTES - Consider patient specific characteristics (weight, CrCl, age, factors likely to alter pharmacokinetic/dynamic profile of digoxin) when dosing; see package insert for alterations based on weight & renal function. Adjust dose based on response and therapeutic serum levels (range from 0.8-2.0 ng/mL). Heart failure may respond at lower levels (≥0.5 ng/mL) while A-fib may need higher. Serum digoxin concentration of 0.5-0.8 ng/mL (compared to higher serum concentrations) is associated with decreased mortality in men with stable heart failure and ejection fraction ≤45%. Toxicity exacerbated by hypokalemia. 100 mcg Lanoxicaps = 125 mcg tabs or elixir. Avoid IM route due to severe local irritation. Elimination prolonged with renal impairment, monitor levels carefully. Many drug and herb interactions.

digoxin immune Fab (Digibind, Digifab) ▶K ♀C ▶? $$$$$

ADULT - Digoxin toxicity: 2-20 vials IV, one formula is: Number vials = (serum dig level in ng/mL) x (kg) / 100.

PEDS - Same as adult.

NOTES - Do not draw serum digoxin concentrations after administering digoxin-immune Fab; levels will be falsely elevated for several days. One vial binds approximately 0.5 mg digoxin.

disopyramide (Norpace, Norpace CR, ✱Rythmodan, Rythmodan-LA) ▶KL ♀C ▶+ $$$$

WARNING - Proarrhythmic. Increased mortality in patients with non-life threatening ventricular arrhythmias and structural heart disease (i.e. MI, LV dysfunction).

ADULT - Rarely indicated, consult cardiologist. Ventricular arrhythmia: 400-800 mg PO daily in divided doses (immediate-release, q6h or extended-release, q12h). With cardiomyopathy or possible cardiac decompensation, limit initial dose to 100 mg of immediate-release q6-8h; do not give a loading dose. With liver disease or moderate renal impairment (CrCl>40): 400 mg/day PO in divided doses. Use immediate release form when CrCl ≤40 mg/dL: CrCl 30-40 mg/dL: 100 mg q8h; CrCl 15-30 mg/dL: 100 mg q12h; CrCl <15 mg/dL: 100 mg q24h.

PEDS - Ventricular arrhythmia: Divide dose q6h. <1 yr, 10-30 mg/kg/day; 1-4 yrs, 10-20 mg/kg/day; 4-12 yrs, 10-15 mg/kg/day; 12-18 yrs, 6-15 mg/kg/day.

UNAPPROVED ADULT - Maintain sinus rhythm with A-fib: 400-750 mg/day in divided doses.

FORMS - Generic/Trade: Caps, immediate-release, 100,150 mg; extended-release 150 mg. Trade only: extended-release 100 mg.

NOTES - Consider inpatient rhythm monitoring during initiation of therapy, especially when treating life-threatening arrhythmias. Anticholinergic side effects (dry mouth, constipation, blurred vision, urinary hesitancy) commonly occur. Reduce dose in patients with CrCl <40 mL/min. Initiate as an outpatient with extreme caution. May start 6-12 hrs after last dose of quinidine, or 3-6 hrs after last dose of procainamide. May start extended release form 6 hrs after last dose of immediate release form.

dofetilide (*Tikosyn*) ▶KL ♀C ▶- $$$$

WARNING - Rarely indicated; available only to hospitals and prescribers who have received appropriate dosing and treatment initiation education. Contraindicated if CrCl is <20 mL/min or QTc interval >440 msec, or >500 msec in patients with ventricular conduction abnormalities. Must be initiated or re-initiated in a facility that can provide CrCl calculation, ECG monitoring, and cardiac resuscitation; monitor there for ≥3 days. Do not discharge if ≤12 h since electrical or pharmacological conversion to sinus rhythm.

ADULT - Conversion of A-fib/flutter: Specialized dosing based on CrCl and QTc interval.

PEDS - Not approved in children.

FORMS - Trade only: Caps, 0.125,0.25,0.5 mg.

NOTES - Use with heart rate <50 bpm has not been studied. Serum K+, Mg++ should be within normal range prior to initiating and during therapy. Monitor K+ and Mg++ (low levels increase risk of arrhythmias). Assess CrCl and QTc prior to first dose. Continuously monitor ECG during hospital initiation and adjust dose based on QTc interval. Effects may be increased by known cytochrome P450 3A4 inhibitors and drugs that inhibit renal elimination. Contraindicated with HCTZ (alone or with triamterene), trimethoprim, verapamil, cimetidine, prochlorperazine, megestrol, and ketoconazole. Using with phenothiazines, cisapride, tricyclic antidepressants, macrolides, fluoroquinolones may increase QTc.

flecainide (*Tambocor*) ▶K ♀C ▶- $$$$

WARNING - Proarrhythmic. Increased mortality in non-life threatening ventricular arrhythmias, structural heart disease (ie, MI, LV dysfunction); do not use with chronic atrial fibrillation.

ADULT - Prevention of paroxysmal atrial fib/flutter or PSVT, with symptoms & no structural heart disease: Start 50 mg PO q12h, may increase by 50 mg bid q4 days, max 300 mg/day. Life-threatening ventricular arrhythmias without structural heart disease: Start 100 mg PO q12h, may increase by 50 mg bid q 4 days, max 400 mg/day. With severe renal impairment (CrCl<35 mL/min): Start 50 mg PO bid.

PEDS - Consult pediatric cardiologist.

UNAPPROVED ADULT - Cardioversion of recent onset atrial fib: 300 mg PO single dose. Maintain sinus rhythm with A-fib: 200-300 mg/day in divided doses. Outpatient prn therapy for recurrent atrial fib in highly-select patients ("pill-in-the-pocket"): Single dose PO of 300 mg (if ≥70 kg) or 200 mg (if <70 kg).

FORMS - Generic/Trade: Tabs, non-scored 50, scored 100,150 mg.

NOTES - Consider inpatient rhythm monitoring during initiation of therapy, especially when treating life-threatening arrhythmias. Do not use with structural heart disease. Use with AV nodal slowing agent (beta blocker, verapamil, diltiazem) to minimize risk of 1:1 atrial flutter. Reduce dose if QRS widening >20% from baseline or if 2nd/3rd degree AV block. Correct hypo/hyperkalemia before giving. Increases digoxin level 13-19%. Consult cardiologist before using with other antiarrhythmic agents. Reduce dose of flecainide 50% when used with amiodarone. Quinidine, cimetidine may increase levels. Use cautiously with disopyramide, verapamil, or impaired hepatic function. Use cautiously with impaired renal function; will take >4 days to reach new steady state level. Target trough level 0.2-1 mcg/mL.

ibutilide (*Corvert*) ▶K ♀C ▶? $$$$$

WARNING - Proarrhythmic; only administer by trained personnel with continuous ECG monitoring.

ADULT - Recent onset A-fib/flutter: Patients >60 kg: 1 mg (10 mL) IV over 10 mins, may repeat once if no response after 10 additional minutes. Patients <60 kg: 0.01 mg/kg over 10 min, may repeat if no response after 10 additional minutes. Useful in combo with DC cardioversion if DC cardioversion alone is unsuccessful.

PEDS - Not approved in children.

NOTES - Serum K+, Mg++ should be within normal range prior to initiating and during therapy. Monitor K+ and Mg++ (low levels increase risk of arrhythmias). Keep on cardiac monitor ≥4 hours. Caution, if used at all, when QT is >500 ms, severe LV dysfunction, or in patients already using class Ia or III antiarrhythmics. Stop infusion when arrhythmia is terminated.

isoproterenol (*Isuprel*) ▶LK ♀C ▶? $$

ADULT - Refractory bradycardia or third degree

AV block: 0.02-0.06 mg (1-3 mL of a 1:50,000 dilution) IV bolus or IV infusion (2 mg in 250 mL D5W = 8 mcg/mL) at 5 mcg/min; 5 mcg/min = 37 mL/h. General dose range 2-20 mcg/min.

PEDS - Refractory bradycardia or third degree AV block: Start IV infusion 0.05 mcg/kg/min, increase every 5-10 min by 0.1 mcg/kg/min until desired effect or onset of toxicity, max 2 mcg/kg/min. 10 kg: 0.1 mcg/kg/min = 8 mL/h.

lidocaine (*Xylocaine, Xylocard*) ▶LK♀B ▶? $

ADULT - Ventricular arrhythmia: Load 1 mg/kg IV, then 0.5 mg/kg IV q8-10min as needed to max 3 mg/kg. IV infusion: 4 gm in 500 mL D5W (8 mg/mL) at 1-4 mg/min.

PEDS - Ventricular arrhythmia: Loading dose 1 mg/kg IV/intraosseous slowly; may repeat for 2 doses 10-15 minutes apart; max 3-5 mg/kg in one hour. ET tube: Use 2-2.5 times IV dose. IV infusion: 4g in 500 mL D5W (8 mg/mL) at 20-50 mcg/kg/min. 10kg: 40 mcg/kg/min = 3 mL/h.

UNAPPROVED ADULT - ET administration prior to IV access: 2-2.5 x the recommended IV dose in 10 mL of NS or distilled water. Shock refractory VF/pulseless VT: 1-1.5 mg/kg IV push x 1, then 0.5-0.75 mg/kg IV push q5-10 min as needed to max 3 mg/kg.

NOTES - Reduce infusion in heart failure, liver disease, elderly. Not for routine use after acute MI. Monitor for CNS side effects with prolonged infusions.

mexiletine (*Mexitil*) ▶L ♀C ▶- $$$

WARNING - Proarrhythmic. Increased mortality in patients with non-life threatening ventricular arrhythmias and structural heart disease (i.e. MI, LV dysfunction).

ADULT - Rarely indicated, consult cardiologist. Ventricular arrhythmia: Start 200 mg PO q8h with food or antacid, max dose 1,200 mg/day. Patients responding to q8h dosing may be converted to q12h dosing with careful monitoring, max 450 mg/dose q12h.

PEDS - Not approved in children.

FORMS - Generic/Trade: Caps, 150, 200, 250 mg.

NOTES - Patients may require decreased dose with severe liver disease. CNS side effects may limit dose titration. Monitor level when given with phenytoin, rifampin, phenobarbital, cimetidine, fluvoxamine. May increase theophylline level.

moricizine (*Ethmozine*) ▶L ♀B ▶? $$$$

WARNING - Proarrhythmic. Increased mortality in patients with non-life threatening ventricular arrhythmias and structural heart disease (i.e. MI, LV dysfunction).

ADULT - Rarely indicated, consult cardiologist. Ventricular arrhythmia: Start 200 mg PO q8h, max dose 900 mg/day. Patients responding to q8h dosing may be converted to q12h dosing with careful monitoring.

PEDS - Not approved in children.

FORMS - Trade only: Tabs, non-scored 200, 250, 300 mg.

procainamide (*Procanbid, Pronestyl*) ▶LK ♀C ▶? $

WARNING - Proarrhythmic. Increased mortality in non-life threatening ventricular arrhythmias and structural heart disease (i.e. MI, LV dysfunction). Positive ANA titer, blood dyscrasias, and lupus erythematosus-like syndrome.

ADULT - Ventricular arrhythmia: 50 mg/kg/day PO; 250-625 mg PO q3h (immediate-release products), 500-1250 mg PO q6h (SR products), 500-1000 mg PO q12h (Procanbid product). IV dosing: Load 100 mg IV q10 min or 20 mg/min (150 mL/h) until: 1) QRS widens >50%, 2) dysrhythmia suppressed, 3) hypotension, or 4) total of 17 mg/kg or 1000 mg. Infusion 2g in 250 mL D5W (8 mg/mL) at 2-6 mg/min (15-45 mL/h). If rhythm unresponsive, guide therapy by serum procainamide/NAPA levels.

PEDS - Not approved in children.

UNAPPROVED ADULT - Shock responsive VF/pulseless VT: up to 50 mg/min until: 1) QRS widens >50%, 2) dysrhythmia suppressed, 3) hypotension, or 4) total of 17 mg/kg or 1000 mg. Maintain sinus rhythm with A-fib: 1000-4000 mg/day in divided doses. Restoration of sinus rhythm in atrial fibrillation with Wolf-Parkinson-White syndrome (preexcitation) 100 mg IV q10 min or 20 mg/min. until: 1) QRS widens >50%, 2) dysrhythmia suppressed, 3) hypotension, or 4) total of 17 mg/kg or 1000 mg.

UNAPPROVED PEDS - Arrhythmia: 15-50 mg/kg/day PO immediate-release products divided q 3-6 h; 2-6 mg/kg IV over 5 min, max loading dose 100 mg, repeat loading dose every 5-10 min as needed up to max 15 mg/kg; 20-80 mcg/kg/min IV infusion, max dose 2 g/day. Consult peds cardiologist or intensivist.

FORMS - Generic/Trade: Caps, immediate-release 250 mg; tabs, sustained-release, non-scored (Pronestyl SR). Generic only: tabs, sustained-release, non-scored (generic procainamide SR, q6h dosing) 750,1000 mg; caps, immediate-release 500 mg. Trade only: Tabs, immediate-release, non-scored (Pronestyl) 250, 375,500 mg, extended-release, non-scored

(Procanbid, q12h dosing) 500,1000 mg.
NOTES - Do not break or crush SR or XR products. Swallow Tabs whole.

propafenone (*Rythmol, Rythmol SR*) ▶L ♀C ▶? $$$$
WARNING - Proarrhythmic. Increased mortality in patients with non-life threatening ventricular arrhythmias and structural heart disease (ie, MI, LV dysfunction).
ADULT - Prevention of paroxysmal atrial fib/flutter or PSVT, with symptoms & no structural heart disease; or life-threatening ventricular arrhythmias: Start (immediate release) 150 mg PO q8h; may increase after 3-4 days to 225 mg PO q8h; max 900 mg/day. Prolong time to recurrence of symptomatic atrial fib without structural heart disease: 225 mg SR PO q12h, may increase ≥5 days to 325 mg PO q12h, max 425 mg q12h.
PEDS - Not approved in children.
UNAPPROVED ADULT - Cardioversion of recent onset atrial fib: 600 mg PO single dose. Outpatient prn therapy for recurrent atrial fib in highly-select patients ("pill-in-the-pocket"): Single dose PO of 600 mg (if ≥70 kg) or 450 mg (if <70 kg).
FORMS - Generic/Trade: Tabs (immediate release), scored 150, 225, 300 mg; Trade only: SR, capsules 225, 325, 425 mg.
NOTES - Consider inpatient monitoring when starting, especially with life-threatening arrhythmias. Do not use with structural heart disease or for atrial fib ventricular rate control. Consider using with AV nodal slowing agent (beta blocker, verapamil, diltiazem) to minimize risk of 1:1 atrial flutter. Reduce dose if QRS widens >20% from baseline or if 2nd/3rd degree AV block. Correct hypo/hyperkalemia and low magnesium before giving. Consult cardiologist before using with other antiarrhythmics. May increase digoxin level 35-85%. May increase beta blocker, cyclosporine, desipramine, haloperidol, imipramine, theophylline, venlafaxine levels. Increases warfarin activity; monitor INR. Amiodarone, cimetidine, desipramine, erythromycin, ketoconazole, paroxetine, ritonavir, saquinavir, sertraline may increase level and risk of QT prolongation. Instruct patient to report any changes in OTC, prescription, supplement use and symptoms that may be alter electrolytes (prolonged/excessive diarrhea, sweating, vomiting, thirst, appetite loss). Reduce dose 70-80% with impaired hepatic function. Use cautiously with impaired renal function. Bioavail-

ability of 325 mg SR bid = 150 mg immediate release tid. Poorly metabolized by 10% population; reduce dose & monitor for toxicity.

quinidine (❀*Biquin durules*) ▶LK ♀C ▶+ $$-gluconate, $-sulfate
WARNING - Proarrhythmic. Increased mortality in non-life threatening arrhythmias and structural heart disease (i.e. MI, LV dysfunction).
ADULT - Arrhythmia: gluconate, extended-release: 324-648 mg PO q8-12h; sulfate, immediate-release: 200-400 mg PO q6-8h; sulfate, extended-release: 300-600 mg PO q8-12h. Consider inpatient rhythm and QT monitoring during initiation of therapy. Life-threatening malaria: Load with 10 mg/kg (max 600 mg) IV over 1-2h, then 0.02 mg/kg/min for ≥24h. Dose given as quinidine gluconate. When parasitemia <1% and PO meds tolerated, convert to PO quinine to complete 3 days (Africa/South America) or 7 days (Southeast Asia). Also give doxycycline, tetracycline, or clindamycin.
PEDS - Not approved in children.
UNAPPROVED PEDS - Arrhythmia: Test dose (oral sulfate or IM/IV gluconate) 2 mg/kg (max 200 mg). Sulfate: 15-60 mg/kg/day PO divided q6h. Life-threatening malaria: Load with 10 mg/kg IV over 1-2 h, then 0.02 mg/kg/min x ≥24h. Dose given as quinidine gluconate. When parasitemia <1% and PO meds tolerated, convert to PO quinine to complete 3d (Africa/South America) or 7 days (Southeast Asia). Also give doxycycline, tetracycline, or clindamycin.
FORMS - Generic gluconate: Tabs, extended-release non-scored 324 mg; Generic sulfate: Tabs, scored immediate-release 200,300 mg. Generic sulfate: Tabs, ext'd-release 300 mg.
NOTES - QRS widening, QT prolongation (risk increased by hypokalemia, hypomagnesemia, or bradycardia), hypotension, hypoglycemia. Contraindicated with ziprasidone. Monitor EKG and BP. Drug interactions with some anti-arrhythmics, digoxin, phenytoin, phenobarbital, rifampin, verapamil. Do not chew, break, or crush extended-release tabs. Do not use with digitalis toxicity, hypotension, AV/bundle branch block, or myasthenia gravis. Quinidine gluconate 267 mg = quinidine sulfate 200 mg.

sotalol (*Betapace, Betapace AF*, ❀*Rylosol*) ▶K ♀B ▶- $$$$
WARNING - Patients should be in a facility for ≥3 days with ECG monitoring, cardiac resuscitation available, and CrCl calculated when initiating or re-initiating Betapace AF. Do not substitute Betapace for Betapace AF.

ADULT - Ventricular arrhythmia (Betapace), symptomatic A-fib/A-flutter (Betapace AF): Start 80 mg PO bid, usual maintenance dose 160-320 mg/day divided bid, max 640 mg/day.
PEDS - Not approved in children.
FORMS - Generic/Trade: Tabs, scored 80,120, 160,240 mg. Trade only: 80,120,160 mg (Betapace AF).
NOTES - Proarrhythmic. Caution, higher incidence of torsades de pointes with doses >320 mg/day, in women, or heart failure. Adjust dose if CrCl <60 mL/min.

LDL CHOLESTEROL GOALS[1]

Risk Category	LDL Goal	Lifestyle Changes[2]	Also Consider Meds at LDL (mg/dL)[3]
High risk: CHD or equivalent risk,[4,5,6] 10-year risk >20%	<100 (optional < 70)[7]	LDL ≥100[8]	≥100 (<100: consider Rx options)[9]
Moderately-high risk: 2+ risk factors,[10] 10-year risk 10-20%	<130 (optional < 100)	LDL ≥130[8]	≥130 (100-129: consider Rx options)[11]
Moderate risk: 2+ risk factors,[10] 10-year risk <10%	<130 mg/dL	LDL ≥130	≥160
Lower risk: 0 to 1 risk factor[5]	<160 mg/dL	LDL ≥160	≥190 (160-189: Rx optional)

1.CHD=coronary heart disease. LDL=low density lipoprotein. Adapted from NCEP: *JAMA* 2001; 285:2486; NCEP Report: Circulation 2004;110:227-239. All 10-year risks based upon Framingham stratification; calculator available at: http://hin.nhlbi.gov/atpiii/calculator.asp?usertype=prof. 2. Dietary modification, weight reduction, exercise. 3. When using LDL lowering therapy, achieve at least 30-40% LDL reduction. 4. Equivalent risk defined as diabetes, other atherosclerotic disease (peripheral artery disease, abdominal aortic aneurysm, symptomatic carotid artery disease), or ≥2 risk factors such that 10 year risk >20%. 5. Chronic kidney disease=CHD risk equivalent [Am J Kidney Dis 2003 Apr;41 (4 suppl 3):I-IV,S1-91]. 6. History of ischemic stroke or transient ischemic attack=CHD risk equivalents (Stroke 2006;37:577-617). 7. For any patient with atherosclerotic disease, may treat to LDL <70 mg/dL (Circulation 2006;113:2363-72). 8. Regardless of LDL, lifestyle changes are indicated when lifestyle-related risk factors (obesity, physical inactivity, ↑TG, ↓ HDL, or metabolic syndrome) are present. 9. If baseline LDL <100, starting LDL lowering therapy is an option based on clinical trials. With ↑TG or ↓HDL, consider combining fibrate or nicotinic acid with LDL lowering drug. 10. Risk factors: Cigarette smoking, HTN (BP ≥140/90 mmHg or on antihypertensive meds), low HDL (<40 mg/dL), family hx of CHD (1° relative: ♂ <55 yo, ♀ <65 yo), age (♂ ≥45 yo, ♀ ≥55 yo). 11. At baseline or after lifestyle changes - initiating therapy to achieve LDL <100 is an option based on clinical trials.

LIPID REDUCTION BY CLASS / AGENT[1]

Drug class/agent	LDL	HDL	TG
Bile acid sequestrants[2]	↓ 15-30%	↑ 3-5%	No change or ↑
Cholesterol absorption inhibitor[3]	↓ 18%	↑ 1%	↓ 8%
Fibrates[4]	↓ 5-20%	↑ 10-20%	↓ 20-50%
Lovastatin+ext'd release niacin[5]*	↓ 30-42%	↑ 20-30%	↓ 32-44%
Niacin[6]*	↓ 5-25%	↑ 15-35%	↓ 20-50%
Omega 3 fatty acids[7]	No change or ↑	↑ 9%	↓ 45%
Statins[8]	↓18-63%	↑ 5-15%	↓ 7-35%
Simvastatin+ezetimibe[9]	↓ 45-60%	↑ 6-10%	↓ 23-31%

1. LDL=low density lipoprotein. HDL=high density lipoprotein. TG=triglycerides. Adapted from NCEP: *JAMA* 2001; 285:2486 and prescribing information. 2. Cholestyramine (4-16 g), colestipol (5-20 g), colesevelam (2.6-3.8 g). 3. Ezetimibe (10 mg). When added to statin therapy, will ↓ LDL 25%, ↑ HDL 3%, ↓ TG 14% in addition to statin effects. 4. Fenofibrate (145-200 mg), gemfibrozil (600 mg BID). 5. Advicor® (20/1000-40/2000 mg). 6. Extended release nicotinic acid (Niaspan® 1-2 g), immediate release (crystalline) nicotinic acid (1.5-3 g), sustained release nicotinic acid (Slo-Niacin® 1-2 g). 7. Lovasa or Omacor® (4 g) 8. Atorvastatin (10-80 mg), fluvastatin (20-80 mg), lovastatin (20-80 mg), pravastatin (20-80 mg), rosuvastatin (5-40 mg), simvastatin (20-80 mg). 9. Vytorin® (10/10-10/80 mg).
*Lowers lipoprotein a.

CORONARY ARTERY DISEASE 10-YEAR RISK

Framingham model for calculating 10-year risk for coronary artery disease (CAD) in patients without diabetes or clinically evident CAD. Diabetes is considered a CAD risk "equivalent", i.e., the prospective risk of CAD in diabetics is similar to those with established CAD. Automated calculator available at: http://hin.nhlbi.nih.gov/atpiii/calculator.asp?usertype=prof (NCEP, JAMA 2001; 285:2497)

MEN

Age	Points	Age	Points
20-34	-9	55-59	8
35-39	-4	60-64	10
40-44	0	65-69	11
45-49	3	70-74	12
50-54	6	75-79	13

Choles-terol*	Age (years)				
	20-39	40-49	50-59	60-69	70-79
<160	0	0	0	0	0
160-199	4	3	2	1	0
200-239	7	5	3	1	0
240-279	9	6	4	2	1
280+	11	8	5	3	1

*Total in mg/dL

Age (years)	20-39	40-49	50-59	60-69	70-79
Nonsmoker	0	0	0	0	0
Smoker	8	5	3	1	1

HDL mg/dL	Points	HDL mg/dL	Points
60+	-1	40-49	1
50-59	0	<40	2

Systolic BP	If Untreated	If Treated
<120 mmHg	0	0
120-129 mmHg	0	1
130-139 mmHg	1	2
140-159 mmHg	1	2
160+ mmHg	2	3

Point Total	10-Year Risk	Point Total	10-Year Risk
0	1%	9	5%
1	1%	10	6%
2	1%	11	8%
3	1%	12	10%
4	1%	13	12%
5	2%	14	16%
6	2%	15	20%
7	3%	16	25%
8	4%	17+	30+%

WOMEN

Age	Points	Age	Points
20-34	-7	55-59	8
35-39	-3	60-64	10
40-44	0	65-69	12
45-49	3	70-74	14
50-54	6	75-79	16

Choles-terol*	Age (years)				
	20-39	40-49	50-59	60-69	70-79
<160	0	0	0	0	0
160-199	4	3	2	1	1
200-239	8	6	4	2	1
240-279	11	8	5	3	2
280+	13	10	7	4	2

Age (years)	20-39	40-49	50-59	60-69	70-79
Nonsmoker	0	0	0	0	0
Smoker	9	7	4	2	1

HDL mg/dL	Points	HDL mg/dL	Points
60+	-1	40-49	1
50-59	0	<40	2

Systolic BP	If Untreated	If Treated
<120 mmHg	0	0
120-129 mmHg	1	3
130-139 mmHg	2	4
140-159 mmHg	3	5
160+ mmHg	4	6

Point Total	10-Year Risk	Point Total	10-Year Risk
< 9	< 1%	17	5%
9	1%	18	6%
10	1%	19	8%
11	1%	20	11%
12	1%	21	14%
13	2%	22	17%
14	2%	23	22%
15	3%	24	27%
16	4%	25+	30+%

CARDIOVASCULAR: Anti-Hyperlipidemic Agents – Bile Acid Sequestrants

cholestyramine (*Questran, Questran Light, Prevalite, LoCHOLEST, LoCHOLEST Light*) ▶Not absorbed ♀C ▶+ $

ADULT - Elevated LDL cholesterol: Start 4 g PO daily-bid before meals, usual maintenance 12-24 g/day in divided doses bid-qid before meals, max 24 g/day.

PEDS - Not approved in children.

UNAPPROVED ADULT - Cholestasis-associated pruritus: 4-8 g bid-tid. Diarrhea: 4-16 g/day.

UNAPPROVED PEDS - Elevated LDL cholesterol: Start 240 mg/kg/day PO divided tid before meals, usual maintenance 8-16 g/day divided tid.

FORMS - Generic/Trade: Powder for oral suspension, 4 g cholestyramine resin / 9 g powder (Questran, LoCHOLEST), 4 g cholestyramine resin / 5 g powder (Questran Light), 4 g cholestyramine resin / 5.5 g powder (Prevalite, LoCHOLEST Light).

NOTES - Administer other drugs at least 1 hour before or 4-6 h after cholestyramine to avoid decreased absorption of the other agent. BID dosing recommended, but may divide up to 6x/day. Mix powder with 60-180 mL of water, milk, fruit juice, or drink. Avoid carbonated liquids for mixing. GI problems common, mainly constipation. May cause elevated triglycerides; do not use when triglycerides >400 mg/dL.

colesevelam (*Welchol*) ▶Not absorbed ♀B ▶+ $$$$

ADULT - Elevated LDL cholesterol: 3 tabs PO bid with meals or 6 tabs once daily with a meal, max dose 7 tabs/day. Same dose when used with statins or other agents.

PEDS - Not approved in children.

FORMS - Trade: Tabs, non-scored, 625 mg.

NOTES - Take with a full glass of water or other non-carbonated liquid. GI problems common, mainly constipation. May cause elevation of HDL cholesterol and triglycerides; do not use when triglycerides >300 mg/dL. Decreases levels of verapamil SR. TSH may increase when co-administered with thyroid replacement therapy; monitor thyroid function.

colestipol (*Colestid, Colestid Flavored*) ▶Not absorbed ♀B ▶+ $$$

ADULT - Elevated LDL cholesterol: Tabs: Start 2 g PO daily-bid, max 16 g/day. Granules: Start 5 g PO daily-bid, increase by 5 g increments as tolerated at 1-2 month intervals, max 30 g/day.

PEDS - Not approved in children.

UNAPPROVED PEDS - 125-250 mg/kg/day PO divided bid-qid, dose range 10-20 g/day.

FORMS - Generic/Trade: Tab 1 g. Granules for oral suspension, 5 g / 7.5 g powder.

NOTES - Administer other drugs ≥1 hour before or 4-6 h after colestipol to avoid decreased absorption of the other agent. Mix granules in at least 90 mL of water, milk, fruit juice, or drink. Avoid carbonated liquids for mixing. Swallow tabs whole with a full glass of liquid to avoid tab disintegration in the esophagus. GI problems common, mainly constipation. May cause elevated triglycerides; do not use when triglycerides >400 mg/dL.

CARDIOVASCULAR: Ant-Hyperlipidemic Agents – HMG-CoA Reductase Inhibitors ("Statins") and Combinations

NOTE: Hepatotoxicity - monitor LFTs initially, approximately 12 weeks after starting/titrating therapy, then annually or more frequently if indicated. May initiate, continue, or increase dose of statin with modest LFT elevation (<3 times upper limit of normal). Repeat LFTs and rule out other causes with isolated, asymptomatic LFT elevation >3 times upper limit of normal. Consider continuing vs. discontinuing statin or reducing statin dose. Patients with chronic liver disease, nonalcoholic fatty liver, or nonalcoholic steatohepatitis may receive statins. Discontinue statin with objective evidence of liver injury; seek cause; consider referral to gastroenterologist or hepatologist. Evaluate muscle symptoms & creatine kinase before starting therapy. Evaluate muscle symptoms 6-12 weeks after starting/increasing therapy & at each follow-up visit. Obtain creatine kinase when patient complains of muscle soreness, tenderness, weakness, or pain. Teach patients to report promptly unexplained muscle pain, tenderness, or weakness; rule out common causes; discontinue if myopathy diagnosed or suspected. With tolerable muscle complaints or asymptomatic creatine kinase increase <10 times upper limit of normal, continue statin at same/reduced dose; use symptoms to guide continuing/discontinuing statin.

With intolerable muscle symptoms with/without creatine kinase elevation, discontinue statin; when asymptomatic, may restart same/different statin at same/lower dose. With rhabdomyolysis, discontinue statin, provide IV hydration; weigh risk/benefit of statin therapy when recovered. These factors increase risk of myopathy: advanced age (especially >80, women >men); multisystem disease (eg, chronic renal insufficiency, especially due to diabetes); multiple medications; perioperative periods; alcohol abuse; grapefruit juice (>1 quart/day); specific concomitant medications: fibrates (especially gemfibrozil), nicotinic acid (rare), cyclosporine, erythromycin, clarithromycin, itraconazole, ketoconazole, protease inhibitors, nefazodone, verapamil, amiodarone. Weigh potential risk of combination therapy against potential benefit.

Advicor (lovastatin + niacin) ▶LK ♀X ▶- $$$
ADULT - Hyperlipidemia: 1 tab PO qhs with a low-fat snack. Establish dose using extended-release niacin first, or if already on lovastatin substitute combo product with lowest niacin dose.
PEDS - Not approved in children.
FORMS - Trade only: Tabs, non-scored extended release lovastatin/niacin 20/500, 20/750, 20/1000, 40/1000 mg.
NOTES - Do not exceed >40/2000 mg. Do not break, chew, or crush. Swallow whole. Aspirin or NSAID 30 min prior may decrease niacin flushing reaction. Niacin may worsen glucose control, peptic ulcer disease, gout, headaches, and menopausal flushing. Significantly lowers LDL-cholesterol and triglycerides, raises HDL-cholesterol. Do not use with potent inhibitors of cytochrome P450 3A4 enzyme system (clarithromycin, erythromycin, grapefruit juice >1 quart /day, HIV protease inhibitors, itraconazole, ketoconazole, nefazodone, telithromycin); increases risk of myopathy. Do not exceed 20 mg/ day of lovastatin component when used with cyclosporine, danazol, fibrates, or niacin ≥1 g/day; do not exceed 40 mg/day of lovastatin component when used with amiodarone or verapamil. With concomitant cyclosporine or danazol, start with 10 mg daily of lovastatin.

atorvastatin (Lipitor) ▶L ♀X ▶- $$$
ADULT - Hyperlipidemia/prevention of cardiovascular events, including Type 2 DM: Start 10 mg PO daily, 40 mg daily for LDL-C reduction >45%, increase at ≥4-week intervals to a max of 80 mg/day.

PEDS - Hyperlipidemia, ≥10 years: Same as adult.
UNAPPROVED ADULT - Prevention of cardiovascular events & death post-acute coronary syndrome or with stable CAD, or prevention of stroke/cardiovascular events with recent stroke /TIA & no CHD: 80 mg PO daily.
FORMS - Trade only: Tabs, non-scored 10,20,40,80 mg.
NOTES - Metabolism may be decreased by known inhibitors of cytochrome P450 3A4 enzyme system (erythromycin, clarithromycin, cyclosporine, ketoconazole, itraconazole, HIV protease inhibitors, nefazodone, grapefruit and grapefruit juice), increasing risk of myopathy. Increased risk of myopathy and rhabdomyolysis when used with a fibric acid agent or niacin. Give either 1 hour before or 4 hours after colestipol or cholestyramine.

Caduet (amlodipine + atorvastatin) ▶L ♀X ▶- $$$$
ADULT - Simultaneous treatment of HTN and hypercholesterolemia: Establish dose using component drugs first. Dosing interval: daily
PEDS - Not approved in children.
FORMS - Trade only: Tabs, 2.5/10, 2.5/20, 2.5/40, 5/10, 5/20, 5/40, 5/80, 10/10, 10/20, 10/40, 10/80 mg.

fluvastatin (Lescol, Lescol XL) ▶L ♀X ▶- $$$
ADULT - Hyperlipidemia: Start 20 mg PO qhs for LDL-C reduction of <25%, 40-80 mg qhs for LDL-C reduction of ≥25%, max 80 mg/day, give 80 mg daily (Lescol XL) or 40 mg bid. Prevention of cardiac events post percutaneous coronary intervention: 80 mg of extended release PO daily, max 80 mg daily.
PEDS - Hyperlipidemia: Start 20 mg PO qhs, max 80 mg daily (XL) or divided bid.
FORMS - Trade only: Caps, 20, 40 mg; tab, extended-release, non-scored 80 mg.
NOTES - Not metabolized substantially by the cytochrome P450 isoenzyme 3A4, so less potential for drug interactions. Increased risk of myopathy and rhabdomyolysis when used with a fibric acid agent, niacin, or colchicine. Give either 1 hour before or 4 hours after colestipol or cholestyramine.

lovastatin (Mevacor, Altoprev) ▶L ♀X ▶- $$$
ADULT - Hyperlipidemia/prevention of cardiovascular events: Start 20 mg PO daily with the evening meal, increase at ≥4 week intervals to max 80 mg/day (daily or divided bid). Altocor dosed daily with max dose 60 mg/day.

PEDS - Hyperlipidemia, ≥10 years: Same as adult.

FORMS - Generic/Trade: Tabs, non-scored 20,40 mg. Trade only: Tabs, extended-release (Altoprev) 20,40,60 mg.

NOTES - Do not use with potent inhibitors of cytochrome P450 3A4 enzyme system (clarithromycin, erythromycin, grapefruit juice >1 quart /day, HIV protease inhibitors, itraconazole, ketoconazole, nefazodone, telithromycin); increases risk of myopathy. Do not exceed 20 mg/ day when used with cyclosporine, danazol, fibrates, or niacin ≥1 g/day; do not exceed 40 mg/day when used with amiodarone or verapamil. With concomitant cyclosporine or danazol, start with 10 mg daily. Give either 1 hour before or 4 hours after colestipol or cholestyramine. Measure LFTs prior to starting if history of liver disease or if using ≥40 mg/day.

pravastatin (*Pravachol*) ▶L ♀X ▶- $$$

ADULT - Hyperlipidemia/prevention of cardiovascular events: Start 40 mg PO daily, increase at ≥4-week intervals to max 80 mg/day. Renal or hepatic impairment: Start 10 mg PO daily.

PEDS - Hyperlipidemia, 8-13 yo: 20 mg PO daily. 14-18 yo: 40 mg PO daily.

FORMS - Generic/Trade: Tabs, non-scored 10, 20, 40, 80 mg. Generic only: Tabs 30 mg.

NOTES - Not metabolized substantially by the cytochrome P450 isoenzyme 3A4, less potential for drug interactions. Increased risk of myopathy and rhabdomyolysis when used with a fibric acid agent. Give either 1 hour before or 4 hours after colestipol or cholestyramine.

rosuvastatin (*Crestor*) ▶L ♀X ▶- $$$

ADULT - Hyperlipidemia: Start 10 mg daily, may adjust dose after 2-4 weeks. Do not start with 40 mg; use 40 mg only with severe hypercholesterolemia when treatment goal not achieved with 20 mg/day. Severe renal impairment: Start 5 mg PO daily, max 10 mg/day. With predisposing factors for myopathy (renal impairment, advanced age, hypothyroidism): Start 5 mg PO daily. Asians: Start 5 mg PO daily, max 20 mg daily.

PEDS - Canada only: May use with age >8 yrs with homozygous familial hypercholesterolemia. Specialist should supervise use.

FORMS - Trade only: Tabs non-scored 5, 10, 20, 40 mg.

NOTES - Do not exceed 10 mg/day with severe renal impairment, gemfibrozil, or the combination of lopinavir and ritonavir. Do not exceed 5 mg/day with cyclosporine. Give aluminum & magnesium containing antacids >2 hours after rosuvastatin. May potentiate effects of warfarin; monitor INR. Proteinuria, with unknown clinical significance, reported with 40 mg/day; consider dose reduction when using 40 mg/day with unexplained persistent proteinuria. May increase levels of ethinyl estradiol & norgestrel. Use cautiously with other drugs that may decrease levels/activity of endogenous steroid hormones (ketoconazole, spironolactone, cimetidine). Asians may have higher blood concentrations & more risk of side effects than Caucasians. Temporarily withhold with acute, serious condition suggestive of myopathy or predisposing to renal failure from rhabdomyolysis (e.g. sepsis, hypotension, dehydration, major surgery, trauma, severe metabolic / endocrine / electrolyte disorders, uncontrolled seizures). Give either 1 hour before or 4 hours after colestipol or cholestyramine.

simvastatin (*Zocor*) ▶L ♀X ▶- $$$$

ADULT - Hyperlipidemia: Start 20-40 mg PO q pm. Reduce cardiovascular mortality/events in high risk for coronary heart disease event (existing coronary heart disease, DM, peripheral vascular disease, history of stroke or cerebrovascular disease): 40 mg q pm. Increase prn at ≥4 week intervals to max 80 mg/day.

PEDS - Hyperlipidemia, ≥10 years: Start 10 mg PO q pm, max 40 mg/day.

FORMS - Generic/Trade: Tabs, non-scored 5, 10, 20, 40, 80 mg.

NOTES - Do not use with potent inhibitors of cytochrome P450 3A4 enzyme system (clarithromycin, erythromycin, grapefruit juice >1 quart /day, HIV protease inhibitors, itraconazole, ketoconazole, nefazodone, telithromycin); increases risk of myopathy. Do not exceed 10 mg/ day when used with gemfibrozil, cyclosporine, danazol; or 20 mg/day when used with amiodarone or verapamil; increased risk of myopathy. Use caution with other fibrates, niacin ≥1 g/ day; increases risk of myopathy. Give either 1 hour before or 4 hours after colestipol or cholestyramine.

Vytorin (ezetimibe + simvastatin) ▶L ♀X ▶- $$$

ADULT - Hyperlipidemia: Start 10/20 mg PO q pm, max 10/80 mg/day. Start 10/40 if need >55% LDL reduction.

PEDS - Not approved in children.

FORMS - Trade only: Tabs, non-scored ezetimibe/simvastatin 10/10, 10/20, 10/40, 10/80 mg.

STATINS*

Minimum Dose for 30-40% LDL Reduction	LDL	LFT Monitoring**
atorvastatin 10 mg	-39%	B, 12 wk, semiannually
fluvastatin 40 mg bid	-36%	B, 12 wk
fluvastatin XL 80 mg	-35%	B, 12 wk
lovastatin 40 mg	-31%	B
pravastatin 40mg	-34%	B
rosuvastatin 5 mg	-45%	B, 12 wk, semiannually
simvastatin 20 mg	-38%	B, ***

*Adapted from *Circulation* 2004;110:227-239. Data taken from prescribing information for primary hypercholesterolemia. B=baseline, LDL=low-density lipoprotein, LFT=liver function tests. Will get ~6% decrease in LDL with every doubling of dose. **From prescribing info; also, when clinically indicated. National Lipid Association schedule for LFT monitoring: baseline, ~12 weeks after starting/titrating therapy, periodically, when clinically indicated. ***Get LFTs prior to & 3 months after dose increase to 80 mg, then semiannually for first year.

CARDIOVASCULAR: Anti-Hyperlipidemic Agents – Other

bezafibrate (✱*Bezalip*) ▶K ♀D ▶- $$$
ADULT - Canada only. Hyperlipidemia/hypertriglyceridemia: 200 mg of immediate release PO bid-tid, or 400 mg of sustained release PO q am or q evening with or after food. Reduce dose in renal insufficiency or dialysis. The 400 mg SR tablet should not be used if CrCl <60 mL/min or creat >1.5 mg/dL.
PEDS - Not approved in children.
FORMS - Trade only: Immediate release tab: 200 mg. Sustained release tab: 400 mg.
NOTES - Increased risk of myopathy and rhabdomyolysis when used with a statin. May increase the effect of warfarin; reduce oral anticoagulant dose by ~50%; monitor INR. Do not use in primary biliary cirrhosis. Take either ≥2 hours before or ≥4 hours after colestipol or cholestyramine.

ezetimibe (*Zetia*, ✱*Ezetrol*) ▶L ♀C ▶? $$$
WARNING - May increase cyclosporine levels.
ADULT - Hyperlipidemia: 10 mg PO daily alone or in combination with statin or fenofibrate.
PEDS - Not approved in children.
FORMS - Trade only: Tabs non-scored 10 mg
NOTES - Take either ≥2 hours before or ≥4 hours after colestipol or cholestyramine. Monitor cyclosporine levels (may increase). When used with statin, monitor LFTs at initiation and then per statin instructions.

fenofibrate (*Tricor, Lipofen, Lofibra, Antara, Triglide, ✱Lipidil Micro, Lipidil Supra, Lipidil EZ*) ▶LK ♀C ▶- $$$
ADULT - Hypertriglyceridemia: Tricor tablets: Start 48-145 mg PO daily, max 145 mg/day. Triglide: 50-160 mg PO daily, max 160 mg/day. Lipofen: 50-150 mg PO daily, max 150 mg/day. Lofibra or generic tablets: 54-160 mg, max 160 mg daily. Lofibra or generic micronized capsules: 67-200 mg PO daily, max 200 mg daily. Antara micronized capsules: 43-130 mg PO daily; max 130 mg daily. Hypercholesterolemia / mixed dyslipidemia: Tricor tablets: 145 mg PO daily. Triglide: 160 mg daily. Lipofen: 150 mg daily. Generic tablets: 160 mg daily. Lofibra or generic micronized capsules: 200 mg PO daily. Antara micronized capsules: 130 mg PO daily. Renal impairment, elderly: Tricor tablets: Start 48 mg PO daily; Triglide: Start 50 mg PO daily; Lipofen: Start 50 mg daily; Antara micronized capsules: Start 43 mg PO daily.
PEDS - Not approved in children.
FORMS - Generic only: Tabs, non-scored 54, 160 mg. Generic/Trade (Lofibra) micronized caps, 67, 134, 200 mg. Trade: Tricor tabs, non-scored 48,145 mg. Triglide tabs, non-scored 50, 160 mg. Antara micronized caps 43, 130 mg. Lipofen non-scored tabs 50,100,150 mg.
NOTES - Micronized capsules should be taken with food to increase plasma concentrations. Conversion between forms: Lofibra or generic 200 mg cap with food = 145 mg Tricor; Antara 130 mg = 200 mg Lofibra or generic under low-fat fed conditions; Lipofen 150 mg with food = Tricor 160 mg with food. Monitor LFTs, dose related hepatotoxicity. Increased risk of myopathy and rhabdomyolysis when used with a statin. May increase the effect of warfarin, monitor INR. Tricor 48 mg and 145 mg replaces Tricor 54 mg and 160 mg.

gemfibrozil (*Lopid*) ▶LK ♀C ▶? $$
ADULT - Hypertriglyceridemia / primary prevention of artery heart disease: 600 mg PO bid 30

minutes before meals.
PEDS - Not approved in children.
FORMS - Generic/Trade: Tabs, scored 600 mg.
NOTES - Increased risk of myopathy and rhabdomyolysis when used with a statin or with moderate/severe renal dysfunction. May increase the effect of warfarin, monitor INR. Avoid with repaglinide; increased risk of hypoglycemia. Avoid itraconazole with combined gemfibrozil and repaglinide.

CARDIOVASCULAR: Antihypertensive Combinations

BY TYPE: ACE Inhibitor/Diuretic: *Accuretic, Capozide, Inhibace Plus, Lotensin HCT, Monopril HCT, Prinzide, Uniretic, Vaseretic, Zestoretic.* ACE Inhibitor/Calcium Channel Blocker: *Lexxel, Lotrel, Tarka.* Angiotensin Receptor Blocker/Diuretic: *Atacand HCT, Avalide, Benicar HCT, Diovan HCT, Hyzaar, Micardis HCT, Teveten HCT.* Angiotensin Receptor Blocker/Calcium Channel Blocker: *Exforge.* Betablocker/Diuretic: *Corzide, Dutoprol, Inderide, Lopressor HCT, Tenoretic, Timolide, Ziac.* Diuretic combinations: *Aldactazide, Dyazide, Maxzide, Moduretic, Triazide.* Diuretic/miscellaneous antihypertensive: *Aldoril, Apresazide, Clorpres, Minizide.*

NOTE: Dosage should first be adjusted by using each drug separately. See component drugs for metabolism, pregnancy, and lactation. None are approved in children.

Accuretic **(quinapril + hydrochlorothiazide) $$**
ADULT - HTN: Dosing interval: daily.
FORMS - Generic/Trade: Tabs, 10/12.5, 20/12.5, 20/25.

Aldactazide **(spironolactone + hydrochlorothiazide) $$**
ADULT - HTN: Dosing interval: daily-bid.
FORMS - Generic/Trade: Tabs, non-scored 25/25, scored 50/50 mg.

Aldoril **(methyldopa + hydrochlorothiazide) $$**
ADULT - HTN: Dosing interval: bid.
FORMS - Generic/Trade: Tabs, non-scored, 250/15 (Aldoril-15), 250/25 mg (Aldoril-25). Trade only: Tabs, non-scored, 500/30 (Aldoril D30), 500/50 mg (Aldoril D50).

Apresazide **(hydralazine + hydrochlorothiazide) $$**
ADULT - HTN: Dosing interval: bid.
FORMS - Generic only: Caps 25/25, 50/50 mg.

Atacand HCT **(candesartan + hydrochlorothiazide, ✿ Atacand Plus) $$$**
ADULT - HTN: Dosing interval: daily.
FORMS - Trade only: Tab, non-scored 16/12.5, 32/12.5 mg.

Avalide **(irbesartan + hydrochlorothiazide) $$$**
ADULT - HTN: Dosing interval: daily.
FORMS - Trade only: Tabs, non-scored 150/12.5, 300/12.5, 300/25 mg.

Benicar HCT **(olmesartan + hydrochlorothiazide) $$$**
ADULT - HTN: Dosing interval: daily.
FORMS - Trade only: Tabs, non-scored 20/12.5, 40/12.5, 40/25

Capozide **(captopril + hydrochlorothiazide) $$**
ADULT - HTN: Dosing interval: bid-tid.
FORMS - Generic/Trade: Tabs, scored 25/15, 25/25, 50/15, 50/25 mg.

Clorpres **(clonidine + chlorthalidone) $$$**
ADULT - HTN: Dosing interval: bid-tid.
FORMS - Trade only: Tabs, scored 0.1/15, 0.2/15, 0.3/15 mg.

Corzide **(nadolol+bendroflumethiazide)$$$**
ADULT - HTN: Dosing interval: daily.
FORMS - Generic/Trade: Tabs 40/5, 80/5 mg.

Diovan HCT **(valsartan + hydrochlorothiazide) $$$**
ADULT - HTN: Dosing interval: daily.
FORMS - Trade only: Tabs, non-scored 80/12.5, 160/12.5, 160/25, 320/12.5, 320/25 mg.

Dutoprol **(metoprolol + hydrochlorothiazide) $$**
ADULT - HTN: Dosing interval: daily.
FORMS - Trade only: Tabs, non-scored 25/12.5, 50/12.5 mg. Tabs, scored 100/12.5 mg

Dyazide **(triamterene + hydrochlorothiazide) $**
ADULT - HTN: Dosing interval: daily.
FORMS - Generic/Trade: Caps, (Dyazide) 37.5/25, (generic only) 50/25 mg.
NOTES - Dyazide 37.5/25 cap same combination as Maxzide-25 tab.

Exforge **(amlodipine + valsartan) $$$$**
ADULT - HTN: Dosing interval: daily.
FORMS - Trade only: Tabs, non-scored 5/160, 5/320, 10/160, 10/320 mg.

Hyzaar **(losartan+hydrochlorothiazide) $$$**

ADULT - Dosing interval: daily. Severe HTN: Start 50/12.5 PO daily, may increase to 100/25 PO daily after 2-4 weeks. Stroke risk reduction in HTN & left ventricular hypertrophy (stroke risk reduction may not occur in Blacks).
FORMS - Trade only: Tabs, non-scored 50/12.5, 100/12.5, 100/25 mg.

Inderide (propranolol + hydrochlorothiazide) $$
ADULT - HTN: Dosing interval: daily-bid.
FORMS - Generic/Trade: Tabs, scored 40/25, 80/25.
NOTES - Do not crush or chew cap contents. Swallow whole.

Inhibace Plus (cilazapril + hydrochlorothiazide) $$
ADULT - Canada only: Dosing interval daily.
FORMS - Trade only: Scored tabs 5 mg cilazapril + 12.5 mg HCTZ.

Lexxel (enalapril + felodipine) $$
ADULT - HTN: Dosing interval: daily.
FORMS - Trade: Tabs non-scored 5/2.5, 5/5mg.
NOTES - Do not crush or chew, swallow whole.

Lopressor HCT (metoprolol + hydrochlorothiazide) $$$
ADULT - HTN: Dosing interval: daily-bid.
FORMS - Generic/Trade: Tabs, scored 50/25, 100/25, 100/50 mg.

Lotensin HCT (benazepril + hydrochlorothiazide) $$
ADULT - HTN: Dosing interval: daily.
FORMS - Generic/Trade: Tabs, scored 5/6.25, 10/12.5, 20/12.5, 20/25 mg.

Lotrel (amlodipine + benazepril) $$$
ADULT - HTN: Dosing interval: daily.
FORMS - Generic/Trade: Cap, 2.5/10, 5/10, 5/20, 10/20 mg. Trade: Cap, 5/40, 10/40 mg.

Maxzide (triamterene + hydrochlorothiazide, ✦*Triazide*) $
ADULT - HTN: Dosing interval: daily.
FORMS - Generic/Trade: Tabs, scored (Maxzide-25) 37.5/25 (Maxzide) 75/50 mg.

Maxzide-25 (triamterene + hydrochlorothiazide) $
ADULT - HTN: Dosing interval: daily.
FORMS - Generic/Trade: Tabs, scored (Maxzide-25) 37.5/25 (Maxzide) 75/50 mg.

Micardis HCT (telmisartan + hydrochlorothiazide, ✦*Micardis Plus*) $$$
ADULT - HTN: Dosing interval: daily.
FORMS - Trade only: Tabs, non-scored 40/12.5, 80/12.5, 80/25 mg.
NOTES - Swallow tabs whole, do not break or crush. Caution in hepatic insufficiency.

Minizide (prazosin + polythiazide) $$$
ADULT - HTN: Dosing interval: bid-tid.
FORMS - Trade: cap, 1/0.5, 2/0.5, 5/0.5 mg.

Moduretic (amiloride + hydrochlorothiazide, ✦*Moduret*) $
ADULT - HTN: Dosing interval: daily.
FORMS - Generic/Trade: Tabs, scored 5/50 mg.

Monopril HCT (fosinopril + hydrochlorothiazide) $$
ADULT - HTN: Dosing interval: daily.
FORMS - Generic/Trade: Tabs, non-scored 10/12.5, scored 20/12.5 mg.

Prinzide (lisinopril + hydrochlorothiazide) $$
ADULT - HTN: Dosing interval: daily.
FORMS - Generic/Trade: Tabs, non-scored 10/12.5, 20/12.5, 20/25 mg.

Tarka (trandolapril + verapamil) $$$
ADULT - HTN: Dosing interval: daily.
FORMS - Trade only: Tabs, non-scored 2/180, 1/240, 2/240, 4/240 mg.
NOTES - Contains verapamil extended release; do not chew or crush, swallow whole.

Tenoretic (atenolol + chlorthalidone) $$
ADULT - HTN: Dosing interval: daily.
FORMS - Generic/Trade: Tabs, scored 50/25, non-scored 100/25 mg.

Teveten HCT (eprosartan + hydrochlorothiazide) $$
ADULT - HTN: Dosing interval: daily.
FORMS - Trade only: Tabs, non-scored 600/12.5, 600/25 mg.

Timolide (timolol + hydrochlorothiazide) $$
ADULT - HTN: Dosing interval: daily-bid.
FORMS - Trade: Tabs, non-scored 10/25 mg.

Uniretic (moexipril + hydrochlorothiazide) $$
ADULT - HTN: Dosing interval: daily-bid.
FORMS - Generic/Trade: Tabs, scored 7.5/12.5, 15/12.5, 15/25 mg.

Vaseretic (enalapril + hydrochlorothiazide) $$
ADULT - HTN: Dosing interval: daily-bid.
FORMS - Generic/Trade: Tabs, non-scored 5/12.5, 10/25 mg.

Zestoretic (lisinopril + hydrochlorothiazide) $$
ADULT - HTN: Dosing interval: daily.
FORMS - Generic/Trade: Tabs, non-scored 10/12.5, 20/12.5, 20/25 mg.

Ziac (bisoprolol + hydrochlorothiazide) $$
ADULT - HTN: Dosing interval: daily.
FORMS - Generic/Trade: Tabs, non-scored 2.5/6.25, 5/6.25, 10/6.25 mg.

CARDIOVASCULAR: Antihypertensives – Other

aliskiren (*Tekturna*) ▶LK ♀- ▶-? $$$
ADULT - HTN: 150 mg PO daily, max 300 mg/day.
PEDS - Not approved in children.
FORMS - Trade only: Tabs, non-scored 150, 300 mg.
NOTES - Not studied with severe renal impairment (creat ≥1.7 mg/dL for women, ≥2.0 mg/dL for men, and/or estimated GFR <30 mL/min), heart failure, or with max doses of ACEIs. Best absorbed on empty stomach. High fat meals decrease absorption. May decrease effects of furosemide. Monitor potassium and renal function when given with related medications (ie. ACEIs, ARBs). May increase creatine kinase, uric acid levels.

diazoxide (*Hyperstat, Proglycem*) ▶L ♀C ▶- $$$$$
ADULT - Severe HTN: 1-3 mg/kg (up to 150 mg) IV q5-15 min until BP is controlled. Hypoglycemia: initially 3 mg/kg/day PO divided equally q8h, usual maintenance 3-8 mg/kg/day divided equally q8-12 hours, max 10-15 mg/kg/day.
PEDS - Severe HTN: same as adult. Hypoglycemia: neonates and infants, initially 10 mg/kg/day divided equally q8h, usual maintenance dose 8-15 mg/kg/day divided equally q8-12h; children, same as adult.
UNAPPROVED ADULT - Preeclampsia/eclampsia: 30 mg IV every few minutes until control of BP is achieved.
FORMS - Trade only: Susp 50 mg/mL (30 mL).
NOTES - Severe hyperglycemia possible. Monitor for edema and heart failure exacerbation during administration; consider diuretics.

fenoldopam (*Corlopam*) ▶LK ♀B ▶? $$$$$
ADULT - Severe HTN: 10 mg in 250 mL D5W (40 mcg/mL), start at 0.1 mcg/kg/min for 70 kg adult = 11 mL/h), titrate q15 min, usual effective dose 0.1-1.6 mcg/kg/min. Lower initial doses (0.03-0.1 mcg/kg/min) associated with less reflex tachycardia.
PEDS - Reduce BP: Start 0.2 mcg/kg/min, increase by up to 0.3-0.5 mcg/kg/min q 20–30 min. Max infusion 0.8 mcg/kg/min. Administer in hospital by continuous infusion pump; use max 4 hrs; monitor BP & HR continuously. Refer to package insert for dilution instructions & infusion rates.
UNAPPROVED ADULT - Prevention of contrast nephropathy in those at risk (conflicting evidence of efficacy): Start 0.03 mcg/kg/min infusion 60 min prior to dye. Titrate infusion q15 min up to 0.1 mcg/kg/min if BP tolerates. Maintain infusion (with concurrent saline) up to 4-6 hours after procedure.
NOTES - Avoid use with beta blockers; if must be done, watch for sudden hypotension. Patients at high-risk for contrast nephropathy include age >70, creat >1.5 mg/dL, HTN, DM, heart failure. Use cautiously with glaucoma or increased intraocular HTN. Concurrent acetaminophen may increase fenoldopam levels.

hydralazine (*Apresoline*) ▶LK ♀C ▶+ $
ADULT - HTN: Start 10 mg PO bid-qid for 2-4 days, increase to 25 mg bid-qid, then 50 mg bid-qid if necessary, max 300 mg/day. Hypertensive emergency: 10-50 mg IM or 10-20 mg IV. Use lower doses initially & repeat prn to control BP. Preeclampsia/eclampsia: 5-10 mg IV initially, followed by 5-10 mg IV every 20-30 min as needed to control BP.
PEDS - Not approved in children.
UNAPPROVED ADULT - Heart failure: Start 10-25 mg PO tid, target dose 75 mg tid, max 100 mg tid. Use in combination with isosorbide dinitrate for patients intolerant to ACE inhibitors
UNAPPROVED PEDS - HTN: Start 0.75-1 mg/kg/day PO divided bid-qid, increase slowly over 3-4 weeks up to 7.5 mg/kg/day; initial IV dose 1.7-3.5 mg/kg/day divided in 4-6 doses. HTN urgency: 0.1-0.2 mg/kg IM/IV q4-6h as needed. Max single dose, 25 mg PO and 20 mg IV.
FORMS - Generic/Trade: Tabs, non-scored 10,25,50,100 mg.
NOTES - Headache, nausea, dizziness, tachycardia, peripheral edema, lupus-like syndrome. Usually used in combination with diuretic and beta-blocker to counter side effects.

mecamylamine (*Inversine*) ▶K ♀C ▶- $$$$$
ADULT - Severe HTN: Start 2.5 mg PO bid, increase as needed by 2.5 mg increments no sooner than every 2 days, usual maintenance dose 25 mg/day divided bid-qid.
PEDS - Not approved in children.
FORMS - Trade only: Tabs, scored, 2.5 mg.
NOTES - Orthostatic hypotension, especially during dosage titration. Monitor BP standing and supine. Rebound, severe hypertension with sudden drug withdrawal. Discontinue slowly and use other antihypertensives.

metyrosine (*Demser*) ▶K ♀C ▶? $$$$$

ADULT - Pheochromocytoma: Start 250 mg PO qid, increase by 250-500 mg/day as needed, max dose 4 g/day.

PEDS - Pheochromocytoma >12 yo: Same as adult.

FORMS - Trade only: Caps, 250 mg.

minoxidil (Loniten) ▶K ♀C ▶+ $$

ADULT - Refractory HTN: Start 2.5-5 mg PO daily, increase at no less than 3 day intervals, usual dose 10-40 mg daily, max 100 mg/day.

PEDS - Not approved in children <12 yo.

UNAPPROVED PEDS - HTN: Start 0.2 mg/kg PO daily, increase q3 days prn up to 0.25-1 mg/kg/day daily or divided bid; max 50 mg/day.

FORMS - Generic/Trade: Tabs, scored, 2.5,10 mg.

NOTES - Edema, weight gain, hypertrichosis, may exacerbate heart failure. Usually used in combination with a diuretic and a beta-blocker to counteract side effects .

nitroprusside (Nipride, Nitropress) ▶RBC's ♀C ▶- $

WARNING - May cause significant hypotension. Reconstituted solution must be further diluted before use. Cyanide toxicity may occur, especially with high infusion rates (10 mcg/kg/min), hepatic/renal impairment, and prolonged infusions (>3-7 days). Protect from light.

ADULT - Hypertensive emergency: 50 mg in 250 mL D5W (200 mcg/mL), start at 0.3 mcg/kg/min (for 70 kg adult = 6 mL/h) via IV infusion, titrate slowly, usual range 0.3-10 mcg/kg/min, max 10 mcg/kg/min.

PEDS - Severe HTN: Same as adult.

NOTES - Discontinue if inadequate response to 10 mcg/kg/min after 10 minutes. Cyanide toxicity with high doses, hepatic/renal impairment, and prolonged infusions, check thiocyanate levels. Protect IV infusion minibag from light.

phenoxybenzamine (Dibenzyline) ▶KL ♀C ▶? $$$$$

ADULT - Pheochromocytoma: Start 10 mg PO bid, increase slowly qod as needed, usual dose 20-40 mg bid-tid, max 120 mg/day.

PEDS - Not approved in children.

UNAPPROVED PEDS - Pheochromocytoma: 0.2 mg/kg/day PO daily, initial dose ≤10 mg, increase slowly qod as needed, usual dose 0.4-1.2 mg/kg/day.

FORMS - Trade only: Caps, 10 mg.

NOTES - Patients should be observed after each dosage increase for symptomatic hypotension and other adverse effects. Do not use for essential HTN.

phentolamine (Regitine, Rogitine) ▶Plasma ♀C ▶? $$

ADULT - Diagnosis of pheochromocytoma: 5 mg IV/IM. Rapid IV administration is preferred. An immediate, marked decrease in BP should occur, typically, 60 mm Hg SBP and 25 mm Hg DBP decrease in 2 minutes. HTN during pheochromocytoma surgery: 5 mg IV/IM 1-2h pre-op, 5 mg IV during surgery prn.

PEDS - Diagnosis of pheochromocytoma: 0.05-0.1 mg/kg IV/IM, up to 5 mg per dose. Rapid IV administration is preferred. An immediate, marked decrease in BP should occur, typically, 60 mmHg SBP and 25 mmHg DBP decrease in 2 minutes. HTN during pheochromocytoma surgery: 0.05-0.1 mg/kg IV/IM 1-2h pre-op, repeat q2-4h prn.

UNAPPROVED ADULT - IV extravasation of catecholamines: 5-10 mg in 10 mL NS, inject 1-5 mL SC (in divided doses) around extravasation site. Hypertensive crisis: 5-15 mg IV.

UNAPPROVED PEDS - IV extravasation of catecholamines: neonates, 2.5-5 mg in 10 mL NS, inject 1 mL SC (in divided doses) around extravasation site; children, same as adult.

NOTES - Weakness, flushing, hypotension; priapism with intracavernous injection. Use within 12h of extravasation. Distributed to hospital pharmacies, at no charge, only for use in life-threatening situations, call (888) 669-6682.

CARDIOVASCULAR: Antiplatelet Drugs

abciximab (ReoPro) ▶Plasma ♀C ▶? $$$$$

ADULT - Platelet aggregation inhibition, prevention of acute cardiac ischemic events associated with PTCA: 0.25 mg/kg IV bolus over 1 min via separate infusion line 10-60 min before procedure, then 0.125 mcg/kg/min up to 10 mcg/min infusion for 12h. Unstable angina not responding to standard therapy when percutaneous coronary intervention (PCI) is planned within 24h: 0.25 mg/kg IV bolus over 1 min via separate infusion line, followed by 10 mcg/min IV infusion for 18-24h, concluding 1h after PCI.

PEDS - Not approved in children.

NOTES - Thrombocytopenia possible. Discontinue abciximab, heparin, and aspirin if uncontrollable bleeding occurs.

Aggrenox (aspirin + dipyridamole) ▸LK ♀D ▸? $$$$

ADULT - Prevention of stroke after TIA/stroke: 1 cap PO bid.

PEDS - Not approved in children.

FORMS - Trade only: Caps, 25 mg aspirin/ 200 mg extended-release dipyridamole.

NOTES - Do not crush or chew Caps. May need supplemental aspirin for prevention of MI.

clopidogrel (*Plavix*) ▸LK ♀B ▸? $$$$

WARNING - Rarely may cause life-threatening thrombotic thrombocytopenia purpura (TTP), usually during the first 2 weeks of therapy.

ADULT - Reduction of thrombotic events after recent AMI, recent stroke, established peripheral arterial disease: 75 mg PO daily. Acute coronary syndrome, non-ST segment elevation: 300 mg loading dose, then 75 mg PO daily in combination with aspirin. ST segment elevation MI: Start with/without 300 mg loading dose, then 75 mg PO daily in combination with aspirin, with/without thrombolytics.

PEDS - Not approved in children.

UNAPPROVED ADULT - Before percutaneous coronary intervention: 300 mg PO ≥6 hrs before procedure. Post percutaneous coronary intervention: 75 mg daily in combination with aspirin for ≥1 month after bare metal stent placement, ≥3 months after sirolimus-eluting stent placement, ≥6 months after paclitaxel-eluting stent placement, & preferably up to 12 months in patients not at high risk for bleeding. Post percutaneous coronary brachytherapy: 75 mg daily in combination with aspirin indefinitely. Post ST-elevation MI with aspirin allergy: 75 mg PO daily. Reduction of thrombotic events in high-risk patient after TIA: 75 mg PO daily.

FORMS - Generic/Trade: Tab, non-scored 75 mg.

NOTES - Prolongs bleeding time. Discontinue use 7 days before surgery, except in first year post-coronary stent implantation. Loading dose 300 mg PO >6 hours prior to procedure may be used for prevention of cardiac stent occlusion. Contraindicated with active pathologic bleeding (peptic ulcer or intracranial bleed). Concomitant ASA increases bleeding risk. Cardiovascular (but not stroke) patients may receive additional benefit when given with ASA. Should not be used with aspirin for primary prevention of cardiovascular events.

dipyridamole (*Persantine*) ▸L ♀B ▸? $

ADULT - Prevention of thromboembolic complications of cardiac valve replacement: 75-100 mg PO qid in combination with warfarin.

PEDS - Not approved in children <12 yo.

UNAPPROVED ADULT - Platelet aggregation inhibition: 150-400 mg/day PO divided tid-qid.

FORMS - Generic/Trade: Tabs, non-scored 25, 50, 75 mg.

NOTES - Not effective for angina; may cause chest pain when used in CAD.

eptifibatide (*Integrilin*) ▸K ♀B ▸? $$$$$

ADULT - Acute coronary syndrome (unstable angina/non-ST-segment elevation MI): Load 180 mcg/kg IV bolus, then IV infusion 2 mcg/kg/min for up to 72 hr. If percutaneous coronary intervention (PCI) occurs during the infusion, continue infusion for 18-24 hr after procedure. PCI: Load 180 mcg/kg IV bolus just before procedure, followed by infusion 2 mcg/kg/min and a second 180 mcg/kg IV bolus 10 min after the first bolus. Continue infusion for up to 18-24 hr (minimum 12 hr) after the procedure. Renal impairment (CrCl <50 mL/min): No change in bolus dose; decrease infusion to 1 mcg/kg/min. Obese patient (>121 kg): Max bolus dose 22.6 mg; max infusion rate 15 mg/hr. Renal impairment and obese: Max bolus dose 22.6 mg; max infusion rate 7.5 mg/hr.

PEDS - Not approved in children.

NOTES - Discontinue infusion prior to CABG. Thrombocytopenia possible. Concomitant aspirin & heparin/enoxaparin use recommended, unless contraindicated. Contraindicated in dialysis patients.

ticlopidine (*Ticlid*) ▸L ♀B ▸? $$$$

WARNING - May cause life-threatening neutropenia, agranulocytosis, and thrombotic thrombocytopenia purpura (TTP). TTP usually occurs during the first two weeks of treatment. Monitor CBC routinely.

ADULT - Due to adverse effects, clopidogrel preferred. Platelet aggregation inhibition/reduction of thrombotic stroke: 250 mg PO bid with food. Prevention of cardiac stent occlusion: 250 mg PO bid in combo with aspirin 325 mg daily for up to 30 days post stent implantation.

PEDS - Not approved in children.

UNAPPROVED ADULT - Due to adverse effects, clopidogrel preferred. Prevention of graft occlusion with CABG: 250 mg PO bid.

FORMS - Generic/Trade: Tab, non-scored 250 mg.

NOTES - Check CBC every 2 weeks during the first 3 months of therapy. Neutrophil counts usually return to normal within 1-3 weeks following discontinuation. Loading dose 500 mg

PO on day 1 may be used for prevention of cardiac stent occlusion.

tirofiban (*Aggrastat*) ▸K ♀B ▸? $$$$$
ADULT - Acute coronary syndromes (unstable angina and non-Q wave MI): Start 0.4 mcg/kg/min IV infusion for 30 mins, then decrease to 0.1 mcg/kg/min for 48-108 hr or until 12-24 hr after coronary intervention.

PEDS - Not approved in children.
NOTES - Thrombocytopenia possible. Concomitant aspirin & heparin/enoxaparin use recommended, unless contraindicated. Dose heparin to keep PTT twice normal. Decrease bolus dose and rate of infusion by 50% in patients with CrCl <30 mL/min. Dilute concentrate solution before using.

CARDIOVASCULAR: Beta Blockers

NOTE: See also antihypertensive combinations. Not first-line for HTN unless to treat angina, post-MI, left ventricular dysfunction. Abrupt discontinuation may precipitate angina, myocardial infarction, arrhythmias, or rebound hypertension; discontinue by tapering over 2 weeks. Avoid using nonselective beta-blockers and use agents with beta-1 selectivity cautiously in asthma/COPD. Beta-1 selectivity diminishes at high doses. Avoid in decompensated heart failure, sick sinus syndrome, and severe peripheral artery disease. Avoid agents with intrinsic sympathomimetic activity post-AMI. May mask hypoglycemic response. Cross sensitivity between beta blockers can occur. Discontinue beta-blocker several days before discontinuing concomitant clonidine to minimize the risk of rebound hypertension. In pheochromocytoma, give beta blocker only after initiating alpha blocker; using beta blocker alone may increase blood pressure due to the attenuation of beta-mediated vasodilatation in skeletal muscle. Some inhalation anesthetics may increase the cardiodepressant effect of beta-blockers. Concomitant digoxin or non-dihydropyridine calcium channel blockers may increase risk of bradycardia.

acebutolol (*Sectral*, ✚*Rhotral*) ▸LK ♀B ▸- $
ADULT - HTN: Start 400 mg PO daily or 200 mg PO bid, usual maintenance 400-800 mg/day, max 1200 mg/day. Twice daily dosing appears to be more effective than daily dosing.
PEDS - Not approved in children <12.
UNAPPROVED ADULT - Angina: Start 200 mg PO bid, increase as needed up to 800 mg/day.
FORMS - Generic/Trade: Caps, 200,400 mg.
NOTES - Has mild intrinsic sympathomimetic activity (partial beta agonist activity). Beta1 receptor selective.

atenolol (*Tenormin*) ▸K ♀D ▸- $
WARNING - Avoid abrupt cessation in coronary heart disease or HTN.
ADULT - Acute MI: 5 mg IV over 5 min, repeat in 10 min, follow with 50 mg PO 10 min after IV dosing in patients tolerating the total IV dose, increase as tolerated to 100 mg/day given daily or divided bid. HTN: Start 25-50 mg PO daily or divided bid, maximum 100 mg/day. Renal impairment, elderly: Start 25 mg PO daily, increase as needed. Angina: Start 50 mg PO daily or divided bid, increase as needed to max of 200 mg/day.
PEDS - Not approved in children.
UNAPPROVED ADULT - Reduce perioperative cardiac events (death) in high risk patients undergoing noncardiac surgery: Start 5-10 mg IV prior to anesthesia, then 50-100 mg PO daily during hospitalization (max 7 days). Maintain HR between 55-65 bpm. Hold dose for HR <55 bpm and SBP <100 mm Hg. Reentrant PSVT associated w/ ST-elevation MI (after carotid massage, IV adenosine): 2.5-5 mg over 2 min to 10 mg max over 10-15 min. Rate control of atrial fibrillation/flutter: Start 25 mg PO daily, titrate to desired heart rate.
UNAPPROVED PEDS - HTN: 1-1.2 mg/kg/dose PO daily, max 2 mg/kg/day.
FORMS - Generic/Trade: Tabs, non-scored 25, 100; scored, 50 mg.
NOTES - Doses >100 mg/day usually do not provide further BP lowering. Beta1 receptor selective. Risk of hypoglycemia to neonates born to mothers using atenolol at parturition or while breastfeeding. May be less effective for HTN than other beta-blockers.

betaxolol (*Kerlone*) ▸LK ♀C ▸? $$
ADULT - HTN: Start 5-10 mg PO daily, max 20 mg/day. Renal impairment, elderly: Start 5 mg PO daily, increase as needed.
PEDS - Not approved in children.
FORMS - Trade only: Tabs, scored 10, non-scored 20 mg.
NOTES - Beta1 receptor selective.

bisoprolol (*Zebeta*, ✚*Monocor*) ▸LK ♀C ▸? $$

ADULT - HTN: Start 2.5-5 mg PO daily, max 20 mg/day. Renal impairment: Start 2.5 PO daily, increase as needed.

PEDS - Not approved in children.

UNAPPROVED ADULT - Compensated heart failure: Start 1.25 mg PO daily, double dose every 2 weeks as tolerated to max 10 mg/day. Reduce perioperative cardiac events (death, MI) in high risk patients undergoing noncardiac surgery: Start 5 mg PO daily, at least 1 week prior to surgery, increase to 10 mg daily to maintain HR <60 bpm, continue for 30 days postop. Hold dose for HR <50 bpm or SBP <100 mm Hg.

FORMS - Generic/Trade: Tabs, scored 5, non-scored 10 mg.

NOTES - Monitor closely for heart failure exacerbation and hypotension when titrating dose. Avoid in decompensated heart failure (i.e. NYHA class IV heart failure or pulmonary edema). Stabilize dose of digoxin, diuretics, and ACEI before starting bisoprolol. Beta1 receptor selective.

carvedilol (*Coreg, Coreg CR*) ▶L♀C ▶? $$$$
ADULT - Heart failure: immediate release: Start 3.125 mg PO bid, double dose q2 weeks as tolerated up to max of 25 mg bid (if <85 kg) or 50 mg bid (if >85 kg). Heart failure, sustained release: Start 10 mg PO daily, double dose q2 weeks as tolerated up to max of 80 mg/day. Reduce cardiovascular risk in post-MI with LV dysfunction, immediate release: Start 6.25 mg PO bid, double dose q 3-10 days as tolerated to max of 25 mg bid. LV dysfunction post-MI, sustained release: Start 20 mg PO daily, double dose q 3-10 days as tolerated to max of 80 mg/day. HTN, immediate release: Start 6.25 mg PO bid, double dose q7-14 days as tolerated to max 50 mg/day. HTN, sustained release: Start 20 mg PO daily, double dose q7-14 days as tolerated to max 80 mg/day.

PEDS - Not approved in children.

FORMS - Trade only: Tabs, immediate-release non-scored 3.125, 6.25, 12.5, 25 mg. Caps, extended-release 10, 20, 40, 80 mg.

NOTES - Avoid in asthma, hepatic impairment, and acute decompensated heart failure (i.e. requiring IV inotropes or pulmonary edema). Monitor closely for heart failure exacerbation and hypotension (particularly orthostatic) when titrating dose. Stabilize dose of digoxin, diuretics, and ACEI before starting carvedilol. Reduce the dose with bradycardia (<55 beats/minute). May reversibly elevate LFTs. Take

with food to decrease orthostatic hypotension. Separate Coreg CR and alcohol (including medications containing alcohol) by at least 2 hours. Give Coreg CR in the morning. The contents of Coreg CR may be sprinkled over applesauce and consumed immediately. Dosing conversion from immediate release to sustained release: 3.125 bid=10 mg CR; 6.25 mg bid=20 mg CR; 12.5 mg bid=40 mg CR; 25 mg bid=80 mg CR.

esmolol (*Brevibloc*) ▶K♀C ▶? $$
ADULT - SVT/HTN emergency: Mix infusion 5 g in 500 mL (10 mg/mL), load with 500 mcg/kg IV over 1 minute (70 kg: 35 mg or 3.5 mL) then IV infusion 50 mcg/kg/min for 4 min (70 kg: 100 mcg/kg/min = 40 mL/h). If optimal response is not attained, repeat IV load and increase IV infusion to 100 mcg/kg/min for 4 min. If necessary, additional boluses (500 mcg/kg/min over 1 min) may be given followed by IV infusion with increased dose by 50 mcg/kg/min for 4 min. Max IV infusion rate 200 mcg/kg/min.

PEDS - Not approved in children.

UNAPPROVED PEDS - Same schedule as adult except loading dose 100-500 mcg/kg IV over 1 min and IV infusion 25-100 mcg/kg/min. IV infusions may be increased by 25-50 mcg/kg/min every 5-10 min. Titrate dose based on patient response.

NOTES - Hypotension. Beta1 receptor selective. Half-life = 9 minutes.

labetalol (*Trandate*) ▶LK♀C ▶+ $$$
ADULT - HTN: Start 100 mg PO bid, usual maintenance dose 200-600 mg bid, max 2400 mg/day. HTN emergency: Start 20 mg slow IV injection, then 40-80 mg IV q10min as needed up to 300 mg total cumulative dose or start 0.5-2 mg/min IV infusion, adjust rate as needed up to total cumulative dose 300 mg.

PEDS - Not approved in children.

UNAPPROVED PEDS - HTN: 4 mg/kg/day PO divided bid, increase as needed up to 40 mg/kg/day. IV: Start 0.3-1 mg/kg/dose (max 20 mg) slow IV injection q10 min or 0.4-1 mg/kg/h IV infusion up to 3 mg/kg/hr.

FORMS - Generic/Trade: Tabs, scored 100,200, 300 mg.

NOTES - Hypotension. Contraindicated in asthma/COPD. Alpha1, beta1, and beta2 receptor blocker.

metoprolol (*Lopressor, Toprol-XL, ✦Betaloc*) ▶L♀C ▶? $$
WARNING - Avoid abrupt cessation in ischemic heart disease or HTN.

ADULT - Acute MI: 5 mg IV q5-15 min up to 15 mg, then start 50 mg PO q6h for 48h, then 100 mg PO bid as tolerated. If usual IV dose is not tolerated, start 25-50 mg PO q6h. If early IV therapy is contraindicated, patient should be titrated to 100 mg PO bid as soon as possible. HTN (immediate release): Start 100 mg PO daily or in divided doses, increase as needed up to 450 mg/day; may require multiple daily doses to maintain 24 hour BP control. HTN (extended release): Start 25-100 mg PO daily, increase as needed q 1 wk up to 400 mg/day. Heart failure: Start 12.5-25 mg (extended-release) PO daily, double dose every 2 weeks as tolerated up to max 200 mg/day. Angina: Start 50 mg PO bid (immediate release) or 100 mg PO daily (extended-release), increase as needed up to 400 mg/day.

PEDS - HTN ≥6 yo: Start 1 mg/kg, max 50 mg/daily. Not recommended <6 yo.

UNAPPROVED ADULT - Heart failure: Start 6.25 PO bid, max 75 mg bid. Atrial tachyarrhythmia, except with Wolff-Parkinson-White syndrome: 2.5-5 mg IV q2-5 min as needed to control rapid ventricular response, max 15 mg over 10-15 min. Reentrant PSVT (after carotid massage, IV adenosine): 2.5-5 mg q 2-5 min to 15 mg max over 10-15 min. Reduce perioperative cardiac events (death) in high-risk patients undergoing noncardiac surgery: Start 100 mg (extended release) 2 hours prior to anesthesia, then 50-100 mg (extended release) PO daily or 2.5-5 mg IV q6 hours during hospitalization (max 7 days). Maintain HR between 55-65 bpm. Hold dose for HR <55 bpm and SBP <100 mm Hg. Rate control of atrial fibrillation/flutter: Start 25 mg PO bid, titrate to desired heart rate.

FORMS - Generic/Trade: Tabs, scored 50,100 mg, extended-release 25, 50, 100, 200 mg. Generic only: Tabs, scored 25 mg.

NOTES - Monitor closely for heart failure exacerbation and hypotension when titrating dose. Avoid in decompensated heart failure (i.e. NYHA class IV heart failure or pulmonary edema. Stabilize dose of digoxin, diuretics, and ACEI before starting metoprolol. Beta1 receptor selective. Extended-release tabs may be broken in half, but do not chew or crush. Avoid using extended release tabs with verapamil, diltiazem, or peripheral vascular disease. May need lower doses in elderly. Monitor BP with potent CYP 2D6 inhibitors that may increase levels (eg, bupropion, cimetidine, diphenhydra-mine, fluoxetine, hydroxychloroquine, paroxetine, propafenone, quinidine, thioridazine, ritonavir, terbinafine). Take with food.

nadolol (*Corgard*) ▶K ♀C ▶- $$
ADULT - HTN: Start 20-40 mg PO daily, usual maintenance dose 40-80 mg/day, max 320 mg/day. Renal impairment: Start 20 mg PO daily, adjust dosage interval based on CrCl - CrCl 31-50 mL/min, q24-36h; CrCl 10-30 mL/min, q24-48h; CrCl <10 mL/min, q40-60h. Angina: Start 40 mg PO daily, usual maintenance dose 40-80 mg/day, max 240 mg/ day.

PEDS - Not approved in children.

UNAPPROVED ADULT - Prevent rebleeding esophageal varices: 40-160 mg/day PO. Titrate dose to reduce heart rate to 25% below baseline. Ventricular arrhythmia: 10-640 mg/day.

FORMS - Generic/Trade: Tabs, scored 20,40, 80,120,160 mg.

NOTES - Beta1 and beta2 receptor blocker.

oxprenolol (♣*Trasicor, Slow-Trasicor*) ▶L ♀D ▶- $$
ADULT - Canada only. Mild to moderate HTN, usually in combination with a thiazide-type diuretic: Regular release: Initially 20 mg PO tid, titrate upwards prn to usual maintenance 120-320 mg/day divided bid-tid. Alternatively, may substitute an equivalent daily dose of sustained release product; do not exceed 480 mg/day.

PEDS - Not approved in children.

FORMS - Trade only: Regular release tabs: 40, 80 mg. Sustained release tabs: 80, 160 mg.

NOTES - Caution in bronchospasm, diabetes, or heart failure. Has mild intrinsic sympathomimetic activity (partial beta agonist activity). No dose adjustment in impaired renal function. Empty matrix of sustained release tablet may be excreted and found in the feces.

penbutolol (*Levatol*) ▶LK ♀C ▶? $$$
ADULT - HTN: Start 20 mg PO daily, usual maintenance dose 20-40 mg, max 80 mg/day.

PEDS - Not approved in children.

FORMS - Trade only: Tabs, scored 20 mg.

NOTES - Has mild intrinsic sympathomimetic activity (partial beta agonist activity). Beta1 and beta2 receptor blocker.

pindolol (♣*Visken*) ▶K ♀B ▶? $$$
ADULT - HTN: Start 5 mg PO bid, usual maintenance dose 10-30 mg/day, max 60 mg/day.

PEDS - Not approved in children.

UNAPPROVED ADULT - Angina: 15-40 mg/day PO in divided doses tid-qid.

FORMS - Generic only: Tabs, scored 5,10 mg.

NOTES - Has intrinsic sympathomimetic activity

(partial beta agonist activity). Beta1 and beta2 blocker. Contraindicated with thioridazine.

propranolol (*Inderal, Inderal LA, InnoPran XL*) ▶L ♀C ▶+ $$

WARNING - Avoid abrupt cessation in coronary heart disease or HTN.

ADULT - HTN: Start 20-40 mg PO bid, usual maintenance dose 160-480 mg/day, max 640 mg/day; extended-release (Inderal LA): start 60-80 mg PO daily, usual maintenance dose 120-160 mg/day, max 640 mg/day; extended-release (InnoPran XL): start 80 mg qhs (10 PM), max 120 mg qhs. Angina: Start 10-20 mg PO tid/qid, usual maintenance 160-240 mg/day, max 320 mg/day; extended-release (Inderal LA): start 80 mg PO daily, same usual dosage range and max for HTN. Migraine prophylaxis: Start 40 mg PO bid or 80 mg PO daily (extended-release), max 240 mg/day. Supraventricular tachycardia or rapid atrial fibrillation/flutter: 10-30 mg PO tid-qid. MI: 180-240 mg/day PO in divided doses bid-qid. Pheochromocytoma surgery: 60 mg PO in divided doses bid-tid beginning 3 days before surgery, use in combination with an alpha blocking agent. IV: reserved for life-threatening arrhythmia, 1-3 mg IV, repeat dose in 2 min if needed, additional doses should not be given in <4h. Not for use in HTN emergency. Essential tremor: Start 40 mg PO bid, titrate prn to 120-320 mg/day.

PEDS - HTN: Start 1 mg/kg/day PO divided bid, usual maintenance dose 2-4 mg/kg/day PO divided bid, max 16 mg/kg/day.

UNAPPROVED ADULT - Prevent rebleeding esophageal varices: 20-180 mg PO bid. Titrate dose to reduce heart rate to 25% below baseline. Control heart rate with A-fib: 80-240 mg/day daily or in divided doses.

UNAPPROVED PEDS - Arrhythmia: 0.01-0.1 mg/kg/dose (max 1 mg/dose) by slow IV push. Manufacturer does not recommend IV propranolol in children.

FORMS - Generic/Trade: Tabs, scored 10, 20, 40, 60, 80. Caps, extended-release 60, 80, 120, 160 mg. Generic only: Solution 20, 40 mg/5 mL. Concentrate 80 mg/mL. Trade only: (InnoPran XL qhs) 80, 120 mg.

NOTES - Beta1 and beta2 receptor blocker. Do not substitute extended-release for immediate-release product on mg-for-mg basis. Dosage titration may be necessary with extended-release product when converting from immediate-release Tabs. Extended-release Caps (Inderal LA) may be opened, and the contents sprinkled on food for administration. Cap contents should be swallowed whole without crushing or chewing. Contraindicated with thioridazine. InnoPran XL is a chronotherapeutic product; give at bedtime to blunt early morning surge in BP. Concomitant use of alcohol may increase propranolol levels.

timolol (*Blocadren*) ▶LK ♀C ▶+ $$

ADULT - HTN: Start 10 mg PO bid, usual maintenance 20-40 mg/day, max 60 mg/day. MI: 10 mg PO bid, started 1-4 weeks post-MI. Migraine headaches: Start 10 mg PO bid, use 20 mg/day daily or divided bid for prophylaxis, increase as needed up to max 60 mg/day. Stop therapy if satisfactory response not obtained after 6-8 weeks of max dose.

PEDS - Not approved in children.

UNAPPROVED ADULT - Angina: 15-45 mg/day PO divided tid-qid.

FORMS - Generic/Trade: Tabs, non-scored 5, scored 10,20 mg.

NOTES - Beta1 and beta2 receptor blocker.

CARDIOVASCULAR: Calcium Channel Blockers (CCBs) - Dihydropyridines

NOTE: See also antihypertensive combinations. Peripheral edema, especially with higher doses. Extended / controlled / sustained-release tabs should be swallowed whole; do not chew or crush. Avoid concomitant grapefruit / grapefruit juice, which may enhance effect. Avoid in decompensated heart failure.

amlodipine (*Norvasc*) ▶L ♀C ▶? $$$

ADULT - HTN: Start 2.5 to 5 mg PO daily, max 10 daily. Coronary artery disease: Start 5 mg PO daily, usual maintenance dose 10 mg daily.

PEDS - HTN (6-17 yo): 2.5-5 mg PO daily.

UNAPPROVED PEDS - HTN: Start 0.1-0.2 mg/kg/day PO daily, max 0.3 mg/kg/day.

FORMS - Generic/Trade: Tabs, non-scored 2.5, 5, 10 mg.

felodipine (*Plendil,* ✱*Renedil*) ▶L ♀C ▶? $$

ADULT - HTN: Start 2.5-5 mg PO daily, usual maintenance 5-10 mg/day, max 10 mg/day.

PEDS - Not approved in children.

FORMS - Generic/Trade: Tabs, extended-release, non-scored 2.5, 5, 10 mg.

NOTES - Extended-release tab. May increase tacrolimus concentration; monitor level.

isradipine (DynaCirc, DynaCirc CR) ►L ♀C ►? $$$

ADULT - HTN: Start 2.5 mg PO bid, usual maintenance 5-10 mg/day, max 20 mg/day divided bid (max 10 mg/day in elderly). Controlled-release (DynaCirc CR): Start 5 mg daily, usual maintenance 5-10 mg/day, max 20 mg/day.

PEDS - Not approved in children.

FORMS - Generic/Trade: Immediate release caps 2.5 mg. Generic: Immediate release caps 5 mg. Trade: Tabs, controlled-release 5,10 mg.

nicardipine (Cardene, Cardene SR) ►L ♀C ►? $$

ADULT - HTN: sustained-release (Cardene SR), Start 30 mg PO bid, usual maintenance dose 30-60 mg PO bid, max 120 mg/day; immediate-release, Start 20 mg PO tid, usual maintenance dose 20-40 mg PO tid, max 120 mg/day. Hypertensive emergency/short-term management of acute HTN: Begin IV infusion at 5 mg/h, titrate infusion rate by 2.5 mg/h q15min as needed, max 15 mg/h. Angina: immediate-release, Start 20 mg PO tid, usual maintenance dose 20-40 mg tid.

PEDS - Not approved in children.

UNAPPROVED PEDS - HTN: 0.5-3 mcg/kg/min IV infusion.

FORMS - Generic/Trade: caps, immediate-release 20,30 mg. Trade only: caps, sustained-release 30,45,60 mg.

NOTES - Hypotension, especially with immediate-release Caps and IV. Decrease dose if hepatically impaired. Use sustained-release Caps for HTN only, not for angina.

nifedipine (Procardia, Adalat, Procardia XL, Adalat CC, ♥Adalat XL, Adalat PA) ►L ♀C ►+ $$

ADULT - HTN: extended-release, Start 30-60 mg PO daily, max 120 mg/day. Angina: extended-release, Start 30-60 mg PO daily, max 120 mg/day; immediate-release, Start 10 mg tid, usual 10-20 mg tid, max 120 mg/day.

PEDS - Not approved in children.

UNAPPROVED ADULT - Preterm labor: loading dose 10 mg PO q20-30 min if contractions persist up to 40 mg within the first hour. After contractions are controlled, maintenance dose: 10-20 mg PO q4-6h or 60-160 mg extended-release PO daily. Duration of treatment has not been established.

UNAPPROVED PEDS - HTN: 0.25-0.5 mg/kg/dose PO q4-6 h as needed, max 10 mg/dose or 3 mg/kg/day. Doses <0.25 mg/kg may be effective.

FORMS - Generic/Trade: Caps, 10,20 mg. Tabs, extended-release 30,60,90 mg.

NOTES - Immediate-release cap should not be chewed and swallowed or given sublingually; may cause excessive hypotension, stroke. Do not use immediate-release caps for treating HTN, hypertensive emergencies, or ST-elevation MI. Extended-release tabs can be substituted for immediate-release caps at the same dose in patients whose angina is controlled.

nisoldipine (Sular) ►L ♀C ►? $$

ADULT - HTN: Start 20 mg PO daily, usual maintenance 20-40 mg/day, max 60 mg/day. Impaired hepatic function, elderly: Start 10 mg PO daily, titrate as needed.

PEDS - Not approved in children.

FORMS - Trade only: Tabs, extended-release 10,20,30,40 mg.

CARDIOVASCULAR: Calcium Channel Blockers (CCBs) – Other

NOTE: See also antihypertensive combinations. Avoid in decompensated heart failure or 2nd/3rd degree heart block.

diltiazem (Cardizem, Cardizem SR, Cardizem LA, Cardizem CD, Cartia XT, Dilacor XR, Diltiazem CD, Diltia XT, Diltzac, Tiazac, Taztia XT) ►L ♀C ►+ $$

ADULT - Atrial fibrillation/flutter, PSVT: 20 mg (0.25 mg/kg) IV bolus over 2 min. If needed and patient tolerated IV bolus with no hypotension, rebolus 15 min later with 25 mg (0.35 mg/kg). IV infusion: Start 10 mg/h, increase by 5 mg/h (usual range 5-15 mg/h). Once daily, extended-release (Cardizem CD, Cartia XT, Dilacor XR, Diltia XT, Taztia XT, Tiazac), HTN: Start 120-240 mg PO daily, usual maintenance range 240-360 mg/day, max 540 mg/day. Once daily, graded extended-release (Cardizem LA), HTN: Start 180-240 mg, max 540 mg/day. Twice daily, sustained-release (Cardizem SR), HTN: Start 60-120 mg PO bid, max 360 mg/day. Immediate-release, angina: Start 30 mg PO qid, max 360 mg/day divided tid-qid. Extended-release, angina: 120-180 mg PO daily, max 540 mg/day. Once daily, graded extended-release (Cardizem LA), angina: Start 180 mg PO daily, doses >360 mg may provide no additional benefit.

PEDS - Not approved in children. Injection contains benzyl alcohol; avoid in neonates.

UNAPPROVED ADULT – A-fib heart rate control: 120-360 mg/day daily or in divided doses.

UNAPPROVED PEDS – HTN: Start 1.5-2 mg/kg/day PO divided tid-qid, max 3.5 mg/kg/day.

FORMS - Generic/Trade: Immediate-release tabs, non-scored (Cardizem) 30, scored 60, 90, 120 mg; extended-release caps (Cardizem CD, Taztia XT daily) 120, 180, 240, 300, 360 mg, (Cartia XT, Dilt-CD daily) 120, 180, 240, 300, (Tiazac daily) 120, 180, 240, 300, 360, 420 mg, (Dilacor XR, Diltia XT daily) 120, 180, 240 mg, (Diltzac) 120,180,240,300,360 mg. Trade only: Sustained-release caps (Cardizem SR q12h) 60,90,120 mg; ext'd-release graded tabs (Cardizem LA daily) 120,180,240,300,360,420 mg.

NOTES - Contraindicated in acute MI and pulmonary congestion, hypotension, sick sinus syndrome without pacemaker, second or third degree AV block without pacemaker, Wolff-Parkinson-White syndrome with rapid A-fib/flutter. Contents of extended-release caps may be sprinkled over food. Do not chew or crush cap contents. May accumulate with hepatic impairment; dose based on clinical response. Cardizem LA is a chronotherapeutic product; give at bedtime to blunt early morning surge in BP. May increase levels of buspirone, quinidine.

verapamil (*Isoptin, Calan, Covera-HS, Verelan, Verelan PM, ♣Veramil*) ▶L ♀C ▶+ $$

ADULT - SVT: 5-10 mg (0.075-0.15 mg/kg) IV over 2 min. A second dose of 10 mg IV may be given 15-30 min later if needed. PSVT/rate control with atrial fibrillation: 240-480 mg/day PO divided tid-qid. Angina: Start 40-80 mg PO tid-qid, max 480 mg/day; sustained-release (Isoptin SR, Calan SR, Verelan), start 120-240 mg PO daily, max 480 mg/day (use bid dosing for doses >240 mg/day with Isoptin SR and Calan SR); extended-release (Covera-HS), start 180 mg PO qhs, max 480 mg/day. HTN: Same as angina, except (Verelan PM) start 100-200 mg PO qhs, max 400 mg/day; (Covera-HS) start 180 mg PO qhs, max 480 mg/day; avoid immediate-release tabs when treating HTN.

PEDS - SVT: (1-15 yo) 2-5 mg (0.1-0.3 mg/kg) IV, max dose 5 mg. Repeat dose once in 30 min if needed, max second dose 10 mg. Immediate-release and sustained-release tabs not approved in children.

FORMS - Generic/Trade: tabs, immediate-release, scored 40,80,120 mg; sustained-release, non-scored (Calan SR, Isoptin SR) 120, scored 180,240 mg; caps, sustained-release (Verelan) 120,180,240,360 mg. Trade: tabs, ext'd-release (Covera HS) 180, 240 mg; caps, ext'd-release (Verelan PM) 100,200,300 mg.

NOTES - Contraindicated in severe LV dysfunction, hypotension, sick sinus syndrome, second or third degree AV block without pacemaker, A-fib/flutter conducted via accessory pathway (ie, Wolff-Parkinson-White). Avoid concomitant grapefruit juice (enhances effect). Scored, sustained-release tabs (Calan SR, Isoptin SR) may be broken and each piece swallowed whole, do not chew or crush. Other extended-release tabs (Covera HS) should be swallowed whole. Contents of sustained-release caps may be sprinkled on food (eg, apple sauce). Do not chew or crush cap contents. Coadministration with aspirin may increase bleeding times. Use cautiously with impaired renal/hepatic function. Covera-HS and Verelan PM are chronotherapeutic products; give at bedtime to blunt early morning surge in BP.

CARDIOVASCULAR: Diuretics – Carbonic Anhydrase Inhibitors

acetazolamide (*Diamox*) ▶LK ♀C ▶+ $

ADULT - Glaucoma: 250 mg PO up to qid (immediate release) or 500 mg PO up to bid (sustained release). Max 1g/day. Acute glaucoma: 250 mg IV q4h or 500 mg IV initially with 125-250 mg q4h, followed by oral therapy. Mountain sickness prophylaxis: 125-250 mg PO bid-tid, beginning 1-2 days prior to ascent and continuing ≥5 days at higher altitude. Edema: Rarely used, start 250-375 mg IV/PO qam given intermittently (qod or 2 consecutive days followed by none for 1-2 days) to avoid loss of diuretic effect.

PEDS - Diuretic: 5 mg/kg PO/IV qam.

UNAPPROVED PEDS - Glaucoma: 8-30 mg/kg/day PO, divided tid. Acute glaucoma: 5-10 mg/kg IV every 6h.

FORMS - Generic only: Tabs, 125,250 mg; Trade only: cap, sustained-release 500 mg.

NOTES - A suspension (250 mg/5 mL) can be made by crushing and mixing tabs in flavored syrup. The susp is stable for 7 days at room temperature. One tab may be softened in 2 teaspoons of hot water, then add to 2 teaspoons of honey or syrup, and swallowed at once. Tabs and compounded susp may have a bitter taste. Use cautiously in sulfa allergy. Prompt descent is necessary if severe forms of high altitude sickness occur (eg, pulmonary or cerebral edema). Test the drug for tolerance/ allergies 1-2 weeks before initial dosing prior to ascent.

CARDIOVASCULAR: Diuretics – Loop

NOTE: Give second dose of bid schedule in mid afternoon to avoid nocturia. Rare hypersensitivity in patients allergic to sulfa-containing drugs, except ethacrynic acid.

bumetanide (*Bumex*, ♥*Burinex*) ▶K ♀C▶? $
ADULT - Edema: 0.5-2 mg PO daily, repeat doses at 4-5 hr intervals prn until desired response is attained, max 10 mg/day; 0.5-1 mg IV/IM, repeat doses at 2-3 hr intervals prn until desired response is attained, max 10 mg/day. Dosing for 3-4 consecutive days followed by no drug for 1-2 days is acceptable. BID dosing may enhance diuretic effect. IV injections should be over 1-2 min. An IV infusion may be used, change bag every 24 hours.
PEDS - Not approved in children.
UNAPPROVED PEDS - Edema: 0.015-0.1 mg/kg/dose PO/IV/IM daily or qod.
FORMS - Generic/Trade: Tabs, scored 0.5,1,2 mg.
NOTES - 1 mg bumetanide is roughly equivalent to 40 mg oral furosemide. IV administration is preferred when GI absorption is impaired.

ethacrynic acid (*Edecrin*) ▶K ♀B ▶? $$
ADULT - Edema: 0.5-1 mg/kg IV, max 100 mg/ dose; 25 mg PO daily on day one, followed by 50 mg PO bid on day two, followed by 100 mg PO in the morning and 50-100 mg PO in the evening depending on the response to the morning dose, max 400 mg/day.
PEDS - Not approved in children.
UNAPPROVED ADULT - HTN: 25 mg PO daily, max 100 mg/day divided bid-tid.
UNAPPROVED PEDS - Edema: 1 mg/kg IV; 25 mg PO daily, increase slowly by 25 mg increments as needed. Ethacrynic acid should not be administered to infants.
FORMS - Trade only: Tabs, scored 25
NOTES - Rarely used. Ototoxicity possible. No sulfonamide group, so may be useful in the sulfa-allergic. Do not administer SC or IM due to local irritation. IV ethacrynic acid should be reconstituted to a concentration of 50 mg/mL and given slowly by IV infusion over 20-30 min. May increase lithium levels.

furosemide (*Lasix*) ▶K ♀C ▶? $
ADULT - Edema: Start 20-80 mg IV/IM/PO, increase dose by 20-40 mg every 6-8h until desired response is achieved, max 600 mg/day. Give maintenance dose daily or divided bid. IV infusion: 0.05 mg/kg/h, titrate rate to desired response. HTN: Start 20-40 mg bid, adjust dose as needed based on BP response. Use lower doses in elderly. Thiazide diuretics generally preferred for HTN.
PEDS - Edema: 0.5-2 mg/kg/dose IV/IM/PO q6-12h, max 6 mg/kg dose. IV infusion: 0.05 mg/ kg/h, titrate rate to achieve desired response.
FORMS - Generic/Trade: Tabs, non-scored 20, scored 40,80 mg. Generic only: Oral solution 10 mg/mL, 40 mg/5 mL.
NOTES - Loops are diuretic of choice with decreased renal function (CrCl <30 mL/min or creat >2.5 mg/dL). Oral absorption may decrease in acute heart failure exacerbation. Bioequivalence of oral form is 50% of IV dose. Monitor renal function in elderly.

torsemide (*Demadex*) ▶LK ♀B ▶? $
ADULT - Edema: Start 5-20 mg IV/PO daily, double dose as needed to desired response, max 200 mg as a single dose. HTN: Start 5 mg PO daily, increase as needed every 4-6 weeks, max 100 mg PO daily or divided bid. Thiazide diuretics generally preferred for HTN.
PEDS - Not approved in children.
FORMS - Generic/Trade: Tabs, scored 5,10,20, 100 mg.
NOTES - Loop diuretics are agent of choice for edema with decreased renal function (CrCl <30 mL/min or creat >2.5 mg/dl).

CARDIOVASCULAR: Diuretics – Potassium Sparing

NOTE: See also antihypertensive combinations and aldosterone antagonists. Beware of hyperkalemia. Use cautiously with other agents that may cause hyperkalemia (ie. ACEIs, ARBs).

amiloride (*Midamor*) ▶LK ♀B ▶? $$
ADULT - Diuretic-induced hypokalemia: Start 5 mg PO daily, increase prn, max 20 mg/day. Edema/HTN: Start 5 mg PO daily in combination with another diuretic, usually a thiazide for HTN, increase prn, max 20 mg/day. Other diuretics may be needed when treating edema.
PEDS - Not approved in children.
UNAPPROVED ADULT - Hyperaldosteronism: 10-40 mg PO daily. Do not use combo product (Moduretic) for hyperaldosteronism.
UNAPPROVED PEDS - Edema: 0.625 mg/kg daily for children weighing 6-20 kg.
FORMS - Generic/Trade: Tabs, non-scored 5 mg.

NOTES - Spironolactone is generally preferred for treating primary hyperaldosteronism.

triamterene (*Dyrenium*) ▶LK ♀B ▶- $$$
ADULT - Edema (cirrhosis, nephrotic syndrome, heart failure): Start 100 mg PO bid, max 300 mg/day. Most patients can be maintained on 100 mg PO daily or qod after edema is controlled. Other diuretics may be needed.
PEDS - Not approved in children.
UNAPPROVED PEDS - Edema: 4 mg/kg/day divided bid after meals, increase to 6 mg/kg/day if needed, max 300 mg/day.
FORMS - Trade only: Caps, 50,100 mg.
NOTES - Combo product with HCTZ (eg, Dyazide, Maxzide) available for HTN.

CARDIOVASCULAR: Diuretics – Thiazide Type

NOTE: See also antihypertensive combinations. Possible hypersensitivity in sulfa allergy. Should be used for most HTN, alone or combined with other anti-hypertensives. Thiazides are not recommended for pregnancy-induced HTN. Coadministration with NSAIDs, including selective COX-2 inhibitors, may reduce the antihypertensive, diuretic, and natriuretic effects of thiazides.

chlorothiazide (*Diuril*) ▶L ♀C, D if used in pregnancy-induced HTN ▶+ $
ADULT - HTN: Start 125-250 mg PO daily or divided bid, max 1000 mg/day divided bid. Edema: 500-2000 mg PO/IV daily or divided bid. Dosing on alternate days or for 3-4 consecutive days followed by no drug for 1-2 days is acceptable.
PEDS - Edema: Infants: Start 10-20 mg/kg/day PO daily or divided bid, up to 30 mg/kg/day divided bid. Children 6 mo-2 yo: 10-20 mg/kg/day PO daily or divided bid, max 375 mg/day. Children 2-12 yo: start 10-20 mg/kg/day PO daily or divided bid, up to 1g/day. IV formulation not recommended for infants or children.
FORMS - Trade only: Susp 250 mg/5 mL. Generic only: Tabs, scored 250, 500 mg.
NOTES - Do not administer SC or IM.

chlorthalidone (*Thalitone*) ▶L ♀B, D if used in pregnancy-induced HTN ▶+ $
ADULT - HTN: For generics, start 12.5-25 mg PO daily, usual maintenance dose 12.5-50 mg/day, max 50 mg/day. For Thalitone, start 15 mg PO daily, usual maintenance 30-45 mg/day, max 50 mg/day. Edema: For generics, start 50-100 mg PO daily after breakfast or 100 mg qod or 100 mg 3 times/week, usual maintenance dose 150-200 mg/day, max 200 mg/day. For Thalitone, start 30-60 mg PO daily or 60 mg qod, usual maintenance dose 90-120 mg PO daily or qod.
PEDS - Not approved in children.
UNAPPROVED ADULT - Nephrolithiasis: 25-50 mg PO daily.
UNAPPROVED PEDS - Edema: 2 mg/kg PO 3 times weekly.
FORMS - Trade only: Tabs, non-scored (Thalitone) 15 mg. Generic only: Tabs non-scored 25,50 mg.
NOTES - Thalitone has greater bioavailability than generic forms, do not interchange. Doses greater than 50 mg/day for HTN are usually associated with hypokalemia with little added BP control.

hydrochlorothiazide (*HCTZ, Esidrix, Oretic, Microzide, HydroDiuril*) ▶L ♀B, D if used in pregnancy-induced HTN ▶+ $
ADULT - HTN: Start 12.5-25 mg PO daily, usual maintenance dose 12.5-25 mg/day, max 50 mg/day. Edema: 25-100 mg PO daily or in divided doses or 50-100 mg PO qod or 3-5 days/week, max 200 mg/day.
PEDS - Edema: 1-2 mg/kg/day PO daily or divided bid, max 37.5 mg/day in infants up to 2 yo, max 100 mg/day in children 2-12 yo.
UNAPPROVED ADULT - Nephrolithiasis: 50-100 mg PO daily.
FORMS - Generic/Trade: Tabs, scored 25, 50 mg; Cap 12.5 mg.
NOTES - Doses as low as 6.25 mg daily may be effective in combination with other antihypertensives. Doses ≥50 mg/day for HTN may

cause hypokalemia with little added BP control.

indapamide (Lozol, ✦Lozide) ▶L ♀B, D if used in pregnancy-induced HTN ▶? $

ADULT - HTN: Start 1.25-2.5 mg PO daily, max 5 mg/day. Edema/Heart failure: 2.5-5 mg PO q am.

PEDS - Not approved in children.

FORMS - Generic/Trade: Tabs, non-scored 1.25, 2.5 mg.

methyclothiazide (Enduron) ▶L ♀B, D if used in pregnancy-induced HTN ▶? $

ADULT - HTN: Start 2.5 mg PO daily, usual maintenance dose 2.5-5 mg/day. Edema: Start 2.5 mg PO daily, usual maintenance dose 2.5-10 mg/day.

PEDS - Not approved in children.

FORMS - Generic/Trade: Tabs, scored, 5 mg.

NOTES - May dose qod or 3-5 days/week as maintenance therapy to control edema.

metolazone (Zaroxolyn) ▶L ♀B, D if used in pregnancy-induced HTN ▶? $$$

ADULT - Edema (heart failure, renal disease): 5-10 mg PO daily, max 10 mg/day in heart failure, 20 mg/day in renal disease. If used with loop diuretic, start with 2.5 mg PO daily. Reduce to lowest effective dose as edema resolves. May be given qod as edema resolves.

PEDS - Not approved in children.

UNAPPROVED PEDS - Edema: 0.2-0.4 mg/kg/day daily or divided bid.

FORMS - Generic/Trade: Tabs 2.5,5,10 mg.

NOTES - Generally used for heart failure, not HTN. When used with furosemide or other loop diuretics, administer metolazone 30 min before IV loop diuretic. Cross-allergy may occur if allergic to sulfonamides or thiazides.

CARDIOVASCULAR: Nitrates

NOTE: Avoid if systolic BP <90 mmHg or ≥30 mmHg below baseline, severe bradycardia (<50 bpm), tachycardia (>100 bpm) or right ventricular infarction. Avoid in those who have received erectile dysfunction therapy in the last 24 (sildenafil, vardenafil) to 48 (tadalafil) hours.

isosorbide dinitrate (Isordil, Dilatrate-SR, ✦Cedocard SR, Coronex) ▶L ♀C ▶? $

ADULT - Acute angina: 2.5-10 mg SL or chewed immediately, repeat as needed every 5-10 minutes up to 3 doses in 30 min. SL and chew Tabs may be used prior to events likely to provoke angina. Angina prophylaxis: Start 5-20 mg PO tid (7 am, noon, & 5 pm), max 40 mg tid. Sustained-release (Dilatrate SR): Start 40 mg PO bid, max 80 mg PO bid (8 am & 2 pm).

PEDS - Not approved in children.

UNAPPROVED ADULT - Heart failure: 10-40 mg PO tid, max 80 mg tid. Use in combination with hydralazine.

FORMS - Generic/Trade: Tabs, scored 5,10,20, 30,40, chewable, scored 5,10, sublingual tabs, non-scored 2.5,5,10 mg. Trade only: cap, sustained-release (Dilatrate-SR) 40 mg. Generic only: tab, sustained-release 40 mg.

NOTES - Headache possible. Use SL or chew Tabs for an acute angina attack. Extended-release tab may be broken, but do not chew or crush, swallow whole; do not use for acute angina. Allow for a nitrate-free period of 10-14 h each day to avoid nitrate tolerance.

isosorbide mononitrate (ISMO, Monoket, **Imdur)** ▶L ♀C ▶? $$

ADULT - Angina: 20 mg PO bid (8 am and 3 pm). Extended-release (Imdur): Start 30-60 mg PO daily, max 240 mg/day.

PEDS - Not approved in children.

FORMS - Generic/Trade: Tabs, non-scored (ISMO, bid dosing) 20, scored (Monoket, bid dosing) 10,20, extended-release, scored (Imdur, daily dosing) 30,60, non-scored 120 mg.

NOTES - Headache. Extended-release tab may be broken, but do not chew or crush, swallow whole. Do not use for acute angina.

nitroglycerin intravenous infusion (Tridil) ▶L ♀C ▶? $

ADULT - Perioperative HTN, acute MI/heart failure, acute angina: mix 50 mg in 250 mL D5W (200 mcg/mL), start at 10-20 mcg/min IV (3-6 mL/h), then titrate upward by 10-20 mcg/min every 3-5 min until desired effect is achieved.

PEDS - Not approved in children.

UNAPPROVED ADULT - Hypertensive emergency: Start 10-20 mcg/min IV infusion, titrate up to 100 mcg/min. Antihypertensive effect is usually evident in 2-5 min. Effect may persist for only 3-5 min after infusion is stopped.

UNAPPROVED PEDS - IV infusion: start 0.25-0.5 mcg/kg/min, increase by 0.5-1 mcg/kg/min q3-5 min as needed, max 5 mcg/kg/min.

FORMS - Brand name "Tridil" no longer manufactured, but retained for name recognition.

NOTES - Nitroglycerin migrates into polyvinyl chloride (PVC) tubing. Use lower initial doses

(5 mcg/min) with non-PVC tubing. Use with caution in inferior/right ventricular myocardial infarction. Nitroglycerin-induced venodilation can cause severe hypotension.

nitroglycerin ointment (*Nitrol, Nitro-BID*) ▶L ♀C ▶? $

ADULT - Angina prophylaxis: Start 0.5 inch q8h applied to non-hairy skin area, maintenance 1-2 inches q8h, maximum 4 inches q4-6h.

PEDS - Not approved in children.

FORMS - Trade only: Ointment, 2%, tubes 1,30,60g (Nitro-BID).

NOTES - 1 inch ointment is approximately 15 mg nitroglycerin. Allow for a nitrate-free period of 10-14 h each day to avoid nitrate tolerance. Generally change to oral tabs or transdermal patch for long-term therapy. Do not use topical therapy (ointment, transdermal system) for acute angina.

nitroglycerin spray (*Nitrolingual, Nitro-Mist*) ▶L ♀C ▶? $$$

ADULT - Acute angina: 1-2 sprays under the tongue at the onset of attack, repeat as needed, max 3 sprays in 15 min. A dose may be given 5-10 mins before activities that might provoke angina.

PEDS - Not approved in children.

FORMS - Trade only: Nitrolingual solution, 4.9,12 mL. 0.4 mg/spray (60 or 200 sprays/canister); NitroMist aerosol 0.4 mg/spray (230 sprays/canister)

NOTES - May be preferred over SL tabs in patients with dry mouth. Patient can see how much medicine is left in the upright bottle. Nitrolingual: replace bottle when fluid is below level of center tube; NitroMist: replace bottle when fluid reaches the bottom of the hole in the side of the container. Before initial use, prime pump: Nitrolingual - spray 5 times into air (away from self and others); NitroMist – spray 10 times into air (away from self and others). Prime at least once every 6 weeks if not used: Nitrolingual spray 1 time into the air (away from self and others); NitroMist spray 2 times into the air (away from self and others). Do not shake NitroMist before using.

nitroglycerin sublingual (*Nitrostat, Nitro-Quick*) ▶L ♀C ▶? $

ADULT - Acute angina: 0.4 mg under tongue or between the cheek and gum, repeat dose every 5 min as needed up to 3 doses in 15 min. A dose may be given 5-10 min before activities that might provoke angina.

PEDS - Not approved in children.

FORMS - Generic/Trade: Sublingual tabs, non-scored 0.3,0.4,0.6 mg; in bottles of 100 or package of 4 bottles with 25 tabs each.

NOTES - Headache. May produce a burning/tingling sensation when administered, although this should not be used to assess potency. Store in original glass bottle to maintain potency/stability. Traditionally, unused Tabs should be discarded 6 months after the original bottle is opened; however the Nitrostat product is stable for 24 months after the bottle is opened or until the expiration date on the bottle, whichever is earlier. If used rarely, prescribe package with 4 bottles with 25 Tabs each.

nitroglycerin sustained release ▶L ♀C ▶? $

ADULT - Angina prophylaxis: Start 2.5 mg PO bid-tid, then titrate upward as needed.

PEDS - Not approved in children.

FORMS - Generic only: cap, extended-release 2.5, 6.5, 9 mg.

NOTES - Headache. Extended-release tab may be broken, but do not chew or crush, swallow whole. cap should be swallowed whole. Do not use extended-release Tabs or Caps for acute angina attack. Allow for a nitrate-free period of 10-14 h each day to avoid nitrate tolerance.

nitroglycerin transdermal (*Minitran, Nitro-Dur,* ✿*Trinipatch*) ▶L ♀C ▶? $$$

ADULT - Angina prophylaxis: Start with lowest dose and apply 1 patch for 12-14 h each day to non-hairy skin.

PEDS - Not approved in children.

FORMS - Trade only: Transdermal system, doses in mg/h: Nitro-Dur 0.1, 0.2, 0.3, 0.4, 0.6, 0.8; Minitran 0.1, 0.2, 0.4, 0.6. Generic only: Transdermal system, doses in mg/h: 0.1, 0.2, 0.4, 0.6.

NOTES - Do not use topical therapy (ointment, transdermal system) for acute angina attack. Allow for a nitrate-free period of 10-14 h each day to avoid nitrate tolerance. Elderly are at more risk of hypotension and falling; start at lower doses.

nitroglycerin transmucosal (*Nitroguard*) ▶L ♀C ▶? $$$

ADULT - Acute angina and prophylaxis: 1-3 mg PO, between lip and gum or between cheek and gum, q 3-5 h while awake.

PEDS - Not approved in children.

FORMS - Trade only: Tabs, controlled-release 2,3 mg.

NOTES - May cause headache and flushing. Allow for a nitrate-free period of 10-14 h each day to avoid nitrate tolerance.

CARDIAC PARAMETERS AND FORMULAS	Normal
Cardiac output (CO) = heart rate x stroke volume	4-8 l/min
Cardiac index (CI) = CO/BSA	2.8-4.2 l/min/m2
MAP (mean arterial press) = [(SBP - DBP)/3] + DBP	80-100 mmHg
SVR (systemic vasc resis) = (MAP - CVP)x(80)/CO	800-1200 dyne/sec/cm5
PVR (pulm vasc resis) = (PAM - PCWP)x(80)/CO	45-120 dyne/sec/cm5
QT_C = QT / square root of RR [calculate using both measures in sec]	≤0.44
Right atrial pressure (central venous pressure)	0-8 mmHg
Pulmonary artery systolic pressure (PAS)	20-30 mmHg
Pulmonary artery diastolic pressure (PAD)	10-15 mmHg
Pulmonary capillary wedge pressure (PCWP)	8-12 mmHg (post-MI ~16 mmHg)

CARDIOVASCULAR: Pressors / Inotropes

dobutamine (*Dobutrex*) ▶Plasma ♀D ▶- $
ADULT - Inotropic support (heart failure, surgical procedures): 2-20 mcg/kg/min. 70 kg: 5 mcg/kg/min with 1 mg/mL concentration (eg, 250 mg in 250 mL D5W) = 21 mL/h; 5 mcg/kg/min with 2 mg/mL concentration (eg, 200 mg in 100 mL D5W) = 10.5 mL/h.
PEDS - Not approved in children.
UNAPPROVED PEDS - Same as adult.
NOTES - For short-term use, up to 72 hours.

dopamine (*Intropin*) ▶Plasma ♀C ▶- $
ADULT - Pressor: Start 5 mcg/kg/min, increase as needed by 5-10 mcg/kg/min increments at 10 min intervals, max 50 mcg/kg/min. 70 kg: 5 mcg/kg/min with 1600 mcg/mL concentration (eg, 400 mg in 250 mL D5W) = 13 mL/h; 5 mcg/kg/min with 3200 mcg/mL concentration (eg, 320 mg in 100 mL D5W) = 6.5 mL/h.
PEDS - Not approved in children.
UNAPPROVED ADULT - Symptomatic bradycardia unresponsive to atropine: 5-20 mcg/kg/min IV infusion.
UNAPPROVED PEDS - Pressor: same as adult.
NOTES - Doses in mcg/kg/min: 2-4 = (traditional renal dose; recent evidence suggests ineffective) dopaminergic receptors; 5-10 = (cardiac dose) dopaminergic and beta1 receptors; >10 = dopaminergic, beta1, and alpha1 receptors.

ephedrine ▶K ♀C ▶? $
ADULT - Pressor: 10-25 mg slow IV slow, repeat every 5-10 min prn, max 150 mg/day. Orthostatic hypotension: 25 mg PO daily-qid. Bronchospasm: 25-50 mg PO q3-4h prn.
PEDS - Not approved in children.
UNAPPROVED PEDS - Pressor: 3 mg/kg/day SC or IV in 4-6 divided doses.
FORMS - Generic only: Caps, 50 mg.

epinephrine (*EpiPen, EpiPen Jr, Twinject, adrenalin*) ▶Plasma ♀C ▶- $

ADULT - Cardiac arrest: 1 mg (1:10,000 solution) IV, repeat every 3-5 minutes if needed; infusion 1 mg in 250 mL D5W (4 mcg/mL) at 1-4 mcg/min (15-60 mL/h). Anaphylaxis: 0.1-0.5 mg SC/IM (1:1,000 solution), may repeat SC dose q10-15 minutes for anaphylactic shock. Acute asthma & hypersensitivity reactions: 0.1 to 0.3 mg of 1:1,000 soln SC or IM. Hypersensitivity reactions: 0.01 mg/kg SC autoinjector.
PEDS - Cardiac arrest: 0.01 mg/kg IV/intraosseous (IO) (max 1 mg/dose) or 0.1 mg/kg ET (max 10 mg/dose), repeat 0.1-0.2 mg/kg IV/IO/ET q3-5 minutes if needed. Neonates: 0.01-0.03 mg/kg IV (preferred) or up to 0.1 mg/kg ET, repeat every 3-5 minutes if needed; IV infusion start 0.1 mcg/kg/min, increase in increments of 0.1 mcg/kg/min if needed, max 1 mcg/kg/min. Anaphylaxis: 0.01 mg/kg (0.01 mL/kg of 1:1000 injection) SC, may repeat SC dose at 20 minute to 4 hour intervals depending on condition severity. Acute asthma: 0.01 mL/kg (up to 0.5 mL) of 1:1,000 soln SC or IM; repeat q15 min x 3-4 doses prn. Hypersensitivity reactions: 0.01 mg/kg SC autoinjector.
UNAPPROVED ADULT - Symptomatic bradycardia unresponsive to atropine: 2-10 mcg/min IV infusion. ET administration prior to IV access: 2-2.5 x the recommended IV dose in 10 mL of NS or distilled water.
FORMS - Soln for injection: 1,10,000 (1 mg/mL in 10 mL syringe), 1:1,000 (1 mg/mL in 1 mL amps). EpiPen Auto-injector delivers 0.3 mg (1:1,000 soln) IM dose. EpiPen Jr. Autoinjector delivers 0.15 mg (1:2,000 solution) IM dose. Twinject Auto-injector delivers 0.15, 0.3 mg IM/SQ dose.
NOTES - Cardiac arrest: ADULT: Use the 1:10,000 injectable solution for IV use (10 mL = 1 mg); PEDS: use 1:10,000 for initial IV dose,

then 1:1,000 for subsequent dosing or ET doses. Anaphylaxis: Use the 1:1000 injectable solution for SC/IM (0.1 mL = 0.1 mg);. consider EpiPen Jr. in patients weighing <30 kg. Directions for injectable kit use: Remove cap. Place black tip end on thigh & push down to inject. Hold in place for 10 seconds. May be injected directly through clothing.

inamrinone (*Amrinone*) ▸K ♀C ▸? $$$$$

ADULT - Heart failure (NYHA class III,IV): 0.75 mg/kg bolus IV over 2-3 min, then infusion 100 mg in 100 mL NS (1 mg/mL) at 5-10 mcg/kg/min. 70 kg: 5 mcg/kg/min = 21 mL/h. An additional IV bolus of 0.75 mg/kg may be given 30 min after initiating therapy if needed. Total daily dose should not exceed 10 mg/kg.

PEDS - Not approved in children.

UNAPPROVED ADULT - CPR: 0.75 mg/kg bolus IV over 2-3 min, then 5-15 mcg/kg/ min.

UNAPPROVED PEDS - Inotropic support: 0.75 mg/kg IV bolus over 2-3 minutes, followed by 3-5 mcg/kg/min (neonates) or 5-10 mcg/kg/min (children) maintenance infusion.

NOTES - Thrombocytopenia possible. Children may require higher bolus doses, 3-4.5 mg/kg. Name changed from "amrinone".

mephentermine (*Wyamine*) ▸Plasma ♀C ▸- $$$$

ADULT - Hypotension during anesthesia: 0.5 mg/kg/dose, usually 15-30 mg IM, max 80 mg/ dose. Spinal anesthesia: 30-45 mg IV, repeat 30 mg dose prn to maintain BP. Spinal anesthesia in cesarean section: 15 mg IV, repeat dose prn to maintain BP.

PEDS - Not approved in children.

UNAPPROVED PEDS - Hypotension during anesthesia: 0.4 mg/kg/dose IM.

metaraminol (*Aramine*) ▸Plasma ♀C ▸- $

ADULT - Hypotension during spinal anesthesia: Dilute 15-100 mg in 250-500 mL D5W or normal saline, give 5 mcg/kg/min IV infusion, adjust rate of infusion based on blood pressure. Prevention of hypotension: 2-10 mg IM/ SC, wait 10 min. before dose increase.

PEDS - Not approved in children.

UNAPPROVED PEDS - Acute hypotension during spinal anesthesia: 0.1 mg/kg SC/IM, wait at least 10 min before repeat dose. Severe hypotension/shock: 0.01 mg/kg IV and, if needed, continue with IV infusion 0.4 mg/kg diluted and administered at a rate to maintain BP.

midodrine (*Orvaten*, *ProAmatine*, ✜*Amatine*) ▸LK ♀C ▸? $$$$$

WARNING - May cause significant HTN. Clinical benefits (ie, improved activities of daily living) have not been verified. Use in patients when nonpharmacological treatment fails.

ADULT - Orthostatic hypotension: Start 10 mg PO tid while awake, increase dose as needed to max 40 mg/day. Renal impairment: Start 2.5 mg tid while awake, increase dose as needed.

PEDS - Not approved in children.

FORMS - Generic/Trade: Tabs, scored 2.5,5,10 mg.

NOTES - The last daily dose should be no later than 6 pm to avoid supine HTN during sleep.

milrinone (*Primacor*) ▸K ♀C ▸? $$$$$

ADULT - Systolic heart failure (NYHA class III,IV): Load 50 mcg/kg IV over 10 min, then begin IV infusion of 0.375-0.75 mcg/kg/min. Renal impairment: reduce IV infusion rate (mcg/kg/min) as follows, CrCl 50-41 mL/min, 0.43; CrCl 40-31 mL/min, 0.38; CrCl 30-21 mL/min, 0.33; CrCl 20-11 mL/min, 0.28; CrCl 10-6 mL/min, 0.23; CrCl ≤5 mL/min, 0.2.

PEDS - Not approved in children.

UNAPPROVED PEDS - Inotropic support: Limited data, 50 mcg/kg IV bolus over 10 minutes, followed by 0.5-1 mcg/kg/min IV infusion, titrate to effect within dosing range.

norepinephrine (*Levophed*) ▸Plasma ♀C ▸? $

ADULT - Acute hypotension: 4 mg in 500 mL D5W (8 mcg/mL), start IV infusion 8-12 mcg/ min, ideally through central line, adjust rate to maintain BP, average maintenance dose 2-4 mcg/min. 3 mcg/min = 22.5 mL/h.

PEDS - Not approved in children.

UNAPPROVED PEDS - Acute hypotension: Start 0.05-0.1mcg/kg/min IV infusion, titrate to desired effect, max dose 2 mcg/kg/min.

NOTES - Avoid extravasation, do not administer IV push or IM.

phenylephrine (*Neo-Synephrine*) ▸Plasma ♀C ▸- $

ADULT - Mild to moderate hypotension: 0.1-0.2 mg slow IV injection, do not exceed 0.5 mg in initial dose, repeat dose prn no less than every 10-15 min; 1-10 mg SC/IM, initial dose should not exceed 5 mg. Infusion for severe hypotension: 20 mg in 250 mL D5W (80 mcg/mL), start 100-180 mcg/min (75-135 mL/h), usual dose once BP is stabilized 40-60 mcg/min.

PEDS - Not approved in children.

UNAPPROVED PEDS - Mild to moderate hypotension: 5-20 mcg/kg IV bolus q10-15 min prn; 0.1-0.5 mcg/kg/min IV infusion, titrate.

NOTES - Avoid SC or IM administration during shock, use IV route to ensure drug absorption.

CARDIOVASCULAR: Pulmonary Arterial Hypertension

bosentan (*Tracleer*) ▶L ♀X ▶-? $$$$$
WARNING - Hepatotoxicity; monitor LFTs prior to starting therapy & monthly thereafter. Contraindicated in pregnancy due to birth defects; women of child bearing age must use reliable contraception & have pregnancy tests monthly and before each refill. Oral, injectable, transdermal, and implanted contraception must be supplemented with another method.
ADULT - Pulmonary arterial hypertension: Start 62.5 mg PO bid for 4 weeks, increase to 125 mg bid maintenance dose.
PEDS - Not approved in children.
FORMS - Trade: Tabs, non-scored 62.5,125mg.
NOTES - Available only through access program by calling 866-228-3546. Concomitant glyburide contraindicated due to increased risk of hepatotoxicity. Ketoconazole and cyclosporine inhibit metabolism via cytochrome P450 3A4; concomitant cyclosporine contraindicated. Induces metabolism of other drugs (eg, contraceptives, simvastatin, lovastatin, atorvastatin). Do not use with both CYP2C9 inhibitor (eg, amiodarone, fluconazole) and CYP3A4 inhibitor (eg, ketoconazole, itraconazole, ritonavir); may increase levels of bosentan. May decrease warfarin plasma concentration; monitor INR. Discontinue with signs of pulmonary edema. Monitor hemoglobin after 1 and 3 months of therapy, then q3 months.

epoprostenol (*Flolan*) ▶Plasma ♀B ▶? $$$$$
ADULT - Pulmonary arterial hypertension: Acute dose ranging, 2 ng/kg/min increments via IV infusion until symptomatic intolerance (mean maximal dose without symptoms 8.6 ng/kg/min), start continuous IV infusion at 4 ng/kg/min or less than the patient's maximum-tolerated infusion (MTI) rate for acute dose ranging. If the MTI rate is <5 ng/kg/min, start chronic IV infusion at one-half the MTI.
PEDS - Not approved in children.
NOTES - Administer by central venous catheter, with peripheral infusions temporarily only.

iloprost (*Ventavis*) ▶L ♀C ▶? $$$$$
ADULT - Pulmonary arterial hypertension: Start 2.5 mcg/dose by inhalation (as delivered at

mouthpiece); if well tolerated increase to 5 mcg/ dose by inhalation (as delivered at mouthpiece). Use 6-9 times daily (not > than q2h) during waking hours.
PEDS - Not approved in children.
NOTES - Only administer with Prodose or I-neb AAD Systems. Each single-use ampule delivers 20 mcg to medication chamber of nebulizer and 2.5 or 5 mcg to the mouthpiece; discard remaining solution after each inhalation. Do not mix with other medications. Avoid contact with skin/eyes or oral ingestion. Monitor vital signs when initiating therapy. Do not initiate therapy if SBP < 85 mm Hg. Do not use in patients with moderate to severe hepatic impairment and/or 3x upper limit of transaminase or patients on dialysis. May potentiate bleeding risk for patients on anticoagulants. May potentiate hypotensive effects of other medications.

treprostinil (*Remodulin*) ▶KL ♀B ▶? $$$$$
ADULT - Continuous subcutaneous (preferred) or central IV infusion in pulmonary arterial HTN with NYHA Class II to IV symptoms: Start 1.25 ng/kg/minute based on ideal body weight. Reduce to 0.625 ng/kg/minute if initial dose not tolerated. Dose based on clinical response & tolerance. Increase by no more than 1.25 ng/kg /minute/week in first 4 weeks, then increase by no more than 2.5 ng/kg/minute/week. Max 40 ng/kg/minute. Transitioning from epoprostenol: Must be done in hospital; initiate at 10% epoprostenol dose; gradually increase dose as epoprostenol dose is decreased (see chart in package insert).
PEDS - Not approved in children.
NOTES - Use cautiously in the elderly and those with liver or renal dysfunction. Initiate in setting with personnel & equipment for physiological monitoring & emergency care. Administer by continuous infusion using infusion pump. Patient must have access to backup infusion pump and infusion sets. Must dilute prior to giving IV; see package insert for details. May potentiate bleeding risk for patients on anticoagulants. May potentiate hypotensive effects of other medications.

CARDIOVASCULAR: Thrombolytics

**alteplase (*tpa, t-PA, Activase, Cathflo,
❖Activase rt-PA*)** ▶L ♀C ▶? $$$$$

ADULT - Acute MI: (patients >67 kg) 15 mg IV bolus, then 50 mg IV over 30 min, then 35 mg

IV over the next 60 min; (patients ≤67 kg) 15 mg IV bolus, then 0.75 mg/kg (not to exceed 50 mg) IV over 30 min, then 0.5 mg/kg (not to exceed 35 mg) IV over the next 60 min. Concurrent heparin infusion. Acute ischemic stroke with symptoms ≤3h: 0.9 mg/kg (max 90 mg); give 10% of total dose as an IV bolus, and the remainder IV over 60 min. Multiple exclusion criteria. Acute pulmonary embolism: 100 mg IV over 2h, then restart heparin when PTT ≤twice normal. Occluded central venous access device: 2 mg/mL in catheter for 2 hr. May use second dose if needed.

PEDS - Occluded central venous access device: ≥10 kg and <30 kg: Dose equal to 110% of the internal lumen volume, not to exceed 2 mg/2 mL. Other uses not approved in children.

NOTES - Must be reconstituted. Solution must be used within 8h after reconstitution.

reteplase (*Retavase*) ▶L ♀C ▶? $$$$$
ADULT - Acute MI: 10 units IV over 2 minutes; repeat one dose in 30 min.
PEDS - Not approved in children.
NOTES - Must be reconstituted with sterile water for injection to 1 mg/mL concentration. Solution must be used within 4 h after reconstitution.

streptokinase (*Streptase, Kabikinase*) ▶L ♀C ▶? $$$$$
ADULT - Acute MI: 1.5 million units IV over 60 min. Pulmonary embolism: 250,000 units IV loading dose over 30 min, followed by 100,000 units/h IV infusion for 24 h (maintain infusion for 72 h if concurrent DVT suspected). DVT: 250,000 units IV loading dose over 30 min, followed by 100,000 units/h IV infusion for 24 hours. Occluded arteriovenous catheter: 250,000 units instilled into the catheter, remove solution containing 250,000 units of drug from

catheter after 2 h using a 5-mL syringe.
PEDS - Not approved in children.
NOTES - Must be reconstituted. Solution must be used within 8 h of reconstitution. Do not shake vial. Do not repeat use in less than one year. Do not use with history of severe allergic reaction.

tenecteplase (*TNKase*) ▶L ♀C ▶? $$$$$
ADULT - Acute MI: Single IV bolus dose over 5 seconds based on body weight; <60 kg, 30 mg; 60-69 kg, 35 mg; 70-79 kg, 40 mg; 80-89 kg, 45 mg; ≥90kg, 50 mg.
PEDS - Not approved in children.
NOTES - Must be reconstituted. Solution must be used within 8h after reconstitution.

urokinase (*Kinlytic*) ▶L ♀B ▶? $$$$$
ADULT - Pulmonary embolism: 4400 units/kg IV loading dose over 10 min, followed by IV infusion 4400 units/kg/h for 12 hours. Occluded IV catheter: 5000 units instilled into the catheter with a tuberculin syringe, remove solution containing 5000 units of drug from catheter after 5 min using a 5-mL syringe. Aspiration attempts may be repeated q5min. If unsuccessful, cap catheter and allow 5000 unit solution to remain in catheter for 30-60 min before again attempting to aspirate solution and residual clot.
PEDS - Not approved in children.
UNAPPROVED ADULT - Acute MI: 2-3 million units IV infusion over 45-90 min. Give one-half the total dose as a rapid initial IV injection over 5 min.
UNAPPROVED PEDS - Arterial or venous thrombosis: 4400 units/kg IV loading dose over 10 minutes, followed by 4400 units/kg/hr for 12-72 hours. Occluded IV catheter: same as adult.
NOTES - Must be reconstituted. Do not shake vial.

THROMBOLYTIC THERAPY FOR ACUTE MI (if high-volume cath lab unavailable)
Indications: Clinical history & presentation strongly suggestive of MI within 12 hours plus ≥1 of the following: 1 mm ST↑ in ≥2 contiguous leads; new left BBB; or 2 mm ST↓ in V1-4 suggestive of true posterior MI. *Absolute contraindications*: Previous cerebral hemorrhage, known cerebral aneurysm or arteriovenous malformation, known intracranial neoplasm, recent (<3 months) ischemic stroke (except acute ischemic stroke <3 hours), aortic dissection, active bleeding or bleeding diathesis (excluding menstruation), significant closed head or facial trauma (<3 months). *Relative contraindications*: Severe uncontrolled HTN (>180/110 mmHg) on presentation or chronic severe HTN; prior ischemic stroke (>3 months), dementia, other intracranial pathology; traumatic/prolonged (>10 minutes) cardiopulmonary resuscitation; major surgery (<3 weeks); recent (within 2-4 weeks) internal bleeding; puncture of noncompressible vessel; pregnancy; active peptic ulcer disease; current use of anticoagulants. For streptokinase/anistreplase: prior exposure (>5 days ago) or prior allergic reaction.

Circulation 2004;110:588-636

CARDIOVASCULAR: Volume Expanders

albumin (*Albuminar, Buminate, Albumarc, ♣Plasbumin*) ▶L ♀C ▶? $$$$
ADULT - Shock, burns: 500 mL of 5% solution (50 mg/mL) infused as rapidly as tolerated. Repeat infusion in 30 min if response is inadequate. 25% solution may be used with or without dilution if necessary. Undiluted 25% solution should be infused at 1 mL/min to avoid too rapid plasma volume expansion.
PEDS - Shock, burns: 10-20 mL/kg IV infusion at 5-10 mL/min using 50 mL of 5% solution.
UNAPPROVED PEDS - Shock/hypovolemia: 1 g/kg/dose IV rapid infusion. Hypoproteinemia: 1 g/kg/dose IV infusion over 30-120 min.
NOTES - Fever, chills. Monitor for volume overload (dyspnea, fluid in lungs, abnormal increase in BP or CVP). Less likely to cause hypotension than plasma protein fraction, more purified. In treating burns, large volumes of crystalloid solutions (0.9% sodium chloride) are co-administered to maintain plasma volume. Use 5% solution in children (25% if volume restrictions).

dextran (*Rheomacrodex, Gentran, Macrodex*) ▶K ♀C ▶? $$$$
ADULT - Shock/hypovolemia: Dextran 40, Dextran 70 and 75, up to 20 mL/kg during the first 24 hours, up to 10 mL/kg/day thereafter, do not continue for longer than 5 days. The first 500 mL may be infused rapidly with CVP monitoring. DVT/PE prophylaxis during surgery: Dextran 40, 50-100 g IV infusion the day of surgery, continue for 2-3 days post-op with 50 g/day. 50 g/day may be given every 2nd or 3rd day thereafter up to 14 days.
PEDS - Total dose should not exceed 20 mL/kg.
UNAPPROVED ADULT - DVT/PE prophylaxis during surgery: Dextran 70 and 75 solutions have been used. Other uses: to improve circulation with sickle cell crisis, prevention of nephrotoxicity with radiographic contrast media, toxemia of late pregnancy.
NOTES - Monitor for plasma volume overload (dyspnea, fluid in lungs, abnormal increase in BP or CVP) and anaphylactoid reactions. May impair platelet function. Less effective that other agents for DVT/PE prevention.

hetastarch (*Hespan, Hextend*) ▶K ♀C ▶? $$$
ADULT - Shock/hypovolemia: 500-1000 mL IV infusion, total daily dose usually should not exceed 20 mL/kg (1500 mL). Renal impairment: CrCl <10 mL/min, usual initial dose followed by 20-25% of usual dose.
PEDS - Not approved in children.
UNAPPROVED PEDS - Shock/hypovolemia: 10 mL/kg/dose; do not exceed 20 mL/kg/day.
NOTES - Monitor for plasma volume overload (dyspnea, fluid in lungs, abnormal increase in BP or CVP). Little or no antigenic properties compared to dextran.

plasma protein fraction (*Plasmanate, Protenate, Plasmatein*) ▶L ♀C ▶? $$$
ADULT - Shock/hypovolemia: Adjust initial rate according to clinical response and BP, but rate should not exceed 10 mL/min. As plasma volume normalizes, infusion rate should not exceed 5-8 mL/min. Usual dose 250-500 mL. Hypoproteinemia: 1000-1500 mL/day IV infusion.
PEDS - Shock/hypovolemia: Initial dose 6.6-33 mL/kg infused at a rate of 5-10 mL/min.
NOTES - Fever, chills, hypotension with rapid infusion. Monitor for plasma volume overload (dyspnea, fluid in lungs, abnormal increase in BP or CVP). Less pure than albumin products.

CARDIOVASCULAR: Other

BiDil (hydralazine + isosorbide dinitrate) ▶LK ♀C ▶? $$$$$
ADULT - Heart Failure (adjunct to standard therapy in black patients): Start 1 tab PO tid, increase as tolerated to max 2 tabs bid. May decrease to ½ tab tid with intolerable side effects; try to increase dose when side effects subside.
PEDS - Not approved in children.
FORMS - Trade only: Tabs, scored 37.5/20 mg.
NOTES - See component drugs

cilostazol (*Pletal*) ▶L ♀C ▶? $$$
WARNING - Contraindicated in heart failure of any severity.
ADULT - Intermittent claudication: 100 mg PO bid on empty stomach. 50 mg PO bid with CYP P450 3A4 inhibitors (like ketoconazole, itraconazole, erythromycin, diltiazem) or cytochrome P450 2C19 inhibitors (like omeprazole). Beneficial effect may take up to 12 weeks.
PEDS - Not approved in children.
FORMS - Generic/Trade: Tabs 50, 100 mg.
NOTES - Avoid grapefruit juice. Caution with

moderate/severe liver impairment or CrCl <25 mL/min. Give with other antiplatelet therapy (aspirin/clopidogrel) when treating lower extremity peripheral arterial disease to reduce cardiovascular risk.

isoxsuprine (Vasodilan) ▶KL ♀C ▶? $
ADULT - Adjunctive therapy for cerebral vascular insufficiency and PVD: 10-20 mg PO tid-qid.
PEDS - Not approved in children.
FORMS - Generic/Trade: Tabs, 10,20 mg.
NOTES - Drug has questionable benefit.

nesiritide (Natrecor) ▶K,plasma ♀C ▶? $$$$$
ADULT - Hospitalized patients with decompensated heart failure with dyspnea at rest: 2 mcg/kg IV bolus over 60 seconds, then 0.01 mcg/kg/min IV infusion for up to 48 hours. Do not initiate at higher doses. Limited experience with increased doses: 0.005 mcg/kg/min increments, preceded by 1 mcg/kg bolus, no more frequently than q3h up to max infusion dose 0.03 mcg/kg/min. 1.5 mg vial in 250mL D5W (6 mcg/mL). 70 kg: 2 mcg/kg bolus = 23.3 mL, 0.01 mcg/kg/min infusion = 7 mL/h.
PEDS - Not approved in children.
NOTES - May increase mortality; meta-analysis showed non-statistically significant increased death risk within 30 days post-treatment compared with non-inotropic control group. Not indicated for outpatient infusion, for scheduled repetitive use, to improve renal function, or to enhance diuresis. Contraindicated as primary therapy for cardiogenic shock and when SBP <90 mmHg. Discontinue if dose-related symptomatic hypotension occurs and support BP prn. May restart infusion with dose reduced by 30% (no bolus dose) once BP stabilized. Do not shake reconstituted vial, and dilute vial prior to administration. Incompatible with most injectable drugs; administer agents using separate IV lines. Do not measure BNP levels while infusing; may measure BNP at least 2-6 hrs after infusion completion.

papaverine ▶LK ♀C ▶? $
ADULT - Cerebral & peripheral ischemia: Start 150 mg PO bid, increase to max 300 mg bid if needed. Start 30 mg IV/IM, dose range 30-120 mg q3h prn. Give IV doses over 1-2 min.
PEDS - Not approved in children.
FORMS - Generic only: cap, extended-release, 150 mg.

pentoxifylline (Trental) ▶L ♀C ▶? $$$
ADULT - Intermittent claudication: 400 mg PO tid with meals. For CNS/GI adverse effects, decrease dose to 400 mg PO bid. Beneficial effect may take up to 8 weeks. May be less effective in relieving cramps, tiredness, tightness, and pain during exercise.
PEDS - Not approved in children.
FORMS - Generic/Trade: Tabs 400 mg.
NOTES - Contraindicated with recent cerebral/retinal bleed. Increases theophylline levels. Increases INR with warfarin.

ranolazine (Ranexa) ▶LK ♀C ▶? $$$$$
ADULT - Chronic angina: 500 mg PO bid, increase to 1000 mg PO bid prn based on symptoms, max 2000 mg daily. Reserve for angina not controlled with other antianginal drugs; use with amlodipine, beta blockers, or nitrates.
PEDS - Not approved in children.
FORMS – Trade: Tabs, ext'd release 500 mg.
NOTES - Get baseline and follow-up EKGs; evaluate effects on QT interval. Contraindicated with pre-existing QT prolongation, hepatic impairment, QT prolonging drugs (e.g. Class Ia /III antiarrhythmics, erythromycin, thioridazine, ziprasidone), potent/moderately potent CYP 3A4 inhibitors (e.g. ketoconazole, HIV protease inhibitors, macrolides, diltiazem, verapamil), grapefruit juice/products, severe renal impairment. May need to reduce doses of co-administered simvastatin, digoxin, or P-gp substrates. Swallow whole; do not crush, break, or chew. May be less effective in women. Instruct patients to report palpitations or fainting spells.

CONTRAST MEDIA: MRI Contrast – Gadolinium-based

NOTE: Avoid gadolinium-based contrast agents if severe renal insufficiency (GFR <30 mL/min/1.73 m^2) due to risk of nephrogenic systemic fibrosis / nephrogenic fibrosing dermopathy. Similarly avoid in acute renal insufficiency of any severity due to hepatorenal syndrome or during the perioperative phase of liver transplant.

gadobenate (MultiHance) ▶K ♀C ▶? $$$$

ADULT - Non-iodinated, non-ionic IV contrast for MRI.
PEDS - Not approved in children.

gadodiamide (Omniscan) ▶K ♀C ▶? $$$$
ADULT, PEDS - Non-iodinated, non-ionic IV contrast for MRI.
NOTES - Use caution if renal disease. May falsely lower serum calcium.

gadopentetate (*Magnevist*) ▶K ♀C ▶? $$$
ADULT - Non-iodinated IV contrast for MRI.
PEDS - >2 yo: Non-iodinated IV MRI contrast.
NOTES - Caution in sickle cell, renal disease.

gadoteridol (*Prohance*) ▶K ♀C ▶? $$$$
ADULT - Non-iodinated, non-ionic IV contrast for MRI.

PEDS - >2 yo: Non-iodinated, non-ionic IV contrast for MRI.
NOTES - Caution in sickle cell, renal disease.

gadoversetamide (*OptiMARK*) ▶K♀C▶- $$$$
ADULT - Non-iodinated IV contrast for MRI.
PEDS - Not approved in children.
NOTES - Caution in sickle cell, renal disease.

CONTRAST MEDIA: MRI Contrast – Other

ferumoxides (*Feridex*) ▶L ♀C ▶? $$$$
ADULT - Non-iodinated, non-ionic, iron-based IV contrast for hepatic MRI.
PEDS - Not approved in children.
NOTES - Contains dextran.

ferumoxsil (*GastroMARK*) ▶L ♀B ▶? $$$$

ADULT - Non-iodinated, non-ionic, iron-based, oral GI contrast for MRI.
PEDS - Not approved in children <16 yo.

mangafodipir (*Teslascan*) ▶L ♀- ▶- $$$$
ADULT - Non-iodinated manganese IV contrast.
PEDS - Not approved in children.

CONTRAST MEDIA: Radiography Contrast

NOTE: Beware of allergic or anaphylactoid reactions. Avoid IV contrast in renal insufficiency or dehydration. Hold metformin (Glucophage) prior to or at the time of iodinated contrast dye use and for 48 h after procedure. Restart after procedure only if renal function is normal.

barium sulfate ▶Not absorbed ♀? ▶+ $
ADULT, PEDS - Non-iodinated GI (eg, oral, rectal) contrast.
NOTES - Contraindicated if suspected esophageal, gastric or intestinal perforation. Use with caution in GI obstruction. May cause abdominal distention, cramping, and constipation with oral use.

diatrizoate (*Cystografin, Gastrografin, Hypaque, MD-Gastroview, RenoCal, Reno-DIP, Reno-60, Renografin*) ▶K ♀C ▶? $
WARNING - Not for intrathecal or epidural use.
ADULT, PEDS - Iodinated, ionic, high osmolality IV or GI contrast.
NOTES - High osmolality contrast may cause tissue damage if infiltrated/extravasated. IV: Hypaque, Renografin, Reno-DIP, RenoCal. GI: Gastrografin, MD-Gastroview.

iodixanol (*Visipaque*) ▶K ♀B ▶? $$$
ADULT, PEDS - Iodinated, non-ionic, iso-

osmolar IV contrast.
NOTES - Not for intrathecal use.

iohexol (*Omnipaque*) ▶K ♀B ▶? $$$
ADULT, PEDS - Iodinated, non-ionic, low osmolality IV and oral/body cavity contrast.

iopamidol (*Isovue*) ▶K ♀? ▶? $$
ADULT, PEDS - Iodinated, non-ionic, low osmolality IV contrast.

iopromide (*Ultravist*) ▶K ♀B ▶? $$$
ADULT, PEDS - Iodinated, non-ionic, low osmolality IV contrast.

iothalamate (*Conray*, ♥*Vascoray*) ▶K ♀B ▶- $
ADULT, PEDS - Iodinated, ionic, high osmolality IV contrast.
NOTES - High osmolality contrast may cause tissue damage if infiltrated/extravasated.

ioversol (*Optiray*) ▶K ♀B ▶? $$
ADULT, PEDS - Iodinated, non-ionic, low osmolality IV contrast.

ioxaglate (*Hexabrix*) ▶K ♀B ▶- $$$
ADULT, PEDS - Iodinated, ionic, low osmolality IV contrast.

ioxilan (*Oxilan*) ▶K ♀B ▶- $$$
ADULT, PEDS - Iodinated, non-ionic, low osmolality IV contrast.

DERMATOLOGY: Acne Preparations

NOTE: For topical agents, wash area prior to application. Wash hands before & after application; avoid eye area.

adapalene (*Differin*) ▶Bile ♀C ▶? $$

ADULT - Acne: apply qhs.
PEDS - Not approved in children.
UNAPPROVED PEDS - Acne: apply qhs.
FORMS - Trade only: gel 0.1% & 0.3% (15,45 g)

cream 0.1% (15,45 g), soln 0.1% pad (30 mL).

NOTES - During early weeks of therapy, acne exacerbation may occur. May cause erythema, scaling, dryness, pruritus, and burning in up to 40% of patients. Results take 8-12 weeks.

azelaic acid (*Azelex, Finacea, Finevin*) ►K ♀B ▶? $$$

ADULT - Acne (Azelex, Finevin): apply bid. Rosacea (Finacea): apply bid.

PEDS - Not approved in children.

UNAPPROVED ADULT - Melasma: apply bid.

UNAPPROVED PEDS - Acne: apply qhs.

FORMS - Trade only: cream 20%, 30g, 50g (Azelex, Finevin), gel 15% 30g (Finacea).

NOTES - Improvement of acne occurs within 4 weeks. Monitor for hypopigmentation esp. in patients with dark complexions. Avoid use of occlusive dressings.

BenzaClin **(clindamycin + benzoyl peroxide)** ►K ♀C ▶+ $$$

ADULT - Acne: apply bid.

PEDS - Not approved in children.

UNAPPROVED PEDS - Acne: apply qhs.

FORMS - Trade only: gel clindamycin 1% + benzoyl peroxide 5%; 25, 50 g, gel pump clindamycin 1% + benzoyl peroxide 5%; 50 g.

NOTES - Expires 10 weeks after mixing.

Benzamycin **(erythromycin base + benzoyl peroxide)** ►LK ♀C ▶? $$$

ADULT - Acne: apply bid.

PEDS - Not approved in children.

UNAPPROVED PEDS - Acne: apply qhs.

FORMS - Generic/Trade: gel erythromycin 3% + benzoyl peroxide 5%; 23.3, 46.6 g.

NOTES - Must be refrigerated, expires 3 months after pharmacy dispensing.

benzoyl peroxide (*Benzac, Benzagel 10%, Desquam, Clearasil, ✚Solugel, Benoxyl*) ►LK ♀C ▶? $

ADULT - Acne: Cleansers: wash daily-bid. Creams/gels/lotion: apply daily initially, gradually increase to bid-tid if needed.

PEDS - Not approved in children.

UNAPPROVED PEDS - Acne: Cleansers: wash daily-bid. Creams/gels/lotion: apply daily initially, gradually increase to bid-tid if needed.

FORMS - OTC & Rx generic: liquid 2.5, 5, 10%, bar 5,10%, mask 5%, lotion 5,5.5,10%, cream 5,10%, cleanser 10%, gel 2.5,4,5, 6,10, 20%.

NOTES - If excessive drying or peeling occurs, reduce frequency of application. Use with PABA-containing sunscreens may cause transient skin discoloration. May bleach fabric.

Clenia **(sulfacetamide + sulfur)** ►K♀C ▶? $$

ADULT - Acne, rosacea, seborrheic dermatitis: apply cream/gel daily-tid, foaming wash daily-bid.

PEDS - Not approved in children.

FORMS - Generic only: lotion (sodium sulfacetamide 10% & sulfur 5%) 25 g. Trade only (sodium sulfacetamide 10% & sulfur 5%): cream 28 g, foaming wash 170,340 g.

NOTES - Avoid with sulfa allergy, renal failure.

clindamycin (*Cleocin T, ClindaMax, Evoclin, ✚Dalacin T*) ►L ♀B ▶- $

ADULT - Acne: apply daily (Evoclin) or bid (Cleocin T).

PEDS - Not approved in children.

UNAPPROVED ADULT - Rosacea: apply lotion bid.

UNAPPROVED PEDS - Acne: apply bid.

FORMS - Generic/Trade: gel 1% 7.5, 30g, lotion 1% 60 mL, solution 1% 30,60 mL. Trade only: foam 1% 50 g (Evoclin).

NOTES - Concomitant use with erythromycin may decrease effectiveness. Most common adverse effects dryness, erythema, burning, peeling, oiliness and itching. Pseudomembranous colitis has been reported with topical use.

Diane-35 **(cyproterone + ethinyl estradiol)** ►L ♀X ▶- $$

WARNING - Not recommended in women who smoke. Increased risk of thromboembolism, stroke, MI, hepatic neoplasia & gallbladder disease. Nausea, breast tenderness, & breakthrough bleeding are common, transient side effects. Nighttime dosing may minimize nausea. Effectiveness is reduced by hepatic enzyme-inducing drugs such as certain anticonvulsants and barbiturates, rifampin, rifabutin, griseofulvin & protease inhibitors. Antibiotics or St. John's wort may reduce efficacy.

ADULT - Canada only. In women, severe acne unresponsive to oral antibiotics and other treatments, with associated symptoms of androgenization, including seborrhea and mild hirsutism: 1 tab PO daily for 21 consecutive days, stop for 7 days, repeat cycle.

PEDS - Not approved in children.

FORMS - Rx trade: blister pack of 21 tabs 2 mg/ 0.035 mg cyproterone acetate/ethinyl estradiol.

NOTES - Higher thromboembolic risk than other oral contraceptives, therefore only indicated for acne, and not solely for contraception (although effective for the latter). Same warnings, precautions, and contraindications as other oral contraceptives.

Duac **(clindamycin + benzoyl peroxide,**

♣*Clindoxyl)* ▶K ♀C ▶+ $$$$
ADULT - Acne: apply qhs.
PEDS - Not approved in children.
UNAPPROVED PEDS - Acne: apply qhs.
FORMS - Trade only: gel clindamycin 1% + benzoyl peroxide 5%; 45 g.
NOTES - Expires 2 months after pharmacy dispensing.

erythromycin (Eryderm, Erycette, Erygel, A/T/S, ♣Sans-Acne, Erysol) ▶L ♀B ▶? $$
ADULT - Acne: apply bid.
PEDS - Not approved in children.
UNAPPROVED PEDS - Acne: apply bid.
FORMS - Generic only: solution 1.5% 60 mL, 2% 60,120 mL, pads 2%, gel 2% 30,60 g, ointment 2% 25 g.
NOTES - May be more irritating when used with other acne products. Concomitant use with clindamycin may decrease effectiveness.

isotretinoin (Accutane, Amnesteem, Claravis, Sotret, ♣Clarus) ▶LK ♀X ▶- $$$$$
WARNING - Physicians pharmacists, and patients must register with the iPledge program in order to prescribe, dispense or take isotretinoin. Contraindicated in pregnant women or in women who may become pregnant. If used in a woman of childbearing age, patient must have severe, disfiguring acne, be reliable, comply with mandatory contraceptive measures, receive written and oral instructions about hazards of taking during pregnancy, have 2 negative pregnancy tests prior to beginning therapy. Must use 2 forms of effective contraception, unless absolute abstinence is chosen or patient has undergone a hysterectomy, from 1 month prior until 1 month after discontinuation of therapy. Men should not father children. May cause depression, suicidal thought, and aggressive or violent behavior; monitor for symptoms. Obtain written informed consent. Write prescription for no more than a 1 month supply. Informed consent documents available from the manufacturer.
ADULT - Severe, recalcitrant cystic acne: 0.5-2 mg/kg/day PO divided bid for 15-20 weeks. Typical target dose is 1 mg/kg/day. May repeat 2nd course after >2 months off therapy.
PEDS - Not approved in children.
UNAPPROVED ADULT - Prevention of second primary tumors in patients treated for squamous cell carcinoma of the head and neck: 50-100 mg/m^2/day PO. Also been used in keratinization disorders.
UNAPPROVED PEDS - Severe, recalcitrant cystic acne: 0.5-2 mg/kg/day PO divided bid for 15-20 weeks. Typical target dose is 1 mg/kg/day. Maintenance therapy for neuroblastoma: 100-250 mg/m^2/day PO in 2 divided doses.
FORMS - Generic/Trade: caps 10, 20, 40 mg. Generic only (Sotret & Claravis): caps 30 mg.
NOTES - Prescription must have iPledge "qualification sticker" attached and can be for max 1 month supply. May cause headache, cheilitis, drying of mucous membranes including eyes, nose, mouth, hair loss, abdominal pain, pyuria, joint and muscle pain/ stiffness, conjunctivitis, elevated ESR, and changes in serum lipids and LFTs. Effect on bone loss unknown; caution if predisposed to osteoporosis. In children with incomplete skeletal growth, do not exceed the recommended dose. Pseudotumor cerebri has occurred; avoid concomitant vitamin A, tetracycline, minocycline. May cause corneal opacities, decreased night vision, inflammatory bowel disease. May decrease carbamazepine levels. Avoid excessive exposure to sunlight.

Rosula (sulfacetamide + sulfur) ▶K ♀C ▶? $$
ADULT - Acne, rosacea, seborrheic dermatitis: apply cream / gel / aqueous cleanser daily-tid, foaming wash daily-bid.
PEDS - Not approved in children.
FORMS - Generic only: lotion (sodium Sulfacetamide 10% & sulfur 5%) 25 g. Trade only: gel (sodium sulfacetamide 10% & sulfur 5%) 45 mL, aqueous cleanser (sodium sulfacetamide 10% & sulfur 5%) 355 mL.
NOTES - Avoid with sulfa allergy or renal failure.

salicylic acid (Akurza, Clearasil Cleanser, Stridex Pads) ▶Not absorbed ♀? ▶? $
ADULT - Acne (OTC): apply/wash area up to three times daily. Removal of excessive keratin in hyperkeratotic disorders (Rx): apply to affected area at bedtime and cover. Hydrate skin before application.
PEDS - Acne: apply/wash area up to three times daily.
FORMS - Generic/Trade: OTC: pads, foam, mask scrub, 0.5%, 1%, 2%. Rx/Trade: cream 6%, 12 oz. (Akurza), lotion 6%, 12 oz. (Akurza)

sulfacetamide (Klaron) ▶K ♀C ▶? $$
ADULT - Acne: apply bid.
PEDS - Not approved in children.
FORMS - Generic/Trade: lotion 10% 59,118 mL.
NOTES - Cross-sensitivity with sulfa allergy.

Sulfacet-R (sulfacetamide + sulfur) ▶K ♀C ▶? $$
ADULT - Acne, rosacea, seborrheic dermatitis:

apply cream/gel daily-tid, foaming wash daily-bid.

PEDS - Not approved in children.

FORMS - Trade (Sulfacet-R) and generic: lotion (sodium sulfacetamide 10% & sulfur 5%) 25 g.

NOTES - Avoid with sulfa allergy or renal failure.

tazarotene (*Tazorac, Avage*) ▶L ♀X ▶? $$$$

ADULT - Acne (Tazorac): apply 0.1% cream qhs. Palliation of fine facial wrinkles, mottled hyper- and hypopigmentation, benign facial lentigines (Avage): apply qhs. Psoriasis: apply 0.05% cream qhs, increase to 0.1% prn.

PEDS - Not approved in children.

UNAPPROVED PEDS - Acne: apply 0.1% cream qhs. Psoriasis: apply 0.05% cream qhs.

FORMS - Trade only (Tazorac): Cream 0.05% and 0.1% - 30, 60g, Gel 0.05% and 0.1% - 30, 100g. Trade (Avage): Cream 0.1% 15, 30g.

NOTES - In psoriasis, may reduce irritation and improve efficacy by using topical corticosteroid in morning and tazarotene at bedtime. Desquamation, burning, dry skin, erythema, pruritus may occur in up to 30% of patients. May cause photosensitivity.

tretinoin (*Retin-A, Retin-A Micro, Renova, Retisol-A, ✦Stieva-A, Rejuva-A, Vitamin A Acid Cream*) ▶LK ♀C ▶? $$

ADULT - Acne (Retin A, Retin-A Micro): apply qhs. Wrinkles, hyperpigmentation, tactile roughness (Renova): apply qhs.

PEDS - Not approved in children.

UNAPPROVED ADULT - Used in skin cancer and lamellar ichthyosis, mollusca contagiosa, verrucae plantaris, verrucae planae juvenilis, hyperpigmented lesions in black individuals, ichthyosis vulgaris, and pityriasis rubra pilaris.

FORMS - Generic/Trade: cream 0.025% 20,45 g, 0.05% 20,45 g, 0.1% 20,45 g, gel 0.025% 15,45 g, 0.1% 15,45 g, liquid 0.05% 28 mL. Trade: Renova cream 0.02% & 0.05% 40,60 g, Retin-A Micro gel 0.04%, 0.1% 20,45 g.

NOTES - May induce erythema, peeling. Minimize sun exposure. Concomitant use with sulfur, resorcinol, benzoyl peroxide, or salicylic acid may result in skin irritation. Gel preps are flammable.

Ziana (clindamycin + tretinoin) ▶LK ♀C ▶? $$$$

ADULT - Acne: Apply qhs.

PEDS - ≥12 yo: Use adult dose.

FORMS - Trade only: gel clindamycin 1.2% + tretinoin 0.025% 30, 60 g.

NOTES - May induce erythema, peeling. Minimize sun exposure.

DERMATOLOGY: Actinic Keratosis Preparations

aminolevulinic acid (*Levulan Kerastick*) ▶Not absorbed ♀C ▶? $$$

ADULT - Non-hyperkeratotic actinic keratoses: apply solution to lesions on scalp or face; expose to special light source 14-18 h later.

PEDS - Not approved in children.

FORMS - Trade only: 20% solution single use ampules.

NOTES - Should be applied by healthcare personnel. Advise patients to avoid sunlight during 14-18 h period before blue light illumination.

diclofenac (*Solaraze*) ▶L ♀B ▶? $$$$

ADULT - Actinic/solar keratoses: apply bid to lesions x 60-90 days.

PEDS - Not approved in children.

FORMS - Trade only: gel 3% 50, 100 g.

NOTES - Avoid exposure to sun and sunlamps. Use caution in aspirin-sensitive patients.

fluorouracil (*5-FU, Carac, Efudex, Fluoroplex*) ▶L ♀X ▶- $$$$$

WARNING - Contraindicated in pregnancy or in women who plan to get pregnant during therapy. Avoid application to mucous membranes.

ADULT - Actinic or solar keratoses: apply bid to lesions x 2-6 wks. Superficial basal cell carcinomas: apply 5% cream/solution bid.

PEDS - Not approved in children.

UNAPPROVED ADULT - Condylomata acuminata: a 1% solution in 70% ethanol and the 5% cream has been used.

FORMS - Trade: Cream 0.5% 30 g (Carac), 5% 25, 40 g (Efudex), 1% 30 g (Fluoroplex). Generic/Trade: Soln 2% & 5% 10 mL (Efudex).

NOTES - May cause severe irritation & photosensitivity. Contraindicated in women who are or who may become pregnant during therapy. Avoid application to mucous membranes.

methylaminolevulinate (*Metvixia*) ▶Not absorbed ♀C ▶? ?

ADULT - Non-hyperkeratotic actinic keratoses of face/scalp: Apply cream 1 mm thick (max 1 g) to lesion and 5 mm surrounding area; cover with dressing for 3h; remove dressing and cream and perform illumination therapy. Repeat in 7 days.

PEDS - Not approved in children.

FORMS - Trade only: cream: 16.8%, 2 g.
NOTES - Use in immunocompetent individuals. Lesion debridement should be performed prior to application of cream. Formulated in peanut and almond oil; has not been tested in patients allergic to peanuts.

DERMATOLOGY: Antibacterials (Topical)

bacitracin (✽*Baciguent*) ▶Not absorbed ♀C ▶? $
ADULT - Minor cuts, wounds, burns or skin abrasions: apply daily-tid.
PEDS - Not approved in children.
UNAPPROVED PEDS - Minor cuts, wounds, burns or skin abrasions: apply daily-tid.
FORMS - OTC Generic/Trade: ointment 500 units/g 1,15,30g.
NOTES - May cause contact dermatitis or anaphylaxis.

fusidic acid (✽*Fucidin*) ▶L ♀? ▶? $
ADULT, PEDS - Canada only. Skin infections: Apply tid-qid.
FORMS - Canada trade only: cream 2% fusidic acid 5,15,30 g, ointment 2% sodium fusidate 5,15,30 g.
NOTES - Contains lanolin; possible hypersensitivity.

gentamicin (*Garamycin*) ▶K ♀D ▶? $
ADULT - Skin infections: apply tid-qid.
PEDS - Skin infections >1 yo: apply tid-qid.
FORMS - Generic/Trade: ointment 0.1% 15,30 g, cream 0.1% 15,30 g.

mafenide (*Sulfamylon*) ▶LK ♀C ▶? $$$
ADULT, PEDS - Adjunctive treatment of burns: apply daily-bid.
FORMS - Trade only: cream 37, 114, 411 g, 5% topical solution 50 g packets.
NOTES - Can cause metabolic acidosis. Contains sulfonamides.

metronidazole (*Noritate*, *MetroCream*, *MetroGel*, *MetroLotion*, ✽*Rosasol*) ▶KL ♀B(- in 1st trimester) ▶- $$$
ADULT - Rosacea: apply daily (1%) or bid (0.75%).
PEDS - Not approved in children.
UNAPPROVED ADULT - A 1% solution prepared from the oral tabs has been used in the treatment of infected decubitus ulcers.
FORMS - Trade only: Gel (MetroGel) 1% 45,60 g, Cream (Noritate) 1% 30,60 g. Generic/Trade: Gel 0.75% 29g. Cream 0.75% 45 g. Lotion (MetroLotion) 0.75% 59 mL.
NOTES - Results usually noted within 3 weeks, with continuing improvement through 9 weeks. Avoid using vaginal prep on face due to irritation because of formulation differences.

mupirocin (*Bactroban, Centany*) ▶Not absorbed ♀B ▶? $$$
ADULT - Impetigo: apply tid x 3-5 days. Infected wounds: apply tid x 10 days. Nasal methicillin-resistant Staph aureus eradication: 0.5 g in each nostril bid x 5 days.
PEDS - Impetigo (mupirocin cream/ointment): apply tid. Infected wounds: apply tid x 10 days. Nasal form not approved in children <12 yo.
FORMS - Generic/Trade: cream/ointment 2% 15, 22, 30 g, 2% nasal ointment 1 g single-use tubes (for MRSA eradication).

Neosporin cream (neomycin + polymyxin) ▶K ♀C ▶? $
ADULT - Minor cuts, wounds, burns or skin abrasions: apply daily-tid.
PEDS - Not approved in children.
UNAPPROVED PEDS - Minor cuts, wounds, burns or skin abrasions: apply daily-tid.
FORMS - OTC Trade: neomycin 3.5 mg/g + polymyxin 10,000 units/g 15 g & unit dose 0.94 g.
NOTES - Neomycin component can cause contact dermatitis.

Neosporin ointment (bacitracin + neomycin + polymyxin) ▶K ♀C ▶? $
ADULT - Minor cuts, wounds, burns or skin abrasions: apply daily-tid.
PEDS - Not approved in children.
UNAPPROVED PEDS - Minor cuts, wounds, burns or skin abrasions: apply daily-tid.
FORMS - OTC Generic/Trade: bacitracin 400 units/g + neomycin 3.5 mg/g + polymyxin 5,000 units/g 2.4,9.6,14.2,15,30 g & unit dose 0.94 g.
NOTES - Also known as triple antibiotic ointment. Neomycin can cause contact dermatitis.

Polysporin (bacitracin + polymyxin, ✽*Polytopic*) ▶K ♀C ▶? $
ADULT - Minor cuts, wounds, burns or skin abrasions: apply daily-tid.
PEDS - Not approved in children.
UNAPPROVED PEDS - Minor cuts, wounds, burns or skin abrasions: apply daily-tid.
FORMS - OTC Trade only: ointment 15,30 g and unit dose 0.9 g, powder 10 g, aerosol 90 g.
NOTES - May cause allergic contact dermatitis and rarely contact anaphylaxis.

retapamulin (*Altabax*) ▶Not absorbed ♀B ▶? $$$
ADULT - Impetigo: apply bid for 5 days.
PEDS - Impetigo (9 months or older): apply bid for 5 days.
FORMS - Trade only: ointment 1% 5, 10, 15 g.
silver sulfadiazine (*Silvadene*, ♥*Dermazin, Flamazine, SSD*) ▶LK ♀B ▶- $
ADULT - Burns: apply daily-bid.
PEDS - Not approved in children.
UNAPPROVED ADULT - Has been used for pressure ulcers.
UNAPPROVED PEDS - Burns: apply daily-bid.
FORMS - Generic/Trade: cream 1% 20,50,85, 400,1000g.
NOTES - Avoid in sulfa allergy. Leukopenia (primarily neutrophils) in up to 20%. Significant absorption may occur and sulfa concentrations approach therapeutic levels. Avoid in G6PD deficiency. Use caution in pregnancy nearing term, premature infants, infants ≤2 months and in patients with renal or hepatic dysfunction.

DERMATOLOGY: Antifungals

butenafine (*Lotrimin Ultra, Mentax*) ▶L ♀B ▶? $
ADULT - Tinea pedis treatment: apply daily for 4 weeks or bid x 7 days. Tinea corporis, tinea versicolor, or tinea cruris: apply daily x 2 wks.
PEDS - Not approved in children.
FORMS - Trade. Rx: cream 1% 15,30 g (Mentax). OTC: cream 1% 12,24 g (Lotrimin Ultra).
NOTES - Most common adverse effects include contact dermatitis, burning, and worsening of condition. If no improvement in 4 weeks, re-evaluate diagnosis.
ciclopirox (*Loprox, Penlac*, ♥*Stieprox shampoo*) ▶K ♀B ▶? $$$$
ADULT - Tinea pedis, cruris, corporis, and versicolor, candidiasis (cream, lotion): apply bid. Onychomycosis of fingernails/toenails (nail solution): apply daily to affected nails; apply over previous coat; remove with alcohol every 7 days. Seborrheic dermatitis (Loprox shampoo): shampoo twice/week x 4 weeks.
PEDS - Onychomycosis of fingernails/toenails in children ≥12 yo (nail solution): apply daily to affected nails; apply over previous coat; remove with alcohol every 7 days (Penlac). Not approved in children <12 yo.
FORMS - Trade only: gel (Loprox) 0.77% 30,45 g, shampoo (Loprox) 1% 120 mL, nail solution (Penlac) 8% 6.6 mL. Generic/Trade: cream (Loprox) 0.77% 15,30,90 g, lotion (Loprox) 0.77% 30,60 mL.
NOTES - Tinea improvement usually within first week. Patients with tinea versicolor usually exhibit clinical and mycological clearing after 2 weeks. If no improvement in 4 weeks, reevaluate diagnosis. Do not get shampoo in eyes. No safety information available in diabetes or immunocompromise. Shampoo may affect hair color in those with light-colored hair. For nail solution, infected portion of each nail should be removed by health care professional as frequently as monthly. Oral antifungal therapy is more effective for onychomycosis than Penlac.
clotrimazole (*Lotrimin, Mycelex*, ♥*Canesten, Clotrimaderm*) ▶L ♀B ▶? $
ADULT, PEDS - Treatment of tinea pedis, cruris, corporis, and versicolor, and cutaneous candidiasis: apply bid.
FORMS - Note that Lotrimin brand cream, lotion, solution are clotrimazole, while Lotrimin powders & liquid spray are miconazole. OTC & Rx generic/Trade: cream 1% 15, 30, 45, 90 g, solution 1% 10,30 mL. Trade: lotion 1% 30 mL.
NOTES - If no improvement in 4 weeks, reevaluate diagnosis.
econazole (*Spectazole*) ▶Not absorbed ♀C ▶? $$
ADULT - Treatment of tinea pedis, cruris, corporis, and versicolor: apply daily. Cutaneous candidiasis: apply bid.
PEDS - Not approved in children.
FORMS - Generic/Trade: cream 1% 15,30,85g.
NOTES - Treat candidal infections, tinea cruris and tinea corporis for 2 weeks and tinea pedis for 1 month to reduce risk of recurrence.
ketoconazole (*Extina, Nizoral, Xolegel*, ♥*Ketoderm*) ▶L ♀C ▶? $$
ADULT - Shampoo (2%): Tinea versicolor: apply to affected area, leave on for 5 min, rinse. Cream: cutaneous candidiasis, tinea corporis, cruris, and versicolor: apply daily. Seborrheic dermatitis: apply cream (2%) bid for 4 weeks or gel daily for 2 weeks or foam bid for 4 weeks. Dandruff: apply shampoo (1%) twice a week.
PEDS - Not approved in children <12 years.
UNAPPROVED ADULT - Seborrheic dermatitis: apply cream (2%) daily.
UNAPPROVED PEDS - Shampoo (2%): Tinea

versicolor: apply to affected area, leave on for 5 min, rinse. Cream: cutaneous candidiasis, tinea corporis, cruris, and versicolor: apply daily. Seborrheic dermatitis: apply cream (2%) bid. Dandruff: apply shampoo (1%) twice a week.

FORMS - Generic/Trade: cream 2% 15, 30, 60 g, shampoo 2% (120 mL). Trade only: shampoo 1% (OTC), gel 2%, 15g (Rx, Xolegel) foam 2%, 50, 100 g (Rx, Extina).

NOTES - Treat candidal infections, tinea cruris, corporis and versicolor for 2 weeks. Treat seborrheic dermatitis for 4 weeks. Treat tinea pedis for 6 weeks.

miconazole (*Monistat-Derm, Micatin, Lotrimin*) ▶L ♀+ ▶? $

ADULT - Tinea pedis, cruris, corporis, and versicolor, cutaneous candidiasis: apply bid.

PEDS - Not approved in children.

UNAPPROVED PEDS - Tinea pedis, cruris, corporis, and versicolor, cutaneous candidiasis: apply bid.

FORMS - Note that Lotrimin brand cream, lotion, solution are clotrimazole, while Lotrimin powders and liquid spray are miconazole. OTC generic: ointment 2% 29 g, spray 2% 105 mL, soln 2% 7.39, 30 mL. Generic/Trade: cream 2% 15,30,90 g, powder 2% 90 g, spray powder 2% 90,100 g, spray liquid 2% 105,113 mL.

NOTES - Symptomatic relief generally occurs in 2-3 days. Treat candida, tinea cruris, tinea corporis for 2 weeks, tinea pedis for 1 month to reduce risk of recurrence.

naftifine (*Naftin*) ▶LK ♀B ▶? $$$

ADULT - Tinea pedis, cruris, and corporis: apply daily (cream) or bid (gel).

PEDS - Not approved in children.

FORMS - Trade only: cream 1% 15,30,60 g, gel 1% 20,40, 60 g.

NOTES - If no improvement in 4 weeks, re-evaluate diagnosis.

nystatin (*Mycostatin, ✚Nilstat, Nyaderm, Candistatin*) ▶Not absorbed ♀C ▶? $

ADULT, PEDS - Cutaneous or mucocutaneous Candida infections: apply bid-tid.

FORMS - Generic/Trade: cream 100,000 units/g 15,30,240 g, ointment 100,000 units/g 15,30 g,

powder 100,000 units/g 15 g.

NOTES - Ineffective for dermatophytes/tinea. For fungal infections of the feet, dust feet and footwear with powder.

oxiconazole (*Oxistat, Oxizole*) ▶? ♀B▶? $$$

ADULT - Tinea pedis, cruris, and corporis: apply daily-bid. Tinea versicolor (cream only): apply daily.

PEDS - Cream: Tinea pedis, cruris, and corporis: apply daily-bid. Tinea versicolor: apply daily.

FORMS - Trade only: cream 1% 15, 30, 60 g, lotion 1% 30 mL.

sertaconazole (*Ertaczo*) ▶Not absorbed ♀C ▶? $$

ADULT - Tinea pedis: apply bid.

PEDS - Not approved for children <12 yo.

FORMS - Trade only: cream 2% 15, 30, 60 g.

terbinafine (*Lamisil, Lamisil AT*) ▶L ♀B ▶? $$$

ADULT - Tinea pedis: apply bid. Tinea cruris and corporis: apply daily-bid. Tinea versicolor (solution): apply bid.

PEDS - Not approved in children.

UNAPPROVED ADULT - Cutaneous candidiasis.

UNAPPROVED PEDS - Tinea pedis: apply bid. Tinea cruris and corporis: apply daily-bid. Tinea versicolor (solution): apply bid.

FORMS - Trade only: cream 1% 15,30 g, gel 1% 5,15,30 g OTC: Trade (Lamisil AT): cream 1% 12,24 g, spray pump solution 1% 30 mL.

NOTES - In many patients, improvement noted within 3-4 days, but therapy should continue for a minimum of 1 week, maximum of 4 weeks. Topical therapy not effective for nail fungus.

tolnaftate (*Tinactin, ✚ZeaSorb AF*) ▶♀▶? $

ADULT - Tinea pedis, cruris, corporis, and versicolor: apply bid. Prevention of tinea pedis (powder and aerosol): apply prn.

PEDS - >2 yo: Tinea pedis, cruris, corporis, and versicolor: apply bid. Prevention of tinea pedis (powder and aerosol): apply prn.

FORMS - OTC Generic/Trade: cream 1% 15,30 g, solution 1% 10,15 mL, powder 1% 45,90 g, spray powder 1% 100,105,150 g, spray liquid 1% 60,120 mL. Trade only: gel 1% 15 g.

DERMATOLOGY: Antiparasitics (Topical)

A-200 (pyrethrins + piperonyl butoxide, ✚R&C) ▶L ♀C ▶? $

ADULT, PEDS - Lice: Apply shampoo, wash after 10 min. Reapply in 5-7 days.

FORMS - OTC Generic/Trade: shampoo (0.33% pyrethrins, 4% piperonyl butoxide) 60,120,240 mL.

NOTES - Use caution if allergic to ragweed.

Avoid contact with mucous membranes.

crotamiton (*Eurax*) ▶? ♀C ▶? $$

ADULT - Scabies: massage cream/lotion into entire body from chin down, repeat 24 h later, bathe 48 h later. Pruritus: massage into affected areas prn.

PEDS - Not approved in children.

UNAPPROVED PEDS - Scabies: massage cream/lotion into entire body from chin down, repeat 24h later, bathe 48h later. Pruritus: massage into affected areas prn.

FORMS - Trade only: cream 10% 60 g, lotion 10% 60,480 mL.

NOTES - Patients with scabies should change bed linen and clothing in am after second application and bathe 48h after last application. Consider treating entire family.

lindane (✚*Hexit*) ▶L ♀B ▶? $

WARNING – Use only if other agents have failed. Seizures and deaths have been reported with repeat or prolonged use. Use caution with infants, children, elderly, those who weigh <50 kg. Contraindicated in premature infants and patients with uncontrolled seizures.

ADULT - Head/crab lice: Lotion: apply 30-60 mL to affected area, wash off after 12h. Shampoo: apply 30-60 mL, wash off after 4 min. Scabies (lotion): apply 30-60 mL to total body from neck down, wash off after 8-12h.

PEDS - Lindane penetrates human skin and has potential for CNS toxicity. Studies indicate potential toxic effects of topical lindane are greater in young. Max dose if <6 yo is 30 mL.

FORMS - Generic/Trade: lotion 1% 30,60,480 mL, shampoo 1% 30,60,480 mL.

NOTES - For lice, reapply if living lice noted after 7 days. After shampooing, comb with fine tooth comb to remove nits. Consider treating entire family.

malathion (*Ovide*) ▶? ♀B ▶? $$

ADULT - Head lice: apply to dry hair, let dry naturally, wash off in 8-12 hrs.

PEDS - Head lice in children >6 yo: apply to dry hair, let dry naturally, wash off in 8-12 hrs.

FORMS - Trade only: lotion 0.5% 59 mL.

NOTES - Do not use hair dryer; flammable. Avoid contact with eyes. Use a fine tooth comb to remove nits and dead lice. Application may be repeated in 7-9 days.

permethrin (*Elimite, Acticin, Nix*, ✚*Kwellada-P*) ▶L ♀B ▶? $$

ADULT - Scabies (cream): massage cream into entire body (avoid mouth, eyes, nose), wash off after 8-14h. 30 g is typical adult dose. Head lice (liquid): apply to clean, towel-dried hair, saturate hair and scalp, wash off after 10 min.

PEDS - Scabies (cream) >2 mo: massage cream into entire body (avoid mouth, eyes, nose), wash off after 8-14h. Head lice (liquid) in children >2 yo: saturate hair and scalp, wash off after 10 min.

FORMS - Trade only: cream (Elimite, Acticin) 5% 60 g. OTC Generic/Trade: liquid creme rinse (Nix) 1% 60 mL.

NOTES - If necessary, may repeat application in 7 days. Consider treating entire family.

RID (pyrethrins + piperonyl butoxide) ▶L ♀C ▶? $

ADULT, PEDS - Lice: Apply shampoo/mousse, wash after 10 min. Reapply in 5-10 days.

FORMS - OTC Generic/Trade: shampoo 60, 120,240 mL. Trade only: mousse 5.5 oz.

NOTES - Use caution if allergic to ragweed. Avoid contact with mucus membranes. Available alone or as part of a RID 1-2-3 kit containing shampoo, egg and nit comb-out gel and home lice control spray for non-washable items.

DERMATOLOGY: Antipsoriatics

acitretin (*Soriatane*) ▶L ♀X ▶- $$$$$

WARNING - Contraindicated in pregnancy and avoid pregnancy for 3 years following medication discontinuation. Major human fetal abnormalities have been reported. Females of child bearing age must avoid alcohol while on medication and for 2 months following therapy since alcohol prolongs elimination of a teratogenic metabolite. Use in reliable females of reproductive potential only if they have severe, unresponsive psoriasis, have received written and oral warnings of the teratogenic potential, are using 2 reliable forms of contraception, and have 2 negative pregnancy tests within 1 week prior to starting therapy. It is unknown whether residual acitretin in seminal fluid poses a risk to the fetus while a male patient is taking the drug or after it is discontinued.

ADULT - Severe psoriasis: initiate at 25-50 mcg PO daily.

PEDS - Not approved in children.

UNAPPROVED ADULT - Lichen planus: 30 mg/

day PO for 4 weeks, then titrate to 10-50 mg/day for 12 weeks total. Sjogren-Larsson syndrome: 0.47 mg/kg/day PO. Also used in Darier's disease, palmoplantar pustulosis, non-bullous & bullous ichthyosiform erythroderma, lichen sclerosus et atrophicus of the vulva, palmoplantar lichen nitidus & chemoprevention for high-risk immunosuppressed patients with history of squamous cell carcinomas of the skin.

UNAPPROVED PEDS - Has been used in children with lamellar ichthyosis. Pediatric use is not recommended. Adverse effects on bone growth are suspected.

FORMS - Trade only: cap 10,25 mg.

NOTES - Transient worsening of psoriasis may occur, and full benefit may take 2-3 mo. Elevated LFTs may occur in 1/3 of patients; monitor LFTs at 1-2 week intervals until stable and then periodically thereafter. Monitor serum lipid concentrations every 1-2 weeks until response to drug is established. May decrease tolerance to contact lenses due to dry eyes. Avoid prolonged exposure to sunlight. May cause hair loss. May cause depression. May cause bone changes, especially with use >6 months. Many adverse drug reactions.

alefacept (Amevive) ▶? ♀B ▶? $$$$$
ADULT - Moderate to severe psoriasis: 7.5 mg IV or 15 mg IM once weekly x 12 doses. May repeat with 1 additional 12-week course after 12 weeks have elapsed from last dose.

PEDS - Not approved in children.

NOTES - Monitor CD4+ T lymphocyte cells weekly; withhold therapy if count <250/mcL and stop altogether if <250/mcL for one month. Do not give to HIV-positive patients or with other immunosuppressives or phototherapy.

anthralin (Anthra-Derm, Drithocreme, ♣Anthrascalp, Anthranol, Anthraforte, Dithranol) ▶? ♀C ▶- $$
ADULT - Chronic psoriasis: apply daily.

PEDS - Not approved in children.

UNAPPROVED PEDS - Chronic psoriasis: apply daily.

FORMS - Trade only: ointment 0.1% 42.5 g, 0.25% 42.5 g, 0.4% 60 g, 0.5% 42.5 g, 1% 42.5 g, cream 0.1% 50 g, 0.2% 50 g, 0.25% 50 g, 0.5% 50 g. Generic/Trade: cream 1% 50 g.

NOTES - Short contact periods (i.e. 15-20 minutes) followed by removal with an appropriate solvent (soap or petrolatum) may be preferred. May stain fabric, skin, or hair.

calcipotriene (Dovonex) ▶L ♀C ▶? $$$
ADULT - Moderate plaque psoriasis: apply bid.

PEDS - Not approved in children.

UNAPPROVED ADULT - Has been used for vitiligo.

UNAPPROVED PEDS - Moderate plaque psoriasis: apply bid. Has been used for vitiligo.

FORMS - Trade only: ointment 0.005% 30,60, 100 g, cream 0.005% 30,60,100 g, scalp solution 0.005% 60 mL.

NOTES - Avoid contact with face. Do not exceed 100 g/week to minimize risk of hypercalcemia, hypercalciuria. Burning, itching, and skin irritation may occur in 10-15% of patients.

efalizumab (Raptiva) ▶L ♀C ▶? $$$$$
WARNING - Can cause serious infections or reactivate latent chronic infections. Discontinue if serious infection. Caution if high risk for / history of malignancy. Monitor CBC; can cause severe thrombocytopenia and hemolytic anemia. Can cause worsening of psoriasis during or after treatment.

ADULT - Moderate to severe plaque psoriasis: 0.7 mg/kg SC x 1 then 1 mg/kg SC q week.

PEDS - Not approved in children.

FORMS - Trade only: single use vials, 125 mg.

NOTES - Monitor platelets upon initiation and monthly thereafter. May decrease to every 3 months with continued therapy.

methoxsalen (8-MOP, Oxsoralen-Ultra) ▶Skin ♀C ▶? $$$$$
ADULT - Psoriasis: dose based on weight (0.4 mg/kg/dose), 1½ to 2 hours before ultraviolet light exposure.

PEDS - Not approved in children.

FORMS - Trade only: soft gelatin cap 10 mg (Oxsoralen-Ultra), hard gelatin cap 10 mg (8-MOP).

NOTES - Oxsoralen-Ultra (soft gelatin cap) cannot be interchanged with 8-MOP (hard gelatin cap) due to significant bioavailability differences and photosensitization onset times. Take with food or milk. Wear ultraviolet light blocking glasses and avoid sun exposure after ingestion and for remainder of day.

Taclonex (calcipotriene + betamethasone) ▶L ♀C ▶? $$$$$
ADULT - Psoriasis vulgaris: Apply daily for up to 4 weeks.

PEDS - Not approved in children.

FORMS - Trade only: ointment calcipotriene 0.005% + betamethasone dipropionate 0.064% ointment 15, 30, 60g.

NOTES - Do not exceed 100g per week. Do not use on more than 30% of body surface area. Do not apply to face, groin, or axillae.

DERMATOLOGY: Antivirals (Topical)

acyclovir (*Zovirax*) ▶K ♀C ▶? $$$$$
ADULT - Initial episodes of herpes genitalis: apply oint q3h (6 times/d) x 7 days. Non-life threatening mucocutaneous herpes simplex in immunocompromised patients: apply oint q3h (6 times/d) x 7 days. Recurrent herpes labialis: apply cream 5 times/day for 4 days.
PEDS - <12 yo: Not approved. ≥12 yo: Recurrent herpes labialis: apply cream 5 times/day for 4 days.
UNAPPROVED PEDS - Initial episodes of herpes genitalis: apply oint q3h (6 times/d) x 7 days. Non-life threatening mucocutaneous herpes simplex in immunocompromised patients: apply oint q3h (6 times/d) x 7 days.
FORMS - Trade only: ointment 5% 15 g, cream 5% (2 & 5 g).
NOTES - Use finger cot or rubber glove to apply ointment to avoid dissemination. Burning/stinging may occur in up to 28% of patients. Oral form more effective than topical for herpes genitalis.

docosanol (*Abreva*) ▶Not absorbed ♀B ▶? $
ADULT - Oral-facial herpes (cold sores): apply 5x/day until healed.
PEDS - Oral-facial herpes (cold sores), ≥12 yo: Use adult dose.
FORMS - OTC: Trade only: cream 10% 2 g.

imiquimod (*Aldara*) ▶Not absorbed ♀C ▶? $$$$$
ADULT - External genital and perianal warts: apply 3 times weekly at bedtime for up to 16 weeks. Wash off after 8 hours. Nonhyperkeratotic, nonhypertrophic actinic keratoses on face/scalp in immunocompetent adults: apply to face or scalp (but not both) 2 times weekly for up to 16 weeks. Wash off after 8 hours. Primary superficial basal cell carcinoma: apply 5 times weekly for 6 weeks. Wash off after 8 hours.
PEDS - Children >11 yo: External genital and perianal warts: apply 3 times/week at bedtime. Wash off after 6-10 hours.
UNAPPROVED ADULT - Molluscum contagiosum: apply 3 times weekly for 6-10 hours.
UNAPPROVED PEDS - Molluscum contagiosum
FORMS - Trade only: cream 5% 250 mg single use packets.
NOTES - May weaken condoms and diaphragms. Avoid sexual contact while cream is

on when used for genital/perianal warts. Most common adverse effects include erythema, itching, erosion, burning, excoriation, edema and pain. Discard partially used packets.

penciclovir (*Denavir*) ▶Not absorbed ♀B ▶? $$
ADULT - Recurrent herpes labialis (cold sores): apply q2h while awake x 4 days.
PEDS - Not approved in children.
UNAPPROVED PEDS - Recurrent herpes labialis: apply q2h while awake x 4 days.
FORMS - Trade only: cream 1% tubes 1.5 g.
NOTES - Start therapy as soon as possible during prodrome. For moderate to severe cases of herpes labialis, systemic treatment with famciclovir or acyclovir may be preferred.

podofilox (*Condylox*, ✦*Condyline, Wartec*) ▶? ♀C ▶? $$$
ADULT - External genital warts (gel and solution) and perianal warts (gel only): apply bid for 3 consecutive days of a week and repeat for up to 4 weeks.
PEDS - Not approved in children.
FORMS - Generic/Trade: Solution 0.5% 3.5 mL. Trade only: Gel 0.5% 3.5 g.

podophyllin (*Podocon-25, Podofin, Podofilm*) ▶? ♀- ▶- $$$
ADULT - Genital wart removal: Initial application: apply to wart and leave on for 30-40 min to determine patient's sensitivity. Thereafter, use minimum contact time necessary (1-4h depending on result). Remove dried podophyllin with alcohol or soap and water.
PEDS - Not approved in children.
FORMS - Not to be dispensed to patients. For hospital/clinic use; not intended for outpatient prescribing. Trade only: Liquid 25% 15 mL
NOTES - Not to be dispensed to patients. Do not treat large areas or numerous warts all at once. Contraindicated in diabetics, pregnancy, patients using steroids or with poor circulation, and on bleeding warts.

sinecatechins (*Veregen*) ▶Unknown ♀C ▶? ?
ADULT - Apply tid to external genital warts for up to 16 weeks.
PEDS - Not approved in children.
FORMS - Trade only: ointment 15% 15g.
NOTES - Botanical drug product. Contains a partially purified fraction of the water extract of green tea leaves. Generic name used to be kunecatechins.

DERMATOLOGY: Atopic Dermatitis

NOTE: Potential risk of cancer. Should only be used as 2nd-line agent for short-term and intermittent treatment of atopic dermatitis in those unresponsive to or intolerant of other treatments. Long-term safety has not been established. Avoid use in immunocompromise and if <2 yo. Use minimum amount to control symptoms.

pimecrolimus (*Elidel*) ▶L ♀C ▶? $$$$
ADULT - Atopic dermatitis: apply bid.
PEDS - Atopic dermatitis: ≥2 yo: apply bid. Don't use if <2 yo.
FORMS - Trade only: cream 1% 30, 60, 100 g.
NOTES - Long term safety unclear.

tacrolimus (*Protopic*) ▶Minimal absorption ♀C ▶? $$$$
ADULT - Atopic dermatitis: apply bid.
PEDS - Children <2 yo: not approved. Children 2-15 yo: Atopic dermatitis: apply 0.03% oint bid.
UNAPPROVED ADULT - Vitiligo: apply 0.1% bid. Chronic allergic contact dermatitis (i.e. nickel-induced): apply 0.1% oint bid.
FORMS - Trade only: ointment 0.03% 30, 60, 100 g, 0.1% 30, 60, 100 g.
NOTES - Do not use with an occlusive dressing. Continue for 1 week after symptom clearing.

DERMATOLOGY: Corticosteroids (Topical)

NOTE: After long-term use, do not discontinue abruptly; switch to a less potent agent or alternate corticosteroids and emollient products. Monitor for hyperglycemia / adrenal suppression if used for long period of time or over a large area of the body, especially in children. Chronic administration may cause skin atrophy and interfere with pediatric growth & development.

alclometasone dipropionate (*Aclovate*) ▶L ♀C ▶? $$
ADULT - Inflammatory and pruritic manifestations of corticosteroid-responsive dermatoses: apply sparingly 2-3 times/day.
PEDS - Inflammatory & pruritic manifestations of corticosteroid-responsive dermatoses, ≥1 yo: apply sparingly 2-3 times/day. Safety and efficacy for >3 weeks have not been established.
FORMS - Generic/Trade: Ointment & cream 0.05% 15, 45, 60 g.

amcinonide (*Cyclocort*) ▶L ♀C ▶? $$
ADULT, PEDS - Inflammatory and pruritic manifestations of corticosteroid-responsive dermatoses: apply sparingly 2-3 times/day.
FORMS - Generic only: Cream & ointment 0.1% 15, 30, 60 g, Lotion 0.1% 60 mL.

augmented betamethasone dipropionate (*Diprolene, Diprolene AF, ✚Topilene Glycol*) ▶L ♀C ▶? $$
ADULT - Inflammatory and pruritic manifestations of corticosteroid-responsive dermatoses: apply sparingly 1-2 times/day.
PEDS - Not approved in children <12 yo.
FORMS - Generic/Trade: Diprolene: Ointment 0.05% 15, 50 g, Lotion 0.05% 30, 60 mL. Diprolene AF: Cream 0.05% 15, 50 g. Generic only: Gel 0.05% 15, 50 g.
NOTES - Do not use occlusive dressings. Do not use for longer than 2 consecutive weeks and do not exceed a total dose of 45-50 g/week or 50 mL/week of the lotion.

betamethasone dipropionate (*Diprosone, Maxivate, ✚Propaderm, TARO-sone*) ▶L ♀C ▶? $
ADULT, PEDS - Inflammatory and pruritic manifestations of corticosteroid-responsive dermatoses: apply sparingly 1-2 times/day.
FORMS - Generic only: Ointment & cream 0.05% 15, 45 g, Lotion 0.05% 60 mL.
NOTES - Do not use occlusive dressings.

betamethasone valerate (*Luxiq foam, Veta-Val, ✚Betaderm*) ▶L ♀C ▶? $
ADULT - Inflammatory and pruritic manifestations of corticosteroid-responsive dermatoses: apply sparingly 1-2 times/day. Dermatoses of scalp: apply small amount of foam to scalp bid.
PEDS - Inflammatory and pruritic manifestations of corticosteroid-responsive dermatoses: apply sparingly 1-2 times/day.
FORMS - Generic only: Ointment & cream 0.1% 15, 45 g, Lotion 0.1% 60 mL. Trade only: Foam (Luxiq) 0.12% 50,100,150 g.

clobetasol (*Temovate, Olux, Clobex, Cormax, ✚Dermovate*) ▶L ♀C ▶? $$
ADULT - Inflammatory and pruritic manifestations of corticosteroid-responsive dermatoses: apply sparingly 2 times/day. For scalp apply foam 2 times/day.
PEDS - Not approved in children.

FORMS - Generic/Trade: Cream & ointment 0.05% 15, 30, 45, 60 g, Scalp application 0.05% 25, 50 mL, Gel 0.05% 15, 30, 60 g. Trade (Olux): Foam 0.05% 50,100g. Trade only (Clobex): Lotion 0.05% 30, 60,120 mL, Spray 0.05% 60 mL, Shampoo 0.05% 120 mL.

NOTES - Adrenal suppression at doses as low as 2 g/day. Do not use occlusive dressings. Do not use for longer than 2 consecutive weeks and do not exceed a total dose of 50 g/week.

clocortolone pivalate (Cloderm) ▶L ♀C ▶? $$$

ADULT, PEDS - Inflammatory and pruritic manifestations of corticosteroid-responsive dermatoses: apply sparingly 3 times/day.

FORMS - Trade only: Cream 0.1% 15, 45, 90 g.

desonide (DesOwen, Desonate, Tridesilon, Verdeso) ▶L ♀C ▶? $

ADULT, PEDS - Inflammatory and pruritic manifestations of corticosteroid-responsive dermatoses: apply sparingly 2-3 times/day.

FORMS - Generic/Trade: Cream and Ointment 0.05%, 15, 60 g, Lotion 0.05%, 60,120 mL. Trade only: Gel (Desonate) 0.05% 60 g, Foam (Verdeso) 0.05%, 50,100 g.

NOTES - Do not use with occlusive dressings.

desoximetasone (Topicort, Topicort LP, ✦Desoxi) ▶L ♀C ▶? $$

ADULT - Inflammatory and pruritic manifestations of corticosteroid-responsive dermatoses: apply sparingly 2 times/day.

PEDS - Safety and efficacy have not been established for Topicort 0.25% ointment. For inflammatory and pruritic manifestations of corticosteroid-responsive dermatoses (cream and gel): apply sparingly 2 times/day.

FORMS - Generic/Trade: Cream and Gel 0.05% 15, 60 g, Cream and Ointment 0.25%15, 60 g.

diflorasone (Psorcon E, Maxiflor) ▶L ♀C ▶? $$

ADULT - Inflammatory and pruritic manifestations of corticosteroid-responsive dermatoses: apply sparingly 1-3 times/day.

PEDS - Not approved in children.

FORMS - Generic/Trade: Cream and Ointment 0.05% 15, 30, 60 g.

NOTES - Doses of 30 g/day of diflorasone 0.05% cream for 1 week resulted in adrenal suppression in some psoriasis patients.

fluocinolone (Synalar, Capex, Derma-Smoothe/FS, ✦Caprex) ▶L ♀C ▶? $

ADULT - Inflammatory and pruritic manifestations of corticosteroid-responsive dermatoses: apply sparingly 2-4 times/day. Psoriasis of the scalp (Derma-Smoothe/FS): Massage into scalp, cover with shower cap and leave on ≥4 h or overnight and then wash off.

PEDS - Inflammatory and pruritic manifestations of corticosteroid-responsive dermatoses: apply sparingly 2-4 times/day.

FORMS - Generic/Trade: Cream and Ointment 0.025% 15, 30, 60 g, Solution 0.01% 20, 60 mL. Generic only: Cream 0.01% 15, 60 g. Trade (Derma-Smoothe/FS): Topical oil 0.01% 120 mL, (Capex) Shampoo 0.01% 120 mL.

fluocinonide (Lidex, Lidex-E, Vanos, ✦Lidemol, Topsyn, Tiamol) ▶L ♀C ▶? $

ADULT - Inflammatory and pruritic manifestations of corticosteroid-responsive dermatoses: apply sparingly 2-4 times/day. Plaque-type psoriasis: apply 0.1% cream (Vanos) daily-bid x 2 consecutive weeks only; no more than 60 g/week. Atopic dermatitis: apply 0.1% cream (Vanos) once daily.

PEDS - Inflammatory and pruritic manifestations of corticosteroid-responsive dermatoses: apply sparingly 2-4 times/day.

FORMS - Generic/Trade: Cream, Ointment, and Gel 0.05% 15, 30, 60, Solution 0.05% 20, 60 mL. Trade: Cream 0.1% 30, 60, 120 g (Vanos).

flurandrenolide (Cordran, Cordran SP) ▶L ♀C ▶? $$$

ADULT, PEDS - Inflammatory and pruritic manifestations of corticosteroid-responsive dermatoses: apply sparingly 2-3 times/day.

FORMS - Trade only: Ointment and Cream 0.05% 15, 30, 60 g. Lotion 0.05% 15, 60 mL. Tape 4 mcg/cm².

fluticasone (Cutivate, ✦Flixonase, Flixotide) ▶L ♀C ▶? $$

ADULT - Eczema: apply sparingly 1-2 times/day. Other inflammatory and pruritic manifestations of corticosteroid-responsive dermatoses: apply sparingly 2 times/day.

PEDS - Children >3 mo old: Eczema: apply sparingly 1-2 times/day. Other inflammatory & pruritic manifestations of corticosteroid-responsive dermatoses: apply sparingly 2 times/day.

FORMS - Generic/Trade: Cream 0.05% 15,30, 60 g, Ointment 0.005% 15,30,60 g. Trade only: Lotion 0.05% 60 mL

NOTES - Do not use with an occlusive dressing.

halcinonide (Halog) ▶L ♀C ▶? $$

ADULT, PEDS - Inflammatory and pruritic manifestations of corticosteroid-responsive dermatoses: apply sparingly 2-3 times/day.

FORMS - Trade only: Cream and Ointment 0.1% 15, 30, 60 g Solution 0.1% 20, 60 mL.

CORTICOSTEROIDS – TOPICAL*

	Agent	Strength/Formulation*	Freq
Low Potency	alclometasone dipropionate (Aclovate)	0.05% C O	bid-tid
	clocortolone pivalate (Cloderm)	0.1% C	tid
	desonide (DesOwen, Tridesilon)	0.05% C L O G F (Verdeso)	bid-tid
	hydrocortisone (Hytone, others)	0.5% C L O; 1% C L O; 2.5% C L O	bid-qid
	hydrocortisone acetate (Cortaid, Corticaine)	0.5% C O, 1% C O SP	bid-qid
Medium Potency	betamethasone valerate (Luxiq)	0.1% C L O; 0.12% F(Luxiq)	qd-bid
	desoximetasone‡ (Topicort)	0.05% C	bid
	fluocinolone (Synalar)	0.01% C S; 0.025% C O	bid-qid
	flurandrenolide (Cordran)	0.05% CLO; T	bid-qid
	fluticasone propionate (Cutivate)	0.005% O; 0.05% C L	qd-bid
	hydrocortisone butyrate (Locoid)	0.1% C O S	bid-tid
	hydrocortisone valerate (Westcort)	0.2% C O	bid-tid
	mometasone furoate (Elocon)	0.1% C L O	qd
	triamcinolone‡ (Kenalog)	0.025% CLO; 0.1% CLO; SP	bid-tid
High Potency	amcinonide (Cyclocort)	0.1% C L O	bid-tid
	betamethasone dipropionate‡ (Maxivate, others)	0.05% C L O (non-Diprolene)	qd-bid
	desoximetasone‡ (Topicort)	0.05% G; 0.25% C O	bid
	diflorasone diacetate (Psorcon E)	0.05% C O	bid
	fluocinonide (Lidex)	0.05% C G O S	bid-qid
	halcinonide (Halog)	0.1% C O S	bid-tid
	triamcinolone‡ (Kenalog)	0.5% C O	bid-tid
Very high	betamethasone dipropionate‡ (Diprolene, Diprolene AF)	0.05% C G L O	qd-bid
	clobetasol (Temovate, Cormax, Olux)	0.05% C G O L S SH SP F (Olux)	bid
	halobetasol propionate (Ultravate)	0.05% C O	qd-bid

*C-cream, G-gel, L-lotion, O-ointment, S-solution, SH-shampoo, T-tape, F-foam, SP-spray; bolded items have available generics. Potency based on vasoconstrictive assays, which may not correlate with efficacy. Not all available products are listed, including those lacking potency ratings. ‡These drugs have formulations in more than once potency category.

halobetasol propionate (Ultravate) ▶L ♀C ▶? $$
ADULT - Inflammatory and pruritic manifestations of corticosteroid-responsive dermatoses: apply sparingly 1-2 times/day.
PEDS - Not approved in children.
FORMS - Generic/Trade: Cream and Ointment 0.05% 15, 50 g.
NOTES - Do not use occlusive dressings. Do not use for >2 consecutive weeks and do not exceed a total dose of 50 g/week.

hydrocortisone (Cortizone, Hycort, Hytone, Tegrin-HC, Dermolate, Synacort, Anusol-HC, Proctocream HC, Cortifoam, ✿Cortoderm, Prevex-HC, Cortate, Emo-Cort) ▶L ♀C ▶? $
ADULT, PEDS - Inflammatory and pruritic manifestations of corticosteroid-responsive dermatoses: apply sparingly 2-4 times/day. External

anal itching (adult only): apply cream tid-qid prn or supp bid or rectal foam daily-bid.
FORMS - Products available OTC & Rx depending on labeling. 2.5% preparation available Rx only. Generic: ointment 0.5% 30 g, ointment 1% 15, 20,30,60,120 g, ointment 2.5% 20,30 g, cream 0.5% 15,30,60 g, cream 1% 20,30,60, 90,120 g, cream 2.5% 15,20,30,60,120 g, lotion 0.25% 120 mL, lotion 0.5% 30,60,120 mL, lotion 1% 60,120 mL, lotion 2% 30 mL, lotion 2.5% 60 mL. Anal preparations: Generic/Trade: cream 1% (Anusol HC-1), 2.5% g (Anusol HC, Proctocream HC), suppository 25 mg (Anusol HC), 10% rectal foam (Cortifoam) 15g.

hydrocortisone acetate (Cortaid, Corticaine, Micort-HC Lipocream, ✿Hyderm, Cortamed) ▶L ♀C ▶? $
ADULT, PEDS - Inflammatory and pruritic manifestations of corticosteroid-responsive derma-

toses: apply sparingly 2-4 times/day.
FORMS - OTC Generic/Trade: Ointment 0.5% 15 g, Ointment 1% 15, 30g, Cream 0.5% 15 g, Cream 1% 15, 30, 60 g. Topical spray 1% 60 mL. Rx Trade only: Cream 2.5% 30 g (Micort-HC Lipocream).

hydrocortisone butyrate (*Locoid, Locoid Lipocream*) ▶L ♀C ▶? $$
ADULT, PEDS - Inflammatory and pruritic manifestations of corticosteroid-responsive dermatoses: apply sparingly 2-3 times/day. Seborrheic dermatitis (soln only): apply 2-3 x /day.
FORMS - Generic/Trade: Cream and Ointment 0.1% 15, 45 g, Solution 0.1% 20, 60 mL. Trade only: Cream 0.1% (Lipocream) 15, 45, 60 g.

hydrocortisone probutate (*Pandel*) ▶L ♀C ▶? $$
ADULT - Inflammatory and pruritic manifestations of corticosteroid-responsive dermatoses: apply sparingly 1-2 times/day.
PEDS - Not approved in children.
FORMS - Trade only: Cream 0.1% 15, 45, 80 g.

hydrocortisone valerate (*Westcort, ♥Hydroval*) ▶L ♀C ▶? $$
ADULT - Inflammatory and pruritic manifestations of corticosteroid-responsive dermatoses: apply sparingly 2-3 times/day.
PEDS - Safety and efficacy of Westcort ointment have not been established in children. Inflammatory and pruritic manifestations of corticosteroid-responsive dermatoses (cream only): apply sparingly 2-3 times/day.
FORMS - Generic/Trade: Cream and Ointment 0.2% 15, 45, 60 g.

mometasone (*Elocon, ♥Elocom*) ▶L ♀C ▶? $
ADULT - Inflammatory and pruritic manifestations of corticosteroid-responsive dermatoses:

apply sparingly once daily.
PEDS - Inflammatory and pruritic manifestations of corticosteroid-responsive dermatoses ≥2 yo: apply sparingly once daily. Safety and efficacy for >3 weeks have not been established.
FORMS - Generic/Trade: Cream and Ointment 0.1% 15, 45 g, Lotion 0.1% 30, 60 mL.
NOTES - Do not use an occlusive dressing. Not for ophthalmic use.

prednicarbate (*Dermatop*) ▶L ♀C ▶? $$
ADULT - Inflammatory and pruritic manifestations of corticosteroid-responsive dermatoses: apply sparingly 2 times/day.
PEDS - Inflammatory and pruritic manifestations of corticosteroid-responsive dermatoses, ≥1 yo: apply sparingly 2 times/day. Safety and efficacy for >3 weeks have not been established.
FORMS - Generic/Trade: Cream and Ointment 0.1% 15, 60 g.

triamcinolone (*Kenalog, Kenalog in Orabase, ♥Oracort, Triaderm*) ▶L ♀C ▶? $
ADULT - Inflammatory and pruritic manifestations of corticosteroid-responsive dermatoses: apply sparingly 3-4 times/day. Oral paste: Aphthous ulcers: Using finger, apply about 1/2 cm of paste to oral lesion and a thin film will develop. Apply paste bid-tid, ideally pc & qhs.
PEDS - Inflammatory and pruritic manifestations of corticosteroid-responsive dermatoses: apply sparingly 3-4 times/day.
FORMS - Generic/Trade: Cream and Ointment 0.1% 15, 60, 80 g, Cream 0.5% 20 g, Lotion 0.025% and 0.1% 60 mL, Oral paste (in Orabase) 0.1% 5 g. Generic only: Cream and Ointment 0.025% 15, 80 g, Cream and Ointment 0.5% 15 g. Trade only: Aerosol topical spray 0.147 mg/g-63 g.

DERMATOLOGY: Corticosteroid / Antimicrobial Combinations

Cortisporin **(neomycin + polymyxin + hydrocortisone)** ▶LK ♀C ▶? $$$
ADULT - Corticosteroid-responsive dermatoses with secondary infection: apply bid-qid.
PEDS - Not approved in children.
UNAPPROVED PEDS - Corticosteroid-responsive dermatoses with secondary infection: apply bid-qid.
FORMS - Trade: Cream 7.5 g, Ointment 15 g.
NOTES - Due to concerns about neomycin nephrotoxicity and ototoxicity, do not use over wide areas or for prolonged periods of time.

Fucidin H **(fusidic acid + hydrocortisone)**

▶L ♀? ▶? $$
ADULT - Atopic dermatitis: apply tid.
PEDS - >3 yo, atopic dermatitis: apply tid.
FORMS - Canada trade only: cream 2% fusidic acid, 1% hydrocortisone acetate 30 g.

Locacorten Vioform **(flumethasone + cloquinol)** ▶? ♀? ▶? $
ADULT - Canada only. Skin: Apply 2-3 times daily. Otic drops: 2-3 gtts bid.
PEDS - Canada only. Children ≥ 2 yo: Skin: Apply 2-3 times daily. Otic drops: 2-3 gtts bid.
FORMS - Trade only: Cream 0.02% flumethasone & 3% cloquinol. Otic drops 0.02% flu-

methasone & 1% cloquinol, 10 mL.
NOTES - May stain clothing.

Lotrisone (clotrimazole + betamethasone, ✚Lotriderm) ▶L ♀C ▶? $$$

ADULT - Tinea pedis, cruris, corporis: apply bid.
PEDS - Not approved in children.
FORMS - Generic/Trade: cream (clotrimazole 1%+betamethasone 0.05%) 15,45g, lotion (clotrimazole 1% + betamethasone 0.05%) 30 mL.
NOTES - Treat tinea cruris and corporis for 2 weeks and tinea pedis for 4 weeks. Do not use for diaper dermatitis.

Mycolog II (nystatin + triamcinolone) ▶L ♀C ▶? $

ADULT - Cutaneous candidiasis: apply bid.
PEDS - Not approved in children.
UNAPPROVED PEDS - Sometimes used for diaper dermatitis, but this is not recommended due to risk of adrenal suppression.
FORMS - Generic/Trade: cream 15,30,60,120 g, ointment 15,30,60,120 g.
NOTES - Avoid occlusive dressings.

DERMATOLOGY: Hemorrhoid Care

dibucaine (Nupercainal) ▶L ♀? ▶? $

ADULT - Hemorrhoids or other anorectal disorders: apply tid-qid prn.
PEDS - Not approved in children.
UNAPPROVED PEDS - Hemorrhoids or other anorectal disorders; children >2yo or >35 pounds: apply tid-qid prn.
FORMS - OTC Generic/Trade ointment 1% 30g.
NOTES - Do not use if <2 yo or <35 pounds.

pramoxine (Anusol Hemorrhoidal Ointment, Fleet Pain Relief, Proctofoam NS) ▶Not absorbed ♀+ ▶+ $

ADULT - Hemorrhoids: apply ointment, pads, or foam up to 5 times/day prn.
PEDS - Not approved in children.
FORMS - OTC Trade only: ointment (Anusol Hemorrhoidal Ointment), pads (Fleet Pain Relief), aerosol foam (ProctoFoam NS).

Proctofoam HC (pramoxine + hydrocortisone) ▶L ♀C ▶? $$$

ADULT, PEDS - Inflammatory / pruritic manifestations of corticosteroid-responsive dermatoses of the anal region: apply 3 to 4 times a day.
FORMS - Trade only: Topical aerosol foam (1% pramoxine + 1% hydrocortisone) 10g

starch (Anusol Suppositories) ▶Not absorbed ♀+ ▶+ $

ADULT - Hemorrhoids: 1 suppository PR up to 6 times/day prn or after each bowel movement.
PEDS - Not approved in children.
FORMS - OTC Trade only: suppositories (51% topical starch; soy bean oil, tocopheryl acetate).

witch hazel (Tucks) ▶? ♀+ ▶+ $

ADULT - Hemorrhoids: Apply to anus/perineum up to 6 times/day prn.
PEDS - Not approved in children.
FORMS - OTC Generic/Trade: pads, gel.

DERMATOLOGY: Other Dermatologic Agents

alitretinoin (Panretin) ▶Not absorbed ♀D ▶- $$$$$

WARNING - May cause fetal harm if significant absorption were to occur. Women of child-bearing age should be advised to avoid becoming pregnant during treatment.
ADULT - Cutaneous lesions of AIDS-related Kaposi's sarcoma: apply bid-qid.
PEDS - Not approved in children.
FORMS - Trade only: gel 0.1%, 60 g.

aluminum chloride (Drysol, Certain Dri) ▶K ♀? ▶? $

ADULT - Hyperhidrosis: apply qhs. For maximum effect, cover area with plastic wrap held in place with tight shirt and wash area following morning. Once excessive sweating stopped, use once or twice weekly.
PEDS - Not approved in children.
FORMS - Rx: Generic/Trade: solution 20%: 37.5 mL bottle, 35, 60 mL bottle with applicator. OTC: Trade only (Certain Dri): solution 12.5%: 36 mL bottle.
NOTES - To prevent irritation, apply to dry area.

becaplermin (Regranex) ▶Minimal absorption ♀C ▶? $$$$$

ADULT - Diabetic neuropathic ulcers: apply daily and cover with saline-moistened gauze for 12 hours. Rinse after 12 h and cover with saline gauze without medication.
PEDS - Not approved in children.
FORMS - Trade only: gel 0.01% 2, 15 g.
NOTES - Length of gel to be applied calculated by size of wound (length x width x 0.6 = amount of gel in inches). If ulcer does not de-

crease by 30% in size by 10 weeks, or complete healing has not occurred by 20 weeks, continued therapy should be reassessed. Ineffective for stasis ulcers and pressure ulcers.

calamine ▶? ♀? ▶? $

ADULT, PEDS >2 yo - Itching due to poison ivy/oak/sumac, insect bites, or minor irritation: apply up to tid-qid prn.

FORMS - OTC Generic: lotion 120,240,480 mL.

***Capital Soleil 15* (avobenzone + ecamsule + octocrylene)** ▶? ♀? ▶? $

ADULT, PEDS - Apply sunscreen prn.

FORMS - OTC Trade: Cream, 2% avobenzone + 3% ecamsule + 10% octocrylene 120 mL.

NOTES - Broad spectrum, UVA and UVB protection. Also known as mexoryl.

capsaicin (*Zostrix, Zostrix-HP*) ▶? ♀? ▶? $

ADULT, PEDS >2 yo - Pain due to rheumatoid arthritis, osteoarthritis, and neuralgias such as zoster or diabetic neuropathies: apply to affected area up to tid-qid.

UNAPPROVED ADULT - Psoriasis and intractable pruritus, postmastectomy/ postamputation neuromas (phantom limb pain), vulvar vestibulitis, apocrine chromhidrosis and reflex sympathetic dystrophy.

FORMS - OTC Generic/Trade: cream 0.025% 45,60 g, 0.075% 30,60 g, lotion 0.025% 59 mL, 0.075% 59 mL, gel 0.025% 15,30 g, 0.05% 43 g, roll-on 0.075% 60 mL.

NOTES - Burning occurs in ≥30% but diminishes with continued use. Pain more commonly occurs when applied <3-4 times/day. Wash hands immediately after application.

***Carmol HC* (hydrocortisone acetate + urea)** ▶L ♀C ▶? $

ADULT, PEDS - Inflammatory and pruritic manifestations of corticosteroid-responsive dermatoses: apply sparingly 2-4 times/day.

FORMS - Trade only: hydrocortisone acetate 1% + urea 10% cream 30,90g.

coal tar (*Polytar, Tegrin, Cutar, Tarsum*) ▶? ♀? ▶? $

ADULT, PEDS >2 yo - Dandruff, seborrheic dermatitis: apply shampoo at least twice a week. Psoriasis: apply to affected areas daily to qid or use shampoo on affected areas.

FORMS - OTC Generic/Trade: shampoo, conditioner, cream, ointment, gel, lotion, soap, oil.

NOTES - May cause photosensitivity for up to 24 h after application.

DEET (*Off, Cutter, Repel, Ultrathon, n-n-diethyl-m-toluamide*) ▶L ♀+ ▶+ $

ADULT - Mosquito repellant: 10% to 50% q2-6h.

Higher concentration products do not work better, but have a longer duration of action.

PEDS - Infants and children ≥2 months: up to 30% spray/lotion every 2 to 6 hours.

FORMS - OTC: spray, lotion, towelette: 4.75% to 100%

NOTES - Duration of action varies by concentration. For example, 23.8% DEET provides about 5 hours of protection from mosquito bites, 20% DEET approximately 4 hours, 6.65% DEET about 2 hours, and 4.75% DEET about 1.5 hours. Apply sunscreen prior to application of DEET-containing products.

doxepin (*Zonalon*) ▶L ♀B ▶- $

ADULT - Pruritus associated with atopic dermatitis, lichen simplex chronicus, eczematous dermatitis: apply qid for up to 8 days.

PEDS - Not approved in children.

FORMS - Trade only: cream 5% 30,45 g.

NOTES - Systemic toxicity risk if applied to >10% of body. Can cause contact dermatitis.

eflornithine (*Vaniqa*) ▶K ♀C ▶? $$$

ADULT - Reduction of facial hair: apply to face bid at least 8 h apart.

PEDS - Not approved in children.

FORMS - Trade only: cream 13.9% 30 g.

NOTES - Takes ≥4-8 weeks to see an effect.

***EMLA* (prilocaine + lidocaine - topical)** ▶LK ♀B ▶? $$

ADULT - Topical anesthesia for minor dermal procedures (eg, IV cannulation, venipuncture) apply 2.5 g over 20-25 cm^2 area or 1 disc ≥1 hour prior to procedure, for major dermal procedures (ie, skin grafting harvesting) apply 2 g per 10 cm^2 area ≥2h prior to procedure.

PEDS - Prior to circumcision in infants >37 wks gestation: apply a max dose 1g over a max of 10 cm^2. Topical anesthesia: age 1-3 mo or <5 kg: apply a max 1 g over max of 10 cm^2; age 4-12 mo and >5kg: apply max 2 g over a max of 20 cm^2; age 1-6 yo and >10kg: apply max 10g over max of 100 cm^2; age 7-12 yo and >20kg: apply max 20g over max of 200 cm^2.

FORMS - Trade only: cream (2.5% lidocaine + 2.5% prilocaine) 5 g, disc 1 g. Generic/Trade: cream (2.5% lidocaine + 2.5% prilocaine) 30 g.

NOTES - Cover cream with an occlusive dressing. Do not use in children <12 mo if receiving methemoglobin-inducing agents. Do not use on open wounds. Methemoglobinemia risk with glucose-6-phosphate deficiencies. Use caution with amiodarone, bretylium, sotalol, dofetilide; possible additive cardiac effects. Dermal analgesia increases for up to 3 h under occlusive dressings, and persists for 1-2 h after removal.

finasteride (*Propecia*) ▶L ♀X ▶- $$$

ADULT - Androgenetic alopecia in men: 1 mg PO daily.

PEDS - Not approved in children.

UNAPPROVED ADULT - Androgenetic alopecia in postmenopausal women (no evidence of efficacy): 1 mg PO daily.

FORMS - Generic/Trade: tab 1 mg.

NOTES - May require ≥3 months before benefit seen. Monitor PSA before therapy; finasteride will decrease PSA by 50% in patients with BPH, even with prostate cancer. Contraindicated in pregnancy or possible pregnancy. Women should not handle crushed or broken tabs if they are or could be pregnant.

hyaluronic acid (*Restylane*) ▶? ♀? ▶? $$$$$

ADULT - Moderate to severe facial wrinkles: inject into wrinkle/fold.

PEDS - Not approved in children.

FORMS - Rx: 0.4 mL and 0.7 mL syringe.

NOTES - Do not use >1.5 mL per treatment area. Contains trace amounts of gram positive bacterial proteins; contraindicated if history of anaphylaxis or severe allergy.

hydroquinone (*Eldopaque, Eldoquin, Eldoquin Forte, EpiQuin Micro, Esoterica, Glyquin, Lustra, Melanex, Solaquin, Claripel, ♣Ultraquin*) ▶? ♀C ▶? $$$

ADULT - Temporary bleaching of hyperpigmented skin conditions (ie, chloasma, melasma, freckles, senile lentigines, ultraviolet-induced discoloration from oral contraceptives, pregnancy, or hormone therapy): apply bid to affected area.

PEDS - Not approved in children.

FORMS - OTC Generic/Trade: cream 1.5%, lotion 2%. Rx Generic/Trade: solution 3%, gel 4%, cream 4%.

NOTES - Response may take 3 weeks to 6 months. Use a sunscreen on treated, exposed areas.

lactic acid (*Lac-Hydrin, Amlactin, ♣Dermalac*) ▶? ♀? ▶? $$

ADULT, PEDS >2 yo - Ichthyosis vulgaris and xerosis (dry, scaly skin): apply bid to affected area.

FORMS - Trade only: lotion 12% 150,360 mL. Generic/OTC: cream 12% 140,385 g. AmLactin AP is lactic acid (12%) with pramoxine (1%).

NOTES - Frequently causes irritation in non-intact skin.

lidocaine (*Xylocaine, Lidoderm, Numby Stuff, LMX, Zingo, ♣Maxilene*) ▶LK ♀B ▶+ $$

WARNING - Contraindicated in allergy to amide-type anesthetics.

ADULT - Topical anesthesia: apply to affected area prn. Dose varies with anesthetic procedure, degree of anesthesia required and individual patient response. Post-herpetic neuralgia (patch): apply up to 3 patches to affected area at once for up to 12h within a 24h period.

PEDS - Topical anesthesia: apply to affected area prn. Dose varies with anesthetic procedure, degree of anesthesia required and individual response. Max 3 mg/kg/dose, do not repeat dose within 2 hours. Intradermal powder injection for venipuncture / IV cannulation, 3-18 yo (Zingo): 0.5 mg to site 1-10 minutes prior.

UNAPPROVED PEDS - Topical anesthesia prior to venipuncture: apply 30 min prior to procedure (ELA-Max 4%).

FORMS - For membranes of mouth and pharynx: spray 10%, ointment 5%, liquid 5%, solution 2,4%, dental patch. For urethral use: jelly 2%. Patch (Lidoderm) 5%. Intradermal powder injection system: 0.5 mg (Zingo). OTC: Trade only: liposomal lidocaine 4% (ELA-Max).

NOTES - Apply patches only to intact skin to cover the most painful area. Patches may be cut into smaller sizes w/scissors prior to removal of the release liner. Store and dispose out of the reach of children & pets to avoid possible toxicity from ingestion.

minoxidil (*Rogaine, Rogaine Forte, Rogaine Extra Strength, Minoxidil for Men, Theroxidil Extra Strength, ♣Minox, Apo-Gain*) ▶K ♀C ▶- $$

ADULT - Androgenetic alopecia in men or women: 1 mL to dry scalp bid.

PEDS - Not approved in children.

UNAPPROVED ADULT - Alopecia areata.

UNAPPROVED PEDS - Alopecia: Apply to dry scalp bid.

FORMS - OTC Trade only: solution 2%, 60 mL, 5%, 60 mL, 5% (Rogaine Extra Strength, Theroxidil Extra Strength - for men only) 60 mL, foam 5% 60g.

NOTES - 5% strength for men only. Alcohol content may cause burning and stinging. Evidence of hair growth usually takes ≥4 months. If treatment is stopped, new hair will be shed in a few months.

monobenzone (*Benoquin*) ▶Minimal absorption ♀C ▶? $$

ADULT - Extensive vitiligo: apply bid-tid.

PEDS - Not approved if <12 yo.

FORMS - Trade only: cream 20% 35.4 g.

NOTES - Avoid prolonged exposure to sunlight. May take 1-4 months for depigmentation to occur. Depigmentation is permanent and can cause lifelong increase in photosensitivity.

oatmeal (*Aveeno***)** ▶Not absorbed ♀? ▶? $

ADULT, PEDS - Pruritus from poison ivy/oak, varicella: apply lotion qid prn. Also available in packets to be added to bath.

FORMS - OTC Generic/Trade: lotion, packets.

Panafil **(papain + urea + chlorophyllin copper complex)** ▶? ♀? ▶? $$$

ADULT - Debridement of acute/chronic lesions: apply to clean wound and cover daily-bid.

PEDS - Not approved in children.

FORMS - Trade: Ointment: 6,30 g, spray 33 mL.

NOTES - Longer redressings (2-3 days) are acceptable. May be applied under pressure dressings. Hydrogen peroxide inactivates papain; avoid concomitant use.

Pliagis **(tetracaine + lidocaine)** ▶Minimal absorption ♀B ▶? $$

WARNING - Contraindicated in allergy to amide-type anesthetics.

ADULT - Prior to venipuncture, intravenous cannulation, superficial dermatological procedure: apply 20-30 min prior to procedure (60 min for tattoo removal).

PEDS - Not approved in children.

FORMS - Trade only: cream lidocaine 7% + tetracaine 7%.

poly-L-lactic acid (*Sculptra***)** ▶Not absorbed ♀? ▶? $$$$$

ADULT - Restoration of facial fat loss due to HIV lipoatrophy: dose based on degree of correction needed.

PEDS - Not approved in children <18 yo.

Pramosone **(pramoxine + hydrocortisone, ✤***Pramox HC***)** ▶Not absorbed ♀C ▶? $$$

ADULT - Inflammatory and pruritic manifestations of corticosteroid-responsive dermatoses: Apply tid-qid.

PEDS - Apply bid-tid.

FORMS - Trade only: 1% pramoxine/1% hydrocortisone acetate: cream 30, 60 g, oint 30 g, lotion 60, 120, 240 mL. 1% pramoxine/2.5% hydrocortisone acetate: cream 30, 60 g, oint 30 g, lotion 60, 120 mL.

NOTES - Monitor for hyperglycemia / adrenal suppression if used for long period of time or over a large area of the body, especially in children. Chronic administration may interfere with pediatric growth & development.

selenium sulfide (*Selsun, Exsel, Versel***)**

▶? ♀C ▶? $

ADULT, PEDS - Dandruff, seborrheic dermatitis: Massage 5-10 mL of shampoo into wet scalp, allow to remain 2-3 minutes, rinse. Apply twice a week for 2 weeks. For maintenance, less frequent administration needed. Tinea versicolor: Apply 2.5% shampoo/lotion to affected area, allow to remain on skin 10 min, rinse. Repeat daily x 7 days.

FORMS - OTC Generic/Trade: lotion/shampoo 1% 120,210,240, 330 mL, 2.5% 120 mL. Rx Generic/Trade: lotion/shampoo 2.5% 120 mL.

Solag **(mequinol + tretinoin, ✤***Solage***)** ▶Not absorbed ♀X ▶? $$$$

ADULT - Solar lentigines: apply bid separated by at least 8 hrs.

PEDS - Not approved in children.

FORMS - Trade only: soln 30 mL (mequinol 2% + tretinoin 0.01%).

NOTES - Use in non-Caucasians has not been evaluated. Avoid in patients taking photosensitizers. Minimize exposure to sunlight.

Synera **(tetracaine + lidocaine)** ▶Minimal absorption ♀B ▶? $$

WARNING - Contraindicated in allergy to amide-type anesthetics.

ADULT, PEDS ≥3 yo - Prior to venipuncture, IV cannulation, superficial dermatological procedure: apply 20-30 min prior to procedure.

FORMS - Trade only: patch lidocaine 70 mg + tetracaine 70 mg.

NOTES - Do not cut patch or remove top cover.

thalidomide (*Thalomid***)** ▶Plasma ♀X▶?$$$$$

WARNING - Pregnancy category X. Has caused severe, life-threatening human birth defects. Available only through special restricted distribution program. Prescribers and pharmacists must be registered in this program in order to prescribe or dispense.

ADULT - Erythema nodosum leprosum: 100-400 mg PO qhs. Use low end of dose range for initial episodes and patients <50 kg.

PEDS - Not approved in children.

UNAPPROVED PEDS - Clinical trials show beneficial effects when combined with dexamethasone in multiple myeloma.

FORMS - Trade only: cap 50, 100, 150, 200 mg.

Tri-Luma **(fluocinolone + hydroquinone + tretinoin)** ▶Minimal absorption ♀C ▶? $$$

ADULT - Melasma of the face: apply qhs x 4-8 weeks.

PEDS - Not approved in children.

FORMS - Trade only: soln 30 g (fluocinolone 0.01% + hydroquinone 4% + tretinoin 0.05%).

NOTES - Minimize exposure to sunlight. Not intended for melasma maintenance therapy.

urea (*Carmol 40*) ▶? ♀B ▶? $

ADULT, PEDS - Debridement of hyperkeratotic surface lesions: apply 2 times/day.

FORMS - Trade only: urea 40% cream 30, 90, 200g, lotion 8 oz, gel 15 mL.

Vusion (miconazole + zinc oxide + white petrolatum) ▶Minimal absorption ♀C ▶? $$$$

ADULT - Not approved in adults.

PEDS - Apply to affected diaper area with each change for 7 days.

FORMS - Trade only: 50 g.

NOTES - Use only in documented candidiasis.

ENDOCRINE & METABOLIC: Androgens / Anabolic Steroids

NOTE: Monitor LFTs & lipids. See OB/GYN section for other hormones.

fluoxymesterone (*Halotestin*) ▶L ♀X ▶? ©III $$$$

ADULT - Palliative treatment of androgen-responsive recurrent breast cancer in women who are 1-5 years postmenopausal: 5-10 mg PO bid-qid x 1-3 months. Hypogonadism in men: 5-20 mg PO daily.

PEDS - Delayed puberty in males: 2.5-10 mg PO daily x 4-6 months.

FORMS - Trade only: Tabs (scored) 2, 5, 10 mg. Generic only: Tabs 10 mg.

NOTES - Transdermal or injectable therapy preferred for hypogonadism. Pediatric use by specialists who monitor bone maturation q6 months. Prolonged high-dose use may cause hepatic adenomas, hepatocellular carcinoma, and peliosis hepatitis.

methyltestosterone (*Android, Methitest, Testred, Virilon*) ▶L ♀X ▶? ©III $$$

ADULT - Advancing inoperable breast cancer in women who are 1-5 years postmenopausal: 50-200 mg/day PO in divided doses. Hypogonadism in men: 10-50 mg PO daily.

PEDS - Delayed puberty in males: 10 mg PO daily x 4-6 months.

FORMS - Generic: Caps 10 mg, Tabs 10, 25 mg.

NOTES - Transdermal or injectable therapy preferred to oral for hypogonadism. Pediatric use by specialists who monitor bone maturation q6 months. Prolonged high-dose use may cause hepatic adenomas, hepatocellular carcinoma, and peliosis hepatitis.

nandrolone (*Deca-Durabolin*) ▶L ♀X ▶- ©III $$

WARNING - Peliosis hepatitis, liver cell tumors, and lipid changes have occurred secondary to anabolic steroid use.

ADULT - Anemia of renal insufficiency: women 50-100 mg IM q wk, men 100-200 mg IM q wk.

PEDS - Anemia of renal disease age 2- 13 yo: 25- 50 mg IM q3-4 weeks.

FORMS - Generic: Injection 50,100,200 mg/mL.

NOTES - Pediatric use by specialists who monitor bone maturation q6 months. Long-term use may cause hepatic adenomas, hepatocellular carcinoma, and peliosis hepatitis.

oxandrolone (*Oxandrin*) ▶L ♀X ▶? ©III $$$$$

WARNING - Peliosis hepatitis, liver cell tumors, and lipid changes have occurred secondary to anabolic steroid use.

ADULT - To promote weight gain following extensive surgery, chronic infection, or severe trauma; in some patients who fail to gain or maintain weight without a physiologic cause; to offset protein catabolism associated with long-term corticosteroid therapy: 2.5 mg PO bid-qid for 2-4 wks. Max 20 mg/day. May repeat therapy intermittently as indicated.

PEDS - Weight gain: ≤0.1 mg/kg or ≤0.045 mg/pound PO divided bid-qid for 2-4 wks. May repeat therapy intermittently as indicated.

FORMS - Generic/Trade: Tabs 2.5, 10 mg.

NOTES - Contraindicated in known or suspected prostate/breast cancer. Not shown to enhance athletic ability. Associated with dyslipidemia. Pediatric use by specialists who monitor bone maturation q6 months. Long-term use may cause hepatic adenomas, hepatocellular carcinoma, and peliosis hepatitis. May increase anticoagulant effects of warfarin.

testosterone (*Androderm, AndroGel, Delatestryl, Depo-Testosterone, Striant, Testim, Testopel, Testro AQ, ♣Andriol*) ▶L ♀X ▶? ©III $$$$$

ADULT – Male hypogonadism: injectable enanthate or cypionate- 50-400 mg IM q2-4 weeks. Androderm- 5 mg patch qhs to clean, dry area of skin on back, abdomen, upper arms, thighs. Non-virilized start with 2.5 mg patch qhs. AndroGel 1%: Apply 5 g from gel pack or 4 pumps (5 g) from dispenser daily to clean, dry, intact skin of the shoulders, upper arms, or abdomen. May increase dose to 7.5-10 g after 2 weeks. Testim: One tube (5 g) daily to the clean, dry intact skin of the shoulders or upper arms. May increase dose to 2 tubes (10 g) after 2 weeks. Testopel: 2-6 pellets (150-450 mg testosterone) pellets SC q 3-6 months. 2 pellets for each 25 mg testosterone propionate required weekly. Buccal- Striant: 30 mg q12 hours on upper gum above the incisor tooth; alternate sides for each application.

PEDS - Not approved in children.

FORMS - Trade only: Patch 2.5 & 5 mg/24hr (Androderm). Gel 1% 2.5, 5 g packet & 75 g multi-dose pump (AndroGel). Gel 1%, 5 g tube (Testim). Pellet 75 mg (Testopel). Buccal: blister packs - 30 mg (Striant). Generic/Trade: Injection 100, 200 mg/mL (cypionate), 200 mg/mL (ethanate).

NOTES - Do not apply Androderm or AndroGel to scrotum. Do not apply Testim to the scrotum or abdomen. Pellet implantation is less flexible for dose adjustment, therefore, take great care when estimating the amount. For testosterone gel form, obtain serum testosterone level 2 weeks after initiation, then increase dose if necessary. Inject IM formulations slowly into gluteal muscle; rare reports of cough or respiratory distress following injection. Prolonged high-dose use may cause hepatic adenomas, hepatocellular carcinoma, and peliosis hepatitis. May promote the development of prostatic hyperplasia or prostate cancer. Monitor PSA, hemoglobin to detect polycythemia. Advise patient to regularly inspect the gum region where Striant is applied and report any abnormality; refer for dental consultation as appropriate.

ENDOCRINE & METABOLIC: Bisphosphonates

NOTE: Supplemental Vit D and calcium are recommended for osteoporosis prevention & treatment. Osteonecrosis of the jaw has been reported in patients on bisphosphonates; generally associated with tooth extraction and/or local infection with delayed healing.

alendronate (*Fosamax, Fosamax Plus D, ✦Fosavance*) ▶K ♀C ▶- $$$

ADULT - Postmenopausal osteoporosis prevention (5 mg PO daily or 35 mg PO weekly) & treatment (10 mg daily, 70 mg PO weekly or 70 mg/vit D3 2800 IU PO weekly). Treatment of glucocorticoid-induced osteoporosis in men & women: 5 mg PO daily or 10 mg PO daily (postmenopausal women not taking estrogen). Treatment of osteoporosis in men: 10 mg PO daily, 70 mg PO weekly, or 70 mg/vit D3 2800 IU PO weekly. Paget's disease in men & women: 40 mg PO daily x 6 months.

PEDS - Not approved in children.

UNAPPROVED ADULT - Prevention of glucocorticoid-induced osteoporosis men & women: 5 mg PO daily or 35 mg PO weekly; 10 mg PO daily or 70 mg PO weekly (postmenopausal women not taking estrogen). Treatment of glucocorticoid-induced osteoporosis in men & women: 35 mg weekly or 70 mg weekly (postmenopausal women not taking estrogen).

FORMS - Trade only (Fosamax): Tabs 5, 10, 35, 40, 70 mg. Oral soln 70 mg/75 mL (single dose bottle). Fosamax Plus D: 70 mg + either 2800 or 5600 units of vitamin D3.

NOTES - May cause esophagitis, esophageal ulcers and esophageal erosions, occasionally with bleeding and rarely followed by stricture or perforation. Monitor frequently for dysphagia, odynophagia, and retrosternal pain. Take 30 minutes before first food, beverage, or medication of the day with a full glass of water only. Remain in upright position for ≥30 minutes following dose. Caution if CrCl <35 mL/min.

clodronate (*✦Ostac, Bonefos*) ▶K ♀D ▶- $$$$$

ADULT - Canada only. Hypercalcemia of malignancy; management of osteolysis resulting from bone metastases of malignant tumors: IV single dose - 1500 mg slow infusion over ≥4 hours. IV multiple dose - 300 mg slow infusion daily over 2-6 hours up to 10 days. Oral - following IV therapy, maintenance 1600-2400 mg/ day in single or divided doses. Max PO dose 3200 mg/day; therapy duration usually 6 mon.

PEDS - Not approved in children.

FORMS - Generic/Trade: Capsules 400 mg.

NOTES - Contraindicated if creat >5 mg/dl or if severe GI tract inflammation. Avoid rapid bolus which may cause severe local reactions, thrombophlebitis, or renal failure. Do not mix with calcium-containing infusions. Ensure adequate hydration prior to infusion. Normocalcemia usually occurs within 2-5 days after initiation of therapy with multiple dose infusion. Monitor calcium, renal function in those with renal insufficiency, LFTs & CBC.

etidronate (*Didronel*) ▶K ♀C ▶? $$$$

ADULT - Paget's disease: 5-10 mg/kg PO daily

x 6 months or 11-20 mg/kg daily x 3 months. Heterotopic ossification with hip replacement: 20 mg/kg/day PO x 1 month before and 3 months after surgery. Heterotopic ossification with spinal cord injury: 20 mg/kg/day PO x 2 weeks, then 10 mg/kg/day PO x 10 weeks.

PEDS - Not approved in children.

FORMS - Generic/Trade: Tabs 200, 400 mg.

NOTES - Divide dose if GI discomfort occurs. Avoid food, vitamins with minerals, or antacids within 2 h of dose.

ibandronate (*Boniva*) ▶K ♀C ▶? $$$
ADULT - Treatment/Prevention of postmenopausal osteoporosis. Oral: 2.5 mg PO daily or 150 mg PO q month. IV: 3 mg IV q 3 months.

PEDS - Not approved in children.

FORMS - Trade only: 2.5, 150 mg tabs.

NOTES - May cause esophagitis. Avoid if CrCl <30 mL/min. Oral: Take 1 hr before first food/ beverage with a full glass of plain water; remain in upright position 1 hr after taking. IV: Administer over 15-30 seconds.

pamidronate (*Aredia*) ▶K ♀D ▶? $$$$$
WARNING - Single dose should not exceed 90 mg due to risk of renal impairment/failure.

ADULT - Hypercalcemia of malignancy, moderate (corrected Ca= 12-13.5 mg/dl): 60-90 mg IV single dose infused over 2-24 h. Hypercalcemia of malignancy, severe (Ca >13.5 mg/dl): 90 mg IV single dose infused over 2-24 h. Wait ≥7 days before considering retreatment. Paget's disease: 30 mg IV over 4h daily x 3 days. Osteolytic bone lesions: 90 mg IV over 4 h once monthly. Osteolytic bone metastases: 90 mg IV over 2 h q3-4 weeks.

PEDS - Not approved in children.

UNAPPROVED ADULT - Mild hypercalcemia: 30 mg IV single dose over 4 h. Osteoporosis treatment: 30 mg IV q 3 months. Prevention of bone loss during androgen deprivation treatment for prostate cancer: 60 mg IV q12 weeks.

UNAPPROVED PEDS - Osteogenesis imperfecta: 3.0 mg/kg IV over 4 hr q4-6 month.

NOTES - Fever occurs in >20%. Monitor creatinine (prior to each dose), lytes, calcium, phosphate, magnesium and Hb (regularly). Avoid in severe renal impairment and hold if worsening renal function. Longer infusions (>2 h) may reduce renal toxicity. Maintain adequate hydration. Avoid invasive dental procedures.

risedronate (*Actonel, Actonel Plus Calcium*) ▶K ♀C ▶? $$$
ADULT - Paget's disease: 30 mg PO daily x 2 months. Prevention & treatment of postmeno-

pausal osteoporosis: 5 mg PO daily, 35 mg PO weekly, or 75 mg on 2 consecutive days each month. Treatment of male osteoporosis: 35 mg PO weekly. Prevention & treatment of glucocorticoid-induced osteoporosis: 5 mg PO daily.

PEDS - Not approved in children.

UNAPPROVED ADULT - Prevention & treatment of glucocorticoid-induced osteoporosis: 35 mg PO weekly.

FORMS - Trade only: Tabs 5, 30, 35, 75 mg; 35/1250 mg (calcium).

NOTES - May cause esophagitis, monitor frequently for dysphagia, odynophagia, and retrosternal pain; take 30 minutes before first food, beverage, or medication of the day with a full glass of water only. Remain in upright position for ≥30 minutes following dose.

tiludronate (*Skelid*) ▶K ♀C ▶? $$$$$
ADULT - Paget's disease: 400 mg PO daily x 3 months.

PEDS - Not approved in children.

FORMS - Trade only: Tabs 200 mg.

NOTES - May cause esophagitis; take 30 minutes before first food, beverage, or medication of the day with a full glass of water only. Remain in upright position for ≥30 minutes following dose.

zoledronic acid (*Reclast, Zometa*, ✚*Aclasta*) ▶K ♀D ▶? $$$$$
ADULT - Postmenopausal osteoporosis: 5 mg (Reclast) once yearly IV infusion over ≥15 min. Hypercalcemia of malignancy (corrected Ca ≥12 mg/dL, Zometa): 4 mg single dose IV infusion over ≥15 min. Wait ≥7 days before considering retreatment. Paget's Disease (Reclast): 5 mg IV single dose. Multiple myeloma and metastatic bone lesions from solid tumors (Zometa): 4 mg (CrCl >60 mL/min), 3.5mg (CrCl 50-60 mL/min), 3.3 mg (CrCl 40-49 mL/min) or 3 mg (CrCl 30-39 mL/min) IV infusion over >=15 min q3-4 weeks.

PEDS - Not approved in children.

UNAPPROVED ADULT - Osteoporosis: 4 mg (Zometa) once yearly IV infusion over ≥15 min. Paget's Disease (Zometa; approved in Canada): 5 mg IV single dose. Treatment of hormone–refractory prostate cancer metastatic to bone (Zometa): 4 mg IV q 3-4 weeks. Prevention of bone loss during androgen-deprivation treatment for non-metastatic prostate cancer (Zometa): 4 mg IV q3 months for 1 year.

NOTES - Avoid in severe renal impairment (CrCl <35 mL/min) and hold dosing with worsening renal function. Monitor creatinine (before each dose), lytes, calcium, phosphate, magnesium and Hb/HCT (regularly). Avoid single doses >4 mg (Zometa) or > 5 mg (Reclast), infusions <15 min. Fever occurs in >15%. In treatment of Paget's disease, correct pre-existing hypocalcemia with calcium and vitamin D before therapy. Maintain adequate hydration for those with hypercalcemia of malignancy, and give 500 mg calcium supplement and vitamin D 400 IU PO daily to those with multiple myeloma or metastatic bone lesions. Avoid invasive dental procedures.

CORTICOSTEROIDS	Approximate equivalent dose (mg)	Relative anti-inflammatory potency	Relative mineralocorticoid potency	Biologic Half-life (hours)
betamethasone	0.6-0.75	20-30	0	36-54
cortisone	25	0.8	2	8-12
dexamethasone	0.75	20-30	0	36-54
fludrocortisone	--	10	125	18-36
hydrocortisone	20	1	2	8-12
methylprednisolone	4	5	0	18-36
prednisolone	5	4	1	18-36
prednisone	5	4	1	18-36
triamcinolone	4	5	0	12-36

ENDOCRINE & METABOLIC: Corticosteroids

NOTE: See also dermatology, ophthalmology.

betamethasone (Celestone, Celestone Soluspan, ♥Betaject) ▶L ♀C ▶- $$$$$
ADULT - Anti-inflammatory/Immunosuppressive: 0.6-7.2 mg/day PO divided bid-qid or up to 9 mg/day IM. 0.25-2.0 mL intraarticular depending on location and size of joint.
PEDS - Dosing guidelines not established.
UNAPPROVED ADULT - Fetal lung maturation, maternal antepartum between 24 & 34 weeks gestation: 12 mg IM q24h x 2 doses.
UNAPPROVED PEDS - Anti-inflammatory/ Immunosuppressive: 0.0175-0.25 mg/kg/day PO divided tid-qid. Fetal lung maturation, maternal antepartum: 12 mg IM q24h x 2 doses.
FORMS - Trade only: Syrup 0.6 mg/5 mL.
NOTES - Avoid prolonged use in children due to possible bone growth retardation. If such therapy necessary monitor growth & development.

cortisone (Cortone) ▶L ♀D ▶- $
ADULT - Adrenocortical insufficiency: 25-300 mg PO daily.
PEDS - Dosing guidelines not established.
UNAPPROVED PEDS - Adrenocortical insufficiency: 0.5-0.75 mg/kg/day PO divided q8h.
FORMS - Generic only: Tabs 5, 10, 25 mg.

dexamethasone (Decadron, Dexpak, ♥Dexasone) ▶L ♀C ▶- $
ADULT - Anti-inflammatory/Immunosuppressive: 0.5-9 mg/day PO/IV/IM divided bid-qid. Cerebral edema: 10-20 mg IV load, then 4 mg IM q6h (off-label IV use common) or 1-3 mg PO tid.
PEDS - Dosage in children <12 yo of age has not been established.
UNAPPROVED ADULT - Initial treatment of immune thrombocytopenic purpura: 40 mg PO daily x 4 days. Fetal lung maturation, maternal antepartum between 24 & 34 weeks gestation: 6 mg IM q12h x 4 doses. Bacterial meningitis (controversial): 0.15 mg/kg IV q6h x 2-4 days; start 10-15 minutes before the first dose of antibiotic. Antiemetic, prophylaxis: 8 mg IV or 12 mg PO prior to chemotherapy; 8 mg PO daily x 2-4 days. Antiemetic, treatment: 10-20 mg PO/IV q4-6h.
UNAPPROVED PEDS - Anti-inflammatory/immunosuppressive: 0.08-0.3 mg/kg/day PO/IV/IM divided q6-12h. Croup: 0.6 mg/kg PO/IV/IM x 1. Bacterial meningitis: 0.15 mg/kg/dose IV q6h x 16 doses. Bacterial meningitis (controversial): 0.15 mg/kg IV q6h x 2-4 days; start 10-15 minutes before the first dose of antibiotic. Bronchopulmonary dysplasia in preterm infants: 0.5 mg/kg PO/IV divided q12h x 3 days, then taper. Acute asthma: >2 yo: 0.6 mg/kg to max 16 mg PO daily x 2 days.
FORMS - Generic/Trade: Tabs 0.5, 0.75. Generic only: Tabs 0.25, 1.0, 1.5, 2, 4, 6 mg; elixir 0.5 mg/5 mL; solution 0.5 mg/5 mL, 1 mg/1 mL (concentrate). Trade only: Dexpak (51 total 1.5 mg tabs for a 13 day taper).

NOTES - Avoid prolonged use in children due to possible bone growth retardation. If such therapy necessary monitor growth & development.

fludrocortisone (*Florinef*) ▶L ♀C ▶? $

ADULT - Adrenocortical insufficiency/ Addison's disease: 0.1 mg PO 3 times weekly to 0.2 mg PO daily. Salt-losing adrenogenital syndrome: 0.1-0.2 mg PO daily.

PEDS - Not approved in children.

UNAPPROVED ADULT - Postural hypotension: 0.05-0.4 mg PO daily.

UNAPPROVED PEDS - Adrenocortical insufficiency: 0.05-0.2 mg PO daily.

FORMS - Generic only: Tabs 0.1 mg.

NOTES - Usually given in conjunction with cortisone or hydrocortisone for adrenocortical insufficiency.

hydrocortisone (*Cortef, Cortenema, Solu-Cortef*) ▶L ♀C ▶- $

ADULT - Adrenocortical insufficiency: 20-240 mg/day PO divided tid-qid or 100-500 mg IV/IM q2-10h prn (sodium succinate). Ulcerative colitis: 100 mg retention enema qhs (laying on side for ≥1 hour) for 21 days. May use for 2-3 months for severe cases; when course extends >3 weeks then discontinue gradually by decreasing to every other night for 2-3 weeks.

PEDS - Dosing guidelines not established.

UNAPPROVED PEDS - Chronic adrenocortical insufficiency: 0.5-0.75 mg/kg/day PO divided q8h or 0.25-0.35 mg/kg/day IM daily. Acute adrenocortical insufficiency: infants & young children 1-2 mg/kg IV bolus, then 25-150 mg/day divided q6-8 hours. Older children 1-2 mg/kg IV bolus, then 150-250 mg/day IV q6-8 hrs.

FORMS - Generic/Trade: Tabs 5, 10, 20 mg, Enema 100 mg/60 mL.

NOTES - Agent of choice for adrenocortical insufficiency because of mixed glucocorticoid & mineralocorticoid properties at doses >100 mg/day.

methylprednisolone (*Solu-Medrol, Medrol, Depo-Medrol*) ▶L ♀C ▶- $

ADULT - Anti-inflammatory/ Immunosuppressive: Parenteral (Solu-Medrol) 10- 250 mg IV/IM q4h prn. Oral (Medrol) 4- 48 mg PO daily. Medrol Dosepak tapers 24 to 0 mg PO over 7d. IM/ joints (Depo-Medrol) 4- 120 mg IM q1-2 weeks. Multiple sclerosis flare: 200 mg PO/IV daily x 1 week followed by 80 mg PO daily x 1 month.

PEDS - Dosing guidelines not established.

UNAPPROVED ADULT - Optic neuritis: 1 g IV daily (or in divided doses) x 3 days, then PO prednisone 1 mg/kg/day x 11 days (followed by a 3-day taper). Multiple sclerosis flare: 1 g IV daily (or in divided doses) x 3-5 days. May follow with PO prednisone 1 mg/kg/day for 14 days, then taper off. Spinal cord injury: 30 mg/kg IV over 15 minutes, followed in 45 minutes by 5.4 mg/kg/h IV infusion for 23 hours (if initiated within 3 hours of injury) or for 47 hours (if initiated 3-8h after injury).

UNAPPROVED PEDS - Anti-inflammatory/ Immunosuppressive: 0.5-1.7 mg/kg/day PO/IV/IM divided q6-12h. Spinal cord injury: 30 mg/kg IV over 15 minutes, followed in 45 minutes by 5.4 mg/kg/hour IV infusion x 23 hours.

FORMS - Trade only: Tabs 2, 16, 32 mg. Generic/Trade: Tabs 4, 8 mg. Medrol Dosepak (4 mg-21 tabs).

NOTES - Other dosing regimens have been used for MS and optic neuritis. Avoid initial treatment of optic neuritis with oral steroids, as it may increase the risk of new episodes.

prednisolone (*Prelone, Pediapred, Orapred, Orapred ODT*) ▶L ♀C ▶+ $$

ADULT - Anti-inflammatory/ Immunosuppressive: 5- 60 mg/day PO/IV/IM.

PEDS - Dosing guidelines not established.

UNAPPROVED PEDS - Anti-inflammatory/ Immunosuppressive: 0.1-2 mg/kg/day PO divided daily-qid or 0.04-0.25 mg/kg/day IV/IM divided daily-bid. Early active rheumatoid arthritis: 10 mg/day PO.

FORMS - Generic/Trade: Syrup 15 mg/5 mL (Prelone; wild cherry flavor). Solution 15 mg/5 mL (Orapred; grape flavor). Trade only: orally disintegrating tabs 10, 15, 30 mg (Orapred ODT). Generic only: Tabs 5 mg. Syrup & Solution 5 mg/5 mL.

prednisone (*Deltasone, Sterapred, ✦Winpred*) ▶L ♀C ▶+ $

ADULT - Anti-inflammatory/ Immunosuppressive: 5-60 mg/day PO daily or divided bid-qid.

PEDS - Dosing guidelines not established.

UNAPPROVED PEDS - Anti-inflammatory/ Immunosuppressive: 0.05-2 mg/kg/day divided daily-qid.

FORMS - Trade only: Sterapred (5 mg tabs: tapers 30 to 5 mg PO over 6d or 30 to 10 mg over 12d), Sterapred DS (10 mg tabs: tapers 60 to 10 mg over 6d, or 60 to 20 mg PO over 12d) taper packs. Generic only: Tabs 1, 2.5, 5, 10, 20, 50 mg. Solution 5 mg/5 mL & 5 mg/mL (Prednisone Intensol).

NOTES - Conversion to prednisolone may be impaired in liver disease.

triamcinolone (*Aristocort, Kenalog, Aristospan*) ▶L ♀C ▶- $$$$
ADULT - Anti-inflammatory/Immunosuppressive: 4-48 mg/day PO divided daily-qid. 2.5-60 mg IM daily (Kenalog). 40 mg IM q wk (Aristospan)
PEDS - Dosing guidelines not established.
UNAPPROVED PEDS - Anti-inflammatory/Immunosuppressive: 0.117-1.66 mg/kg/day PO divided qid.
FORMS - Trade: Tabs 4 mg. Injection 10 mg/mL & 40 mg/mL (Kenalog), 5 mg/mL & 20 mg/mL (Aristospan), 25 & 40 mg/mL (Aristocort).
NOTES - Parenteral form not for IV use. Do not use in neonates; contains benzyl alcohol.

ENDOCRINE & METABOLIC: Diabetes-Related – Alphaglucosidase Inhibitors

acarbose (*Precose*, ♥*Glucobay*) ▶Gut/K ♀B ▶- $$$
ADULT - Diabetes: initiate therapy with 25 mg PO tid with the first bite of each meal. Start with 25 mg PO daily to minimize GI adverse effects. May increase to 50 mg PO tid after 4-8 weeks. Usual range is 50-100 mg PO tid. Maximum dose for patients ≤60 kg is 50 mg tid, >60 kg is 100 mg tid.
PEDS - Not approved in children.
UNAPPROVED ADULT - Type 2 DM prevention: 100 mg PO tid or to max tolerated dose.
FORMS - Trade only: Tabs 25, 50, 100 mg.
NOTES - Acarbose alone should not cause hypoglycemia. If hypoglycemia occurs, treat with oral glucose rather than sucrose (table sugar). Adverse GI effects (eg, flatulence, diarrhea, abdominal pain) may occur with initial use.

miglitol (*Glyset*) ▶K ♀B ▶- $$$
ADULT - Diabetes: Initiate therapy with 25 mg PO tid with the first bite of each meal. Use 25 mg PO daily to start if GI adverse effects. May increase dose to 50 mg PO tid after 4-8 weeks, max 300 mg/day.
PEDS - Not approved in children.
FORMS - Trade only: Tabs 25, 50, 100 mg.
NOTES - Miglitol administered alone should not cause hypoglycemia. If hypoglycemia occurs, treat with oral glucose rather than sucrose (table sugar). Adverse GI effects (i.e. flatulence, diarrhea, abdominal pain) may occur with initial therapy.

ENDOCRINE & METABOLIC: Diabetes-Related – Combinations

NOTE: Metformin-containing products may cause life-threatening lactic acidosis, usually in setting of decreased tissue perfusion, hypoxia, hepatic dysfunction, or impaired renal clearance. Hold prior to IV contrast agents and for 48 h after. Avoid if ethanol abuse, heart failure (requiring treatment), hepatic or renal insufficiency (creat ≥1.4 mg/dl in women, ≥1.5 mg/dl in men), or hypoxic states (cardiogenic shock, septicemia, acute MI). Glitazone-containing products may cause edema, weight gain, new heart failure, or exacerbate existing heart failure (avoid in NYHA Class III or IV). Monitor for signs of heart failure (rapid weight gain, dyspnea, edema) following initiation or dose increase. If occurs, manage fluid retention and consider discontinuation or dosage decrease. Avoid if liver disease or ALT >2.5 x normal. Monitor LFTs before therapy & periodically thereafter. Discontinue if ALT >3x upper normal limit. Full effect may not be apparent for up to 12 weeks. May cause resumption of ovulation in premenopausal anovulatory women; recommend contraception use.

ACTOPLUS Met (pioglitazone + metformin) ▶KL ♀C ▶? $$$$
ADULT - Type 2 DM: 1 tab PO daily-bid. If inadequate control with metformin monotherapy, start 15/500 or 15/850 PO daily-bid. If inadequate control with pioglitazone monotherapy, start 15/500 bid or 15/850 daily. Max 45/2550 mg/day.
PEDS - Not approved in children.
FORMS - Trade only: Tabs 15/500, 15/850 mg.
NOTES - Initial GI upset may be minimized by starting with lower dose of metformin component. Reports of fracture risk in women.

Avandamet (rosiglitazone + metformin) ▶KL ♀C ▶? $$$$$
ADULT - Type 2 DM, initial therapy (drug naive): Start 2/500 mg PO daily or bid. If inadequate control with metformin alone, select strength based on adding 4 mg/day rosiglitazone to existing metformin dose. If inadequate control with rosiglitazone alone, select tab strength based on adding 1000 mg/day metformin to existing rosiglitazone dose. Max 8/2000 mg/day.
PEDS - Not approved in children.

FORMS - Trade only: Tabs 2/500, 4/500, 2/1000, 4/1000 mg.

NOTES - May be given concomitantly with sulfonylureas or insulin. Initial GI upset may be minimized by starting with lower dose of metformin component.

Avandaryl (rosiglitazone + glimepiride) ▶LK ♀C ▶? $$$$

ADULT - Type 2 DM, initial therapy (drug naive): Start 4/1 mg PO daily. If switching from monotherapy with a sulfonylurea or glitazone, consider 4/2 mg PO daily. Max 8/4 mg per day. Give with breakfast or the first main meal of the day. Use low starting dose of 4/1 mg and titrate more slowly in elderly, malnourished and in renal and hepatic impairment.

PEDS - Not approved in children.

FORMS - Trade only: Tabs 4/1, 4/2, 4/4, 8/2, 8/4 mg rosiglitazone/glimepiride.

Duetact (pioglitazone + glimepiride) ▶LK ♀C ▶- $$$$

ADULT - Type 2 DM: Start 30/2 mg PO daily. May start up to 30/4 mg PO daily if prior glimepiride therapy, or up to 30/2 mg PO daily if prior pioglitazone therapy; max 30/4 mg per day. Give with breakfast or the first main meal of the day. In the elderly, the malnourished, or those with renal/hepatic impairment, precede therapy with trial of glimepiride 1 mg/day and then titrate Duetact more slowly.

PEDS - Not approved in children.

FORMS - Trade only: Tabs 30/2, 30/4 mg pioglitazone/glimepiride.

NOTES - Reports of fracture risk in women.

Glucovance (glyburide + metformin) ▶KL ♀B ▶? $$$

ADULT - Type 2 DM, initial therapy (drug naive): Start 1.25/250 mg PO daily or bid with meals; maximum 10/2000 mg daily. Inadequate control with a sulfonylurea or metformin alone: Start 2.5/500 or 5/500 mg PO bid with meals; maximum 20/2000 mg daily.

PEDS - Not approved in children.

FORMS - Generic/Trade: Tabs 1.25/250, 2.5/500, 5/500 mg

NOTES - May add thiazolidinedione if glycemic control is not obtained.

Janumet (sitagliptin + metformin) ▶K ♀B ▶? $$$$

ADULT - Type 2 DM: Start 1 tab PO bid. Individualize based on patient's current therapy. If inadequate control with metformin monotherapy, start 50/500 or 50/1000 bid based on current metformin dose. If inadequate control on sitagliptin monotherapy, start 50/500 bid. Max 100/2000 mg daily. Give with meals.

PEDS - Not approved in children.

FORMS - Trade only: Tabs 50/500, 50/1000 mg sitagliptin/metformin.

NOTES - Not for Type 1 DM or DKA. Assess renal function and CBC prior to initiating and at least annually thereafter.

DIABETES NUMBERS*

Criteria for diagnosis:	Self-monitoring glucose goals	
Pre-diabetes: Fasting glucose 100-125 mg/dL	Preprandial	90-130 mg/dL
Diabetes:† Fasting glucose ≥126 mg/dL,	Postprandial	< 180 mg/dL
random glucose with symptoms: ≥200 mg/dL,	A1C Normal/individualized	
or ≥200 mg/dL 2h after 75 g oral glucose load	goal <6%; general goal <7%	

Complications prevention & management: Aspirin‡ (75–162 mg/day) in Type 1 & 2 adults for primary prevention (those with an increased cardiovascular risk, including >40 yo or with additional risk factors) and secondary prevention (those with any vascular disease) unless contraindicated; statin therapy to achieve 30-40% LDL reduction for >40 yo regardless of baseline LDL; ACE inhibitor or ARB if hypertensive or micro-/macro-albuminuria; pneumococcal vaccine (revaccinate one time if age >64 and previously received vaccine at age <65 and >5 years ago). *At every visit*: Measure weight & BP (goal <130/80 mmHg); visual foot exam; review self-monitoring glucose record; review/adjust meds; review self-management skills, dietary needs, and physical activity; smoking cessation counseling. *Twice a year*: A1C in those meeting treatment goals with stable glycemia (quarterly if not); dental exam. *Annually*: Fasting lipid profile [goal LDL <100 mg/dL; cardiovascular disease consider LDL <70mg/dL, HDL >40 mg/dL (>50 mg/dL in ♀), TG <150 mg/dL], q2 years with low-risk lipid values; creat; albumin to creat ratio spot collection; dilated eye exam; flu vaccine; comprehensive foot exam.

*See recommendations at: care.diabetesjournals.org. Reference: *Diabetes Care* 2007;30 (Suppl 1):S4-S41. Glucose values are plasma. †Confirm diagnosis with glucose testing on subsequent day. ‡Avoid aspirin if <21 yo due to Reye's Syndrome risk; use if <30 yo has not been studied.

Metaglip (glipizide + metformin) ▶KL ♀C ▶? $$$
ADULT - Type 2 DM, initial therapy (drug naive): Start 2.5/250 mg PO daily to 2.5/500 mg PO bid with meals; max 10/2000 mg daily. Inadequate control with a sulfonylurea or metformin alone: Start 2.5/500 or 5/500 mg PO bid with meals; max 20/2000 mg daily.
PEDS - Not approved in children.
FORMS - Generic/Trade: Tabs 2.5/250, 2.5/500, 5/500 mg.
NOTES - May add thiazolidinedione if glycemic control is not obtained.

ENDOCRINE & METABOLIC: Diabetes-Related – "Glitazones" (Thiazolidinediones)

NOTE: May cause edema, weight gain, new heart failure, or exacerbate existing heart failure (contraindicated in NYHA Class III or IV). Monitor for signs of heart failure (rapid weight gain, dyspnea, edema) following initiation or dose increase. If occurs, manage fluid retention and consider discontinuation or dosage decrease. Avoid if liver disease or ALT >2.5 x normal. Monitor LFTs before therapy & periodically thereafter. Discontinue if ALT >3x upper normal limit. Full effect may not be apparent for up to 12 weeks. May cause resumption of ovulation in premenopausal anovulatory women; recommend contraception use.

pioglitazone (*Actos*) ▶L ♀C ▶- $$$$
ADULT - Diabetes monotherapy or in combination with a sulfonylurea, metformin, or insulin: Start 15-30 mg PO daily, may adjust dose after 3 months to max 45 mg/day.
PEDS - Not approved in children.
FORMS - Trade only: Tabs 15, 30, 45 mg.
NOTES - Reports of fracture risk in women.

rosiglitazone (*Avandia*) ▶L ♀C ▶- $$$$
ADULT - Diabetes monotherapy or in combination with metformin, sulfonylurea, insulin: Start 4 mg PO daily or divided bid, may increase after 8-12 weeks to max 8 mg/day as monotherapy or in combo with metformin and/or sulfonylurea. Max 4 mg/day when used with insulin.
PEDS - Not approved in children <18 yo.
FORMS - Trade only: Tabs 2, 4, 8 mg.

INSULINS, INJECTABLE*		Onset (h)	Peak (h)	Duration (h)
Rapid/short-acting:	Insulin aspart (*NovoLog*)	<0.2	1-3	3-5
	Insulin glulisine (*Apidra*)	0.30-0.4	1	4-5
	Insulin lispro (*Humalog*)	0.25-0.5	0.5-2.5	≤ 5
	Regular (*Novolin R, Humulin R*)	0.5-1	2-3	3-6
Intermediate/long-acting:	NPH (*Novolin N, Humulin N*)	2-4	4-10	10-16
	Insulin detemir (*Levemir*)	not available	flat action profile	up to 23†
	Insulin glargine (*Lantus*)	2-4	peakless	24
Mixtures:	Insulin aspart protamine suspension/aspart (*NovoLog Mix 70/30*)	0.25	1-4 (biphasic)	up to 24
	Insulin lispro protamine suspension/insulin lispro (*HumaLog Mix 75/25, HumaLog Mix 50/50*)	<0.25	1-3 (biphasic)	10-20
	NPH/Reg (*Humulin 70/30, Humulin 50/50, Novolin 70/30*)	0.5-1	2-10 (biphasic)	10-20

*These are general guidelines, as onset, peak, and duration of activity are affected by the site of injection, physical activity, body temperature, and blood supply.
† Dose dependent duration of action, range from 6-23 hours.

ENDOCRINE & METABOLIC: Diabetes-Related – Insulins

NOTE: Adjust insulin dosing to achieve glycemic control. See table "diabetes numbers" for goals.
insulin - inhaled (*Exubera*) ▶LK ♀C ▶+ $$$$

ADULT - Diabetes: Initial per meal dose based on patient body weight. 1 mg (30-39.9 kg); 2 mg (40-59.9 kg); 3 mg (60-79.9 kg); 4 mg (80-99.9 kg); 5 mg (100-119.9 kg); 6 mg (120-

139.9 kg). Administer immediately before a meal (within 10 min). In type 1 diabetes, use in combination with long-acting insulin. In type 2 diabetes, may be used alone or in combination with oral agents or long-acting insulins.

PEDS - Not approved in children.

FORMS - Trade only: Combination pack #12 (90 x 1 mg insulin blisters and 90 x 3 mg insulin blisters, 2 release units). Combination pack #15 (180 x 1 mg insulin blisters and 90 x 3 mg insulin blisters, 2 release units).

NOTES - Rapid-acting, peak within 30-90 minutes with duration similar to SC regular insulin. Assess pulmonary function at baseline, at six months, then annually thereafter. Contraindicated in current or recent (<6 months) smokers and in unstable or poorly controlled lung disease. Not recommended in asthma or COPD. Combine 1 mg and 3 mg blisters to use least number of blisters/dose. Approximate equivalence: 1 mg blister of inhaled insulin delivers approximately 3 units of SC regular human insulin; 3 mg blister of inhaled insulin delivers approximately 8 units of SC regular human insulin. Do not substitute three 1 mg unit dose blisters for one 3 mg dose; consecutive inhalation of 1 mg blisters provides higher insulin exposure. Patient will need Exubera CareKit upon initiation (inhaler, replacement chamber and release unit); each patient pack has two additional release units.

insulin - injectable combinations (*Humalog Mix 75/25, Humalog Mix 50/50, Humulin 70/30, Humulin 50/50, Novolin 70/30, Novolog Mix 70/30*) ▶LK ♀B/C ▶+ $$$

ADULT - Doses vary, but typically total insulin 0.3-1 unit/kg/day SC in divided doses (Type 1), and 0.5-1.5 unit/kg/day SC in divided doses (Type 2). Generally, 50% of insulin requirements are provided by basal insulin (intermediate- or long-acting) and the remainder from rapid or short-acting insulin.

PEDS - Not approved in children

UNAPPROVED PEDS - Diabetes: maintenance: insulin 0.5-1 unit/kg/day SC, but doses vary.

FORMS - Trade only: injection insulin lispro protamine suspension / insulin lispro (Humalog Mix 75/25, Humalog Mix 50/50), insulin aspart protamine/insulin aspart (Novolog Mix 70/30) NPH and regular mixtures (Humulin 70/30, Novolin 70/30 or Humulin 50/50). Insulin available in pen form: Novolin 70/30 Innolet, Novolog Mix 70/30 FlexPen, Humulin 70/30, Humalog Mix 75/25, Humalog Mix 50/50.

NOTES - Administer rapid-acting insulin mixtures (Humalog, NovoLog) within 15 min before meals. Administer regular insulin mixtures 30 minutes before meals.

insulin - injectable intermediate / long-acting (*Novolin N, Humulin N, Lantus, Levemir*) ▶LK ♀B/C ▶+ $$$

ADULT - Doses vary, but typically total insulin 0.3-0.5 unit/kg/day SC in divided doses (Type 1), and 1-1.5 unit/kg/day SC in divided doses (Type 2). Generally, 50-70% of insulin requirements are provided by rapid or short-acting insulin and the remainder from intermediate- or long-acting insulin. Lantus: Start 10 units SC daily (same time everyday) in insulin naive patients, adjust to usual dose of 2-100 units/day. When transferring from twice daily NPH human insulin, the initial Lantus dose should be reduced by ~20% from the previous total daily NPH dose, then adjust dose based on response. Levemir: Type 2 DM (inadequately controlled on oral meds): Start 0.1-0.2 units/kg once daily; or 10 units SC daily or BID. When transferring from basal insulin (Lantus, NPH,) in type 1 or 2 DM, change on a unit-to-unit basis; more Levemir may be required than NPH insulin.

PEDS - Diabetes: maintenance: total insulin 0.5-1 unit/kg/day SC, but doses vary. Generally, 50-70% of insulin requirements are provided by rapid-acting insulin and the remainder from intermediate- or long-acting insulin. Age 6-15 yo (Lantus): Start 10 units SC daily (same time everyday) in insulin naive patients, adjust to usual dose of 2-100 units/day. When transferring from twice daily NPH human insulin, the initial Lantus dose should be reduced by ~20% from the previous total daily NPH dose, then adjust dose based on patient response. Levemir (Type 1 DM): When transferring from NPH, change on a unit-to-unit basis; more Levemir may be required than NPH.

FORMS - Trade only: injection NPH (Novolin N, Humulin N), insulin glargine (Lantus), insulin detemir (Levemir). Insulin available in pen form: Humulin N Isophane Insulin Pen, Novolin N Innolet, Lantus OptiClick, Levemir Innolet, Levemir FlexPen. Premixed preparations of NPH and regular insulin also available.

NOTES - May mix NPH with aspart, lispro, glulisine or regular. Draw up rapid/short-acting insulin first. Do not mix Lantus or Levemir with insulins in a syringe.

insulin - injectable short/rapid-acting (*Apidra, Novolin R, NovoLog, Humulin R,*

Humalog, ✚*NovoRapid* ▶LK ♀B/C ▶+ $$$
ADULT - Doses vary, but typically total insulin 0.3-0.5 unit/kg/day SC in divided doses (Type 1), and 1-1.5 unit/kg/day SC in divided doses (Type 2). Generally, 50-70% of insulin requirements are provided by rapid or short-acting insulin and the remainder from intermediate- or long-acting insulin.
PEDS - Diabetes age >3 yo (Humalog) or >2 (NovoLog): Doses vary, but typically total insulin maintenance dose 0.5-1 unit/kg/day SC in divided doses. Generally, 50-70% of insulin requirements are provided by rapid-acting insulin and the remainder from intermediate- or long-acting insulin. Apidra not approved in children.
UNAPPROVED ADULT - Severe hyperkalemia: 5-10 units regular insulin plus concurrent dextrose IV. Profound hyperglycemia (eg, DKA): 0.1 unit/kg regular insulin IV bolus, then begin IV infusion 100 units in 100 mL NS (1 unit/mL) at 0.1 units/kg/hr. 70 kg: 7 units/h (7 mL/h). Titrate to clinical effect.
UNAPPROVED PEDS - Profound hyperglycemia (eg, DKA): 0.1 unit/kg regular insulin IV bolus, then IV infusion 100 units in 100 mL NS (1 unit/mL) at 0.1 units/kg/hr. Titrate to clinical effect. Severe hyperkalemia: 0.1 units/kg regular insulin IV with glucose over 30 min. May repeat in 30-60 min or start 0.1 units/kg/hr.
FORMS - Trade: injection regular, insulin glulisine (Apidra), insulin lispro (Humalog), insulin aspart (NovoLog). Pen form: Novolog FlexPen, Humalog, Novolin R, Apidra OptiClik.
NOTES - Administer rapid-acting insulin (Humalog, NovoLog, Apidra) within 15 min before or immediately after a meal. Administer regular insulin 30 minutes before meals. May mix with NPH. Draw up rapid/short-acting insulin first.

ENDOCRINE & METABOLIC: Diabetes-Related – Meglitinides

nateglinide (*Starlix*) ▶L ♀C ▶? $$$$
ADULT - Diabetes, monotherapy or in combination with metformin or thiazolidinedione: 120 mg PO tid ≤30 min before meals; use 60 mg PO tid in patients who are near goal A1C.
PEDS - Not approved in children.
FORMS - Trade only: Tabs 60, 120 mg.
NOTES - Not for monotherapy in patients inadequately controlled with glyburide or other prior anti-diabetic agents. Hypoglycemia risk if severe renal impairment.
repaglinide (*Prandin*, ✚*Gluconorm*) ▶L ♀C

▶? $$$$
ADULT - Diabetes: 0.5- 2 mg PO tid within 30 minutes before a meal. Allow 1 week between dosage adjustments. Usual range is 0.5-4 mg PO tid-qid, max 16 mg/day.
PEDS - Not approved in children.
FORMS - Trade only: Tabs 0.5, 1, 2 mg.
NOTES - May take dose immediately preceding meal to as long as 30 minutes before the meal. Gemfibrozil and itraconazole increase blood repaglinide levels and may result in an increased risk of hypoglycemia.

ENDOCRINE & METABOLIC: Diabetes-Related – Sulfonylureas – 1st Generation

chlorpropamide (*Diabinese*) ▶LK ♀C ▶- $$
ADULT - Initiate therapy with 100-250 mg PO daily. Titrate after 5-7 days by increments of 50-125 mg at intervals of 3-5 days to obtain optimal control. Max 750 mg/day.
PEDS - Not approved in children.
FORMS - Generic/Trade: Tabs 100, 250 mg.
NOTES - Clinical use in the elderly has not been properly evaluated. Elderly are more prone to hypoglycemia and/or hyponatremia possibly from renal impairment or drug interactions. May cause disulfiram-like reaction with alcohol.
tolazamide (*Tolinase*) ▶LK ♀C ▶? $$
ADULT - Initiate therapy with 100 mg PO daily in patients with FBS <200 mg/dl, and in patients who are malnourished, underweight, or

elderly. Initiate therapy with 250 mg PO daily in patients with FBS >200 mg/dl. Give with breakfast or the first main meal of the day. If daily doses exceed 500 mg, divide the dose bid. Max 1,000 mg/day.
PEDS - Not approved in children.
FORMS - Generic/Trade: Tabs 100, 250, 500 mg.
tolbutamide ▶LK ♀C ▶+ $
ADULT - Start 1g PO daily. Maintenance dose is usually 250 mg to 2 g PO daily. Total daily dose may be taken in the morning, divide doses if GI intolerance occurs. Max 3 g/day.
PEDS - Not approved in children.
FORMS - Generic only: Tabs 500 mg.

ENDOCRINE & METABOLIC: Diabetes-Related – Sulfonylureas – 2nd Generation

gliclazide (❋*Diamicron, Diamicron MR*)
▶KL ♀C ▶? $

ADULT - Canada only, diabetes type 2: Immediate release: Start 80-160 mg PO daily, max 320 mg PO daily (≥160 mg in divided doses). Modified release: Start 30 mg PO daily, max 120 mg PO daily.

PEDS - Not approved in children.

FORMS - Generic/Trade: Tab 80 mg (Diamicron). Trade only: Tabs, modified release 30 mg (Diamicron MR).

NOTES - Immediate and modified release not equipotent; 80 mg of immediate release can be changed to 30 mg of modified release.

glimepiride (*Amaryl*) ▶LK ♀C ▶- $$

ADULT - Diabetes: initiate therapy with 1-2 mg PO daily. Start with 1 mg PO daily in elderly, malnourished patients or those with renal or hepatic insufficiency. Give with breakfast or the first main meal of the day. Titrate in increments of 1-2 mg at 1-2 week intervals based on response. Usual maintenance dose is 1-4 mg PO daily, max 8 mg/day.

PEDS - Not approved in children.

FORMS - Generic/Trade: Tabs 1, 2, 4 mg. Generic only: Tabs 8 mg.

glipizide (*Glucotrol, Glucotrol XL*) ▶LK ♀C ▶? $

ADULT - Diabetes: initiate therapy with 5 mg PO daily. Give 2.5 mg PO daily to geriatric patients or those with liver disease. Adjust dose in increments of 2.5-5 mg to a usual maintenance dose of 10-20 mg/day, max 40 mg/day. Doses

>15 mg should be divided bid. Extended release (Glucotrol XL): initiate therapy with 5 mg PO daily. Usual dose is 5-10 mg PO daily, max 20 mg/day.

PEDS - Not approved in children.

FORMS - Generic/Trade: Tabs 5, 10 mg; Extended release tabs 2.5, 5, 10 mg.

NOTES - Maximum effective dose is generally 20 mg/day.

glyburide (*Micronase, DiaBeta, Glynase PresTab,* ❋*Euglucon*) ▶LK ♀B ▶? $

ADULT - Diabetes: initiate therapy with 2.5-5 mg PO daily. Start 1.25 mg PO daily in elderly, malnourished, or renal or hepatic insufficiency. Give with breakfast or the first main meal of the day. Titrate in increments of ≤2.5 mg at weekly intervals based on response. Usual maintenance dose is 1.25-20 mg PO daily or divided bid, max 20 mg/day. Micronized tabs: initiate therapy with 1.5-3 mg PO daily. Start with 0.75 mg PO daily in elderly, malnourished patients or those with renal or hepatic insufficiency. Give with breakfast or the first main meal of the day. Titrate in increments of ≤1.5 mg at weekly intervals based on response. Usual maintenance dose is 0.75-12 mg PO daily, max 12 mg/day. May divide dose bid if >6 mg/day.

PEDS - Not approved in children.

FORMS - Generic/Trade: Tabs (scored) 1.25, 2.5, 5 mg. micronized Tabs (scored) 1.5, 3, 4.5, 6 mg.

NOTES - Maximum effective dose is generally 10 mg/day.

ENDOCRINE & METABOLIC: Diabetes-Related – Other

A1C home testing (*Metrika A1CNow*) ♀+ ▶+ $

ADULT, PEDS - Use for home A1C testing

FORMS - Fingerstick blood

NOTES - Result displays in 8 minutes.

dextrose (*Glutose, B-D Glucose, Insta-Glucose, Dex-4*) ▶L ♀C ▶? $

ADULT - Hypoglycemia: 0.5-1 g/kg (1-2 mL/kg) up to 25 g (50 mL) of 50% solution by slow IV injection. Hypoglycemia in conscious diabetics: 10-20 g PO q10-20 min prn.

PEDS - Hypoglycemia in neonates: 0.25-0.5 g/kg/dose (5-10 mL of 25% dextrose in a 5 kg infant). Severe hypoglycemia or older infants may require larger doses up to 3 g (12 mL of

25% dextrose) followed by a continuous IV infusion of 10% dextrose. Non-neonates may require 0.5-1.0 g/kg.

FORMS - OTC Generic/Trade: Chewable tablets 4 g (Dex-4), 5 g (Glutose). Trade only: Oral gel 40%.

NOTES - Do not exceed an infusion rate of 0.5 g/kg/hr.

exenatide (*Byetta*) ▶K ♀C ▶? $$$$$

ADULT - Type 2 DM adjunctive therapy when inadequate control on metformin, a sulfonylurea, or a glitazone (alone or in combination): 5 mcg SC bid (within 1 h before the morning and evening meals, or 1 h before the two main meals of the day ≥6h apart). May increase to

10 mcg SC bid after 1 month.

PEDS - Not approved in children.

FORMS - Trade: prefilled pen (60 doses each) 5 mcg/dose, 1.2 mL; 10 mcg/dose, 2.4 mL.

NOTES - Keep refrigerated & protect from light. Discard after 30 days after 1st use. May give SC in upper arm, abdomen, or thigh. Avoid use if renal insufficiency (CrCl <30 mL/min) or severe gastrointestinal disease, including gastroparesis. Do not substitute for insulin in insulindependent. Concurrent insulin, meglitinides or alpha-glucosidase inhibitors has not been studied. Risk of hypoglycemia is higher when used with sulfonylurea, therefore, consider reduction in sulfonylurea dose. Take medications that require rapid gastrointestinal absorption ≥1 h prior to exenatide. May promote slight weight loss. May potentiate warfarin.

glucagon (*GlucaGen*) ▶LK ♀B ▶? $$$

ADULT - Hypoglycemia in adults: 1 mg IV/IM/ SC. If no response within 15 minutes, may repeat dose 1-2 times. Diagnostic aid for GI tract radiography: 1 mg IV/IM/SC.

PEDS - Hypoglycemia in children >20 kg: same as adults. Hypoglycemia in children <20 kg: 0.5 mg IV/IM/SC or 20-30 mcg/kg. If no response in 5-20 minutes, may repeat dose 1-2 times.

UNAPPROVED ADULT - The following indications are based upon limited data. Esophageal obstruction caused by food: 1 mg IV over 1-3 minutes. Symptomatic bradycardia/hypotension, especially with beta blocker therapy: 3-10 mg IV bolus (0.05 mg/kg general recommendation) may repeat in 10 minutes; may be followed by continuous infusion of 1-5 mg/hour or 0.07 mg/kg/hour. Infusion rate should be titrated to the desired response.

FORMS - Trade only: injection 1 mg.

NOTES - Should be reserved for refractory/severe cases or when IV/IM dextrose cannot be administered. Advise patients to educate family members and co-workers how to administer a dose. Give supplemental carbohydrates when patient responds.

glucose home testing (*Accu-Chek Active, Accu-Check Advantage, Accu-Check Compact, Ascencia, FreeStyle, Gluco-Watch, OneTouch InDuo, OneTouch Ultra, OneTouch UltraSmart, Precision Sof-Tact, Precision QID, Precision Xtra, True Track Smart System, Clinistix, Clinitest, Diastix, Tes-Tape*) ▶None ♀+ ▶+ $$

ADULT, PEDS - Home glucose monitoring

FORMS - Plasma: Accu-Check Active, Accu-

Check Advantage, Accu-Check Compact, Ascencia, FreeStyle, OneTouch InDuo, Gluco-Watch Monitor, OneTouch InDuo, OneTouch Ultra, OneTouch UltraSmart, Precision Sof-Tact, Precision QID, Precision Xtra, Precision Sof-Tact, True Track; Urine: Clinistix, Clinitest, Diastix, Tes-Tape

NOTES - GlucoWatch measures q10 min and reports an average of 2 readings q20 min for 12h by sending small electric currents through the skin (a thin plastic sensor is attached to the back of the watch each time it is strapped on to extract glucose from fluid in skin cells). GlucoWatch may cause skin irritation. Accu-Check Active, Accu-Check Compact, Ascensia, FreeStyle, OneTouch InDuo, OneTouch Ultra, OneTouch InDuo, OneTouch UltraSmart, Precision Sof-Tact, and Precision Xtra can be used on alternate site testing (e.g. forearm) prior to or ≥2 hours after meal or exercise.

metformin (*Glucophage, Glucophage XR, Glumetza, Fortamet, Riomet*) ▶K ♀B ▶? $

ADULT - Diabetes: Immediate-release: Start 500 mg PO daily-bid or 850 mg PO daily with meals. Increase by 500 mg q week or 850 mg q other week to a max of 2550 mg/day. Higher doses may be divided tid with meals. Extended release: 500 mg PO daily with evening meal; increase by 500 mg q week to max 2000 mg/ day (may divide 1000 mg PO bid). Fortamet: 500-1000 mg daily with evening meal; increase by 500 mg q week to max 2500 mg/day.

PEDS - Diabetes ≥10 yo: Start 500 mg PO daily-bid (Glucophage) with meals, increase by 500 mg q week to max 2000 mg/day in divided doses (10-16 yo). Glucophage XR & Fortamet are indicated in ≥17 yo.

UNAPPROVED ADULT - Polycystic ovary syndrome: 500 mg PO tid or 850 mg PO bid. Type 2 DM prevention: 850 mg PO daily for 1 month, then increase to 850 mg PO bid.

FORMS - Generic/Trade: Tabs 500, 850, 1000 mg, extended release 500, 750 mg. Trade only, extended release: Fortamet 500, 1000 mg; Glumetza 500, 1000 mg. Trade only: oral soln 500 mg/5 mL (Riomet).

NOTES - May be given concomitantly with sulfonylureas, thiazolidinediones or insulin. May reduce the risk of progression to Type 2 diabetes in those with impaired glucose tolerance, but less effectively than intensive lifestyle modification. Metformin-containing products may cause life-threatening lactic acidosis, usually in setting of decreased tissue perfusion, hypoxia, hepatic dysfunction, unstable congestive heart failure or impaired renal clearance. Hold prior to IV contrast agents and for 48 h after. Avoid if ethanol abuse, hepatic or renal insufficiency (creat ≥1.4 mg/dl in women, ≥1.5 mg/dl in men), or hypoxic states (cardiogenic shock, septicemia, acute MI).

pramlintide (*Symlin*) ▸K ♀C ▸? $$$$
WARNING - May cause severe insulin-induced hypoglycemia especially in Type 1 DM, usually within 3 hours. Avoid if hypoglycemic unawareness, gastroparesis, GI motility medications, alpha-glucosidase inhibitors, A1C >9%, poor compliance, or hypersensitivity to the metacresol preservative. Appropriate patient selection, careful patient instruction and insulin dose adjustments (reduction in pre-meal short-acting insulin of 50%) are critical for reducing the hypoglycemia risk.
ADULT - Type 1 DM with mealtime insulin therapy: Initiate 15 mcg SC immediately before major meals & titrate by 15 mcg increments (if significant nausea has not occurred for ≥3 days) to maintenance 30-60 mcg as tolerated. If significant nausea, decrease to 30 mcg. Type 2 DM with mealtime insulin therapy: Initiate 60 mcg SC immediately before major meals and increase to 120 mcg as tolerated (if significant nausea has not occurred for 3-7 days.) If significant nausea, decrease dose to 60 mcg.
PEDS - Not approved in children.
FORMS - Trade only: 5 mL vials, 0.6 mg/mL.
NOTES - Keep unopened vials refrigerated. Opened vials can be kept at room temperature or refrigerated up to 28 days. May give SC in abdomen or thigh. Take medications that require rapid onset 1 hour prior or 2 hours after. Careful patient selection and skilled health care supervision are critical for safe and effective use. Monitor pre-/post-meal and bedtime glucose. Decrease initial pre-meal short-acting insulin doses by 50% including fixed-mix insulin (i.e. 70/30). Do not mix with insulin. Use new needle & syringe for each dose.

sitagliptin (*Januvia*) ▸K ♀B ▸? $$$$
ADULT - Type 2 DM monotherapy, or in combination with metformin or a glitazone: 100 mg PO daily. If CrCl 30-49 mL/min reduce dose to 50 mg daily; if CrCl <30 mL/min then 25 mg daily.
PEDS - Not approved in children.
FORMS - Trade only: Tabs 25, 50,100 mg.
NOTES - Not for use in Type 1 DM or DKA. Assess renal function periodically.

ENDOCRINE & METABOLIC: Diagnostic Agents

corticotropin (*H.P. Acthar Gel*) ▸K ♀C ▸- $$$
ADULT - Diagnostic testing of adrenocortical function: 80 units IM or SC. Acute exacerbation of multiple sclerosis: 80-120 units IM daily IM x 2-3 weeks.
UNAPPROVED PEDS - Various dosing regimens have been used for infantile spasms.
NOTES - Has limited therapeutic value in conditions responsive to corticosteroids therapy, corticosteroids should be the treatment of choice. Prolonged use in children may inhibit skeletal growth. Cosyntropin preferred for diagnostic testing as it is less allergenic and more potent.

cosyntropin (*Cortrosyn*, ✦*Synacthen*) ▸L ♀C ▸? $
ADULT - Rapid screen for adrenocortical insufficiency: 0.25 mg IM/ IV over 2 min; measure serum cortisol before & 30-60 min after.
PEDS - Rapid screen for adrenocortical insufficiency: 0.25 mg (0.125 mg if <2 yo) IM/IV over 2 min; measure serum cortisol before & 30-60 min after.

metyrapone (*Metopirone*) ▸KL ♀C ▸? $$
WARNING - May cause acute adrenal insufficiency.
ADULT - Diagnostic aid for testing hypothalamic-pituitary adrenocorticotropic hormone (ACTH) function: Specialized single- and multiple-test dose available.
PEDS - Diagnostic aid for testing hypothalamic-pituitary adrenocorticotropic hormone (ACTH) function: Specialized single- and multiple-test dose available.
UNAPPROVED ADULT - Cushing's syndrome: dosing varies.
FORMS - Trade only: Caps 250 mg. Only available from manufacturer due to limited supply: 1-800-988-7768.
NOTES - Ability of adrenals to respond to exogenous ACTH should be demonstrated before metyrapone is employed as a test. In the presence of hypo- or hyperthyroidism, response to the test may be subnormal. May suppress aldosterone synthesis. May cause dizziness & sedation.

ENDOCRINE & METABOLIC: Gout-Related

allopurinol (Aloprim, Zyloprim) ▶K ♀C ▶+ $
ADULT - Mild gout or recurrent calcium oxalate stones: 200-300 mg PO daily (start 100 mg PO daily). Moderately severe gout: 400-600 mg PO daily. Secondary hyperuricemia: 600-800 mg PO daily. Doses >300 mg should be divided. Max 800 mg/day. Reduce dose in renal insufficiency (CrCl 10-20 mL/min= 200 mg/day, CrCl <10 mL/min = 100 mg/day). Prevention of hyperuricemia secondary to chemotherapy and unable to tolerate PO: 200-400 mg/m²/day as a single IV infusion or in equally divided infusions q6-12h. Max 600 mg/day. Reduce dose in renal insufficiency (CrCl 10-20 mL/min = 200 mg/day, CrCl 3-10 mL/min = 100 mg/day, CrCl < 3ml/min 100 mg/day at extended intervals). Initiate 24-48h before chemotherapy.
PEDS - Secondary hyperuricemia, <6 yo = 150 mg PO daily; age 6-10 yo = 300 mg PO daily or 1 mg/kg/day divided q6h to a maximum of 600 mg/day. Prevention of hyperuricemia secondary to chemotherapy and unable to tolerate PO: Initiate with 200 mg/m²/day as a single IV infusion or in equally divided infusions q6-12h.
FORMS - Generic/Trade: Tabs 100, 300 mg.
NOTES - May precipitate acute gout; consider prophylactic NSAIDs or colchicine. Start 100 mg PO daily and increase weekly to target serum uric acid of <6 mg/dL. Risk of rash and hypersensitivity syndrome higher in renal impairment. Discontinue if rash or allergy; do not restart after severe rash. Interacts with warfarin & azathioprine. Normal serum uric acid levels are usually achieved after 1-3 weeks of therapy. Ensure hydration before IV administration.

Colbenemid (colchicine + probenecid) ▶KL ♀C ▶? $$$
ADULT - Chronic gouty arthritis: start 1 tab PO daily x 1 week, then 1 tab PO bid.
PEDS - Not approved in children.
FORMS - Generic only: Tabs 0.5 mg colchicine + 500 mg probenecid.
NOTES - Maintain alkaline urine.

colchicine ▶L ♀C ▶? $
ADULT - Older FDA-approved dosing no longer recommended; see "unapproved adult" section.
PEDS - Not approved in children.
UNAPPROVED ADULT - Rapid treatment of acute gouty arthritis: 0.6 mg PO q1h for up to 3h (max 3 tablets). Gout prophylaxis: 0.6 mg PO bid if CrCl ≥50 ml/min, 0.6 mg PO daily if

CrCl 35-49 ml/min, 0.6 mg PO q2-3 days if CrCl 10-34 ml/min. Familial Mediterranean fever: 1 mg in divided doses daily, may increase to 2-3 mg/day if needed. Acute/recurrent pericarditis in addition to usual therapy: 1 mg PO bid x 1 day, then 0.5 mg PO bid x 3 months; give once daily if <70 kg or intolerance.
FORMS - Generic only: Tabs 0.6 mg.
NOTES - Colchicine is most effective when initiated on the first day of gouty arthritis. IV route no longer recommended due to serious adverse effects including death.

probenecid (✦Benuryl) ▶KL ♀B ▶? $
ADULT - Gout: 250 mg PO bid x 7 days, then 500 mg PO bid. May increase by 500 mg/day q4 weeks not to exceed 2 g/day. Adjunct to penicillin: 2 g/day PO in divided doses. Reduce dose to 1 g/day in renal impairment.
PEDS - Adjunct to penicillin, 2-14 yo: 25 mg/kg PO initially, then 40 mg/kg/day divided qid. Adult dose if >50 kg; don't use if <2 yo.
FORMS - Generic only: Tabs 500 mg.
NOTES - Decrease dose if GI intolerance occurs. Maintain alkaline urine. Begin therapy 2-3 weeks after acute gouty attack subsides.

rasburicase (Elitek, ✦Fasturtec) ▶L ♀C ▶- $$$$$
WARNING - May cause hypersensitivity reactions including anaphylaxis, hemolysis (G6PD-deficient patients), methemoglobinemia, interference with uric acid measurements
ADULT - Not approved in adults.
PEDS - Uric acid elevation prevention in children (1 mo-17 yr) with leukemia, lymphoma, and solid tumor malignancies receiving anti-cancer therapy: 0.15 or 0.20 mg/kg IV over 30 min daily x 5 days. Initiate chemotherapy 4 to 24 hrs after the first dose.
NOTES - Safety and efficacy have been established only for one 5 day treatment course. Hydrate IV if at risk for tumor lysis syndrome. Screen for G6PD deficiency in high risk.

sulfinpyrazone (Anturane, ✦Anturan) ▶K ♀? ▶? $$
ADULT - Gout: start 100-200 mg PO bid with meals, titrate over 1 week to 400-800 mg/day.
PEDS - Not approved in children.
FORMS - Generic: Tabs 100 mg. Caps 200 mg.
NOTES - May precipitate an acute gouty flare; continue treatment throughout exacerbation. Maintain hydration and alkaline urine.

INTRAVENOUS SOLUTIONS (ions in mEq/l)								
Solution	Dextrose	Cal/l	Na	K	Ca	Cl	Lactate	Osm
0.9 NS	0 g/l	0	154	0	0	154	0	310
LR	0 g/l	9	130	4	3	109	28	273
D5 W	50 g/l	170	0	0	0	0	0	253
D5 0.2 NS	50 g/l	170	34	0	0	34	0	320
D5 0.45 NS	50 g/l	170	77	0	0	77	0	405
D5 0.9 NS	50 g/l	170	154	0	0	154	0	560
D5 LR	50 g/l	179	130	4	3	109	28	527

ENDOCRINE & METABOLIC: Minerals

calcium acetate (*PhosLo*) ▶K ♀+ ▶? $$$
ADULT - Hyperphosphatemia in end-stage renal failure: initially 2 tabs/caps PO tid with each meal. Titrate based on serum phosphorus.
PEDS - Not approved in children.
UNAPPROVED PEDS - Titrate to response.
FORMS - Trade only: Gelcaps 667 mg (169 mg elem Ca).
NOTES - Higher doses more effective, but may cause hypercalcemia, especially if given with vitamin D. Most patients require 3-4 tabs/meal.

calcium carbonate (*Caltrate, Mylanta Children's, Os-Cal, Oyst-Cal, Tums, Surpass, Viactiv, ✤Calsan*) ▶K ♀+ (? 1st trimester) ▶? $
ADULT - Supplement: 1-2 g or more elem Ca/ day PO with meals divided bid-qid. Osteoporosis prevention: 1000-1500 mg elem Ca/day PO divided bid-tid with meals. Adequate intake in most is 1000-1200 mg elem Ca /day. Antacid: 1000-3000 mg/day (2-4 tab) PO q2h prn or 1-2 pieces gum chewed prn, max 7000 mg/day.
PEDS - Hypocalcemia: Neonates: 50-150 mg elem Ca/kg/day PO in 4-6 divided doses; Children: 45-65 mg elem Ca/kg/day PO divided qid. Adequate intake for children (in elem calcium): <6 mo: 210 mg/day when fed human milk and 315 mg/day when fed cow's milk; 6-12 mo: 270 mg/day when fed human milk+solid food and 335 mg/day when fed cow's milk + solid food; 1-3 yo: 500 mg/day; 4-8 yo: 800 mg/day; 9-18 yo 1300 mg/day.
UNAPPROVED ADULT - May lower BP in HTN. May reduce PMS symptoms such as fluid retention, pain, and negative affect.
FORMS - OTC Generic/Trade: tab 500, 650, 750, 1000, 1250, 1500 mg, chew tab 400, 500, 750,850, 1000, 1177, 1250 mg, cap 1250 mg, gum 300, 450 mg, susp 1250 mg/5 mL. Calcium carbonate is 40% elem Ca and contains 20 mEq of elem Ca/g calcium carbonate. Not

more than 500-600 mg elem Ca/dose. Available in combination with sodium fluoride, vitamin D and/or vitamin K. Trade examples: Caltrate 600 + D = 600 mg elemental Ca/200 units vit D, Os-Cal 500 + D = 500 mg elemental Ca/200 units vit D, Os-Cal Extra D = 500 mg elemental Ca/400 units vit D, Tums (regular strength) = 200 mg elemental Ca, Tums (ultra) = 400 mg elemental Ca, Viactiv (chew) 500 mg elemental Ca+ 100 units vit D + 40 mcg vit K.
NOTES - Decreases absorption of levothyroxine, tetracycline, and fluoroquinolones.

calcium chloride ▶K ♀+ ▶+ $
ADULT - Hypocalcemia: 500-1000 mg slow IV q1-3 days. Magnesium intoxication: 500 mg IV. Hyperkalemic ECG changes: dose based on ECG.
PEDS - Hypocalcemia: 0.2 mL/kg IV up to 10 mL/day. Cardiac resuscitation: 0.2 mL/kg IV.
UNAPPROVED ADULT - Has been used in calcium channel blocker toxicity and to treat or prevent calcium blocker-induced hypotension.
UNAPPROVED PEDS - Has been used in calcium channel blocker toxicity.
FORMS - Generic only: injectable 10% (1000 mg/10 mL) 10 mL ampules, vials, syringes.
NOTES - Calcium chloride contains 14.4 mEq Ca/g versus calcium gluconate 4.7 mEq Ca/g. For IV use only; do not administer IM or SC. Avoid extravasation. Administer no faster than 0.5-1 mL/min. Use cautiously in patients receiving digoxin; inotropic and toxic effects are synergistic and may cause arrhythmias. Usually not recommended for hypocalcemia associated with renal insufficiency because calcium chloride is an acidifying salt.

calcium citrate (*Citracal*) ▶K ♀+ ▶+ $
ADULT - 1-2 g elem Ca/day or more PO with meals divided bid-qid. Prevention of osteoporosis: 1000-1500 mg elem Ca/day PO divided bid-tid with meals. The adequate intake in most

adults is 1000-1200 mg elem Ca/day.

PEDS - Not approved in children.

FORMS - OTC: Trade only (mg elem Ca): 200 & 250 mg with 200 units vitamin D and 250 mg with 125 units vitamin D and 80 mg of magnesium. Chew tabs 500 mg with 200 units vitamin D. OTC: Generic/Trade: Tabs 200 mg, 315 mg with 200 units vitamin D.

NOTES - Calcium citrate is 21% elem Ca. Not more than 500-600 mg elem Ca/dose. Decreases absorption of levothyroxine, tetracycline and fluoroquinolones.

calcium gluconate ▶K ♀+ ▶+ $

ADULT - Emergency correction of hypocalcemia: 7-14 mEq slow IV prn. Hypocalcemic tetany: 4.5-16 mEq IM prn. Hyperkalemia with cardiac toxicity: 2.25-14 mEq IV while monitoring ECG. May repeat after 1-2 minutes. Magnesium intoxication: 4.5-9 mEq IV, adjust dose based on patient response. If IV not possible, give 2-5 mEq IM. Exchange transfusions: 1.35 mEq calcium gluconate IV concurrent with each 100 mL of citrated blood. Oral calcium gluconate: 1-2 g elem Ca/day or more PO with meals divided bid-qid. Prevention of osteoporosis: 1000-1500 mg elem Ca/day PO with meals in divided doses.

PEDS - Emergency correction of hypocalcemia: Children: 1-7 mEq IV prn. Infants: 1 mEq IV prn. Hypocalcemic tetany: Children: 0.5-0.7 mEq/kg IV tid-qid. Neonates: 2.4 mEq/kg/day IV in divided doses. Exchange transfusions: Neonates: 0.45 mEq IV/100 mL of exchange transfusions. Oral calcium gluconate: Hypocalcemia: Neonates: 50-150 mg elem Ca/kg/day PO in 4-6 divided doses; children: 45-65 mg elem Ca/kg/day PO divided qid.

UNAPPROVED ADULT - Has been used in calcium channel blocker toxicity and to treat or prevent calcium blocker-induced hypotension.

UNAPPROVED PEDS - Has been used in calcium channel blocker toxicity.

FORMS - Generic only: Injectable 10% (1000 mg/10 mL, 4.65mEq/10 mL) 1, 10, 50, 100, 200 mL. OTC Generic only: Tab 50, 500, 650, 975,1000 mg. Chew tab 650 mg.

NOTES - Calcium gluconate is 9.3% elem Ca and contains 4.6 mEq elem Ca/g calcium gluconate. Administer IV no faster than 0.5-2 mL/min. Use cautiously in patients receiving digoxin; inotropic and toxic effects are synergistic and may cause arrhythmias.

ferric gluconate complex (*Ferrlecit*) ▶KL ♀B ▶? $$$$$

WARNING - Potentially fatal hypersensitivity reactions rarely reported with sodium ferric gluconate complex. Facilities for CPR must be available during dosing.

ADULT - Iron deficiency in chronic hemodialysis patients: 125 mg elem iron IV over 10 min or diluted in 100 mL NS IV over 1 h. Most hemodialysis patients require 1 g of elem iron over 8 consecutive hemodialysis session.

PEDS - Iron deficiency in chronic hemodialysis ≥6 yo: 1.5 mg/kg elem iron diluted in 25 mL NS & administered IV over 1 hour at 8 sequential dialysis sessions. Max 125 mg/dose.

UNAPPROVED ADULT - Iron deficiency: 125 mg elem iron IV over 10 min or diluted in 100 mL NS IV over 1 hr.

NOTES - Serious hypotensive events occur in 1.3% of patients.

ferrous gluconate (*Fergon*) ▶K ♀+ ▶+ $

ADULT - Iron deficiency: 800-1600 mg ferrous gluconate (100-200 mg elem iron) PO divided tid. RDA (elem iron): adult males (≥19 yo): 8 mg; adult premenopausal females (19-50 yo) 18 mg; adult females (≥51 yo): 8 mg; pregnancy: 27 mg; lactation: 14-18 yo: 10 mg; 19-50 yo: 9 mg. Upper limit: 45 mg/day.

PEDS - Mild-moderate iron deficiency: 3 mg/kg/day of elem iron PO in 1-2 divided doses; severe iron deficiency: 4-6 mg/kg/day PO in 3 divided doses. RDA (elem iron): <6 mo: 0.27 mg; 7-12 mo: 11 mg; 1-3 yo: 7 mg; 4-8 yo: 10 mg; 9-13 yo: 8 mg; males 14-18 yo: 11 mg; females 14-18 yo: 15 mg.

UNAPPROVED ADULT - Adjunct to epoetin to maximize hematologic response: 200 mg elem iron/day PO.

UNAPPROVED PEDS - Adjunct to epoetin to maximize hematologic response: 2-3 mg/kg elem iron/day PO.

FORMS - OTC Generic/Trade: Tab (ferrous gluconate) 240. Generic: Tab 27,300,324,325 mg.

NOTES - Ferrous gluconate is 12% elem iron. For iron deficiency, 4-6 months of therapy generally necessary to replete stores even after hemoglobin has returned to normal. Do not take within 2 h of antacids, tetracyclines, levothyroxine or fluoroquinolones. May cause black stools, constipation or diarrhea.

ferrous sulfate (*Fer-in-Sol*, *Feosol*, ✦*Fer-odan*, *Slow-Fe*) ▶K ♀+ ▶+ $

ADULT - Iron deficiency: 500-1000 mg ferrous sulfate (100-200 mg elem iron) PO divided tid. Liquid: 5-10 mL tid. For iron supplementation RDA see ferrous gluconate.

PEDS - Mild-moderate iron deficiency: 3 mg/kg/day of elem iron PO in 1-2 divided doses; severe iron deficiency: 4-6 mg/kg/day PO in 3 divided doses. For Iron supplementation RDA see ferrous gluconate.

UNAPPROVED ADULT - Adjunct to epoetin to maximize hematologic response: 200 mg elem iron/day PO.

UNAPPROVED PEDS - Adjunct to epoetin to maximize hematologic response: 2-3 mg/kg elem iron/day PO.

FORMS - OTC Generic/Trade (mg ferrous sulfate): Tabs, extended-release 160 mg; tabs 324 & 325 mg; drops 75 mg/0.6 mL. OTC Generic only: Tabs, extended-release 50 mg; elixir 220 mg/5 mL.

NOTES - Iron sulfate is 20% elem iron. For iron deficiency, 4-6 months of therapy generally necessary. Do not take within 2 h of antacids, tetracyclines, levothyroxine or fluoroquinolones. May cause black stools, constipation or diarrhea.

FLUORIDE: Peds daily dose is based on drinking water fluoride (shown in ppm)			
Age *(years)*	<0.3 *ppm*	0.3-0.6 *ppm*	>0.6 *ppm*
0-0.5	none	none	none
0.5-3	0.25mg	none	none
3-6	0.5mg	0.25mg	none
6-16	1 mg	0.5 mg	none

fluoride (*Luride*, *♥Fluor-A-Day*, *Fluotic*) ▶K ♀? ▶? $

ADULT - Prevention of dental cavities: 10 mL of topical rinse swish and spit daily.

PEDS - Prevention of dental caries: Dose based on chart above.

FORMS - Generic only: chew tab 0.5,1 mg, tab 1 mg, drops 0.125 mg, 0.25 and 0.5 mg/dropperful, lozenges 1 mg, solution 0.2 mg/mL, gel 0.1%, 0.5%, 1.23%, rinse (sodium fluoride) 0.05,0.1,0.2%).

NOTES - In communities without fluoridated water, fluoride supplementation should be used until 13-16 years of age. Chronic overdosage of fluorides may result in dental fluorosis (mottling of tooth enamel) and osseous changes. Use rinses and gels after brushing and flossing and before bedtime.

iron dextran (*InFed, DexFerrum*, *♥Dexiron, Infufer*) ▶KL ♀- ▶? $$$$

WARNING - Parenteral iron therapy has re-

sulted in anaphylactic reactions. Potentially fatal hypersensitivity reactions have been reported with iron dextran injection. Facilities for CPR must be available during dosing. Use only when clearly warranted.

ADULT - Iron deficiency: Dose based on patient weight and hemoglobin. Total dose (ml) = 0.0442 x (desired hgb - observed hgb) x weight (kg) + [0.26 x weight (kg)]. For weight, use lesser of lean body weight or actual body weight. Iron replacement for blood loss: replacement iron (mg) = blood loss (ml) x hematocrit. Maximum daily IM dose 100 mg.

PEDS - Not recommended for infants <4 mo. Iron deficiency in >5 kg: Dose based on patient weight and hemoglobin. Dose (ml) = 0.0442 x (desired hgb - observed hgb) x weight (kg) + [0.26 x weight (kg)]. For weight, use lesser of lean body weight or actual body weight. Iron replacement for blood loss: replacement iron (mg) = blood loss (ml) x hematocrit. Maximum daily IM dose: infants <5 kg: 25 mg; children 5-10 kg: 50 mg; children >10 kg 100 mg.

UNAPPROVED ADULT - Adjunct to epoetin to maximize hematologic response. Total dose (325-1500 mg) as a single, slow (6 mg/min) IV infusion has been used.

UNAPPROVED PEDS - Adjunct to epoetin to maximize hematologic response.

NOTES - A 0.5 mL IV test dose (0.25 mL in infants) over ≥30 seconds should be given at least 1 h before therapy. Infuse ≤50 mg/min. For IM administration, use Z-track technique.

iron polysaccharide (*Niferex, Niferex-150, Nu-Iron 150*) ▶K ♀+ ▶+ $$

ADULT - Iron deficiency: 50-200 mg PO divided daily-tid. For iron supplementation RDA see ferrous gluconate.

PEDS - Mild-moderate iron deficiency: 3 mg/kg/day of elem iron PO in 1-2 divided doses. Severe iron deficiency: 4-6 mg/kg/day PO in 3 divided doses. For iron supplementation RDA see ferrous gluconate.

UNAPPROVED ADULT - Adjunct to epoetin to maximize hematologic response: 200 mg elem iron/day PO.

UNAPPROVED PEDS - Adjunct to epoetin to maximize hematologic response: 2-3 mg/kg elem iron/day PO.

FORMS - OTC Trade only: Cap 60 mg (Niferex). OTC Generic/Trade: Cap 150 mg (Niferex-150, Nu-Iron 150), liquid 100 mg/5 mL (Niferex). 1 mg iron polysaccharide = 1 mg elemental iron.

NOTES - For iron deficiency, 4-6 months of

therapy generally necessary. Do not take within 2 h of antacids, tetracyclines, levothyroxine, or fluoroquinolones. May cause black stools, constipation or diarrhea.

iron sucrose (Venofer) ▶KL ♀B ▶? $$$$$

WARNING - Potentially fatal hypersensitivity reactions have been rarely reported with iron sucrose injection. Facilities for CPR must be available during dosing.

ADULT - Iron deficiency in chronic hemodialysis patients: 5 mL (100 mg elem iron) IV over 5 min or diluted in 100 mL NS IV over ≥15 minutes. Iron deficiency in non-dialysis chronic kidney disease patients: 10 mL (200 mg elem iron) IV over 5 minutes or 500 mg diluted in 250 mL NS IV over 4 hours.

PEDS - Not approved in children.

UNAPPROVED ADULT - Iron deficiency: 5 mL (100 mg elem iron) IV over 5 min or diluted in 100 mL NS IV over ≥15 min.

NOTES - Most hemodialysis patients require 1 g of elem iron over 10 consecutive hemodialysis sessions. Non-dialysis patients require 1 g of elemental iron divided and given over 14 days.

magnesium chloride (Slow-Mag) ▶K♀A▶+ $

ADULT - Dietary supplement: 2 tabs PO daily. RDA (elem Mg): Adult males: 400 mg if 19-30 yo, 420 mg if >30 yo. Adult females: 310 mg if 19-30 yo, 320 mg if >30 yo.

PEDS - Not approved in children.

UNAPPROVED ADULT - Hypomagnesemia: 300 mg elem magnesium PO divided qid.

UNAPPROVED PEDS - Hypomagnesemia: 10-20 mg elem magnesium/kg/dose PO qid. For RDA (elem Mg) see magnesium gluconate.

FORMS - OTC Trade: enteric coated tab 64 mg. 64 mg tab Slow-Mag = 64 mg elem Mg.

NOTES - May cause diarrhea. May accumulate in renal insufficiency.

magnesium gluconate (Almora, Magtrate, Maganate, ✦Maglucate) ▶K ♀A ▶+ $

ADULT - Dietary supplement: 500-1000 mg/day PO divided tid. RDA (elem Mg): Adult males: 19-30 yo: 400 mg; >30 yo: 420 mg. Adult females: 19-30 yo: 310 mg; >30 yo: 320 mg.

PEDS - Not approved in children.

UNAPPROVED ADULT - Hypomagnesemia: 300 mg elem magnesium PO divided qid. Unproven efficacy for oral tocolysis following IV magnesium sulfate.

UNAPPROVED PEDS - Hypomagnesemia: 10-20 mg elem magnesium/kg/dose PO qid. RDA (elem Mg): Age 0-6 mos: 30 mg/day; 7-12 mos: 75 mg/day; 1-3 yo: 80 mg; 4-8 yo: 130 mg; 9-

13 yo: 240 mg; 14-18 yo (males): 410 mg; 14-18 yo (females): 360 mg.

FORMS - OTC Generic only: tab 500 mg, liquid 54 mg elem Mg/5 mL.

NOTES - 500 mg tabs contain 27-29 mg elem magnesium. May cause diarrhea. Use caution in renal failure; may accumulate.

magnesium oxide (Mag-200, Mag-Ox 400) ▶K ♀A ▶+ $

ADULT - Dietary supplement: 400-800 mg PO daily. RDA (elem Mg): Adult males: 19-30 yo: 400 mg;>30 yo 420 mg. Adult females: 19-30 yo: 310 mg; >30yo: 320 mg.

PEDS - Not approved in children.

UNAPPROVED ADULT - Hypomagnesemia: 300 mg elem magnesium PO qid. Has also been used as oral tocolysis following IV magnesium sulfate (unproven efficacy) and in the prevention of calcium-oxalate kidney stones.

UNAPPROVED PEDS - Hypomagnesemia: 10-20 mg elem magnesium/kg/dose PO qid. For RDA (elem Mg) see magnesium gluconate.

FORMS - OTC Generic/Trade: cap 140,250, 400,420,500 mg.

NOTES - Approximately 60% elem magnesium. May accumulate in renal insufficiency.

magnesium sulfate ▶K ♀A ▶+ $

ADULT - Hypomagnesemia: mild deficiency: 1g IM q6h x 4 doses; severe deficiency: 2 g IV over 1 h (monitor for hypotension). Hyperalimentation: maintenance requirements not precisely known; adults generally require 8-24 mEq/day. Seizure prevention in pre-eclampsia or eclampsia: 4-6 g IV over 30 min, then 1-2 g IV per hour. 5 g in 250 mL D5W (20 mg/mL), 2 g/h=100 mL/h. 4-5 g of a 50% soln IM q4h prn.

PEDS - Not approved in children.

UNAPPROVED ADULT - Preterm labor: 6 g IV over 20 minutes, then 1-3 g/h titrated to decrease contractions. Has been used as an adjunctive bronchodilator in very severe acute asthma (2 g IV over 10-20 min), and in chronic fatigue syndrome. Torsades de pointes: 1-2 g IV in D5W over 5-60 minutes.

UNAPPROVED PEDS - Hypomagnesemia: 25-50 mg/kg IV/IM q4-6h for 3-4 doses, maximum single dose 2 g. Hyperalimentation: maintenance requirements not precisely known; infants require 2-10 mEq/day. Acute nephritis: 20-40 mg/kg (in 20% solution) IM prn. Adjunctive bronchodilator in very severe acute asthma: 25-100 mg/kg IV over 10-20 min.

NOTES - 1000 mg contains 8 mEq elem magnesium. Do not give faster than 1.5 mL/min (of

10% solution) except in eclampsia or seizures. Use caution in renal insufficiency; may accumulate. Monitor urine output, patellar reflex, respiratory rate and serum magnesium level. Concomitant use with terbutaline may lead to fatal pulmonary edema. IM administration must be diluted to a 20% soln. If needed, may reverse toxicity with calcium gluconate 1 g IV.

phosphorus (Neutra-Phos, K-Phos) ▶K ♀C ▶? $

ADULT - Dietary supplement: 1 cap/packet (Neutra-Phos) PO qid or 1-2 tab (K-Phos) PO qid after meals and at bedtime. Severe hypophosphatemia (<1 mg/dl): 0.08-0.16 mmol/kg IV over 6 h. In TPN, 310-465 mg/day (10-15 mM) IV is usually adequate, although higher amounts may be necessary in hypermetabolic states. RDA for adults is 800 mg.

PEDS - RDA (elem phosphorus): 0-6 mo: 100 mg; 6-12 mo: 275 mg; 1-3 yo: 460 mg; 4-8 yo: 500 mg; 9-18: 1,250 mg. Severe hypophosphatemia (<1 mg/dl): 0.25-0.5 mmol/kg IV over 4-6 h. Infant TPN: 1.5-2 mmol/kg/day in TPN.

FORMS - OTC: Trade only: (Neutra-Phos, Neutra-Phos K) tab/cap/packet 250 mg (8 mmol) phosphorus. Rx: Trade only: (K-Phos) tab 250 mg (8 mmol) phosphorus.

NOTES - Dissolve caps/tabs/powder in 75 mL water prior to ingestion.

potassium (Cena-K, Effer-K, K+8, K+10, Kaochlor, Kaon, Kaon Cl, Kay Ciel, Kaylixir, K+Care, K+Care ET, K-Dur, K-G Elixir, K-Lease, K-Lor, Klor-con, Klorvess, Klorvess Effervescent, Klotrix, K-Lyte, K-Lyte Cl, K-Norm, Kolyum, K-Tab, K-vescent, Micro-K, Micro-K LS, Slow-K, Ten-K, Tri-K) ▶K ♀C ▶? $

ADULT - Hypokalemia: 20-40 mEq/day or more PO/IV. Intermittent infusion: 10-20 mEq/dose IV over 1-2 h prn. Consider monitoring for infusions >10 mEq/hr. Prevention of hypokalemia: 20-40 mEq/day PO daily-bid.

PEDS - Not approved in children.

UNAPPROVED ADULT - Diuretic-induced hypokalemia: 20-60 mEq/day PO.

UNAPPROVED PEDS - Hypokalemia: 2.5 mEq/ kg/day give IV/PO daily-bid. Intermittent infusion: 0.5-1 mEq/kg/dose IV at 0.3-0.5 mEq/kg/ h prn. Infusions faster than 0.5 mEq/kg/h require continuous monitoring.

FORMS - Injectable, many different products in a variety of salt forms (i.e. chloride, bicarbonate, citrate, acetate, gluconate), available in tabs, caps, liquids, effervescent tabs, packets.

Potassium gluconate is available OTC.

NOTES - Use KCl for hypokalemia associated with alkalosis; use K+ bicarbonate, citrate, acetate, or gluconate when acidosis.

POTASSIUM, oral forms

Effervescent Tablets: 25 mEq (Effer-K, K-Lyte, K-Lyte/Cl, Klor-Con/EF), 50 mEq (K-Lyte DS, K-Lyte/Cl 50)
Liquids: 20 mEq/15 mL (Kay Ciel, Kaon Elixir), 30 mEq/15 mL (Rum-K), 40 mEq/15 mL (generic)
Powders: 20 mEq/pack (Kay Ciel, K-Lor, Klor-Con), 25 mEq/pack (Klor-Con 25)
Tabs/Caps: 8 mEq (Klor-Con 8, Micro-K), 10 mEq (Kaon-Cl 10, Klor-Con 10, Klotrix, K-Tab, K-Dur 10, Micro-K 10), 20 mEq (Klor-Con M20, K-Dur 20)

zinc acetate (Galzin) ▶Min absorption ♀A ▶- $

ADULT - RDA (elemental Zn): Adult males: 11 mg daily. Adult females: 8-12 mg daily. Zinc deficiency: 25-50 mg (elemental) daily. Wilson's disease, previously treated with chelating agent: 25-50 mg (elemental) tid.

PEDS - RDA (elem Zn): Age 7 mos-3 yo: 3 mg/day; 4-8 yo: 5 mg; 9-13 yo: 8 mg; 14-18 yo (males): 8 mg; 14-18 yo (females): 9-14 mg. Zinc deficiency: 0.5-1 mg elemental zinc mg/kg/day divided bid-tid. Wilson's disease (≥10 yo): 25-50 mg (elemental) tid.

FORMS - Trade: cap 25, 50 mg elemental zinc.

NOTES - Poorly absorbed; take 1 hour before or 2-3 hours after meals. Decreases absorption of tetracycline and fluoroquinolones.

zinc sulfate (Orazinc, Zincate) ▶Minimal absorption ♀A ▶- $

ADULT - RDA (elemental Zn): Adult males: 11 mg daily. Adult females: 8-12 mg daily. Zinc deficiency: 25-50 mg (elemental) daily.

PEDS - RDA (elemental Zn): Age 7 mos-3 yo: 3 mg/day; 4-8 yo: 5 mg; 9-13 yo: 8 mg; 14-18 yo (males): 8 mg; 14-18 yo (females): 9-14 mg. Zinc deficiency: 0.5-1 mg elemental zinc mg/ kg/day divided bid-tid.

UNAPPROVED ADULT - Wound healing in zinc deficiency: 200 mg TID.

FORMS - OTC Generic/Trade: tab 66, 110, 200 mg; Rx: cap 220 mg.

NOTES - Zinc sulfate is 23% elemental Zn. Decreases absorption of tetracycline and fluoroquinolones. Poorly absorbed; increased absorption on empty stomach; however administration with food decreases GI upset.

PEDIATRIC REHYDRATION SOLUTIONS (ions in mEq/l)									
Brand	_Glucose_	_Cal/l_	_Na_	_K_	_Cl_	_Citrate_	_Phos_	_Ca_	_Mg_
CeraLyte 50*	0 g/l	160	50	20	40	30	0	0	0
CeraLyte 70*	0 g/l	160	70	20	60	30	0	0	0
CeraLyte 90*	0 g/l	160	90	20	80	30	0	0	0
Infalyte	30 g/l	140	50	25	45	34	0	0	0
Lytren†	20 g/l	80	50	25	45	30	0	0	0
Naturalyte	25 g/l	100	45	20	35	48	0	0	0
Pedialyte‡	25 g/l	100	45	20	35	30	0	0	0
Rehydralyte	25 g/l	100	75	20	65	30	0	0	0
Resol	20 g/l	80	50	20	50	34	5	4	4

*Available in premeasured powder packet. †Canada. ‡and Pedialyte Freezer Pops

ENDOCRINE & METABOLIC: Nutritionals

"banana bag" ▶KL ♀+ ▶+ $

UNAPPROVED ADULT - Alcoholic malnutrition (one formula): Add thiamine 100 mg + folic acid 1 mg + IV multivitamins to 1 liter NS and infuse over 4h. Magnesium sulfate 2g may be added. "Banana bag" is jargon and not a valid drug order; also known as "rally pack"; specify individual components.

fat emulsion (_Intralipid, Liposyn_) ▶L ♀C ▶? $$$$$

WARNING - Deaths have occurred in preterm infants after infusion of IV fat emulsions. Autopsy results showed intravascular fat accumulation in the lungs. Strict adherence to total daily dose and administration rate is mandatory. Premature and small for gestational age infants have poor clearance of IV fat emulsion. Monitor infant's ability to eliminate fat (i.e. triglycerides or plasma free fatty acid levels).

ADULT - Calorie and essential fatty acids source: As part of TPN, fat emulsion should be no more than 60% of total calories; when correcting essential fatty acid deficiency, 8-10% of caloric intake should be supplied by lipids. Initial infusion rate 1 mL/min IV (10% fat emulsion) or 0.5 mL/min (20% fat emulsion) IV for first 15-30 min. If tolerated increase rate. If using 10% fat emulsion infuse 500 mL first day and increase the next day. Maximum daily dose 2.5 g/kg. If using 20% fat emulsion, infuse up to 250 mL (Liposyn II) or up to 500 mL (Intralipid) first day and increase the next day. Maximum daily dose 2.5 g/kg.

PEDS - Calorie and essential fatty acids source: As part of TPN, fat emulsion should be no more than 60% of total calories; when correcting essential fatty acid deficiency, 8-10% of caloric intake should be supplied by lipids. Initial infusion rate 0.1 mL/min IV (10% fat emulsion) or 0.05 mL/min (20% fat emulsion) for first 10-15 min. If tolerated increase rate up to 1 mL/kg/hr (10% fat emulsion) or 0.5 mL/kg/hr (20% fat emulsion). Max daily dose 3g/kg. For premature infants, start at 0.5 g/kg/day and increase based on infant's ability to eliminate fat.

NOTES - Do not use in patients with severe egg allergy; contains egg yolk phospholipids. Use caution in severe liver disease, pulmonary disease, anemia, blood coagulation disorders, when there is the danger of fat embolism or in jaundiced or premature infants. Monitor CBC, blood coagulation, LFTs, plasma lipid profile and platelet count.

formulas - infant (_Enfamil, Similac, Isomil, Nursoy, Prosobee, Soyalac, Alsoy, Nutramigen Lipil_) ▶L ♀+ ▶+ $

ADULT - Not used in adults.

PEDS - Infant meals.

FORMS - OTC: Milk-based (Enfamil, Similac, SMA) or soy-based (Isomil, Nursoy, ProSobee, Soyalac, Alsoy).

levocarnitine (_Carnitor_) ▶KL ♀B ▶? $$$$

ADULT - Prevention of levocarnitine deficiency in dialysis patients: 10-20 mg/kg IV at each dialysis session. Titrate dose based on serum concentration.

PEDS - Prevention of deficiency in dialysis patients: 10-20 mg/kg IV at each dialysis session. Titrate dose based on serum concentration.

FORMS - Generic/Trade: Tabs 330 mg, Oral solution 1 g /10 mL

NOTES - Adverse neurophysiologic effects may occur with long term, high doses of oral levocarnitine in patients with renal dysfunction. Only the IV formulation is indicated in patients receiving hemodialysis.

omega-3 fatty acid (fish oil, Lovaza, Oma-cor, Promega, Cardio-Omega 3, Sea-O-mega, Marine Lipid Concentrate, MAX EPA, SuperEPA 1200) ▶L ♀C ▶? $$

ADULT - Lovaza, adjunct to diet to reduce high triglycerides (≥500 mg/dL): 4 capsules PO daily or divided bid.

PEDS - Not approved in children.

UNAPPROVED ADULT - Hypertriglyceridemia: 2-4 g EPA+DHA content daily under physician's care. Secondary prevention of CHD: 1-2 g EPA+DHA content daily. Adjunctive treatment in rheumatoid arthritis: 20 g/day PO. Psoriasis: 10-15 g/day PO. Prevention of early restenosis after coronary angioplasty in combination with dipyridamole & aspirin: 18 g/day.

FORMS - Trade: Lovaza 1 g cap (total 840 mg EPA+DHA). Generic/Trade: cap, shown as EPA+DHA mg content, 240 (Promega Pearls),

300 (Cardi-Omega 3, Max EPA), 320 (Sea-Omega), 400 (Promega), 500 (Sea-Omega), 600 (Marine Lipid Concentrate, SuperEPA 1200), 875 mg (SuperEPA 2000).

NOTES - Lovaza is only FDA approved fish oil, previously known as Omacor. Dose dependent GI upset, may increase LDL-cholesterol, excessive bleeding, hyperglycemia. Marine Lipid Concentrate, Super EPA 1200 mg cap contains EPA 360 mg + DHA 240 mg, daily dose = 5-8 Caps. Treatment doses lowers triglycerides by 30-50%. Caps may contain omega-6 fatty acids and/or vitamin E; content varies with product. May potentiate warfarin. Monitor sugar in Type 2 diabetes. Caution in seafood allergy.

"rally pack" ▶KL ♀C ▶- $

UNAPPROVED ADULT - Alcoholic malnutrition: See prior page entry for "banana bag". "Rally pack" is jargon and not a valid drug order.

ENDOCRINE & METABOLIC: Phosphate Binders

lanthanum carbonate (Fosrenol) ▶Not absorbed ♀C ▶? $$$$$

ADULT - Hyperphosphatemia in end stage renal disease: Start 750-1500 mg/day PO in divided doses with meals. Titrate dose q2-3 weeks in increments of 750 mg/day until acceptable serum phosphate reached. Most will require 1500-3000 mg/day to reduce phosphate <6.0 mg/dL. Chew tabs completely before swallowing.

PEDS - Not approved in children.

FORMS - Trade only: chewable tabs 250, 500, 750, 1000 mg.

NOTES - Caution if acute peptic ulcer, ulcerative colitis, Crohn's disease or bowel obstruction. Avoid medications known to interact with

antacids within 2 hours. May be radio-opaque enough to appear on abdominal x-ray.

sevelamer (Renagel) ▶Not absorbed ♀C ▶? $$$$$

ADULT - Hyperphosphatemia: 800-1600 mg PO tid with meals, adjust according to serum phosphorus concentration.

PEDS - Not approved in children.

FORMS - Trade only: Tabs 400, 800 mg.

NOTES - Titrate by one tab/cap per meal at 2 week intervals to keep phosphorus ≤6 mg/dl. Anti-arrhythmic & anti-seizure medications may have decreased absorption if not taken 1h before or 3h after sevelamer. Caution in GI motility disorders, including severe constipation.

ENDOCRINE & METABOLIC: Thyroid Agents

levothyroxine (L-Thyroxine, Levolet, Levo-T, Levothroid, Levoxyl, Novothyrox, Synthroid, Thyro-Tabs, Tirosint, Uni-throid, T4, ✚Eltroxin, Euthyrox) ▶L ♀A ▶+ $

WARNING - Do not use for obesity/weight loss.

ADULT - Hypothyroidism: Start 100-200 mcg PO daily (healthy adults) or 12.5-50 mcg PO daily (elderly and CV disease), increase by 12.5-25 mcg/day at 3-8 week intervals. Usual dose 100-200 mcg PO daily, max 300 mcg/day.

PEDS - Hypothyroidism 0-6 months: 8-10 mcg/kg/day PO; 6-12 months: 6-8 mcg/kg/day PO;

1-5 yo: 5-6 mcg/kg/day PO; 6-12 yo: 4-5 mcg/kg/day PO; >12 yo: 2-3 mcg/kg/day PO, max 300 mcg/day.

UNAPPROVED ADULT - Hypothyroidism: 1.6 mcg/kg/day PO; start with lower doses (25 mcg PO daily) in elderly and cardiac disease.

FORMS - Generic/Trade: Tabs 25, 50, 75, 88, 100, 112, 125, 137, 150, 175, 200, 300 mcg. Trade only: Caps: 25, 50, 75, 100, 125, 150 mcg in 7 day blister packs.

NOTES - May crush tabs for infants and children. May give IV or IM at ½ oral dose in adults and ½ - ¾ oral dose in children; then adjust based on tolerance and therapeutic response. Generics are not necessarily bioequivalent to brand products; reevaluate thyroid function when switching.

liothyronine (*T3, Cytomel, Triostat*) ▶L ♀A ▶? $$

WARNING - Do not use for obesity/weight loss.

ADULT - Mild hypothyroidism: 25 mcg PO daily, increase by 12.5-25 mcg/day at 1-2 week intervals to desired response. Usual maintenance dose 25-75 mcg PO daily. Goiter: 5 mcg PO daily, increase by 5-10 mcg/day at 1-2 week intervals. Usual maintenance dose 75 mcg PO daily. Myxedema: 5 mcg PO daily, increase by 5-10 mcg/day at 1-2 week intervals. Usual maintenance dose 50-100 mcg/day.

PEDS - Congenital hypothyroidism: 5 mcg PO daily, increase by 5 mcg/day at 3-4 day intervals to desired response.

FORMS - Trade only: Tabs 5, 25, 50 mcg.

NOTES - Start therapy at 5 mcg/d in children & elderly and increase by 5 mcg increments only. Rapidly absorbed from the GI tract. Monitor T3 and TSH. Elderly may need lower doses due to potential decreased renal function

methimazole (*Tapazole*) ▶L ♀D ▶+ $$$

ADULT - Mild hyperthyroidism: 5 mg PO tid. Moderate hyperthyroidism: 10 mg PO tid. Severe hyperthyroidism: 20 mg PO tid (q8h intervals). Maintenance dose = 5-30 mg/day.

PEDS - Hyperthyroidism: 0.4 mg/kg/day PO divided q8h. Maintenance dose = ½ initial dose, max 30 mg/day.

UNAPPROVED ADULT - Start 10-30 mg PO daily, then adjust.

FORMS - Generic/Trade: Tabs 5, 10. Generic only: Tabs 15, 20 mg.

NOTES - Monitor CBC for evidence of marrow suppression if fever, sore throat, or other signs of infection. Propylthiouracil preferred over methimazole in pregnancy.

potassium iodide (*Iosat, Thyro-Block, Thyrosafe, Thyroshield*) ▶L ♀D ▶- $

WARNING - Do not use for obesity.

ADULT - Thyroidectomy preparation: 50-250 mg PO tid x 10-14 days prior to surgery. Thyroid storm: 1 mL (Lugol's) PO tid at least 1h after initial propylthiouracil or methimazole dose. Thyroid blocking in radiation emergency: 130 mg PO daily x 10 days or as directed by state health officials.

PEDS - Thyroid blocking in radiation emergency age 3-18 years: 65 mg (one-half of a 130 mg tab) PO daily, or 130 mg PO daily in adolescents >70 kg. 1 mo to 3 years: 32 mg (one-quarter of a 130 mg tab) PO daily. Birth to 1 mo: 16 mg (one-eighth of a 130 mg tab) PO daily. Duration is until risk of exposure to radioiodines no longer exists.

FORMS - Trade only OTC: Tabs 130 mg (Iosat, Thyroblock). Generic OTC tab 65 mg (Thyrosafe). Generic only OTC Soln: 65 mg/mL (Thyroshield).

propylthiouracil (*PTU, ♣Propyl Thyracil*) ▶L ♀D (but preferred over methimazole) ▶+ $

ADULT - Hyperthyroidism: 100-150 mg PO tid. Severe hyperthyroidism and/or large goiters: 200-400 mg PO tid. Continue initial dose for ~2 months. Adjust to desired response. Usual maintenance dose 100-150 mg/ day. Thyroid storm: 200 mg PO q4-6h x 1 day, decrease dose gradually to usual maintenance dose.

PEDS – Hyperthyroidism, age 6-10 yo: 50 mg PO daily-tid. Children ≥10 yo: 50-100 mg PO tid. Continue initial dose for 2 months, then maintenance dose is 1/3 to 2/3 initial dose.

UNAPPROVED PEDS - Hyperthyroidism in neonates: 5-10 mg/kg/day PO divided q8h. Children: 5-7 mg/kg/day PO divided q8h.

FORMS - Generic only: Tabs 50 mg.

NOTES - Monitor CBC for marrow suppression if fever, sore throat, or other signs of infection. Vasculitic syndrome with positive anti-neutrophilic cytoplasmic antibodies (ANCA) reported requiring discontinuation. Propylthiouracil preferred over methimazole in pregnancy.

sodium iodide I-131 (*Iodotope, Sodium Iodide I-131 Therapeutic*) ▶K ♀X ▶- $$$$$

ADULT - Specialized dosing for hyperthyroidism and thyroid carcinoma.

PEDS - Not approved in children.

FORMS - Generic/Trade: Capsules & oral soln: radioactivity range varies at calibration.

NOTES - Avoid if preexisting vomiting or diarrhea. Discontinue antithyroid therapy ≥3 days before starting. Low serum chloride or nephrosis may increase uptake; renal insufficiency may decrease excretion and thus increase radiation exposure. Ensure adequate hydration before/after giving. Follow low iodine diet for 1-2 weeks before treatment. Women should have negative pregnancy test prior to treatment and advise not to conceive for ≥6 months.

thyroid - desiccated (*Thyroid USP, Armour Thyroid*) ▶L ♀A ▶? $

WARNING - Do not use for obesity.

ADULT - Obsolete; use thyroxine instead. Hypothyroidism: Start 30 mg PO daily, increase by

15 mg/day at 2-3 week intervals to a maximum dose of 180 mg/day.

PEDS - Congenital hypothyroidism: 15 mg PO daily. Increase at 2 week intervals.

FORMS - Generic/Trade: Tabs 15, 30, 60, 90, 120, 180, 300 mg. Trade only: Tabs 240 mg.

NOTES - 60 mg thyroid desiccated is roughly equivalent to 100 mcg levothyroxine. Combination of levothyroxine (T4) and liothyronine (T3); content varies (range 2:1 to 5:1).

Thyrolar (levothyroxine + liothyronine) ▶L

♀A ▶? $

WARNING - Do not use for obesity.

ADULT - Hypothyroidism: 1 PO daily, starting with small doses initially (¼ - ½ strength), then increase at 2 week intervals.

PEDS - Not approved in children.

FORMS - Trade only: Tabs T4/T3 12.5/3.1 (¼ strength), 50/12.5 (#1), 100/25 (#2), 150/37.5 (#3) mcg.

NOTES - Combination of levothyroxine (T4) and liothyronine (T3).

ENDOCRINE & METABOLIC: Vitamins

ascorbic acid (vitamin C, ✦Redoxon) ▶K ♀C ▶? $

ADULT – Scurvy prevention: 70-150 mg/day PO. Scurvy treatment: 300-1000 mg/day PO. RDA females: 75 mg/day; males: 90 mg/day. Smokers: add 35 mg/day more.

PEDS - Prevention of scurvy: Infants: 30 mg/day PO. Treatment of scurvy: Infants: 100-300 mg/day PO. Adequate daily intake for infants 0-6 mo: 40 mg; 7-12 mo: 50 mg. RDA for children: 1-3 yo: 15 mg; 4-8 yo: 25 mg; 9-13 yo: 45 mg; 14-18 yo: 75 mg (males), 65 mg (females).

UNAPPROVED ADULT - Urinary acidification with methenamine: >2 g/day PO. Idiopathic methemoglobinemia: 150 mg/day or more PO. Wound healing: 300-500 mg/day or more PO for 7-10 days. Severe burns: 1-2 g/day PO.

FORMS - OTC: Generic only: Tabs 25,50,100, 250,500,1000 mg, chew tab 100,250,500 mg, time-released tab 500 mg, 1000,1500 mg, time-released cap 500 mg, lozenge 60 mg, liquid 35 mg/0.6 mL, oral solution 100 mg/mL, syrup 500 mg/5 mL.

NOTES - Use IV/IM/SC ascorbic acid for acute deficiency or when oral absorption is uncertain. Avoid excessive doses in diabetics, patients prone to renal calculi, those undergoing stool occult blood tests (may cause false-negative), those on sodium restricted diets and those taking anticoagulants (may decrease INR). Doses in adults >2 g/day may cause osmotic diarrhea.

calcitriol (Rocaltrol, Calcijex) ▶L ♀C ▶? $$

ADULT - Hypocalcemia in chronic renal dialysis: Oral: 0.25 mcg PO daily, increase by 0.25 mcg q 4-8 weeks until normocalcemia achieved. Most hemodialysis patients require 0.5-1 mcg/day PO. Hypocalcemia and/or secondary hyperparathyroidism in chronic renal dialysis IV: 1-2 mcg, 3 times a week; increase dose by 0.5-

1 mcg every 2-4 weeks. If PTH decreased <30% then increase dose; if PTH decreased 30-60% then maintain current dose; if PTH decreased >60% then decrease dose; if PTH 1.5-3 times the upper normal limit then maintain current dose. Hypoparathyroidism: 0.25 mcg PO qam; increase dose q 2-4 weeks if inadequate response. Most adults respond to 0.5-2 mcg/day PO. Secondary hyperparathyroidism in pre-dialysis patients: 0.25 mcg PO qam; may increase dose to 0.5 mcg qam.

PEDS - Hypoparathyroidism 1-5 yo: 0.25-0.75 mcg PO qam. If ≥6 yo then 0.25 mcg PO qam; increase dose in 2-4 weeks; usually respond to 0.5-2 mcg/day PO. Secondary hyperparathyroidism in pre-dialysis patients ≥ 3 yo: 0.25 mcg qam; may increase dose to 0.5 mcg qam. If <3 yo: 0.01-0.015 mcg/kg/day PO.

UNAPPROVED ADULT - Psoriasis vulgaris: 0.5 mcg/day PO or 0.5 mcg/g petrolatum topically daily.

FORMS - Generic/Trade: Cap 0.25, 0.5 mcg. Oral soln 1 mcg/mL. Injection 1,2 mcg/mL.

NOTES - Calcitriol is the activated form of vitamin D. During titration period, monitor serum calcium at least twice weekly. Successful therapy requires an adequate daily calcium intake. Topical preparation must be compounded (not commercially available).

Cerefolin (L-methylfolate + riboflavin + pyridoxine + cyanocobalamin) ▶KL ♀C ▶+ $$

ADULT - Nutritional supplement for hyperhomocysteinemia: 1-2 tab PO daily.

PEDS - Not approved in children.

FORMS - Trade only: Each tab contains 5.635 mg of L-methylfolate + 5 mg riboflavin + 50 mg pyridoxine + 1 mg cyanocobalamin.

NOTES - Folic acid doses >0.1 mg may obscure pernicious anemia; preventable with the concurrent cyanocobalamin in product.

Cerefolin with NAC (L-methylfolate + methylcobalamin + acetylcysteine) ▶KL ♀B ▶- $$

ADULT - Nutritional supplement for neurovascular oxidative stress or hyperhomocysteinemia: 1 cap PO daily.

PEDS - Not approved in children.

FORMS - Trade only: L-methylfolate 5.6 mg + methylcobalamin 2 mg + N-acetylcysteine 600 mg cap.

NOTES - Folic acid doses >0.1 mg may obscure pernicious anemia; preventable with the concurrent cyanocobalamin in product.

cyanocobalamin (*vitamin B12, CaloMist, Nascobal*) ▶K ♀C ▶+ $

ADULT - See also "unapproved adult" dosing. Maintenance of nutritional deficiency following IM correction: 500 mcg intranasal weekly (Nascobal: 1 spray one nostril once weekly) or 50-100 mcg intranasal daily (CaloMist: 1-2 sprays each nostril daily). Pernicious anemia: 100 mcg IM/SC daily, for 6-7 days, then qod for 7 doses, then q3-4 days for 2-3 weeks, then q month. Other patients with vitamin B12 deficiency: 30 mcg IM daily for 5-10 days, then 100-200 mcg IM q month. RDA for adults is 2.4 mcg.

PEDS - Nutritional deficiency: 100 mcg/24 hr deep IM/SC x 10-15 days then at least 60 mcg/month IM/deep SC. Pernicious anemia: 30-50 mcg/24 hr for ≥14 days to total dose of 1000-5000 mcg deep IM/SC then 100 mcg/month deep IM/SC. Adequate daily intake for infants: 0-6 mo: 0.4 mcg; 7-11 mo: 0.5 mcg. RDA for children: 1-3 yo: 0.9 mcg; 4-8 yo: 1.2 mcg; 9-13 yo: 1.8 mcg; 14-18 yo: 2.4 mcg.

UNAPPROVED ADULT - Pernicious anemia & nutritional deficiency states: 1000-2000 mcg PO daily for 1-2 weeks, then 1000 mcg PO daily. Prevention and treatment of cyanide toxicity associated with nitroprusside.

UNAPPROVED PEDS - Prevention/treatment of nitroprusside-associated cyanide toxicity.

FORMS - OTC Generic only: tab 100, 500, 1000, 5000 mcg; lozenges 100, 250, 500 mcg. Rx Trade: nasal spray 500 mcg/spray (Nascobal 2.3 mL), 25 mcg/spray (CaloMist, 18mL).

NOTES - Prime nasal pump before use per package insert directions. Although official dose for deficiency states is 100-200 mcg IM q month, some give 1000 mcg IM periodically. Oral supplementation is safe & effective for B12 deficiency even when intrinsic factor is not present. Monitor B12, folate, iron and CBC.

Diatx (folic acid + niacinamide + cobalamin + pantothenic acid + pyridoxine + d-biotin + thiamine + ascorbic acid + riboflavin) ▶LK ♀? ▶? $$$

ADULT - Nutritional supplement for renal failure, dialysis, hyperhomocysteinemia or inadequate dietary vitamin intake: 1 tab PO daily.

PEDS - Not approved in children.

FORMS - Trade only: Each tab contains folic acid 5 mg + niacinamide 20 mg + cobalamin 1 mg + pantothenic acid 10 mg + pyridoxine 50 mg + d-biotin 300 mcg + thiamine 1.5 mg + vitamin C 60 mg + riboflavin 1.5 mg. Diatx Fe: adds 100 mg ferrous fumarate per tab. Diatx Zn adds 25 mg of zinc oxide per tab.

NOTES - Cobalamin appears to prevent masking of pernicious anemia by folic acid.

dihydrotachysterol (*DHT*) ▶L ♀C ▶? $$

ADULT - Treatment of acute, chronic, and latent forms of postoperative tetany, idiopathic tetany and hypoparathyroidism: Initial dose 0.75-2.5 mg PO daily for several days, then 0.2-1.75 mg PO daily to maintain normocalcemia.

PEDS - Safe dosing exceeding the RDA and in children undergoing dialysis unclear.

UNAPPROVED PEDS - Hypoparathyroidism: Neonates: 0.05-0.1 mg PO daily; Infants and young children: 1-5 mg PO daily × 4 days, then 0.5-1.5 mg PO daily; Older children: 0.75-2.5 mg PO daily × 4 days, then 0.2-1.5 mg PO daily. Nutritional rickets: 0.5 mg PO for 1 dose or 13-50 mcg/day PO until healing occurs. Renal osteodystrophy: 0.125-0.5 mg PO daily.

FORMS - Generic only: tab 0.125,0.2, 0.4 mg, cap 0.125 mg, oral solution 0.2 mg/mL.

NOTES - Monitor serum calcium. Dose may be supplemented with calcium therapy.

doxercalciferol (*Hectorol*) ▶L ♀B ▶? $$$$

ADULT - Secondary hyperparathyroidism on dialysis: Oral: If PTH >400 pg/ml then start 10 mcg PO 3x/ week; if PTH >300 pg/ml then increase by 2.5 mcg/dose q8 weeks as necessary; if PTH 150-300 pg/ml then maintain current dose; if PTH <100 pg/ml then stop x 1 week, then resume at a dose at least 2.5 mcg lower. Max 60 mcg/week. IV: If PTH >400 pg/ml then 4 mcg IV 3x/ week; if PTH decreased by <50% & >300 pg/ml then increase by 1-2 mcg q8 weeks as necessary; if PTH decreased by >50% & >300 pg/ml then maintain current dose; if PTH 150-300 pg/ml then maintain current dose; if PTH <100 pg/ml then stop x1 week, then resume at a dose that is at least 1 mcg lower. Max 18 mcg/week. Secondary hyperparathyroidism not on dialysis: If PTH >70 pg/ml (Stage 3) or >110 pg/ml (Stage 4) then start 1 mcg PO daily; if PTH >70 pg/ml (Stage 3) or >110 pg/ml (Stage 4) then increase by 0.5 mcg/dose q2 weeks; if PTH 35-70 pg/ml (Stage 3) or 70-110 pg/ml (Stage 4) then maintain current dose; if <35 pg/ml (Stage 3) or <70 pg/ml (Stage 4) then stop x1 week, then resume at a dose that is at least 0.5mcg lower. Max 3.5 mcg/day.

PEDS - Not approved in children.

FORMS - Trade only: Caps 0.5, 2.5 mcg.

NOTES - Monitor PTH, serum calcium and phosphorus weekly during dose titration; may need to monitor patients with hepatic insufficiency more closely.

Folgard (folic acid + cyanocobalamin + pyridoxine) ▶K ♀? ▶? $

ADULT - Nutritional supplement: 1 tab PO daily.

PEDS - Not approved in children.

FORMS - Trade: folic acid 0.8 mg + cyanocobalamin 0.115 mg + pyridoxine 10 mg tab.

NOTES - Folic acid doses >0.1 mg may obscure pernicious anemia, preventable with the concurrent cyanocobalamin.

folic acid (folate, Folvite) ▶K ♀A ▶+ $

ADULT - Megaloblastic anemia: 1 mg PO/IM/IV/ SC daily. When symptoms subside & CBC normalizes, give maintenance dose of 0.4 mg PO daily and 0.8 mg PO daily in pregnant and lactating females. RDA for adults 0.4 mg, 0.6 mg for pregnant females, and 0.5 mg for lactating women. Max recommended daily dose 1 mg.

PEDS - Megaloblastic anemia: Infants: 0.05 mg PO daily, maintenance of 0.04 mg PO daily; Children: 0.5-1 mg PO daily, maintenance of 0.4 mg PO daily. Adequate daily intake for infants: 0-6 mo: 65 mcg; 7-12 mo: 80 mcg. RDA for children: 1-3 yo: 150 mcg; 4-8 yo: 200 mcg; 9-13 yo: 300 mcg, 14-18 yo: 400 mcg.

UNAPPROVED ADULT - Hyperhomocysteinemia: 0.5-1 mg PO daily.

FORMS - OTC Generic only: Tab 0.4,0.8 mg. Rx Generic only.

NOTES - Folic acid doses >0.1 mg/day may obscure pernicious anemia. Prior to conception all women should receive 0.4 mg/day to reduce the risk of neural tube defects in infants. Consider high dose (up to 4 mg) in women with prior history of infant with neural tube defect. Use oral route except in cases of severe intestinal absorption.

Foltx (folic acid + cyanocobalamin + pyridoxine) ▶K ♀A ▶+ $

ADULT - Nutritional supplement for end stage renal failure, dialysis, hyperhomocysteinemia, homocystinuria, nutrient malabsorption or inadequate dietary intake: 1 tab PO daily.

PEDS - Not approved in children.

FORMS - Trade only: folic acid 2.5 mg/ cyanocobalamin 2 mg/ pyridoxine 25 mg tab.

NOTES - Folic acid doses >0.1 mg may obscure pernicious anemia, preventable with the concurrent cyanocobalamin.

Metanx (L-methylfolate + pyridoxal phosphate + methylcobalamin) ▶K ♀C ▶? $$$

ADULT - Nutritional supplement for endothelial dysfunction or hyperhomocysteinemia: 1-2 tab PO daily.

PEDS - Not approved in children.

FORMS - Trade only: Each tab contains 2.8 mg L-methylfolate + 25 mg pyridoxal phosphate + 2 mg methylcobalamin.

NOTES - Folic acid doses >0.1 mg may obscure pernicious anemia; preventable with the concurrent cyanocobalamin in product.

multivitamins (MVI) ▶LK ♀+ ▶+ $

ADULT, PEDS - Dietary supplement: Dose varies by product.

FORMS - OTC & Rx: Many different brands and forms available with and without iron (tab, cap, chew tab, drops, liquid).

NOTES - Do not take within 2 h of antacids, tetracyclines, levothyroxine or fluoroquinolones.

Nephrocap (ascorbic acid + folic acid + niacin + thiamine + riboflavin + pyridoxine + pantothenic acid + biotin + cyanocobalamin) ▶K ♀? ▶? $

ADULT - Nutritional supplement for chronic renal failure, uremia, impaired metabolic functions of the kidney & to maintain levels when the dietary intake of vitamins is inadequate or excretion & loss are excessive: 1 cap PO daily. If on dialysis, take after treatment.

PEDS - Not approved in children.

FORMS - Generic/Trade: vitamin C 100 mg/folic acid 1 mg/ niacin 20 mg/ thiamine 1.5 mg/ riboflavin 1.7 mg/ pyridoxine 10 mg/ pantothenic acid 5 mg/ biotin 150 mcg/ cyanocobalamin 6 mcg

NOTES - Folic acid doses >0.1 mg/day may obscure pernicious anemia (preventable with the concurrent cyanocobalamin).

Nephrovite (ascorbic acid + folic acid + niacin + thiamine + riboflavin + pyridoxine + pantothenic acid + biotin + cyanocobalamin) ▶K ♀? ▶? $

ADULT - Nutritional supplement for chronic renal failure, dialysis, hyperhomocysteinemia or inadequate dietary vitamin intake: 1 tab PO daily. If on dialysis, take after treatment.

PEDS - Not approved in children.

FORMS - Generic/Trade: vitamin C 60 mg/folic acid 1 mg/ niacin 20 mg/ thiamine 1.5 mg/ riboflavin 1.7 mg/ pyridoxine 10 mg/ pantothenic acid 10 mg/ biotin 300 mcg/ cyanocobalamin 6 mcg

NOTES - Folic acid doses >0.1 mg/day may obscure pernicious anemia (preventable with the concurrent cyanocobalamin).

niacin (vitamin B3, nicotinic acid, Niacor, Nicolar, Slo-Niacin, Niaspan) ▶K ♀C ▶? $

ADULT - Niacin deficiency: 100 mg PO daily. Pellagra: up to 500 mg PO daily. RDA is 16 mg for males and 14 mg for females. Hyperlipidemia: Start 50-100 mg PO bid-tid with meals, increase slowly, usual maintenance range 1.5-3 g/day, max 6 g/day. Extended-release (Niaspan): Start 500 mg qhs with a low-fat snack for 4 weeks, increase as needed every 4 weeks to max 2000 mg.

PEDS - Safety and efficacy not established for doses which exceed nutritional requirements. Adequate daily intake for children: 0-6 mo: 2 mg; 7-12 mo: 3 mg. RDA for children: 1-3 yo: 6 mg; 4-8 yo: 8 mg; 9-13 yo: 12 mg; 14-18 yo: 16 mg (males) and 14 mg (females).

FORMS - OTC: Generic only: tab 50,100,250, 500 mg, timed-release cap 125,250,400 mg, timed-release tab 250,500 mg, liquid 50 mg/5 mL. Trade only: 250,500,750 mg (Slo-Niacin). Rx: Trade only: tab 500 mg (Niacor), timed-release cap 500 mg, timed-release tab 500,750,1000 mg (Niaspan, $$$$).

NOTES - Start with low doses and increase slowly to minimize flushing (usually <2h); 325 mg aspirin 30-60 min prior to niacin ingestion will minimize flushing. Caution in diabetes, gout, peptic ulcer, liver, or gallbladder disease. Extended-release formulations not listed here may have greater hepatotoxicity.

paricalcitol (Zemplar) ▶L ♀C ▶? $$$$$

ADULT - Prevention/treatment of secondary hyperparathyroidism with renal insufficiency: If PTH ≤500 pg/mL then start 1 mcg PO daily or 2 mcg PO 3 times/wk. If PTH >500 pg/mL then start 2 mcg PO daily or 4 mcg PO 3 times/wk. Can increase PO dose by 1 mcg daily or 2 mcg 3/week based on PTH in 2-4 week intervals. Prevention/treatment of secondary hyperparathyroidism with renal failure (CrCl <15 mL/min): Initially 0.04-0.1 mcg/kg (2.8-7 mcg) IV 3 times/

week during dialysis. Can increase IV dose 2-4 mcg based on PTH in 2-4 week intervals. PO/IV: If PTH level decreased <30% then increase dose; if PTH level decreased 30-60% then maintain current dose; if PTH level decreased >60% then decrease dose.

PEDS - Prevention/treatment of secondary hyperparathyroidism with renal failure (CrCl<15 mL/min): 0.04-0.1 mcg/kg (2.8-7 mcg) IV 3 times/wk at dialysis; increase dose by 2-4 mcg or 0.04 mcg/kg q 2-4 weeks until desired PTH achieved. Max dose 0.24 mcg/kg (16.8 mcg).

FORMS - Trade only: Caps 1, 2, 4 mcg.

NOTES - Monitor serum PTH, calcium and phosphorus. IV doses up to 0.24 mcg/kg (16.8 mcg) have been administered.

phytonadione (vitamin K, Mephyton, AquaMephyton) ▶L ♀C ▶+ $

WARNING - Severe reactions, including fatalities, have occurred during and immediately after IV injection, even with diluted injection and slow administration. Restrict IV use to situations where other routes are not feasible.

ADULT - Excessive oral anticoagulation: Dose varies based on INR. INR 5-9: 1-2.5 mg PO (≤ 5 mg PO may be given if rapid reversal necessary); INR >9 with no bleeding: 5-10 mg PO; Serious bleeding & elevated INR: 10 mg slow IV infusion. Hypoprothrombinemia due to other causes: 2.5-25 mg PO/IM/SC. Adequate daily intake 120 mcg (males) and 90 mcg (females).

PEDS - Hemorrhagic disease of the newborn: Prophylaxis: 0.5-1 mg IM 1 hr after birth; Treatment: 1 mg SC/IM.

UNAPPROVED PEDS - Nutritional deficiency: Children: 2.5-5m g PO daily or 1-2 mg IM/SC/ IV. Excessive oral anticoagulation: Infants: 1-2 mg IM/SC/IV q4-8 hr; Children: 2.5-10 mg PO/ IM/SC/IV, may be repeated 12-48 hr after PO dose or 6-8 hr after IM/SC/IV dose.

FORMS - Trade only: Tab 5 mg.

NOTES - Excessive doses of vitamin K in a patient receiving warfarin may cause warfarin resistance for up to a week. Avoid IM administration in patients with a high INR.

pyridoxine (vitamin B6) ▶K ♀A ▶+ $

ADULT - Dietary deficiency: 10-20 mg PO daily for 3 weeks. Prevention of deficiency due to isoniazid in high-risk patients: 10-25 mg PO daily. Treatment of neuropathies due to INH: 50-200 mg PO daily. INH overdose (>10 g): Give an equal amount of pyridoxine: 4 g IV followed by 1 g IM q 30 min. RDA for adults: 19-50 yo: 1.3 mg; >50 yo: 1.7 mg (males), 1.5 mg (females). Max recommended: 100 mg/day.

PEDS - Not approved in children. Adequate daily intake for infants: 0-6 mo: 0.1 mg; 7-12 mo: 0.3 mg. RDA for children: 1-3 yo: 0.5 mg; 4-8 yo: 0.6 mg; 9-13 yo: 1 mg; 14-18 yo: 1.3 (boys) and 1.2 mg (girls).

UNAPPROVED ADULT - PMS: 50-500 mg/day PO. Hyperoxaluria type I and oxalate kidney stones: 25-300 mg/day PO. Prevention of oral contraceptive-induced deficiency; 25-40 mg daily. Hyperemesis of pregnancy: 10-50 mg q8h. Has been used in hydrazine poisoning.

UNAPPROVED PEDS - Dietary deficiency: 5-10 mg PO daily for 3 weeks. Prevention of deficiency due to isoniazid: 1-2 mg/kg/day PO daily. Treatment of neuropathies due to INH: 10-50 mg PO daily. Pyridoxine-dependent epilepsy: neonatal: 25-50 mg/dose IV; older infants and children: 100 mg/dose IV for 1 dose then 100 mg PO daily.

FORMS - OTC Generic only: Tab 25,50,100 mg, timed-release tab 100 mg.

riboflavin (*vitamin B2*) ▶K ♀A ▶+ $

ADULT - Deficiency: 5-25 mg/day PO. RDA for adults is 1.3 mg (males) and 1.1 mg (females), 1.4 mg for pregnant women and 1.6 mg for lactating women.

PEDS - Deficiency: 5-10 mg/day PO. Adequate daily intake for infants: 0-6 mo: 0.3 mg; 7-12 mo: 0.4 mg. RDA for children: 1-3 yo: 0.5 mg; 4-8 yo: 0.6 mg; 9-13 yo: 0.9 mg; 14-18 yo: 1.3 mg (males) and 1 mg (females).

UNAPPROVED ADULT - Prevention of migraine headaches: 400 mg PO daily.

FORMS - OTC Generic only: tab 25,50,100 mg.

NOTES - May cause yellow/orange discoloration of urine.

thiamine (*vitamin B1*) ▶K ♀A ▶+ $

ADULT - Beriberi: 10-20 mg IM 3 times/week for 2 weeks. Wet beriberi with myocardial infarction: 10-30 mg IV tid. Wernicke encephalopathy: 50-100 mg IV and 50-100 mg IM for 1 dose then 50-100 mg IM daily until patient resumes normal diet. Give before starting glucose. RDA for adults is 1.2 mg (males) and 1.1 mg (females).

PEDS - Beriberi: 10-25 mg IM daily or 10-50 mg PO daily for 2 weeks then 5-10 mg PO daily for 1 month. Adequate daily intake infants: 0-6 mo: 0.2 mg; 7-12 mo: 0.3 mg. RDA for children: 1-3 yo: 0.5 mg; 4-8 yo: 0.6 mg; 9-13 yo: 0.9 mg; 14-18 yo: 1.2 mg (males), 1.0 mg (females).

FORMS - OTC Generic only: tab 50,100,250, 500 mg, enteric coated tab 20 mg.

tocopherol (*vitamin E*, ✚*Aquasol E*) ▶L ♀A ▶? $

ADULT - RDA is 22 units (natural, d-alpha-tocopherol) or 33 units (synthetic, d,l-alpha-tocopherol) or 15 mg (alpha-tocopherol). Max recommended 1000 mg (alpha-tocopherol).

PEDS - Adequate daily intake (alpha-tocopherol): infants 0-6 mo: 4 mg; 7-12 mo: 6 mg. RDA for children (alpha-tocopherol): 1-3 yo: 6 mg; 4-8 yo: 7 mg; 9-13 yo: 11 mg; 14-18 yo: 15 mg.

UNAPPROVED ADULT - Alzheimer's disease: 1000 units PO bid (controversial based on limited data & efficacy).

UNAPPROVED PEDS - Nutritional deficiency: Neonates: 25-50 units PO daily; Children: 1 unit/kg daily. Cystic fibrosis: 5-10 units/kg daily (use water soluble form), max 400 units/day.

FORMS - OTC Generic only: tab 200,400 units, cap 73.5, 100, 147, 165, 200, 330, 400, 500, 600, 1000 units, drops 50 mg/mL.

NOTES - Natural vitamin E (d-alpha-tocopherol) recommended over synthetic (d,l-alpha-tocopherol). Do not exceed 1500 units natural vit E/day. Higher doses may increase risk of bleeding. Large randomized trials have failed to demonstrate cardioprotective effects.

vitamin A ▶L ♀A (C if exceed RDA, X in high doses) ▶+ $

ADULT - Deficiency states: 100,000 units IM daily x 3 days, then 50,000 units IM daily x 2 weeks. RDA: 1000 mcg RE (males), 800 mcg RE (females). Max recommended daily dose in non-deficiency 3000 mcg (see notes).

PEDS - Deficiency states: Infants: 7,500 - 15,000 units IM daily x 10 days; children 1-8 yo: 17,500 - 35,000 units IM daily x 10 days. Kwashiorkor: 30 mg IM of water-soluble palmitate followed by 5,000-10,000 units PO daily x 2 months. Xerophthalmia: >1 yo: 110 mg retinyl palmitate PO or 55 mg IM plus 110 mg PO next day. Administer another 110 mg PO prior to discharge. Vitamin E (40 units) should be co-administered to increase efficacy of retinol. RDA for children: 0-6 mos: 400 mcg (adequate intake); 7-12 mo: 500 mcg; 1-3 yrs: 300 mcg; 4-8 yrs: 400 mcg; 9-13 yrs: 600 mcg; 14-18 yrs: 900 mcg (males), 700 mcg (females).

UNAPPROVED ADULT - Test for fat absorption: 7000 units/kg (2100 RE/kg) PO x 1. Measure serum vitamin A concentrations at baseline and 4 hr after ingestion. Dermatologic disorders such as follicularis keratosis: 50,000 - 500,000 units PO daily x several weeks.

UNAPPROVED PEDS - Has been tried for reducing malaria episodes in children >12 mo and to reduce the mortality in HIV.

FORMS - OTC: Generic: cap 10,000, 15,000 units. Trade only: tab 5,000 units. Rx: Generic: 25,000 units. Trade only: soln 50,000 units/mL.

NOTES - 1 RE (retinol equivalent) = 1 mcg retinol or 6 mcg beta-carotene. Continued Vitamin A/retinol intake of ≥2000 mcg/d may increase risk of hip fracture in postmenopausal women.

vitamin D (*vitamin D2, ergocalciferol, Calciferol, Drisdol, ♥Osteoforte*) ▸L ♀A (C if exceed RDA) ▸+ $

ADULT - Familial hypophosphatemia (Vitamin D Resistant Rickets): 12,000-500,000 units PO daily. Hypoparathyroidism: 50,000-200,000 units PO daily. Adequate daily intake adults: 19-50 yo: 5 mcg (200 units); 51-70 yo: 10 mcg (400 units); >70 yo: 15 mcg (600 units). Max recommended daily dose in non-deficiency 50 mcg (2000 units).

PEDS - Adequate daily intake infants and children: 5 mcg (200 units). Hypoparathyroidism: 1.25-5 mg PO daily.

UNAPPROVED ADULT - Osteoporosis prevention: 400-800 units PO daily with calcium supplements. Fanconi syndrome: 50,000-200,000 units PO daily. Osteomalacia: 1000-5000 units PO daily. Anticonvulsant-induced osteomalacia: 2000-50,000 units PO daily. Vitamin D deficiency: 50,000 units PO q week to q month.

UNAPPROVED PEDS - Familial hypophosphatemia: 400,000-800,000 units PO daily, increased by 10,000-20,000 units/day q 3-4 mo as needed. Hypoparathyroidism: 50,000-200,000 units PO daily. Fanconi syndrome: 250-50,000 units PO daily.

FORMS - OTC: Trade: soln 8000 units/mL. Rx: Trade: cap 50,000 units, inj 500,000 units/mL.

NOTES - 1 mcg ergocalciferol = 40 units vitamin D. IM or high-dose oral therapy may be necessary if malabsorption exists. Familial hypophosphatemia also requires phosphate supplementation; hypoparathyroidism also requires calcium supplementation.

ENDOCRINE & METABOLIC: Other

aminoglutethimide (*Cytadren*) ▸K♀D▸?$$$$

WARNING - Used only as an interim until more definitive therapy such as surgery can be undertaken; only small numbers of patients have been treated >3 months. Benefits are limited in ACTH-dependent Cushing's syndrome as high levels of ACTH overcome the drug's effect. Avoid alcohol. May cause adrenocortical hypofunction; may give hydrocortisone & mineralocorticoid supplements if indicated; Dexamethasone should not be used. May cause orthostatic hypotension; monitor BP.

ADULT - Cushing's syndrome: 250 mg PO q6h (should be initiated in hospital). Increase dose in increments of 250 mg at intervals of 1-2 weeks if cortisol suppression is inadequate. Max dose 2 g/day.

PEDS - Not approved in children.

UNAPPROVED ADULT - Advanced breast cancer in postmenopausal women: Start 250 mg PO daily, then increase every couple of days to bid, tid, then to qid. Metastatic prostate carcinoma: Start 250 mg PO bid, then increase to 250 mg qid as tolerated. Response may take 4-6 weeks.

FORMS - Trade only: Tab 250 mg

NOTES - Monitor plasma cortisol levels (or to avoid daily variation instead monitor free urinary cortisol or other steroid metabolites) to determine if suppression is adequate. May need glucocorticoid & mineralocorticoid replacement if oversuppression. Dose reduction or temporary discontinuation may be required if adverse effects. Discontinue if skin rash persists >5-8 days or becomes severe; may start at lower dose if rash is mild or moderate. Obtain baseline and monitor periodically CBC, thyroid function tests, LFTs and electrolytes. Decreases effects of warfarin, dexamethasone, digoxin, medroxyprogesterone & theophylline.

Ammonul (sodium phenylacetate + sodium benzoate) ▸KL ♀C ▸? $$$$$

ADULT - Acute hyperammonemia with encephalopathy in urea cycle enzyme deficiency: 55 mL/m² IV over 90-120 min, followed by maintenance 55 mL/m² over 24 hours. Stop when hyperammonemia resolved or oral nutrition and medications are tolerated.

PEDS - Acute hyperammonemia with encephalopathy in urea cycle enzyme deficiency: If ≤20 kg, then 2.5 mL/kg IV over 90-120 min, followed by maintenance 2.5mL/kg over 24 hours. If >20 kg, then 55 mL/m² IV over 90-120 min, followed by maintenance 55 mL/m² over 24 hrs. Consider co-administration of arginine in hyperammonemic infants. Stop when hyperammonemia resolved or oral nutrition and medications are tolerated.

FORMS - Single-use vial 50 mL (10% sodium phenylacetate & 10% sodium benzoate).

NOTES - Administer through a central line. Closely monitor if renal insufficiency. Monitor plasma ammonia level, neurological status, electrolytes, blood pH, blood pC02 and clinical response. May cause hypokalemia. Consider co-administration of antiemetic. Penicillin and probenecid may affect renal secretion.

bromocriptine (*Parlodel*) ▶L ♀B ▶- $$$$$
ADULT - Hyperprolactinemia: Start 1.25-2.5 mg PO qhs, then increase q3-7 days to usual effective dose of 2.5-15 mg/day, max 40 mg/day. Acromegaly: Usual effective dose is 20-30 mg/day, max 100 mg/day. Doses >20 mg/day can be divided bid. Also approved for Parkinson's Disease, but rarely used. Take with food to minimize dizziness and nausea.
PEDS - Not approved in children.
UNAPPROVED ADULT - Neuroleptic malignant syndrome: 2.5-5 mg PO 2-6 times/day. Hyperprolactinemia: 2.5-7.5 mg/day vaginally if GI intolerance occurs with PO dosing.
FORMS - Generic/Trade: Tabs 2.5 mg. Caps 5 mg.
NOTES - Take with food to minimize dizziness and nausea. Ergots have been associated with potentially life-threatening fibrotic complications. Seizures, stroke, HTN, arrhythmias, and MI have been reported. Should not be used for post-partum lactation suppression. Contraindicated in Raynaud's Syndrome. Avoid concomitant use of other ergot medications.

cabergoline (*Dostinex*) ▶L ♀B ▶- $$$$$
ADULT - Hyperprolactinemia: initiate therapy with 0.25 mg PO twice weekly. Increase by 0.25 mg twice weekly at 4 week intervals up to a maximum of 1 mg twice weekly.
PEDS - Not approved in children.
FORMS - Generic/Trade: Tabs 0.5 mg.
NOTES - Monitor serum prolactin levels. Use with caution in hepatic insufficiency.

calcitonin (*Miacalcin, Fortical*, ✚*Calcimar, Caltine*) ▶Plasma ♀C ▶? $$$$
ADULT - Osteoporosis: 100 units SC/IM daily or 200 units (1 spray) intranasal daily (alternate nostrils). Paget's disease: 50-100 units SC/IM daily or 3 times weekly. Hypercalcemia: 4 units/kg SC/IM q12h. May increase after 2 days to maximum of 8 units/kg q6h.
PEDS - Not approved in children.
UNAPPROVED ADULT - Acute osteoporotic

vertebral fracture pain: 100 units SC/IM daily or 200 units intranasal daily (alternate nostrils).
UNAPPROVED PEDS - Osteogenesis imperfecta age 6 mos-15 yo: 2 units/kg SC/IM three times weekly with oral calcium supplements.
FORMS - Trade only: nasal spray 200 units/activation in 3.7 mL bottle (minimum of 30 doses/bottle).
NOTES - Skin test before using injectable product: 1 unit intradermally and observe for local reaction. Hypocalcemic effect diminishes in 2-7 days, therefore, only useful during acute short-term management of hypercalcemia.

cinacalcet (*Sensipar*) ▶LK ♀C ▶? $$$$$
ADULT - Treatment of secondary hyperparathyroidism in dialysis patients: 30 mg PO daily. May titrate q 2-4 weeks through sequential doses of 60, 90, 120 & 180 mg daily to target intact parathyroid hormone level of 150-300 pg/mL. Treatment of hypercalcemia in parathyroid carcinoma: 30 mg PO bid. May titrate q 2-4 weeks through sequential does of 30 mg bid, 60 mg bid, 90 mg bid & 90 mg tid-qid as necessary to normalize serum calcium levels.
PEDS - Not approved in children.
FORMS - Trade only: tab 30, 60, 90 mg
NOTES - Monitor serum calcium & phosphorus 1 week after initiation or dose adjustment, then monthly after established maintenance dose. Intact parathyroid hormone should be checked 1-4 weeks after initiation or dose adjustment, and then 1-3 months after established maintenance dose. For parathyroid carcinoma, monitor calcium within 1 week after initiation or dose adjustment, then q 2 months after established maintenance dose. Withhold if calcium falls below <7.5 mg/dL or if signs & symptoms of hypocalcemia. May restart when calcium level reaches 8.0 mg/dL or when signs & symptoms of hypocalcemia resolve. Re-initiate using the next lowest dose. Use calcium-containing phosphate binder and/or vitamin D to raise calcium if it falls between 7.5-8.4 mg/dL. Reduce dose or discontinue if intact parathyroid hormone level is <150-300 pg/mL to prevent adynamic bone disease. Dose adjustment may be needed when used with ketoconazole, erythromycin & itraconazole. Closely monitor parathyroid hormone & serum calcium if moderate to severe hepatic impairment.

conivaptan (*Vaprisol*) ▶LK ♀C ▶? $$$$$
WARNING - Avoid concurrent use of CYP 3A4 inhibitors (ketoconazole, itraconazole, clarithromycin, ritonavir, indinavir). Discontinue if hypo-

volemia, hypotension, or rapid rise in serum sodium (>12 mEq/L/24 hrs) occurs.
ADULT - Euvolemic or hypervolemic hyponatremia: Load 20 mg IV over 30 minutes, then continuous infusion 20 mg over 24 hours for 1-4 days. Titrate to desired serum sodium. Max dose 40 mg daily as continuous infusion.
PEDS - Not approved in children.
NOTES - Not indicated in heart failure hyponatremia. Requires frequent monitoring of serum sodium, volume, neurologic status. Administer through large veins and change infusion site daily to minimize irritation. May increase digoxin levels.

desmopressin (DDAVP, Stimate, ✚Minirin, Octostim) ▶LK ♀B ▶? $$$$
WARNING - Adjust fluid intake downward in elderly to decrease potential water intoxication and hyponatremia.
ADULT - Diabetes insipidus: 10-40 mcg (0.1-0.4 mL) intranasally daily or divided bid-tid or 0.05-1.2 mg PO daily or divided bid-tid or 0.5-1 mL (2-4 mcg) SC/IV daily in 2 divided doses. Hemophilia A, von Willebrand's disease: 0.3 mcg/kg IV over 15-30 min; 300 mcg intranasally if ≥50 kg (1 spray in each nostril), 150 mcg intranasally if <50 kg (single spray in 1 nostril). Primary nocturnal enuresis: 10-40 mcg (0.1- 0.4 mL) intranasally qhs, administer ½ of dose per nostril or 0.2-0.6 mg PO qhs.
PEDS - Diabetes insipidus 3 mo-12 yo: 5-30 mcg (0.05-0.3 mL) intranasally daily-bid or 0.05 mg PO daily. Hemophilia A, von Willebrand's disease (age ≥3 mo for IV, age ≥11 mo - 12 yo for nasal spray): 0.3 mcg/kg IV over 15-30 min; 300 mcg intranasally if ≥50 kg (1 spray in each nostril), 150 mcg intranasally if <50 kg (single spray in 1 nostril). Primary nocturnal enuresis ≥6 yo: 10-40 mcg (50% of the dose in each nostril) intranasally qhs or 0.2-0.6 mg PO qhs.
UNAPPROVED ADULT - Uremic bleeding: 0.3 mcg/kg IV single dose or q12h (onset 1-2h; duration 6-8h after single dose). Intranasal is 20 mcg/day (onset 24-72 h; duration 14 days during 14-day course).
UNAPPROVED PEDS - Hemophilia A and type 1 von Willebrand' s disease: 2-4 mcg/kg intranasally or 0.2-0.4 mcg/kg IV over 15-30 min.
FORMS - Trade only: Stimate nasal spray 150 mcg/0.1 mL (1 spray), 2.5 mL bottle (25 sprays). Generic/Trade (DDAVP nasal spray): 10 mcg/0.1 mL (1 spray), 5 mL bottle (50 sprays). Note difference in concentration of nasal solutions. Rhinal Tube: 2.5 mL bottle with 2 flexible plastic tube applicators with graduation marks for dosing.
NOTES - Start at lowest dose with diabetes insipidus. Monitor serum sodium. IV/SC doses are approximately 1/10th the intranasal dose. Anaphylaxis reported with both IV and intranasal forms. Avoid excessive fluid intake to prevent water intoxication/hyponatremia. Do not give if type IIB von Willebrand's disease. Changes in nasal mucosa may impair absorption of nasal spray. Refrigerate nasal spray - stable for 3 weeks at room temperature. 10 mcg = 40 units desmopressin.

gallium (Ganite) ▶K ♀C ▶? ?
ADULT - Hypercalcemia of malignancy: 200 mg/m²/day x 5 days. Shorten course if hypercalcemia is corrected. If mild hypercalcemia with few symptoms, consider 100 mg/m²/day x 5 days . Administer as slow IV infusion over 24 h.
PEDS - Not approved in children.
NOTES - Monitor creatinine (contraindicated if >2.5 mg/dL), urine output, calcium and phosphorous. Avoid concurrent nephrotoxic drugs (e.g. aminoglycosides, amphotericin B). Ensure adequate hydration prior to infusion.

mecasermin (Increlex) ▶LK ♀C ▶? $$$$$
ADULT - Not studied in adults.
PEDS - Growth failure with severe primary insulin-like growth factor-1 deficiency or with neutralizing antibodies to growth hormone in gene deletion: Start 0.04 to 0.08 mg/kg SC bid. As tolerated, increase at weekly intervals by 0.04 mg/kg per dose to maximum of 0.12 mg/kg bid. Administer within 20 minutes of meal or snack. Omit dose if patient will skip meal.
FORMS - Trade only: 40 mg multiple dose vial.
NOTES - Monitor pre-prandial glucose at initiation and until stable dose. Reduce dose if hypoglycemia despite adequate food intake. Do not use with closed epiphyses or malignancy. Do not give IV. Contains benzyl alcohol.

nitisinone (Orfadin) ▶? ♀C ▶? $$$$$
WARNING - Elevation of plasma tyrosine level, transient thrombocytopenia and leukopenia.
ADULT, PEDS - Hereditary tyrosinemia type I: 1-2 mg/kg/day PO divided bid.
FORMS - Trade only: capsules 2, 5, 10 mg
NOTES - Orphan drug; keep tyrosine levels <500 micromoles/L; regular liver monitoring by imaging and LFTs, alpha-fetoprotein, serum tyrosine, phenylalanine, and urine succinylacetone (may use to guide dosing).

pegvisomant (Somavert) ▶? ♀B ▶? $$$$$
ADULT - Acromegaly unresponsive to other the-

rapies: Load 40 mg SC on day 1, then maintenance 10 mg SC daily. Max 30 mg/day.
PEDS - Not approved in children.
FORMS - Trade only: 10,15,20 mg single-dose
vials. Available only from manufacturer.
NOTES - Orphan drug. May cause elevations of
growth hormone levels and pituitary tumor
growth; periodically image sella turcica. May
increase glucose tolerance. May cause IGF-1
deficiency, monitor IGF-1 4-6 weeks after initiation or dose change and q6 months after IGF-1
normalizes. May elevate LFTs; obtain baseline
LFTs then check monthly x 6 months, quarterly
for the next 6 months and biannually for the
next year. Refer to manufacturer's guideline
when initiating with abnormal LFTs. Dose adjustment should be every 4-6 weeks in 5-mg
increment and based on IGF-1.

**sodium polystyrene sulfonate (Kayexa-
late)** ▶Fecal excretion ♀C ▶? $$$$
ADULT - Hyperkalemia: 15 g PO daily-qid or 30-
50 g retention enema (in sorbitol) q6h prn. Re-
tain for 30 minutes to several h. Irrigate with
tap water after enema to prevent necrosis.
PEDS - Hyperkalemia: 1 g/kg PO q6h.
UNAPPROVED PEDS - Hyperkalemia: 1 g/kg
PR q2-6h.
FORMS - Generic only: Suspension 15 g/60 mL.
Powdered resin.
NOTES - 1 g binds approximately 1 mEq of K.
Avoid in bowel obstruction or constipation.

**somatropin (*human growth hormone, Ge-
notropin, Humatrope, Norditropin, Norditropin NordiFlex, Nutropin, Nutropin AQ,
Nutropin Depot, Omnitrope, Protropin,
Serostim, Serostim LQ, Saizen, Tev-Tropin, Valtropin, Zorbtive*)** ▶LK ♀B/C ▶?
$$$$$
WARNING - Avoid in patients with Prader-Willi
syndrome who are severely obese, have severe respiratory impairment or sleep apnea, or
unidentified respiratory infection; fatalities have
been reported.
ADULT - Growth hormone deficiency (Genotropin, Humatrope, Nutropin, Nutropin AQ, Norditropin, Nutropin, Nutropin AQ, Omnitrope, Saizen, Valtropin): doses vary according to product. AIDS wasting or cachexia (Serostim, Serostim LQ): 0.1 mg/kg SC daily, max 6 mg daily.
Short bowel syndrome (Zorbtive): 0.1 mg/kg
SC daily, max 8 mg daily.
PEDS - Growth hormone deficiency (Genotropin, Humatrope, Norditropin, Nutropin, Nutropin
AQ, Nutropin Depot, Omnitrope, Tev-Tropin,

Saizen): Doses vary according to product.
Turner syndrome (Genotropin, Humatrope,
Norditropin, Nutropin, Nutropin AQ, Valtropin):
Doses vary according to product used. Growth
failure in Prader-Willi syndrome (Genotropin):
individualized dosing. Long-term treatment of
idiopathic short stature (Humatrope): individualized dosing. SHOX deficiency (Humatrope):
individualized dosing. Short stature in Noonan
syndrome (Norditropin): individualized dosing.
Growth failure in chronic renal insufficiency
(Nutropin, Nutropin AQ): individualized dosing.
FORMS - Single dose vials (powder for injection
with diluent). Tev-Tropin: 5mg vial (powder for
injection with diluent, stable for 14 days when
refrigerated). Genotropin: 1.5, 5.8, 13.8 mg
cartridges. Humatrope: 6, 12, 24 mg pen cartridges, 5mg vial (powder for injection with diluent, stable for 14 days when refrigerated). Nutropin AQ: 10 mg multiple dose vial & 10 mg/
pen cartridges. Norditropin: 5,10,15 mg pen
cartridges. Norditropin NordiFlex: 5, 10, 15 mg
prefilled pens. Omnitrope: 1.5, 5.8 mg vial
(powder for injection with diluent). Saizen: pre-
assembled reconstitution device with autoinjector pen. Serostim: 4, 5, 6 mg single dose vials,
4 & 8.8 mg multidose vials and 8.8 mg cartridges for autoinjector. Valtropin: 5 mg single
dose vials, 5mg prefilled syringe. Zorbtive: 8.8
mg vial (powder for injection with diluent, stable
for 14 days when refrigerated).
NOTES - Do not use in children with closed
epiphyses. Contraindicated in active malignancy or acute critical illness. Monitor glucose for
insulin resistance; use with caution if diabetes
or risk for diabetes. Transient and dose-dependent fluid retention may occur in adults. May
cause hypothyroidism. Monitor thyroid function
periodically. Evaluate patients with Prader-Willi
syndrome for upper airway obstruction and
sleep apnea prior to treatment; control weight
and monitor for signs & symptoms of respiratory infection. Avoid if pre-proliferative or prolif-
erative diabetic retinopathy. Perform fundus-
copic exam initially & then periodically.

teriparatide (*Forteo*) ▶LK ♀C ▶- $$$$$
WARNING - Possibility of osteosarcoma; avoid
in those at risk (eg, Paget's disease, prior
skeletal radiation).
ADULT - Treatment of postmenopausal women
or men with primary or hypogonadal osteoporosis and high risk for fracture: 20 mcg SC daily in thigh or abdomen for ≤2 years.
PEDS - Not approved in children.

FORMS - Trade only: 28-dose pen injector (20 mcg/dose).

NOTES - Take with calcium and vitamin D. Pen-like delivery device requires education, and should be discarded 28 days after first injection even if not empty.

vasopressin (*Pitressin, ADH,* ✦*Pressyn AR*) ▶LK ♀C ▶? $$$$$

ADULT - Diabetes insipidus: 5-10 units IM/SC bid-qid prn

PEDS - Not approved in children.

UNAPPROVED ADULT - Cardiac arrest: 40 units IV; may repeat if no response after 3 min-

utes. Septic shock: 0.01-0.1 units/min IV infusion, usual dose <0.04 units/min. Bleeding esophageal varices: 0.2-0.4 units/min initially (max 0.9 units /min).

UNAPPROVED PEDS - Diabetes insipidus: 2.5-10 units IM/SC bid-qid prn. Bleeding esophageal varices: start 0.002-0.005 units/kg/min IV, increase prn to 0.01 units/kg/min. Growth hormone and corticotropin provocative test: 0.3 units/kg IM, max 10 units.

NOTES - Monitor serum sodium. Injectable form may be given intranasally. May cause tissue necrosis with extravasation.

ENT: Antihistamines – Nonsedating

desloratadine (*Clarinex,* ✦*Aerius*) ▶LK ♀C ▶+ $$$

ADULT - Allergic rhinitis/urticaria: 5 mg PO daily.

PEDS - Allergic rhinitis/urticaria: ≥12 yo: Use adult dose. 6-11 yo: 2.5 mg PO daily. 12 mo - 5 yo: ½ teaspoonful (1.25 mg) PO daily. 6-11 mo: 2 mL (1 mg) PO daily.

FORMS - Trade only: Tabs 5 mg. Fast-dissolve RediTabs 2.5 & 5 mg. Syrup 0.5 mg/mL

NOTES - Increase dosing interval in liver or renal insufficiency to qod. Use a measured dropper for syrup.

fexofenadine (*Allegra*) ▶LK ♀C ▶+ $$$

ADULT - Allergic rhinitis, urticaria: 60 mg PO bid or 180 mg PO daily. 60 mg PO daily if decreased renal function.

PEDS - Allergic rhinitis, urticaria: ≥12 yo: use adult dose. 6-11 yo: 30 mg PO bid or orally disintegrating tab bid. 30 mg PO daily if decreased renal function.

FORMS - Generic/Trade: Tabs 30, 60, 180 mg, Caps 60 mg. Trade only: Susp 30mg/5 mL, orally disintegrating tab 30 mg.

NOTES - Avoid taking with fruit juice due to a large decrease in bioavailability. Do not remove orally disintegrating tab from its blister package until time of administration.

loratadine (*Claritin, Claritin Hives Relief, Claritin RediTabs, Alavert, Tavist ND*) ▶LK ♀B ▶+ $

ADULT - Allergic rhinitis/urticaria: 10 mg PO daily.

PEDS - Allergic rhinitis/urticaria ≥6 yo: Use adult dose. 2-5 yo: 5 mg PO daily (syrup).

FORMS - OTC: Generic/Trade: Tabs 10 mg. Fast-dissolve tabs (Alavert, Claritin RediTabs) 5, 10 mg. Syrup 1 mg/mL. Rx: Trade only: Chew tab 5 mg (Claritin).

NOTES - Decrease dose in liver failure or renal insufficiency. Fast-dissolve tabs dissolve on tongue without water. ND=non-drowsy (Tavist).

ENT: Antihistamines – Other

NOTE: Contraindicated in narrow angle glaucoma, BPH, stenosing peptic ulcer disease, & bladder obstruction. Use half the normal dose in the elderly. May cause drowsiness and/or sedation, which may be enhanced with alcohol, sedatives, and other CNS depressants. Deaths have occurred in children <2 yo attributed to toxicity from cough and cold medications; use in this age group only with extreme caution.

carbinoxamine (*Palgic*) ▶L ♀C ▶- $$$

ADULT - Allergic/vasomotor rhinitis/urticaria: 4-8 mg PO tid-qid.

PEDS - Allergic/vasomotor rhinitis/urticaria: ≥6

yo: 4-6 mg PO tid-qid. 3-6 yo: 2-4 mg PO tid-qid. 2-3 yo: 2 mg PO tid-qid.

FORMS - Trade: Tabs 4 mg. Soln: 4 mg/5 mL.

NOTES - Decrease dose in hepatic impairment.

cetirizine (*Zyrtec,* ✦*Reactine, Aller-Relief*) ▶LK ♀B ▶- $$$

ADULT - Allergic rhinitis/urticaria: 5-10 mg PO daily.

PEDS - Allergic rhinitis/urticaria: 6-11 yo: Use adult dose. 2-5 yo: 2.5 mg PO daily-bid or 5 mg PO daily. 6-23 mo: 2.5 mg PO daily. If >12 mo, may increase to 2.5 mg PO bid.

FORMS - Trade: Tabs 5, 10 mg. Syrup 5 mg/5

mL. Chewable tabs, grape-flavored 5, 10 mg.
NOTES - Decrease dose in renal or hepatic impairment.

chlorpheniramine (*Chlor-Trimeton, Aller-Chlor*) ▶LK ♀B ▶- $
ADULT - Allergic rhinitis: 4 mg PO q4-6h. 8 mg PO q8-12h (timed release) or 12 mg PO q12h (timed release). Max 24 mg/day.
PEDS - Allergic rhinitis ≥12 yo: Use adult dose. 6-11 yo: 2 mg PO q4-6h. Max 12 mg/day.
UNAPPROVED PEDS - Allergic rhinitis 2-5 yo: 1 mg PO q4-6h. Max 6 mg/day. Timed release 6-11 yo: 8 mg PO q12h prn.
FORMS - OTC: Trade only: Tabs, extended-release 12 mg. Generic/Trade: Tabs 4 mg. Syrup 2 mg/5 mL. Tabs, extended release 8 mg.

clemastine (*Tavist-1*) ▶LK ♀B ▶- $
ADULT - Allergic rhinitis: 1.34 mg PO bid. Max 8.04 mg/day. Urticaria/angioedema: 2.68 mg PO daily-tid. Max 8.04 mg/day.
PEDS - Allergic rhinitis ≥12 yo: Use adult dose. 6-12 yo: 0.67 mg PO bid. Max 4.02 mg/day. Urticaria/angioedema ≥12 yo: Use adult dose. 6-12 yo: 1.34 mg PO bid. Max 4.02 mg/day.
UNAPPROVED PEDS - Allergic rhinitis <6 yo: 0.05 mg/kg/day (as clemastine base) PO divided bid-tid. Max dose 1 mg/day.
FORMS - OTC: Generic/Trade: Tabs 1.34 mg. Rx: Generic/Trade: Tabs 2.68 mg, Syrup 0.67 mg/5 mL. Rx: Generic only: Syrup 0.5mg/5 mL.
NOTES - 1.34 mg = 1 mg clemastine base

cyproheptadine (*Periactin*) ▶LK ♀B ▶- $
ADULT - Allergic rhinitis/urticaria: Start 4 mg PO tid, usual effective dose is 12-16 mg/day. Max 32 mg/day.
PEDS - Allergic rhinitis/urticaria: 2-6 yo: Start 2 mg PO bid-tid. Max 12 mg/day. 7-14 yo: Start 4 mg PO bid-tid. Max 16 mg/day.
UNAPPROVED ADULT - Appetite stimulant: 2-4 mg PO tid 1h ac. Prevention of cluster headaches: 4 mg PO qid. Treatment of acute serotonin syndrome: 12 mg PO/NG followed by 2 mg q2h until symptoms clear, then 8 mg q6h maintenance while syndrome remains active.
FORMS - Generic only: Tabs 4 mg. Syrup 2 mg/ 5 mL.

dexchlorpheniramine (*Polaramine*) ▶LK ♀? ▶- $$
ADULT - Allergic rhinitis/urticaria: 2 mg PO q4-6h. Timed release tabs: 4 or 6 mg PO at qhs or q8-10h.
PEDS - Allergic rhinitis/urticaria: Immediate release tabs & syrup: ≥12 years: Use adult dose. 6-11 yo: 1 mg PO q4-6h. 2-5 yo: 0.5 mg PO

q4-6h. Timed Release Tabs: 6-12 yo: 4 mg PO daily, preferably at qhs.
FORMS - Generic: Tabs, immediate release 2 mg, timed release 4, 6 mg. Syrup 2 mg/5 mL.

diphenhydramine (*Benadryl, Banophen, Allermax, Diphen, Diphenhist, Dytan, Siladryl, Sominex, ♣Allerdryl, Nytol*) ▶LK ♀B ▶- $
ADULT - Allergic rhinitis, urticaria, hypersensitivity reactions: 25-50 mg PO/IM/IV q4-6h. Max 300-400 mg/day. Motion sickness: 25-50 mg PO pre-exposure & q4-6h prn. Drug-induced parkinsonism: 10-50 mg IV/IM. Antitussive: 25 mg PO q4h. Max 100 mg/day. EPS: 25-50 mg PO tid-qid or 10-50 mg IV/IM tid-qid. Insomnia: 25-50 mg PO qhs.
PEDS - Hypersensitivity reactions: ≥12 yo: Use adult dose. 6-11 yo: 12.5-25 mg PO q4-6h or 5 mg/kg/day PO/IV/IM divided qid. Max 150 mg/day. Antitussive (syrup): 6-12 yo: 12.5 mg PO q4h. Max 50 mg/day. 2-5 yo: 6.25 mg PO q4h. Max 25 mg/day. EPS: 12.5-25 mg PO tid-qid or 5 mg/kg/day PO/IV/IM divided qid, max 300 mg/day. Insomnia age ≥12 yo: 25-50 mg PO qhs.
FORMS - OTC: Trade only: Tabs 25, 50 mg, Chew tabs 12.5 mg. OTC & Rx: Generic only: Caps 25, 50 mg, softgel cap 25 mg. OTC: Generic/Trade: Solution 6.25 or 12.5 mg per 5 mL. Rx: Trade only: (Dytan) Suspension 25 mg/mL, Chew tabs 25 mg.
NOTES - Anticholinergic side effects are enhanced in the elderly, and may worsen dementia or delirium. Avoid use with donepezil, rivastigmine, galantamine, or tacrine.

hydroxyzine (*Atarax, Vistaril*) ▶L ♀C ▶- $$
ADULT - Pruritus: 25-100 mg IM/PO daily-qid or prn.
PEDS - Pruritus: <6 yo: 50 mg/day PO divided qid. ≥6 yo: 50-100 mg/day PO divided qid.
FORMS - Generic only: Tabs 10, 25, 50, 100 mg, Caps 100 mg, Syrup 10 mg/5 mL. Generic/ Trade: Caps 25, 50 mg, Suspension 25 mg/5 mL (Vistaril). (Caps = Vistaril, Tabs = Atarax)
NOTES - Atarax (hydrochloride salt), Vistaril (pamoate salt).

levocetirizine (*Xyzal*) ▶K ♀B ▶- $$$
ADULT - Allergic rhinitis/urticaria: 5 mg PO daily.
PEDS - Allergic rhinitis/urticaria: 6-11 yo: 2.5 mg PO daily.
FORMS - Trade only: Tabs 5 mg, scored.
NOTES - Decrease dose in renal impairment.

meclizine (*Antivert, Bonine, Medivert, Meclicot, Meni-D, ♣Bonamine*) ▶L ♀B ▶? $

ADULT - Motion sickness: 25-50 mg PO 1 hour prior to travel, then 25-50 mg PO daily.
PEDS - Not approved in children.
UNAPPROVED ADULT - Vertigo: 25 mg PO daily-qid prn.

FORMS - Rx/OTC/Generic/Trade: tabs 12.5, 25 mg. Chew tabs 25 mg. Rx/Trade: tabs 50 mg.
NOTES - FDA classifies meclizine as "possibly effective" for vertigo. May cause dizziness and drowsiness.

ENT: Antitussives / Expectorants

benzonatate (Tessalon, Tessalon Perles) ▶L ♀C ▶? $$
ADULT - Cough: 100-200 mg PO tid. Max 600 mg/day.
PEDS - Cough, >10 yo: Use adult dose.
FORMS - Generic/Trade: Softgel caps: 100, 200 mg.
NOTES - Swallow whole. Do not chew. Numbs mouth; possible choking hazard.

dextromethorphan (Benylin, Delsym, Dexalone, Robitussin Cough, Vick's 44 Cough) ▶L ♀+ ▶+ $
ADULT - Cough: 10- 20 mg PO q4h or 30 mg PO q6-8h. 60 mg PO q12h (Delsym).
PEDS - Cough >12 yo: Use adult dose. 6-12 yo: 5-10 mg PO q4h or 15 mg PO q6-8h. 30 mg PO q12h (sustained action liquid). 2-5 yo: 2.5-5 mg PO q4h or 7.5 mg PO q6-8h. 15 mg PO q12h (sustained action liquid).
FORMS - OTC: Trade only: Caps 15 mg (Robitussin) & 30 mg (DexAlone), Suspension, extended release 30 mg/5 mL (Delsym). Generic/

Trade: Syrup 5, 7.5, 10, 15 mg/5 mL. Generic only: Lozenges 5, 10 mg.
NOTES - Contraindicated with MAOIs due to potential for serotonin syndrome.

guaifenesin (Robitussin, Hytuss, Guiatuss, Mucinex) ▶L ♀C ▶+ $
ADULT - Expectorant: 100-400 mg PO q4h or 600-1200 mg PO q12h (extended release). Max 2.4g/day.
PEDS - Expectorant >12 yo: Use adult dose. 6-11 yo: 100-200 mg PO q4h. Max 1.2g/day. 2-5 yo: 50-100 mg PO q4h. Max 600 mg/day.
UNAPPROVED PEDS - Expectorant: 12-23 mo: 50 mg PO q4h. Max 300 mg/day. 6-11 mo: 25 mg PO q4h. Max 150 mg/day.
FORMS - Rx-Generic/Trade: Extended release tabs 600, 1200 mg. OTC-Generic/Trade: Liquid & Syrup 100 mg/5 mL. OTC-Trade only: Caps 200 mg (Hytuss), Extended release tabs 600 mg (Mucinex). OTC-Generic only: Tabs 100, 200, 400 mg.
NOTES - Lack of documented efficacy.

ENT: Combination Products – OTC (over the counter)

NOTE: Decongestants in some ENT combination products can increase BP, aggravate anxiety or cause insomnia (use caution). Some contain sedating antihistamines. Sedation can be enhanced by alcohol and other CNS depressants. Some states have restricted or ended OTC sale of pseudoephedrine and pseudoephedrine combination products or reclassified it as a scheduled drug due to the potential for diversion to methamphetamine labs. Deaths have occurred in children <2 yo attributed to toxicity from cough and cold medications; use such medications in this age group only with extreme caution.

Actifed Cold & Allergy **(phenylephrine + chlorpheniramine)** ▶L ♀C ▶+ $
ADULT - Allergic rhinitis/nasal congestion: 1 tab PO q4-6h. Max 4 tabs/day.
PEDS - Allergic rhinitis/nasal congestion: >12 yo: Use adult dose. 6-12 yo: 1/2 tab PO q4h. Max 2 tabs/day.

FORMS - OTC: Trade only: Tabs 10 mg phenylephrine/4 mg chlorpheniramine
Actifed Cold & Sinus **(pseudoephedrine + chlorpheniramine + acetaminophen)** ▶L ♀C ▶+ $$
ADULT - Allergic rhinitis/nasal congestion/headache: 2 caplets PO q6h. Max 8 caplets/day.
PEDS - Allergic rhinitis/nasal congestion/headache: >12 yo: Use adult dose.
FORMS - OTC: Trade only: Tabs 30 mg pseudoephedrine /2 mg chlorpheniramine /500 mg acetaminophen.
Alavert D-12 **(pseudoephedrine + loratadine)** ▶LK ♀B ▶- $
ADULT - Allergic rhinitis/nasal congestion: 1 tab PO bid.
PEDS - Not approved in children.
FORMS - OTC: Generic/Trade: Tabs, 12-hour extended release tabs, 120 mg pseudoephedrine /5 mg loratadine.

NOTES - Decrease to 1 tab PO daily with CrCl <30 mL/min. Avoid in hepatic insufficiency.

Aleve Cold & Sinus (naproxen + pseudo-ephedrine) ▶L ♀C (D in 3rd trimester) ▶+ $

ADULT - Nasal/sinus congestion, fever & pain: 1 cap PO q12h.

PEDS - Nasal/sinus congestion, fever & pain: >12 yo: Use adult dose.

FORMS - OTC: Generic/Trade: Extended release caplets: 220 mg naproxen sodium/120 mg pseudoephedrine.

Allerfrim (pseudoephedrine + triprolidine) ▶L ♀C ▶+ $

ADULT - Allergic rhinitis/nasal congestion: 1 tab or 10 mL PO q4-6h. Max 4 tabs or 40 mL/day.

PEDS - Allergic rhinitis/nasal congestion: >12 yo: Use adult dose. 6-12 yo: 1/2 tab or 5 mL PO q4-6h. Max 2 tabs/day or 20 mL/day.

FORMS - OTC: Generic/Trade: Tabs 60 mg pseudoephedrine/2.5 mg triprolidine. Syrup 30 mg pseudoephedrine/1.25 mg triprolidine/5 mL.

Aprodine (pseudoephedrine + triprolidine) ▶L ♀C ▶+ $

ADULT - Allergic rhinitis/nasal congestion: 1 tab or 10 mL PO q4-6h. Max 4 tabs or 40 mL/day.

PEDS - Allergic rhinitis/nasal congestion: >12 yo: Use adult dose. 6-12 yo: 1/2 tab or 5 mL PO q4-6h. Max 2 tabs/day or 20 mL/day.

FORMS - OTC: Trade only: Tabs 60 mg pseudoephedrine/2.5 mg triprolidine. Syrup 30 mg pseudoephedrine/1.25 mg triprolidine/5 mL.

Benadryl Allergy & Cold (phenylephrine + diphenhydramine + acetaminophen) ▶L ♀C ▶- $

ADULT - Allergic rhinitis/nasal congestion/headache: 2 tabs PO q4h. Max 12 tabs/day.

PEDS - Allergic rhinitis/nasal congestion/headache: >12 yo: Use adult dose. 6-12 yo: 1 tab PO q4h. Max 5 tabs/day.

FORMS - OTC: Trade: Tabs 5 / 12.5 / 325 mg of phenylephrine / diphenhydramine / acetamin.

Benadryl-D Allergy & Sinus (phenylephrine + diphenhydramine) ▶L ♀C ▶- $

ADULT - Allergic rhinitis/nasal congestion: 1 tab PO q4h. Max 6 tabs/day.

PEDS - Allergic rhinitis/nasal congestion: >12 yo: Use adult dose.

FORMS - OTC: Trade only: Tabs 10/25 mg phenylephrine/diphenhydramine.

Cheracol D Cough (guaifenesin + dextromethorphan, ✹Benylin DME) ▶L ♀C ▶? $

ADULT - Cough: 10 mL PO q4h

PEDS - Cough ≥12 yo: Use adult dose. 6-11 yo: 5 mL PO q4h. Max 30 mL/day. 2- 5 yo: 2.5 mL

PO q4h. Max 15 mL/day.

FORMS - OTC: Generic/Trade: Syrup 100 mg guaifenesin/10 mg dextromethorphan/5 mL.

Children's Advil Cold (ibuprofen + pseudoephedrine) ▶L ♀C (D in 3rd trimester) ▶+ $

ADULT - Not approved for use in adults

PEDS - Nasal congestion/sore throat/fever: 6-11 yo: 10 mL PO q6h. 2-5 yo: 5 mL PO q6h.

FORMS - OTC: Trade only: Suspension: 100 mg ibuprofen/15 mg pseudoephedrine/5 mL. Grape flavor, alcohol-free.

NOTES - Shake well before using. Do not use for >7 days for cold, sinus, & flu symptoms.

Claritin-D 12 hr (pseudoephedrine + loratadine) ▶LK ♀B ▶+ $

ADULT - Allergic rhinitis/nasal congestion: 1 tab PO bid.

PEDS - Not approved in children.

FORMS - OTC: Generic/Trade: Tabs, 12-hour extended-release tabs: 120 mg pseudoephedrine/5 mg loratadine.

NOTES - Decrease to 1 tab PO daily with CrCl <30 mL/min. Avoid in hepatic insufficiency.

Claritin-D 24 hr (pseudoephedrine + loratadine) ▶LK ♀B ▶+ $

ADULT - Allergic rhinitis/nasal congestion: 1 tab PO daily.

PEDS - Not approved in children.

FORMS - OTC: Generic/Trade: Tabs, 24-hour extended release tabs: 240 mg pseudoephedrine/10 mg loratadine.

NOTES - Decrease to 1 tab PO qod with CrCl <30 mL/min. Avoid in hepatic insufficiency.

Coricidin HBP Congestion & Cough (guaifenesin + dextromethorphan) ▶LK♀B▶+ $$

ADULT - Productive cough: 1-2 softgels PO q4h. Max 12 softgels/day.

PEDS - Productive cough: ≥12 yo: Adult dose.

FORMS - OTC: Trade only: Softgels 200 mg guaifenesin/10 mg dextromethorphan.

Coricidin HBP Cough & Cold (chlorpheniramine + dextromethorphan) ▶LK ♀B ▶+ $

ADULT - Rhinitis/cough: 1 tab q6h. Max 4 doses/day.

PEDS - Rhinitis/cough: ≥12 yo: Use adult dose.

FORMS - OTC: Trade only: Tabs 4 mg chlorpheniramine/30 mg dextromethorphan.

Dimetapp Cold & Allergy (phenylephrine + brompheniramine) ▶LK ♀C ▶- $

ADULT - Allergic rhinitis/nasal congestion: 20 mL PO q4h. Max 4 doses/day.

PEDS - Allergic rhinitis/nasal congestion: ≥12 yo: Use adult dose. 6-11 yo: 10ml PO q4h.

FORMS - OTC: Trade only: Liquid 2.5 mg phen-

ylephrine/1 mg brompheniramine/5 mL.
NOTES - Grape flavor, alcohol-free.

Dimetapp Decongestant Plus Cough Infant Drops (phenylephrine + dextromethorphan) ▶LK ♀C ▶- $
ADULT - Not recommended.
PEDS - Nasal congestion/cough: 2-3 yo: 1.6 mL PO q4h. Max: 6 doses/day.
FORMS – OTC Trade infant drops 1.25 mg phenylephrine/2.5 mg dextromethorphan/0.8 mL.
NOTES - Alcohol-free.

Dimetapp DM Cold & Cough (pseudoephedrine + brompheniramine + dextromethorphan) ▶LK ♀C ▶- $
ADULT - Nasal congestion/cough: 20 mL PO q4h. Max 6 doses/day.
PEDS - Nasal congestion/cough: ≥12 yo: Adult dose. 6-11 yo: 10 mL PO q4h. Max: 6 doses/d.
FORMS - OTC: Trade only: Elixir 2.5 mg phenylephrine/1 mg brompheniramine/5 mg dextromethorphan/5 mL.
NOTES - Red grape flavor, alcohol-free.

Dimetapp Nighttime Flu (phenylephrine + dextromethorphan + acetaminophen + chlorpheniramine) ▶LK ♀C ▶- $
ADULT - Nasal congestion/runny nose/fever/cough/sore throat: 20 mL PO q4h. Max 5 doses/day.
PEDS - Nasal congestion/runny nose/fever/cough/sore throat ≥12 yo: Use adult dose. 6-11 yo: 10 mL PO q4h. Max: 5 doses/day.
FORMS - OTC: Trade only: Syrup 2.5 mg phenylephrine/5 mg dextromethorphan/160 mg acetaminophen/1 mg chlorpheniramine/5 mL.
NOTES - Bubble gum flavor, alcohol-free.

Drixoral Cold & Allergy (pseudoephedrine + dexbrompheniramine) ▶LK ♀C ▶- $
ADULT - Allergic rhinitis/nasal congestion: 1 tab PO q12h.
PEDS - Allergic rhinitis/nasal congestion ≥12 yo: Use adult dose.
FORMS - OTC: Trade only: Tabs, sustained-action 120 mg pseudoephedrine/6 mg dexbrompheniramine.

Guiatuss PE (pseudoephedrine + guaifenesin) ▶L ♀C ▶- $
ADULT - Nasal congestion/cough: 10 mL PO q4h. Max 40 mL/day.
PEDS - Nasal congestion/cough: ≥12 yo: Use adult dose. 6-11 yo: 5 mL PO q4h. 2-5 yo: 2.5 mL PO q4h. Max 4 doses/day.
FORMS - OTC: Trade only: Syrup 30 mg pseudoephedrine/100 mg guaifenesin/5 mL.
NOTES - PE = pseudoephedrine

Mucinex D (guaifenesin + pseudoephedrine) ▶L ♀C ▶? $
WARNING - Multiple strengths; write specific product on Rx.
ADULT - Cough/congestion: 2 tabs (600/60) PO q12h; max 4 tabs/24h. 1 tab (1200/120) PO q12h; max 2 tabs/24h.
PEDS - Cough: ≥12 yo: Use adult dose.
FORMS - OTC: Trade: Tabs, extended release: 600/60 mg guaifenesin/pseudoephedrine.
NOTES - Do not crush, chew or break the tablet. Take with a full glass of water.

Mucinex DM (guaifenesin + dextromethorphan) ▶L ♀C ▶? $
WARNING - Multiple strengths; write specific product on Rx.
ADULT - Cough: 1-2 tabs (600/30) PO q12h; max 4 tabs/24 h. 1 tab (1200/60) PO q12h; max 2 tabs/24 h.
PEDS - Cough: ≥12 yo: Use adult dose.
FORMS - OTC: Trade: Tabs, extended release: 600/30 mg guaifenesin/dextromethorphan.
NOTES - DM = dextromethorphan. Do not crush, chew or break the tablet. Take with a full glass of water.

Robitussin CF (phenylephrine + guaifenesin + dextromethorphan) ▶L ♀C ▶- $
ADULT - Nasal congestion/cough: 10 mL PO q4h.
PEDS - Nasal congestion/cough: ≥12 yo: Use adult dose. 6-11 yo: 5 mL PO q4h. 2-5 yo: 2.5 mL PO q4h.
FORMS - OTC: Generic/Trade: Syrup 5 mg phenylephrine/100 mg guaifenesin/10 mg dextromethorphan/5 mL.
NOTES - CF= cough formula.

Robitussin DM (guaifenesin + dextromethorphan) ▶L ♀C ▶+ $
ADULT - Cough: 10 mL PO q4h. Max 60 mL/day.
PEDS - Cough: ≥12 yo: Use adult dose. 6-11 yo: 5 mL PO q4h. Max 30 mL/day. 2-5 yo: 2.5 mL PO q4h. Max 15 mL/day.
UNAPPROVED PEDS - Cough: 12-23 mo: 2.5 mL PO q8h. Max 7.5 mL/day. 6-11 mo: 1.25 mL PO q8h. Max 3.75 mL/day.
FORMS - OTC: Generic/Trade: Syrup 100 mg guaifenesin/10 mg dextromethorphan/5 mL.
NOTES - Alcohol-free. DM = dextromethorphan.

Robitussin PE (phenylephrine + guaifenesin) ▶L ♀C ▶- $
ADULT - Nasal congestion/cough: 10 mL PO q4h. Max 6 doses/day.
PEDS - Nasal congestion/cough: ≥12 yo: Use

adult dose. 6-11 yo: 5 mL PO q4h. 2-5 yo: 2.5 mL PO q4h. Max 6 doses/day.

FORMS - OTC: Trade only: Syrup 5 mg phenylephrine/100 mg guaifenesin/5 mL.

NOTES - PE = phenylephrine

Triaminic Chest and Nasal Congestion (phenylephrine + guaifenesin) ▶LK♀C ▶- $

ADULT - Child-only preparation.

PEDS - Chest/nasal congestion: Give PO q4h to max 6 doses/24h: 6-12 yo: 10 mL/dose. 2-6 yo: 5 mL/dose.

FORMS - OTC: Yellow label -Trade only: Syrup 2.5 mg phenylephrine/50 mg guaifenesin/5 mL, tropical flavor.

Triaminic Cold & Allergy (phenylephrine + chlorpheniramine) ▶LK♀C ▶- $

ADULT - Child-only preparation.

PEDS - Allergic rhinitis/nasal congestion: 6-12 yo: 10 mL q4h to max 6 doses/24h.

FORMS - OTC: Orange label -Trade only: Syrup 2.5 mg phenylephrine/1 mg chlorpheniramine/5 mL, orange flavor.

Triaminic Cough & Sore Throat (dextromethorphan + acetaminophen) ▶LK♀C▶-$

ADULT - Child-only preparation.

PEDS - Cough/sore throat: Give PO q4h to max 5 doses/24h: 6-12 yo: 10 mL or 2 softchew tabs/dose. 2-6 yo: 5 mL or 1 softchew tab/dose.

FORMS - OTC: Purple label - Trade only: Syrup & softchew tabs 5 mg dextromethorphan/160

mg acetaminophen/5 mL or tab, grape flavor.

Triaminic Day Time Cold & Cough (phenylephrine + dextromethorphan) ▶LK ♀C ▶- $

ADULT - Child-only preparation.

PEDS - Nasal congestion/cough: Give PO q4h to max 6 doses/24h: 6-12 yo: 10 mL or 2 strips per dose. 2-6 yo: 5 mL or 1 strip per dose.

FORMS - OTC: Red label - Trade only: Syrup, thin strips 2.5 mg phenylephrine/5 mg dextromethorphan/5 mL, cherry flavor

NOTES - Allow strips to dissolve on the tongue.

Triaminic Flu Cough and Fever (acetaminophen + chlorpheniramine + dextromethorphan) ▶LK ♀C ▶- $

ADULT - Child-only preparation.

PEDS - Fever/cough: 6-12 yo: 10 mL PO q6h to max 4 doses/24h.

FORMS - OTC: Pink label - Trade: Syrup 160 mg acetaminophen/1 mg chlorpheniramine /7.5 mg dextromethorphan/5 mL, bubble gum.

Triaminic Night Time Cold & Cough (phenylephrine + diphenhydramine) ▶LK ♀C ▶- $

ADULT - Child-only preparation.

PEDS - Nasal congestion/cough: 6-12 yo: 10 mL PO q4h to max 6 doses/24h.

FORMS - OTC: Blue label - Trade only: Syrup 2.5 mg pheynylephrine/6.25 mg diphenhydramine/5 mL, grape flavor.

ENT: Combination Products – Rx Only

NOTE: Decongestants in some ENT combination products can increase BP, aggravate anxiety or cause insomnia (use caution). Some contain sedating antihistamines. Sedation can be enhanced by alcohol and other CNS depressants. Deaths have occurred in children <2 yo attributed to toxicity from cough and cold medications; use such medications in this age group only with extreme caution.

Allegra-D 12-hour (fexofenadine + pseudoephedrine) ▶LK ♀C ▶+ $$$$

ADULT - Allergic rhinitis/nasal congestion: 1 tab PO q12h.

PEDS - Not approved in children.

FORMS - Trade only: Tabs, extended release 60/120 mg fexofenadine/pseudoephedrine.

NOTES - Decrease dose to 1 tab PO daily with decreased renal function. Take on an empty stomach. Avoid taking with fruit juice due to a large decrease in bioavailability.

Allegra-D 24-hour (fexofenadine + pseudoephedrine) ▶LK ♀C ▶+ $$$$

ADULT - Allergic rhinitis/nasal congestion: 1 tab PO daily.

PEDS - Not approved in children.

FORMS - Trade only: Tabs, extended release 180/240 mg fexofenadine / pseudoephedrine.

NOTES - Decrease dose to 1 tab PO qod with decreased renal function. Take on an empty stomach. Avoid taking with fruit juice due to a large decrease in bioavailability.

AlleRx (pseudoephedrine + methscopolamine + chlorpheniramine) ▶LK ♀C ▶- $$$

ADULT - Allergic rhinitis/vasomotor rhinitis/nasal congestion: One yellow AM tab q am and one blue PM tab q pm.

PEDS - Allergic rhinitis/vasomotor rhinitis/nasal congestion: >12 yo: Use adult dose.

FORMS - Trade only: Tabs, AM (yellow): 120 mg pseudophedrine/2.5 mg methscopolamine.

PM (blue): 8 mg chlor/2.5 mg methscop.

NOTES - Contraindicated in severe hypertension, CAD, MAOI therapy, narrow angle glaucoma, urinary retention, & peptic ulcer. Caution in elderly, hepatic and renal disease.

Bromfenex (pseudoephedrine + brompheniramine) ▶LK ♀C ▶- $

ADULT - Allergic rhinitis/nasal congestion: 1 cap PO q12h. Max 2 caps/day.

PEDS - Allergic rhinitis/nasal congestion: >12 yo: Use adult dose. 6-11 yo: 1 cap PO daily.

FORMS - Generic/Trade: Caps, sustained release 120 mg pseudoephedrine/12 mg brompheniramine.

Bromfenex PD (pseudoephedrine + brompheniramine) ▶LK ♀C ▶- $

ADULT - Allergic rhinitis/nasal congestion: 1-2 caps PO q12h. Max 4 caps/day.

PEDS - Allergic rhinitis/nasal congestion: >12 yo: 1 cap PO q12h. Max 2 caps/day.

FORMS - Generic/Trade: Caps, sustained release 60 mg pseudoephedrine/6 mg brompheniramine.

NOTES - PD = pediatric.

Carbodec DM (pseudoephedrine + carbinoxamine + dextromethorphan) ▶L ♀C ▶- $

ADULT - Allergic rhinitis/nasal congestion/cough: 5 mL PO qid.

PEDS - Allergic rhinitis/nasal congestion/cough >6 yo: 5 mL PO qid. 18 mo-5 yo: 2.5 mL PO q6h. Infant drops: Give PO qid: 1-3 mo: 0.25 mL. 4-6 mo: 0.5 mL. 7-9 mo: 0.75 mL. 10 mo-17 mo: 1 mL.

FORMS - Generic only: Syrup, 60/4/15 mg pseudoephedrine / carbinoxamine / dextromethorphan/5 mL. Drops, 25/2/4 mg/mL, grape flavor 30 mL w/dropper, sugar-free.

NOTES - Carbinoxamine has potential for sedation similar to diphenhydramine. DM = dextromethorphan.

Cheratussin AC (guaifenesin + codeine) ▶L ♀C ▶? ©V $

ADULT - Cough: 10 mL PO q4h. Max 60 mL/day.

PEDS - Cough ≥12 yo: Use adult dose. 6-11 yo: 5 mL PO q4h. Max 30 mL/day. 2-5 yo: 2.5-5 mL PO q4h. Max 30 mL/day. 6-23 mo: 1.25-2.5 mL PO q4h. Max 15 mL/day.

FORMS - Generic/Trade: Syrup 100 mg guaifenesin/10 mg codeine/5 mL. Sugar-free.

Cheratussin DAC (pseudoephedrine + guaifenesin + codeine) ▶L ♀C ▶? ©V $

ADULT - Nasal congestion/cough: 10 mL PO q4h. Max 40 mL/day.

PEDS - Nasal congestion/cough ≥12 yo: Adult dose. 6-11 yo: 5 mL PO q4h. Max 20 mL/day.

FORMS - Generic/Trade: Syrup 30 mg pseudoephedrine/100 mg guaifenesin/10 mg codeine/5 mL. Sugar-free.

NOTES - DAC = decongestant and codeine.

Chlordrine SR (pseudoephedrine + chlorpheniramine) ▶LK ♀C ▶- $

ADULT - Allergic rhinitis/nasal congestion: 1 cap PO q12h. Max 2 caps/day.

PEDS - Allergic rhinitis/nasal congestion >12 yo: Use adult dose. 6-11 yo: 1 cap PO daily.

FORMS - Generic: Caps, sustained release 120 mg pseudoephedrine/8 mg chlorpheniramine.

Clarinex-D 12 hour (pseudoephedrine + desloratadine) ▶LK ♀C ▶+ $$$$

ADULT - Allergic rhinitis: 1 tab PO q12h.

PEDS - Allergic rhinitis ≥12 yo: Use adult dose.

FORMS - Trade: Tabs, extended release 120 mg pseudoephedrine/2.5 mg desloratadine.

NOTES - Swallow tablets whole. Avoid with liver or renal insufficiency.

Clarinex-D 24 hour (pseudoephedrine + desloratadine) ▶LK ♀C ▶+ $$$$

ADULT - Allergic rhinitis: 1 tab PO daily.

PEDS - Allergic rhinitis ≥12 yo: Use adult dose.

FORMS - Trade: Tabs, extended release pseudoephedrine+desloratadine 120/2.5, 240/5 mg.

NOTES - Instruct patients to swallow the tablet whole. Increase dosing interval in renal insufficiency to qod. Avoid with liver insufficiency.

Deconamine (pseudoephedrine + chlorpheniramine) ▶LK ♀C ▶- $$

WARNING - Multiple strengths; write specific product on Rx.

ADULT - Allergic rhinitis/nasal congestion: 1 tab or 10 mL PO tid-qid. Max 6 tabs or 60 mL/day. Sust'd release: 1 cap q12h. Max 2 caps/day.

PEDS - Allergic rhinitis/nasal congestion: >12 yo: Use adult dose. 6-11 yo: ½ tab or 5 mL PO tid-qid. Max 3 tabs or 30 mL/day.

FORMS - Trade only: Tabs 60/4 mg pseudoephedrine/chlorpheniramine, scored. Syrup 30/2 mg per 5 mL. Chew tab 15/1 mg. Generic/Trade: Caps, sustained release 120/8 mg (Deconamine SR).

Deconsal II (phenylephrine + guaifenesin) ▶L ♀C ▶- $$

ADULT - Nasal congestion/cough: 1-2 tabs PO q12h. Max 4 tabs/day.

PEDS - Nasal congestion/cough: >12 yo: Adult dose. 6-12 yo: 1 tab PO q12h, max 2 tabs/day. 2-5 yo: ½ tab PO q12h. Max 1 tab/day.

FORMS - Trade only: Caps, sustained release

20 mg phenylephrine/375 mg guaifenesin.

Dimetane-DX Cough Syrup (pseudoephedrine + brompheniramine + dextromethorphan) ▶L ♀C ▶- $$$

ADULT - Nasal congestion/rhinitis/cough: 10 mL PO q4h prn.

PEDS - Nasal congestion/rhinitis/cough: >12 yo: Use adult dose. 6-11 yo: 5 mL PO q4h. 2-5 yo: 2.5 mL PO q4h. 22-40 kg: 2.5 mL PO qid prn. 12-22 kg: 1.25 mL PO qid prn.

FORMS - Trade: Liquid 30 mg pseudoephedrine /2 mg brompheniramine/10 mg dextromethorphan/5 mL, butterscotch flavor. Sugar-free.

Duratuss (phenylephrine + guaifenesin) ▶L ♀C ▶- $

ADULT - Nasal congestion/cough: 1 PO q12h.

PEDS - Nasal congestion/cough: >12 yo: Use adult dose. 6-12 yo: ½ tab PO q12h.

FORMS - Generic/Trade: Tabs, long-acting 25 mg phenylephrine/900 mg guaifenesin.

Duratuss GP (phenylephrine + guaifenesin) ▶L ♀C ▶- $

ADULT - Nasal congestion/cough: 1 PO q12h.

PEDS - Not approved in children.

FORMS - Generic/Trade: Tabs, long-acting 25 mg phenylephrine /1200 mg guaifenesin.

Duratuss HD (hydrocodone + phenylephrine + guaifenesin) ▶L ♀C ▶- ©III $$$

ADULT - Cough/nasal congestion: 10 mL PO q4-6h.

PEDS - Cough/nasal congestion: >12 yo: Use adult dose. 6-12 yo: ½ tab PO q4-6h.

FORMS - Generic/Trade: Elixir 2.5 mg hydrocodone/10 mg phenylephrine /225 mg guaifenesin/5 mL. 5% alcohol.

Entex LA (phenylephrine + guaifenesin) ▶L ♀C ▶- $$

ADULT - Nasal congestion/cough: 1 PO q12h.

PEDS - Nasal congestion/cough: ≥12 yo: Use adult dose. 6-11 yo: ½ tab PO q12h.

FORMS - Generic/Trade: Tabs, long-acting 30/ 600 mg phenylephrine/guaifenesin. Caps, long-acting 30/400 mg.

NOTES - Do not crush or chew.

Entex Liquid (phenylephrine + guaifenesin) ▶L ♀C ▶- $$$

ADULT - Nasal congestion/cough: 5-10 mL PO q4-6h. Max 40 mL/day.

PEDS - Nasal congestion/cough: ≥12 yo: Adult dose. 6-11 yo: 5 mL PO q4-6h. Max 20 mL/ day. 2-5 yo: 2.5 mL q4-6h. Max 10 mL/day.

FORMS - Generic/Trade: Liquid 7.5 mg phenylephrine/100 mg guaifenesin/5 mL. Punch flavor, alcohol-free.

Entex PSE (pseudoephedrine + guaifenesin) ▶L ♀C ▶- $

ADULT - Nasal congestion/cough: 1 PO q12h.

PEDS - Nasal congestion/cough: >12 yo: Use adult dose. 6-12 yo: ½ tab PO q12h.

FORMS - Generic/Trade: Tabs, long-acting 120 mg pseudoephed./600 mg guaifenesin, scored.

NOTES - PSE = pseudoephedrine.

Gani-Tuss NR (guaifenesin + codeine) ▶L ♀C ▶? ©V $

ADULT - Cough: 10 mL PO q4h. Max 60 mL/ day.

PEDS - Cough ≥12 yo: Use adult dose. 6-11 yo: 5 mL PO q4h. Max 30 mL/day. 2-5 yo: 2.5-5 mL PO q4h. Max 30 mL/day. 6-23 mo: 1.25-2.5 mL PO q4h. Max 15 mL/day.

FORMS - Generic/Trade: Syrup 100 mg guaifenesin/10 mg codeine/5 mL. Sugar-free.

Guaifenex DM (guaifenesin + dextromethorphan) ▶L ♀C ▶? $

ADULT - Cough: 1-2 tabs PO q12h. Max 4/day.

PEDS - Cough ≥12 yo: Use adult dose. 6-12 yo: 1 tab PO q12h. Max 2 tabs/day. 2-6 yo: ½ tab PO q12h. Max 1 tab/day.

FORMS - Generic/Trade: Tabs, sustained release 600 mg guaifenesin/30 mg dextromethorphan, scored.

NOTES - DM = dextromethorphan.

Guaifenex PSE (pseudoephedrine + guaifenesin) ▶L ♀C ▶- $

WARNING - Multiple strengths; write specific product on Rx.

ADULT - Nasal congestion/cough: PSE 60: 1-2 tabs PO q12h. Max 4 tabs/day. PSE 120: 1 tab PO q12h.

PEDS - Nasal congestion/cough: PSE 60: >12 yo: Use adult dose. 6-12 yo: 1 tab PO q12h. Max 2 tabs/day. 2-6 yo: ½ tab PO q12h. Max 1 tab/day. PSE 120: >12 yo: Use adult dose. 6-12 yo: ½ tab PO q12h.

FORMS - Generic/Trade: Tabs, extended release 60/600 mg pseudoephedrine/guaifenesin, scored (Guaifenex PSE 60). Trade: Tabs, ext'd release 120/600mg (Guaifenex PSE 120).

NOTES - PSE = pseudoephedrine.

Guaitex II SR/PSE (pseudoephedrine + guaifenesin) ▶L ♀C ▶- $

WARNING - Multiple strengths; write specific product on Rx.

ADULT - Nasal congestion/cough: 1-2 tabs PO q12h. Max 4 tabs/day (Guaitex II SR). 1 tab PO q12h. Max 2 tabs/day (Guaitex PSE).

PEDS - Nasal congestion/cough: >12 yo: Use adult dose. 6-12 yo: 1 tab PO q12h. Max 2 tabs

/day. 2-5 yo: ½ tab PO q12h. Max 1 tab/day (Guaitex II SR). >12 yo: Use adult dose. 6-12 yo: ½ tab PO q12h (Guaitex PSE).

FORMS - Generic/Trade: Tabs, sustained release 60 mg pseudoephedrine/600 mg guaifenesin (Guaitex II SR). Trade only: Tabs, long-acting 120 mg pseudoephedrine/600 mg guaifenesin (Guaitex PSE).

NOTES - PSE=pseudoephedrine.

Guiatuss AC (guaifenesin + codeine) ▶L ♀C ▶? ©V $

ADULT - Cough: 10 mL PO q4h. Max 60 mL/day.

PEDS - Cough ≥12 yo: Use adult dose. 6-11 yo: 5 mL PO q4h. Max 30 mL/day.

FORMS - Generic/Trade: Syrup 100 mg guaifenesin/10 mg codeine/5 mL. Sugar-free.

NOTES - AC = and codeine

Guiatussin DAC (pseudoephedrine + guaifenesin + codeine) ▶L ♀C ▶- ©V $

ADULT - Nasal congestion/cough: 10 mL PO q4h. Max 40 mL/day.

PEDS - Nasal congestion/cough ≥12 yo: Adult dose. 6-11 yo: 5 mL PO q4h. Max 20 mL/day.

FORMS - Generic/Trade: Syrup 30 mg pseudoephedrine/100 mg guaifenesin/10 mg codeine/5 mL. Sugar-free.

NOTES - DAC = decongestant and codeine.

Halotussin AC (guaifenesin + codeine) ▶L ♀C ▶? ©V $

ADULT - Cough: 10 mL PO q4h. Max 60 mL/ d.

PEDS - Cough ≥12 yo: Use adult dose. 6-11 yo: 5 mL PO q4h. Max 30 mL/day.

FORMS - Generic/Trade: Syrup 100 mg guaifenesin/10 mg codeine/5 mL. Sugar-free.

NOTES - AC = and codeine

Halotussin DAC (pseudoephedrine + guaifenesin + codeine) ▶L ♀C ▶- ©V $

ADULT - Nasal congestion/cough: 10 mL PO q4h. Max 40 mL/day.

PEDS - Nasal congestion/cough: ≥12 yo: Adult dose. 6-11 yo: 5 mL PO q4h. Max 20 mL/day.

FORMS - Generic/Trade: Syrup 30 mg pseudoephedrine/100 mg guaifenesin/10 mg codeine/5 mL. Sugar-free.

NOTES - DAC = decongestant and codeine.

Histinex HC (phenylephrine + chlorpheniramine + hydrocodone) ▶L ♀C ▶- ©III $

ADULT - Allergic rhinitis/congestion/cough: 10 mL PO q4h. Max 40 mL/day.

PEDS - Allergic rhinitis/congestion/cough: >12 yo: Use adult dose. 6-12 yo: 5 mL PO q4h. Max 20 mL/day.

FORMS - Generic/Trade: Syrup 5 mg phenyl-

ephrine/2 mg chlorpheniramine/2.5 mg hydrocodone/5 mL. Alcohol- and sugar-free.

Histussin D (pseudoephedrine + hydrocodone) ▶L ♀C ▶- ©III $$

ADULT - Nasal congestion/cough: 5 mL PO qid prn.

PEDS - Nasal congestion/cough: 22-40 kg: 2.5 mL PO qid prn. 12-22 kg: 1.25 mL PO qid prn.

FORMS - Generic/Trade: Liquid 60 mg pseudoephedrine/5 mg hydrocodone/5 mL, cherry / black raspberry flavor.

Histussin HC (phenylephrine + dexbrompheniramine + hydrocodone) ▶L ♀C ▶- ©III $$

ADULT - Allergic rhinitis/congestion/cough: 10 mL PO q4h. Max 40 mL/day.

PEDS - Allergic rhinitis/congestion/cough: >12 yo: Use adult dose. 6-12 yo: 5 mL PO q4h. Max 20 mL/day.

FORMS - Generic/Trade: Syrup 5 mg phenylephrine/1 mg dexbrompheniramine/2.5 mg hydrocodone/5 mL.

Humibid DM (guaifenesin + guaiacolsulfonate + dextromethorphan) ▶L ♀C ▶? $

ADULT - Cough: 1 cap PO q12h. Max 2 caps/day.

PEDS - Cough: ≥12 yo: Use adult dose. 6-12 yo: 1 cap PO daily.

FORMS - Trade only: Caps, sustained release 400 mg guaifenesin/200 mg guaiacolsulfonate/50 mg dextromethorphan.

NOTES - DM = dextromethorphan.

Humibid LA (guaifenesin + guaiacolsulfonate) ▶L ♀C ▶+ $

ADULT - Expectorant: 1 tab PO q12h (extended release). Max 2 tabs/day.

PEDS - Expectorant >12 yo: Use adult dose.

FORMS - Trade only: Tabs, extended release 600 mg guaifenesin/300 mg guaiacolsulfonate.

Hycoclear Tuss (hydrocodone + guaifenesin) ▶L ♀C ▶- ©III $

ADULT - Cough: 5 mL PO pc & qhs. Max 6 doses/day.

PEDS - Cough: >12 yo: Use adult dose. 6-12 yo: 2.5 mL PO pc & qhs. Max 6 doses/day.

FORMS - Generic/Trade: Syrup 5 mg hydrocodone/100 mg guaifenesin/5 mL. Generic is alcohol and sugar free

Hycodan (hydrocodone + homatropine) ▶L ♀C ▶- ©III $

ADULT - Cough: 1 tab or 5 mL PO q4-6h. Max 6 doses/day.

PEDS - Cough >12 yo: Use adult dose. 6-12 yo: 2.5 mg (based on hydrocodone) PO q4-6h prn.

Max 15 mg/day.

FORMS - Generic/Trade: Syrup 5 mg hydrocodone/1.5 mg homatropine methylbromide/5 mL. Tabs 5/1.5 mg.

NOTES - May cause drowsiness/sedation. Dosing based on hydrocodone content.

Hycotuss (hydrocodone + guaifenesin) ▶L ♀C ▶- ⊚III $

ADULT - Cough: 5 mL PO pc & qhs. Max 6 doses/day.

PEDS - Cough: >12 yo: Use adult dose. 6-12 yo: 2.5 mL PO pc & qhs. Max 6 doses/day.

FORMS - Generic/Trade: Syrup 5 mg hydrocodone/100 mg guaifenesin/5 mL. Generic is alcohol and sugar free.

Novafed A (pseudoephedrine + chlorpheniramine) ▶LK ♀C ▶- $

ADULT - Allergic rhinitis/nasal congestion: 1 cap PO q12h. Max 2 caps/day.

PEDS - Allergic rhinitis/nasal congestion: >12 yo: Use adult dose. 6-12 yo: 1 cap PO daily.

FORMS - Generic/Trade: Caps, sustained release 120 mg pseudoephedrine/8 mg chlorph.

Palgic DS (pseudoephedrine + carbinoxamine) ▶L ♀C ▶- $$

ADULT - Allergic rhinitis/nasal congestion: 10 mL PO qid.

PEDS - Allergic rhinitis/nasal congestion: Give up to the following PO qid: 1-3 mo: 1.25 mL. 3-6 mo: 2.5 mL. 6-9 mo: 3.75 mL. 9-18 mo: 3.75-5 mL. 18 mo-6 yo: 5 mL. >6 yo use adult dose.

FORMS - Generic/Trade: Syrup, 25 mg pseudoephedrine/2 mg carbinoxamine/5 mL. Alcohol & sugar-free.

NOTES - Carbinoxamine has potential for sedation similar to diphenhydramine.

Phenergan VC (phenylephrine + promethazine) ▶LK ♀C ▶? $

WARNING - Promethazine contraindicated if <2 yo due to risk of fatal respiratory depression; caution in older children.

ADULT - Allergic rhinitis/congestion: 5 mL PO q4-6h. Max 30 mL/day.

PEDS - Allergic rhinitis/congestion: ≥12 yo: Use adult dose. 6-11 yo: 2.5-5 mL PO q4-6h. Max 20 mL/day. 2-5 yo: 1.25-2.5 mL PO q4-6h. Max 15 mL/day.

FORMS - Generic only: Syrup 6.25 mg promethazine/5 mg phenylephrine/5 mL.

NOTES - VC = vasoconstrictor.

Phenergan VC w/codeine (phenylephrine + promethazine + codeine) ▶LK♀C▶? ⊚V $

WARNING - Promethazine contraindicated if <2 yo due to risk of fatal respiratory depression;

caution in older children.

ADULT - Allergic rhinitis/congestion/cough: 5 mL PO q4-6h. Max 30 mL/day.

PEDS - Allergic rhinitis/congestion/cough: ≥12 yo: Use adult dose. 6-11 yo: 2.5-5 mL PO q4-6h. Max 20 mL/day. 2-5 yo: 1.25-2.5 mL PO q4-6h. Max 10 mL/day.

FORMS - Generic: Syrup 5 mg phenylephrine/6.25 mg promethazine/10 mg codeine/5 mL.

Phenergan with codeine (promethazine + codeine) ▶LK ♀C ▶? ⊚V $

WARNING - Promethazine contraindicated if <2 yo due to risk of fatal respiratory depression; caution in older children.

ADULT - Allergic rhinitis/cough: 5 mL PO q4-6h. Max 30 mL/day.

PEDS - Allergic rhinitis/cough: ≥12 yo: Use adult dose. 6-11 yo: 2.5-5 mL PO q4-6h. Max 20 mL/day. 2-5 yo: 1.25-2.5 mL PO q4-6h. Max 10 mL/day.

FORMS - Trade unavailable. Generic: Syrup 6.25 mg promethazine/10 mg codeine/5 mL.

Phenergan/Dextromethorphan (promethazine + dextromethorphan) ▶LK ♀C ▶? $

WARNING - Promethazine contraindicated if <2 yo due to risk of fatal respiratory depression; caution in older children.

ADULT - Allergic rhinitis/cough: 5 mL PO q4-6h. Max 30 mL/day.

PEDS - Allergic rhinitis/cough: ≥12 yo: Use adult dose. 6-11 yo: 2.5-5 mL PO q4-6h. Max 20 mL/day. 2-5 yo: 1.25-2.5 mL PO q4-6h. Max 10 mL/day.

FORMS - Generic only: Syrup 6.25 mg promethazine/15 mg dextromethorphan/5 mL.

Pseudo-Chlor (pseudoephedrine + chlorpheniramine) ▶LK ♀C ▶- $

ADULT - Allergic rhinitis/nasal congestion: 1 cap PO q12h. Max 2 caps/day.

PEDS - Allergic rhinitis/nasal congestion: >12 yo: Use adult dose.

FORMS - Generic/Trade: Caps, sustained release 120 mg pseudoephedrine/8 mg chlorpheniramine.

Robitussin AC (guaifenesin + codeine) ▶L ♀C ▶? ⊚V $

ADULT, PEDS - The "Robitussin AC" brand is no longer produced; corresponding generics include Cheratussin AC, Gani-Tuss NR, Guiatuss AC, and Halotussin AC.

Robitussin DAC (pseudoephedrine + guaifenesin + codeine) ▶L ♀C ▶- ⊚V $

ADULT, PEDS - The "Robitussin DAC" brand is no longer produced; corresponding generics include Cheratussin DAC, Guiatuss DAC, and Halotussin DAC.

Rondec (phenylephrine + chlorpheniramine) ▶L ♀C ▶- $$

ADULT - Allergic rhinitis/nasal congestion: 5 mL syrup PO qid.

PEDS - Allergic rhinitis/nasal congestion >12 yo: Use adult dose. 6-12 yo: 2.5 mL syrup PO qid. 2-5 yo: 1.25 mL PO qid.

FORMS - Trade only: Syrup 12.5 mg phenylephrine /4 mg chlorpheniramine/5 mL, bubblegum flavor. Alcohol- & sugar-free.

Rondec DM (phenylephrine + chlorpheniramine + dextromethorphan) ▶L ♀C ▶- $$

ADULT - Allergic rhinitis/nasal congestion/cough: 5 mL syrup PO qid.

PEDS - Allergic rhinitis/nasal congestion/cough >12 yo: Use adult dose. 6-12 yo: 2.5 mL syrup PO qid. 2-5 yo: 1.25 mL syrup PO qid.

FORMS - Trade: Syrup 12.5 mg phenylephrine /4 mg chlorpheniramine/15 mg dextromethorphan/5 mL, grape flavor. Alcohol- & sugar-free.

NOTES - DM = dextromethorphan.

Rondec Infant Drops (phenylephrine + chlorpheniramine) ▶L ♀C ▶- $$

PEDS - Allergic rhinitis/nasal congestion: Give PO qid: 6-12 mo: 0.75 mL. 13-24 mo: 1 mL.

FORMS - Trade: Drops 3.5 mg phenylephrine/1 mg chlorpheniramine/mL, bubble-gum flavor, 30 mL. Alcohol- & sugar-free.

Ryna-12 S (phenylephrine + pyrilamine) ▶L ♀C ▶- $$

PEDS - Nasal congestion, allergic rhinitis, sinusitis: >6 yo: 5-10 mL PO q12h. 2-6 yo 2.5-5 mL PO q12h. <2 yo titrate dose individually.

FORMS - Generic/Trade: Susp 5 mg phenylephrine/30 mg pyrilamine/5 mL strawberry-currant flavor with graduated oral syringe.

Rynatan (phenylephrine + chlorpheniramine) ▶LK ♀C ▶- $$

ADULT - Allergic rhinitis/nasal congestion: 1-2 tabs PO q12h.

PEDS - Allergic rhinitis/nasal congestion: ≥12 yo: 1 tab PO q12h.

FORMS - Trade only: Tabs, extended release: 25/9 mg phenylephrine/chlorpheniramine. Chew tabs 5/4.5 mg.

Rynatan Pediatric Suspension (phenylephrine + chlorpheniramine) ▶L ♀C ▶- $$$

PEDS - Nasal congestion, allergic rhinitis, sinusitis >6 yo: 5-10 mL PO q12h. 2-6 yo 2.5-5 mL PO q12h. <2 yo titrate dose individually.

FORMS - Trade only: Suspension 5 mg phenylephrine/4.5 mg chlorpheniramine/5 mL straw-berry-currant flavor.

Semprex-D (pseudoephedrine + acrivastine) ▶LK ♀C ▶- $$

ADULT - Allergic rhinitis/nasal congestion: 1 cap PO q4-6h. Max 4 caps/day.

PEDS - Not approved in children.

FORMS - Trade only: Caps 60 mg pseudoephedrine/8 mg acrivastine.

Tanafed (pseudoephedrine + chlorpheniramine) ▶L ♀C ▶- $$

ADULT - Allergic rhinitis/nasal congestion: 10-20 mL PO q12h. Max 40 mL/day.

PEDS - Allergic rhinitis/nasal congestion: ≥12 yo: Use adult dose. 6-11 yo: 5-10 mL PO q12h. Max 20 mL/day. 2-5 yo: 2.5-5 mL PO q12h. Max 10 mL/day.

FORMS - Generic/Trade: Suspension 75 mg pseudoephedrine/4.5 mg chlorpheniramine/5 mL, strawberry-banana flavor.

Tuss-HC (phenylephrine + chlorpheniramine + hydrocodone) ▶L ♀C ▶- ©III $

ADULT - Allergic rhinitis/congestion/cough: 10 mL PO q4h. Max 40 mL/day.

PEDS - Allergic rhinitis/congestion/cough: >12 yo: Use adult dose. 6-12 yo: 5 mL PO q4h. Max 20 mL/day.

FORMS - Generic/Trade: Syrup 5 mg phenylephrine/2 mg chlorpheniramine/2.5 mg hydrocodone/5 mL.

Tussionex (chlorpheniramine + hydrocodone) ▶L ♀C ▶- ©III $$$

ADULT - Allergic rhinitis/cough: 5 mL PO q12h. Max 10 mL/day.

PEDS - Allergic rhinitis/cough: 6-12 yo: 2.5 mL PO q12h. Max 5 mL/day.

FORMS - Trade: Extended release susp 8 mg chlorpheniramine/10 mg hydrocodone/5 mL.

Zephrex-LA (pseudoephedrine + guaifenesin) ▶L ♀C ▶- $

ADULT - Nasal congestion/cough: 1 PO q12h.

PEDS - Nasal congestion/cough: >12 yo: Use adult dose. 6-12 yo: ½ tab PO q12h.

FORMS - Trade only: Tabs, extended release 120 mg pseudoephedrine/600 mg guaifenesin.

Zyrtec-D (cetirizine + pseudoephedrine) ▶LK ♀C ▶- $$

ADULT - Allergic rhinitis/nasal congestion: 1 tab PO q12h.

PEDS - Not approved in children.

FORMS - Trade only: Tabs, extended release 5 mg cetirizine/120 mg pseudoephedrine.

NOTES - Decrease dose to 1 tablet PO daily with decreased renal or hepatic function. Take on an empty stomach.

ENT: Decongestants

NOTE: See ENT - Nasal Preparations for nasal spray decongestants (oxymetazoline, phenylephrine). Systemic decongestants are sympathomimetic and may aggravate HTN, anxiety and insomnia. Use cautiously in such patients. Some states have restricted or ended OTC sale of pseudoephedrine or reclassified it as schedule III or V drug due to the potential for diversion to methamphetamine labs. Deaths have occurred in children <2 yo attributed to toxicity from cough and cold medications; use such medications in this age group only with extreme caution.

phenylephrine (*Sudafed PE*) ▶L ♀C ▶+ $
ADULT - Nasal congestion: 10 mg PO q4h prn. Max 6 doses/day.
PEDS - Nasal congestion, >12 yo: Adult dose.
FORMS - OTC: Trade only: Tabs 10 mg.
NOTES - Avoid with MAO inhibitors.

pseudoephedrine (*Sudafed, Sudafed 12 Hour, Efidac/24, Dimetapp Decongestant Infant Drops, PediaCare Infants' Decon-gestant Drops, Triaminic Oral Infant Drops*, ♥*Pseudofrin*) ▶L ♀C ▶+ $
ADULT - Nasal Congestion: 60 mg PO q4-6h. 120 mg PO q12h (extended release). 240 mg PO daily (extended release). Max 240 mg/day.
PEDS - Nasal Congestion >12 yo: Use adult dose. 6-11 yo: 30 mg PO q4-6h. Max 120 mg/day. 2-5 yo: 15 mg PO q4-6h. Max 60 mg/day. Dimetapp, PediaCare, & Triaminic Infant Drops: Give PO q4-6h prn. Max 4 doses/day. 2-3 yo: 1.6 mL. 12-23 mo: 1.2 mL. 4-11 mo: 0.8 mL. ≤3 mo: 0.4 mL.
FORMS - OTC: Generic/Trade: Tabs 30, 60 mg, Tabs, extended release 120 mg (12 hour), Infant drops 7.5 mg/0.8 mL, Solution 15 & 30 mg/5 mL. Trade only: Chew tabs 15 mg, Tabs, extended release 240 mg (24 hour).
NOTES - 12 to 24-hour extended release dosage forms may cause insomnia; use a shorter-acting form if this occurs.

ENT: Ear Preparations

Auralgan (benzocaine + antipyrine) ▶Not absorbed ♀C ▶? $
ADULT - Otitis media, adjunct: Instill 2-4 drops (or enough to fill the ear canal) tid-qid or q1-2h prn. Cerumen removal: Instill 2-4 drops (or fill the ear canal) tid x 2-3 days to detach cerumen, then prn for discomfort. Insert cotton plug moistened with soln after instillation.
PEDS - Otitis media, adjunct: Use adult dose. Cerumen removal: Use adult dose.
FORMS - Generic/Trade: Otic soln 10 & 15 mL.

carbamide peroxide (*Debrox, Murine Ear*) ▶Not absorbed ♀? ▶? $
ADULT - Cerumen impaction: Instill 5-10 drops into ear bid x 4 days.
PEDS - Not approved in children.
FORMS - OTC: Generic/Trade: Otic soln 6.5%, 15 & 30 mL.
NOTES - Drops should remain in ear >15 minutes. Do not use for >4 days. Remove excess wax by flushing with warm water using a rubber bulb ear syringe.

Cipro HC Otic (ciprofloxacin + hydrocortisone) ▶Not absorbed ♀C ▶- $$$$
ADULT - Otitis externa: Instill 3 drops into affected ear(s) bid x 7 days.
PEDS - Otitis externa ≥1 yo: Use adult dose.

FORMS - Trade only: Otic suspension 10 mL.
NOTES - Shake well. Contains benzyl alcohol.

Ciprodex Otic (ciprofloxacin + Dexamethasone) ▶Not absorbed ♀C ▶- $$$$
ADULT - Otitis externa: Instill 4 drops into affected ear(s) bid x 7 days.
PEDS - Otitis externa & otitis media w/ tympanostomy tubes, ≥6 mo: Instill 4 drops into affected ear(s) bid x 7 days.
FORMS - Trade: Otic suspension 5 & 7.5 mL.
NOTES - Shake well. Warm by holding bottle in hands for 1-2 minutes before instilling.

Cortisporin Otic (hydrocortisone + polymyxin + neomycin, *Pediotic*) ▶Not absorbed ♀? ▶? $
ADULT - Otitis externa: Instill 4 drops in affected ear(s) tid-qid up to 10 days.
PEDS - Otitis externa: Instill 3 drops in affected ear(s) tid-qid up to 10 days.
FORMS - Generic/Trade: Otic soln or suspension 7.5 & 10 mL.
NOTES - Caveats with perforated TMs or tympanostomy tubes: (1) Risk of neomycin ototoxicity, especially if use prolonged or repeated; (2) Use suspension rather than acidic soln.

Cortisporin TC Otic (hydrocortisone + neomycin + thonzonium + colistin) ▶Not

absorbed ♀? ▶? $$$
ADULT - Otitis externa: Instill 5 drops in affected ear(s) tid-qid up to 10 days.
PEDS - Otitis externa: Instill 4 drops in affected ear(s) tid-qid up to 10 days.
FORMS - Trade only: Otic suspension, 10 mL.
docusate (Colace) ▶Not absorbed ♀+ ▶+ $
ADULT - See gastroenterology section
PEDS - Not approved in children.
UNAPPROVED ADULT, PEDS - Cerumen impaction: Instill 1 mL in affected ear.
FORMS - Generic/Trade: Liquid 150 mg/15 mL.
NOTES - Allow to remain in ear(s) for 10-15 min. Irrigate with 50 mL lukewarm NS if necessary. Use liquid, not syrup.
Domeboro Otic (acetic acid + aluminum acetate) ▶Not absorbed ♀? ▶? $
ADULT - Otitis externa: Instill 4-6 drops in affected ear(s) q2-3h.
PEDS - Otitis externa: Instill 2-3 drops in affected ear(s) q3-4h.
FORMS - Generic only: Otic soln 60 mL.
NOTES - Insert a saturated wick. Keep moist x 24 hours.
fluocinolone - otic (DermOtic) ▶L ♀C ▶? $$
ADULT - Chronic eczematous external otitis: 5 drops in affected ear(s) bid for 7-14 days.
PEDS - Chronic eczematous external otitis: ≥ 2 yo: Use adult dose.
FORMS - Trade only: Otic oil 0.01% 20 mL.
NOTES - Contains peanut oil.
ofloxacin - otic (Floxin Otic) ▶Not absorbed

♀C ▶- $$$
ADULT - Otitis externa: Instill 10 drops in affected ear(s) daily x 7 days. Chronic suppurative otitis media: Instill 10 drops in affected ear(s) bid x 14 days.
PEDS - Otitis externa >12 yo: Use adult dose. 1-12 yo: Instill 5 drops in affected ear(s) daily x 7 days. Chronic suppurative otitis media >12 yo: Use adult dose. Acute otitis media with tympanostomy tubes 1-12 yo: Instill 5 drops in affected ear(s) bid x 10 days.
FORMS - Trade only: Otic soln 0.3% 5, 10 mL, "Singles": single-dispensing containers 0.25 mL (5 drops), 2 per foil pouch.
Swim-Ear (isopropyl alcohol + anhydrous glycerins) ▶Not absorbed ♀? ▶? $
ADULT - Otitis externa, prophylaxis: Instill 4-5 drops in ears after swimming, showering, or bathing.
PEDS - Otitis externa, prophylaxis: Adult dose.
FORMS - OTC: Trade only: Otic soln 30 mL.
VoSol HC (acetic acid + propylene glycol + hydrocortisone) ▶Not absorbed ♀? ▶? $
ADULT - Otitis externa: Instill 5 drops in affected ear(s) tid-qid. Insert cotton plug moistened with 3-5 drops q4-6h for the first 24 hours.
PEDS - Otitis externa >3 yo: Instill 3-4 drops in affected ear(s) tid-qid. Insert cotton plug moistened with 3-4 drops q4-6h for the 1st 24 hours.
FORMS - Generic/Trade: Otic soln 2%-3%-1% 10 mL.
NOTES - VoSol HC adds hydrocortisone 1%.

ENT: Mouth & Lip Preparations

amlexanox (Aphthasol, OraDisc A) ▶LK ♀B ▶? $
ADULT - Aphthous ulcers: Apply ¼ inch paste or mucoadhesive patch to ulcer in mouth qid after oral hygiene for up to 10 days.
PEDS - Aphthous ulcers >12 yo: use adult dose.
FORMS - Trade only: Oral paste 5%, 5 g tube. Mucoadhesive patch 2 mg, #20.
NOTES - Mucoadhesive patch should be applied ≥80 minutes before bedtime to ensure its erosion before sleep. Up to 3 patches may be applied at one time. Avoid food or liquid for 1 hour after application.
cevimeline (Evoxac) ▶L ♀C ▶- $$$$
WARNING - May alter cardiac conduction / heart rate; caution in heart disease. May worsen bronchospasm in asthma / COPD.
ADULT - Dry mouth due to Sjogren's syndrome:

30 mg PO tid.
PEDS - Not approved in children.
FORMS - Trade only: Caps 30 mg.
NOTES - Contraindicated in narrow-angle glaucoma, acute iritis & severe asthma. May potentiate beta-blockers.
chlorhexidine gluconate (Peridex, Periogard, ✦Denticare) ▶Fecal ♀B ▶? $
ADULT - Gingivitis: Bid as an oral rinse, morning & evening after brushing teeth. Rinse with 15 mL of undiluted soln for 30 seconds. Do not swallow. Spit after rinsing.
PEDS - Not approved in children.
FORMS - Generic/Trade: Oral rinse 0.12% 473-480 mL bottles.
Debacterol (sulfuric acid + sulfonated phenolics) ▶Not absorbed ♀C ▶+ $$
ADULT - Aphthous stomatitis, mucositis: Apply

to dry ulcer. Rinse with water.
PEDS - Not approved in children <12 yo.
FORMS - Trade: 1 mL single-use applicator.
NOTES - One application per ulcer treatment.
Dry ulcer area with cotton swab. Apply to ulcer
and ring of normal mucosa around it for 5 to 10
seconds. Rinse and spit. Return of ulcer pain
right after rinsing indicates incomplete application; can be reapplied immediately one time.
Avoid eye contact. If excess irritation, rinse
with dilute bicarbonate soln.

Gelclair (maltodextrin + propylene glycol)
▶Not absorbed ♀+ ▶+ $$$
ADULT - Aphthous ulcers, mucositis, stomatitis:
Rinse mouth with 1 packet tid or prn.
PEDS - Not approved in children.
FORMS - Trade only: 21 packets/box.
NOTES - Mix packet with 3 tablespoons of wa-
ter. Swish for 1 minute, then spit. Do not eat or
drink for 1 hour after treatment.

lidocaine - viscous (Xylocaine) ▶LK♀B ▶+ $
WARNING - Avoid swallowing during oral or la-
bial use due to GI absorption & toxicity. Meas-
ure dose exactly. May apply to small areas in
mouth with a cotton-tipped applicator.
ADULT - Mouth or lip pain: 15-20 mL topically or
swish & spit q3h. Max 8 doses/day.
PEDS - Use lowest effective doses with extreme
caution, as therapeutic doses approach poten-
tially toxic levels. Mouth or lip pain >3 yo: 3.75-
5 mL topically or swish and spit up to q3h.
FORMS - Generic/Trade: soln 2%, 20 mL unit
dose, 100 mL bottle.
NOTES - High risk of adverse effects / overdose
in children. Consider benzocaine as a safer al-
ternative. Clearly communicate the amount,
frequency, max daily dose, & mode of admini-
stration (eg, cotton pledget to individual le-

sions, 1/2 dropper to each cheek q4h, or 20
minutes before meals). Do not prescribe on a
"PRN" basis without specified dosing intervals.

**"magic mouthwash" (diphenhydramine +
Mylanta + sucralfate)** ▶LK ♀B(- in 1st tri-
mester) ▶- $$$
ADULT - See components
PEDS - Not approved in children.
UNAPPROVED ADULT - Stomatitis: 5 mL PO
swish & spit or swish & swallow tid before
meals and prn.
UNAPPROVED PEDS - Stomatitis: Apply small
amounts to lesions prn.
FORMS - Compounded suspension. A standard
mixture is 30 mL diphenhydramine (12.5 mg/5
mL)/60 mL Mylanta or Maalox/4 g Carafate.
NOTES - Variations of this formulation are available. The dose and decision to swish and spit
or swallow may vary with the indication and/or
ingredient. Some preparations may contain:
Kaopectate, nystatin, tetracycline, hydrocortisone, 2% lidocaine, cherry syrup (for children).
Check local pharmacies for customized formulations. Avoid diphenhydramine formulations
with alcohol - may cause stinging of sores.

pilocarpine (Salagen) ▶L ♀C ▶- $$$$
ADULT - Dry mouth due to radiation of head &
neck: 5 mg PO tid. May increase to 10 mg PO
tid. Dry mouth due to Sjogren's syndrome: 5
mg PO qid. Hepatic dysfunction: 5 mg PO bid.
PEDS - Not approved in children.
UNAPPROVED ADULT - Dry mouth due to Sjogren's syndrome: 2% eye drops: Swish & swallow 4 drops diluted in water tid ($).
FORMS - Generic/Trade: Tabs 5, 7.5 mg.
NOTES - Contraindicated in narrow-angle glaucoma, acute iritis & severe asthma. May potentiate beta-blockers.

ENT: Nasal Preparations – Corticosteroids

NOTE: Decrease to the lowest effective dose for
maintenance therapy. Tell patients to prime
pump before 1st use and shake well before each
subsequent use.

**beclomethasone (Vancenase, Vancenase
AQ Double Strength, Beconase AQ)** ▶L
♀C ▶? $$$$
ADULT - Allergic rhinitis/nasal polyp prophylax-
is: Vancenase: 1 spray in each nostril bid-qid.
Beconase AQ: 1-2 spray(s) in each nostril bid.
Vancenase AQ Double Strength: 1-2 spray(s)
in each nostril daily.

PEDS - Allergic rhinitis/nasal polyp prophylaxis:
Vancenase: >12 yo: adult dose. 6-12 yo: 1
spray in each nostril tid. Beconase AQ: >6 yo
1-2 spray(s) in each nostril bid. Vancenase AQ
Double Strength: >6 yo: 1-2 spray(s) in each
nostril daily.
FORMS - Trade: Vancenase 42 mcg/spray, 80
or 200 sprays/bottle. Beconase AQ 42 mcg/
spray, 200 sprays/bottle. Vancenase AQ Double Strength 84 mcg/spray, 120 sprays/bottle.
NOTES - AQ (aqueous) formulation may cause
less stinging.

budesonide (*Rhinocort Aqua*) ▶L ♀B ▶? $$$
ADULT - Allergic rhinitis: 1-4 sprays/nostril daily.
PEDS - Allergic rhinitis ≥6 yo: 1-2 sprays per nostril daily.
FORMS – Trade only: Nasal inhaler 120 sprays/ bottle.
NOTES - CYP3A4 inhibitors such as ketoconazole, erythromycin, ritonavir, etc significantly increase systemic concentrations, possibly causing adrenal suppression.

ciclesonide (*Omnaris*) ▶L ♀C ▶? $
ADULT - Allergic rhinitis: 2 sprays/nostril daily.
PEDS - Allergic rhinitis ≥12 yo: Use adult dose.
FORMS - Trade only: Nasal spray, 50 mcg/ spray, 120 sprays/bottle.
NOTES - Ketoconazole significantly increase systemic concentrations, possibly causing adrenal suppression.

flunisolide (*Nasalide, Nasarel, ✿Rhinalar*) ▶L ♀C ▶? $$
ADULT - Allergic rhinitis: 2 sprays/nostril bid, may increase to tid. Max 8 sprays/nostril/day.
PEDS - Allergic rhinitis 6-14 yo: 1 spray per nostril tid or 2 sprays per nostril bid. Max 4 sprays/ nostril/day.
FORMS - Generic/Trade: Nasal soln 0.025%, 200 sprays/bottle. Nasalide with pump unit. Nasarel with meter pump & nasal adapter.

fluticasone (*Flonase, Veramyst*) ▶L ♀C ▶? $$$
ADULT - Allergic rhinitis: 2 sprays/nostril daily or 1 spray per nostril bid, decrease to 1 spray per nostril daily when appropriate. Seasonal allergic rhinitis alternative: 2 sprays/nostril daily prn.
PEDS - Allergic rhinitis: >4 yo: 1-2 sprays per nostril daily. Max 2 sprays/nostril/day. Seasonal allergic rhinitis alternative: >12 yo: 2 sprays per nostril daily prn.
FORMS - Generic/Trade: Flonase: Nasal spray 0.05%, 120 sprays/bottle. Trade only: (Veramyst): Nasal spray suspension: 27.5 mcg/ spray, 120 sprays/bottle.
NOTES - CYP3A4 inhibitors such as ketoconazole, erythromycin, ritonavir, etc significantly increase systemic concentrations, possibly causing adrenal suppression.

mometasone (*Nasonex*) ▶L ♀C ▶? $$$
ADULT - Allergic rhinitis: 2 sprays/nostril daily.
PEDS - Allergic rhinitis ≥12 yo: Use adult dose. 2-11 yo: 1 spray per nostril daily.
FORMS - Trade: Nasal spray, 120 sprays/bottle.

triamcinolone (*Nasacort AQ, Nasacort HFA, Tri-Nasal*) ▶L ♀C ▶- $$$
ADULT - Allergic rhinitis: Nasacort HFA, Tri-Nasal: Start 2 sprays/nostril daily, may increase to 2 sprays/nostril daily. Max 4 sprays/nostril/day. Nasacort AQ: 2 sprays per nostril daily.
PEDS - Allergic rhinitis: ≥12 yo: Use adult dose. 6-12 yo: 1-2 sprays per nostril daily (Nasacort & Nasacort AQ).
FORMS - Trade only: Nasal inhaler 55 mcg/ spray, 100 sprays/bottle (Nasacort HFA). Nasal spray, 55 mcg/spray, 120 sprays/bottle (Nasacort AQ). Nasal spray 50 mcg/spray, 120 sprays/bottle (Tri-Nasal).
NOTES - AQ (aqueous) formulation may cause less stinging. Decrease to lowest effective dose after allergy symptom improvement.

ENT – Nasal Preparations – Other

NOTE: For ALL nasal sprays except saline, oxymetazoline, & phenylephrine, tell patients to prime pump before 1st use and shake well before each subsequent use.

azelastine (*Astelin*) ▶L ♀C ▶? $$$
ADULT - Allergic/vasomotor rhinitis: 1-2 sprays/ nostril bid.
PEDS - Allergic rhinitis: ≥12 yo: Use adult dose. ≥5 yo: 1 spray/nostril bid. Vasomotor rhinitis ≥12 yo: Use adult dose.
FORMS - Trade only: Nasal spray, 200 sprays/ bottle.

cromolyn (*NasalCrom*) ▶LK ♀B ▶+ $
ADULT - Allergic rhinitis: 1 spray per nostril tid-qid up to 6 times/day.
PEDS - Allergic rhinitis ≥2 yo: Use adult dose.
FORMS - OTC: Generic/Trade: Nasal inhaler 200 sprays/bottle 13 & 26 mL.
NOTES - Therapeutic effects may not be seen for 1-2 weeks.

ipratropium (*Atrovent Nasal Spray*) ▶L ♀B ▶? $$
ADULT - Rhinorrhea due to allergic/non-allergic rhinitis: 2 sprays (0.03%) per nostril bid-tid or 2 sprays (0.06%) per nostril qid. Rhinorrhea due to common cold: 2 sprays (0.06%) per nostril tid-qid.
PEDS - Rhinorrhea due to allergic/non-allergic rhinitis ≥6 yo: Use adult dose (0.03%) or ≥5 yo: Use adult dose (0.06%). Rhinorrhea due to common cold ≥5 yo: 2 sprays (0.06%) per nostril tid.

UNAPPROVED ADULT - Vasomotor rhinitis: 2 sprays (0.06%) in each nostril tid-qid.

FORMS - Generic/Trade: Nasal spray 0.03%, 345 sprays/bottle & 0.06%, 165 sprays/bottle.

levocabastine (✿*Livostin Nasal Spray*) ▶L (but minimal absorption) ♀C ▶- $$

ADULT - Canada only. Allergic rhinitis: 2 sprays per nostril bid; increase prn to 2 sprays per nostril tid-qid.

PEDS - Not approved in children <12 yo.

FORMS - Trade: nasal spray 0.5 mg/mL, plastic bottles of 15 ml. Each spray delivers 50 mcg.

NOTES - Nasal spray is devoid of CNS effects. Unclear safety/efficacy if >65 yo.

oxymetazoline (*Afrin, Dristan 12 Hr Nasal, Nostrilla, Vicks Sinex 12 Hr*) ▶L ♀C ▶? $

ADULT - Nasal congestion: 2-3 sprays or drops (0.05%) per nostril bid prn rhinorrhea for ≤3 days.

PEDS - Nasal congestion ≥6 yo: 2-3 sprays or drops (0.05%) per nostril bid prn rhinorrhea for ≤3 days. 2-5 yo: 2-3 drops (0.025%) per nostril bid x 3 days.

FORMS - OTC: Generic/Trade: Nasal spray 0.05% 15 & 30 mL, Nøse drops 0.025% & 0.05% 20 mL with dropper.

NOTES - Overuse (>3-5 days) may lead to rebound congestion. If this occurs, taper to use in one nostril only, alternating sides, then discontinue. Substituting an oral decongestant or nasal steroid may also be useful.

phenylephrine (*Neo-Synephrine, Vicks Sinex*) ▶L ♀C ▶? $

ADULT - Nasal congestion: 2-3 sprays or drops (0.25 or 0.5%) per nostril q4h prn x 3 days. Use 1% soln for severe congestion.

PEDS - Nasal congestion: >12 yo: Use adult dose. 6-12 yo: 2-3 drops or sprays (0.25%) per nostril q4h prn x 3 days. 1-5 yo: 2-3 drops (0.125% or 0.16%) per nostril q4h prn x 3 days. 6-11 mo: 1-2 drops (0.125% or 0.16%) per nostril q4h prn x 3 days.

FORMS - OTC: Generic/Trade: Nasal drops/spray 0.25, 0.5, 1% (15 mL).

NOTES - Overuse (>3-5 days) may lead to rebound congestion. If this occurs, taper to use in one nostril only, alternating sides, then discontinue. Substituting an oral decongestant or nasal steroid may also be useful.

saline nasal spray (*SeaMist, Entsol, Pretz, NaSal, Ocean, ✿HydraSense*) ▶Not metabolized ♀A ▶+ $

ADULT - Nasal dryness: 1-3 sprays/nostril prn.

PEDS - Nasal dryness: 1-3 drops per nostril prn.

FORMS - Generic/Trade: Nasal spray 0.4, 0.5, 0.65, 0.75%, Nasal drops 0.4 & 0.65%. Trade: Preservative Free-Nasal spray 3% (Entsol).

NOTES – Home preparation: 1/4 teaspoon salt with 8 ounces (1 cup) warm water. Add 1/4 teaspoon baking soda (optional) and put in spray bottle, ear syringe, or any container with a small spout. Discard after one week.

ENT: Other

Cetacaine (benzocaine + tetracaine + butyl aminobenzoate) ▶LK ♀C ▶? $$

WARNING - Do not use on the eyes. Hypersensitivity (rare). Methemoglobinemia (rare).

ADULT - Topical anesthesia of mucous membranes: Spray: Apply for 1 second or less. Liquid or gel: Apply with cotton applicator directly to site.

PEDS - Use adult dose.

FORMS - Trade only: (14%-2%-2%) Spray 56 mL. Topical liquid 56 mL. Hospital gel 29 g.

NOTES - Do not hold cotton applicator in position for extended time due to increased risk of local reactions. Do not use multiple applications. Maximum anesthesia occurs 1 minute after application; duration 30 minutes. May result in potentially dangerous methemoglobinemia; use minimum amount needed.

GASTROENTEROLOGY: Antidiarrheals

bismuth subsalicylate (*Pepto-Bismol, Kaopectate*) ▶K ♀D ▶? $

WARNING - Avoid in children and teenagers with chickenpox or flu due to possible association with Reye's syndrome.

ADULT - Diarrhea: 2 tabs or 30 mL (262 mg/15 mL) PO q 30 min-60 min up to 8 doses/day.

PEDS - Diarrhea: 100 mg/kg/day divided into 5 doses. Age 3-6 yo: 1/3 tab or 5 mL (262 mg/15 mL) every 30 min-60 min prn up to 8 doses/day. 6-9 yo: 2/3 tab or 10 mL (262 mg/15 mL) every 30 min-1 hr prn up to 8 doses/day. 9-12 yo: 1 tab or 15 mL (262 mg/15 mL) every 30 min-1 hr prn up to 8 doses/day.

UNAPPROVED ADULT - Prevention of traveler's diarrhea: 2.1g/day or 2 tab qid before meals and qhs. Has been used as part of a multi-drug regimen for Helicobacter pylori.

UNAPPROVED PEDS - Chronic infantile diarrhea: Age 2-24 mo: 2.5 mL (262 mg/15 mL) PO q4h. 24-48 mo: 5 mL (262 mg/15 mL) q4h. 48-70 mo: 10 mL (262 mg/15 mL) q4h.

FORMS - OTC Generic/Trade: chew tab 262 mg, susp 262,525,750 mg/15 mL. Generic only: susp 130 mg/15 mL. Trade only: caplets 262 mg (Pepto-Bismol), susp 87 mg/5 mL (Kaopectate Children's Liquid), caplets 750mg (Kaopectate).

NOTES - Caution in patients already taking salicylates or warfarin, children recovering from chickenpox or flu. Decreases absorption of tetracycline. May darken stools or tongue.

Imodium Advanced (loperamide + simethicone) ▶L ♀B ▶+ $

ADULT - Diarrhea: 2 caplets PO initially, then 1 caplet PO after each unformed stool to a maximum of 4 caplets/24 h.

PEDS - Diarrhea: 1 caplet PO initially, then ½ caplet PO after each unformed stool to a max of 2 caplets/day (if 6-8 yo or 48-59 lbs) or 3 caplets/day (if 9-11 yo or 60-95 lbs).

FORMS - OTC Generic/trade: caplet & chew tab 2 mg loperamide/125 mg simethicone.

NOTES - Not for pseudomembranous colitis, toxigenic bacterial diarrhea, or most childhood diarrhea (difficult to exclude toxigenic).

Lomotil (diphenoxylate + atropine) ▶L ♀C ▶- ©V $

ADULT - Diarrhea: 2 tabs or 10 mL PO qid.

PEDS - Diarrhea: 0.3-0.4 mg diphenoxylate/kg/24h in 4 divided doses. Age <2 yo: not recommended. 2 yo: 1.5-3 mL PO qid; 3 yo: 2-3 mL PO qid; 4 yo: 2-4 mL qid; 5 yo: 2.5-4.5 mL qid; 6-8 yo: 2.5-5 mL qid; 9-12 yo: 3.5-5 mL qid.

FORMS - Generic/Trade: soln 2.5/0.025 mg diphenox./atropine per 5 mL, tab 2.5/0.025 mg.

NOTES - Give with food to decrease GI upset. May cause atropinism in children, esp. with Down syndrome, even at recommended doses. Can cause delayed toxicity. Has been reported to cause severe respiratory depression, coma, brain damage, death after overdose in children. Do not use for pseudomembranous colitis, toxigenic bacterial diarrhea, or most childhood diarrhea (difficult to exclude toxigenic).

loperamide (Imodium, Imodium AD, ♣Loperacap, Diarr-eze) ▶L ♀B ▶+ $

WARNING - Discontinue if abdominal distention or ileus. Caution in children due to variable response. Diarrhea may need concurrent fluid/electrolyte repletion.

ADULT - Diarrhea: 4 mg PO initially, then 2 mg after each unformed stool to max 16 mg/day.

PEDS - Diarrhea (first day): Age 2-5 yo (13-20 kg): 1 mg PO tid. 6-8 yo (20-30 kg): 2 mg PO bid. 9-12 yo (>30 kg): 2 mg PO tid. After first day, give 1 mg/10 kg PO after each loose stool; daily dose not to exceed daily dose of first day.

UNAPPROVED ADULT - Chronic diarrhea or ileostomy drainage : 4 mg initially then 2 mg after each stool until symptoms are controlled, then reduce dose for maintenance treatment, average adult maintenance dose 4-8 mg daily as a single dose or in divided doses.

UNAPPROVED PEDS - Chronic diarrhea: limited information. Average doses of 0.08-0.24 mg/kg/day PO in 2-3 divided doses.

FORMS - Rx Generic/Trade: cap 2 mg, tab 2 mg. OTC Generic/Trade: tab 2 mg, liquid 1 mg/5 mL.

NOTES - Not for pseudomembranous colitis, toxigenic bacterial diarrhea, or most childhood diarrhea (difficult to exclude toxigenic).

Motofen (difenoxin + atropine) ▶L ♀C ▶- ©IV $

ADULT - Diarrhea: 2 tabs PO initially, then 1 after each loose stool q3-4 h prn. Maximum of 8 tabs/24h.

PEDS - Not approved in children. Contraindicated in children <2 yo.

FORMS - Trade only: tab difenoxin 1 mg + atropine 0.025 mg.

NOTES - Do not use for pseudomembranous colitis, toxigenic bacterial diarrhea, or most childhood diarrhea (difficult to exclude toxigenic). May cause atropinism in children, esp. with Down's syndrome, even at recommended doses. Can cause delayed toxicity. Has been reported to cause severe respiratory depression, coma, brain damage, death after overdose in children. Difenoxin is the primary metabolite of diphenoxylate.

opium (opium tincture, paregoric) ▶L ♀B (D with long-term use) ▶? ©II (opium tincture), III (paregoric) $$

ADULT - Diarrhea: 5-10 mL paregoric PO daily-qid or 0.3-0.6 mL PO opium tincture qid.

PEDS - Diarrhea: 0.25-0.5 mL/kg paregoric PO daily-qid or 0.005-0.01 mL/kg PO opium tincture q3-4h, max 6 doses/day.

FORMS - Trade only: opium tincture 10% (deodorized opium tincture, 10 mg morphine equivalent per mL). Generic only: paregoric (camphorated opium tincture, 2 mg morphine equivalent/5 mL).

NOTES - Opium tincture contains 25 times more morphine than paregoric. Do not use for pseudomembranous colitis, toxigenic bacterial diarrhea, or most childhood diarrhea.

GASTROENTEROLOGY: Antiemetics – 5-HT3 Receptor Antagonists

dolasetron (*Anzemet*) ▶LK ♀B ▶? $$$
ADULT - Prevention of N/V with chemo: 1.8 mg/kg up to 100 mg IV/PO single dose 30 min (IV) or 60 min (PO) before chemo. Prevention/treatment of post-op N/V: 12.5 mg IV as a single dose 15 minutes before end of anesthesia or as soon as N/V starts. Alternative for prevention 100 mg PO 2 h before surgery.
PEDS - Prevention of N/V with chemo in children 2-16 yo: 1.8 mg/kg up to 100 mg IV/PO single dose 30 min (IV) or 60 min (PO) before chemo. Prevention/treatment of post-op N/V in children 2-16 yo: 0.35 mg/kg IV as single dose 15 minutes before end of anesthesia or as soon as N/V starts. Max 12.5 mg. Prevention alternative 1.2 mg/kg PO to max of 100 mg 2 h before surgery.
UNAPPROVED ADULT - N/V due to radiotherapy: 40 mg IV as a single dose. Alternatively, 0.3 mg/kg IV as a single dose.
FORMS - Trade only: tab 50,100 mg.
NOTES - Use caution in patients of any age who have or may develop prolongation of QT interval (i.e. hypokalemia, hypomagnesemia, concomitant antiarrhythmic therapy, cumulative high-dose anthracycline therapy).

granisetron (*Kytril*) ▶L ♀B ▶? $$$
ADULT - Prevention of N/V with chemo: 10 mcg/kg over 5 min IV 30 mins prior to chemo. Oral: 1 mg PO bid x 1 day only. Radiation-induced N/V: 2 mg PO 1 hr before first irradiation fraction of each day. Prevention/treatment post-op N/V: 1 mg IV.
PEDS - Children 2-16 yo: Prevention of N/V with chemo: 10 mcg/kg IV 30 minutes prior to chemo. Oral form not approved in children.
FORMS - Trade only: tab 1 mg, oral soln 2 mg/10 mL (30 mL).

ondansetron (*Zofran*) ▶L ♀B ▶? $$$$$
ADULT - Prevention of N/V with chemo: 32 mg IV as a single dose over 15 min, or 0.15 mg/kg IV 30 minutes prior to chemo and repeated at 4 and 8 hrs after first dose. Alternatively, 8 mg PO 30 min before moderately emetogenic chemo and 8 h later. Can be given q12h for 1-2 days after completion of chemo. For single-day highly emetogenic chemo, 24 mg PO 30 min before chemo. Prevention of post-op nausea: 4 mg IV over 2-5 min or 4 mg IM or 16 mg PO 1 hr before anesthesia. Prevention of N/V associated with radiotherapy: 8 mg PO tid.
PEDS - Prevention of N/V with chemo: IV: Age >6 month: 0.15 mg/kg 30 minutes prior to chemo and repeated at 4 and 8 hrs after first dose. PO: Children 4-11 yo: 4 mg 30 minutes prior to chemo and repeated at 4 and 8 hrs after first dose. Can be given q8h for 1-2 days after completion of chemo. Children ≥12 yo: 8 mg PO 30 min before chemo and 8 h later. Prevention of post-op N/V: 1 month-12 yo: 0.1 mg/kg IV over 2-5 min x 1 if ≤40kg; 4 mg IV over 2-5 min x 1 if >40 kg.
UNAPPROVED ADULT - Has been used in hyperemesis associated with pregnancy.
UNAPPROVED PEDS - <4 yo based on BSA (with caution): <0.3 m²: 1 mg PO tid. 0.3-0.6 m²: 2 mg PO tid. 0.6-1 m²: 3 mg PO tid. >1 m²: 4 mg PO tid. Caution if <6 months of age.
FORMS - Generic/Trade: Tab 4, 8, 24 mg, orally disintegrating tab 4, 8 mg, solution 4 mg/5 mL. Generic only: Tab 16 mg, orally disintegrating tab 16, 24 mg.
NOTES - Max oral dose if severe liver disease is 8 mg/day. Use following abdominal surgery or in those receiving chemotherapy may mask a progressive ileus or gastric distension.

palonosetron (*Aloxi*) ▶L ♀B ▶? $$$$$
ADULT - Prevention of N/V with chemo: 0.25 mg IV over 30 seconds, 30 min prior to chemo.
PEDS - Not approved in children.
NOTES - Caution with cardiac conduction delay propensity, especially prolonged QTc.

GASTROENTEROLOGY: Antiemetics – Other

aprepitant (*Emend*) ▶L ♀B ▶? $$$$$
ADULT - Prevention of N/V with moderately to highly emetogenic chemo, in combination with dexamethasone and ondansetron: 125 mg PO

on day 1 (1 h prior to chemo), then 80 mg PO q am on days 2 & 3. Prevention of postoperative N/V: 40 mg PO <3 hours prior to anesthesia.

PEDS - Not approved in children.

FORMS - Trade only: cap 40, 80, 125 mg.

NOTES - Use caution with other medications metabolized by CYP3A4 hepatic enzyme system and an inducer of the CYP2C9 hepatic enzyme system. Contraindicated with pimozide. May decrease efficacy of oral contraceptives; women should use alternate/back-up method. Monitor INR in patients receiving warfarin.

Diclectin (doxylamine + pyridoxine) ▶LK ♀A ▶? $

ADULT - Canada only. Nausea / vomiting in pregnancy. 2 tabs PO qhs. May add 1 tab in am and 1 tab in afternoon, if needed.

PEDS - Not approved in children.

FORMS - Trade only: delayed-release tab doxylamine 10 mg + pyridoxine 10 mg.

dimenhydrinate (Dramamine, ✦Gravol) ▶LK ▶- $

ADULT - Nausea: 50-100 mg/dose PO/IM/IV q4-6h prn. Maximum PO dose 400 mg/24h, maximum IM dose 300 mg/24h.

PEDS - Nausea: Age <2 yo: not recommended. 2-6 yo: 12.5-25 mg PO q6-8h or 5 mg/kg/24h divided q6h. Max daily PO dose: 75 mg/24h. Children 6-12 yo: 25-50 mg PO q6-8h. Max daily PO dose 150 mg/24h.

FORMS - OTC: Generic/Trade: tab 50 mg. Trade only: chew tab 50 mg. Generic only: solution 12.5 mg/5ml.

NOTES - May cause drowsiness. Use with caution in conditions which may be aggravated by anticholinergic effects (i.e. prostatic hypertrophy, asthma, narrow-angle glaucoma).

domperidone (✦Motilium) ▶L ♀? ▶- $

ADULT - Canada only. Postprandial dyspepsia: 10-20 mg PO tid-qid, 30 min before a meal.

PEDS - Not approved in children.

UNAPPROVED ADULT - Has been used for diabetic gastroparesis, chemotherapy/radiation induced N/V. Has also been used to increase milk production in lactating mothers although this is not considered safe.

UNAPPROVED PEDS - Use in children not recommended except for chemotherapy or radiation-induced N/V: 200-400 mcg/kg PO q4-8h.

FORMS - Canada only. Trade/generic: tabs 10, 20 mg.

NOTES - Similar in efficacy to metoclopramide but less likely to cause EPS.

doxylamine (Unisom Nighttime Sleep Aid, *others)* ▶L ♀A ▶? $

PEDS - Not approved in children.

UNAPPROVED ADULT - Nausea and vomiting associated with pregnancy: 12.5 mg PO bid; often used in combination with pyridoxine.

FORMS - OTC Generic/Trade: tab 25 mg.

dronabinol (Marinol) ▶L ♀C ▶- ©III $$$$$

ADULT - Nausea with chemo: 5 mg/m² PO 1-3 h before chemo then 5 mg/m²/dose q2-4h after chemo for 4-6 doses/day. Dose can be increased to max 15 mg/m². Anorexia associated with AIDS: Initially 2.5 mg PO bid before lunch and dinner. Maximum 20 mg/day.

PEDS - Not approved in children.

UNAPPROVED PEDS - Nausea with chemo: 5 mg/m² PO 1-3 h before chemo then 5 mg/m²/dose q2-4h after chemo for 4-6 doses/day. Dose can be increased to max 15 mg/m².

FORMS - Trade only: cap 2.5, 5, 10 mg.

NOTES - Patient response varies; individualize dosing (start low in elderly). Additive CNS effects with alcohol, sedatives, hypnotics, psychomimetics. Caution if history of seizures.

droperidol (Inapsine) ▶L ♀C ▶? $

WARNING - Cases of fatal QT prolongation and/or torsades de pointes have occurred at or below recommended doses (some without risk factors for QT prolongation). Reserve for non-response to other treatments, and ECG monitor prior to administration and 2-3 hours after. Use with extreme caution (if at all) if prolonged baseline QT.

ADULT - Antiemetic premedication: 0.625-2.5 mg IV or 2.5 mg IM then 1.25 mg prn.

PEDS - Preop: Age 2-12 yo: 0.088-0.165 mg/kg IV. Post-op antiemetic: 0.01-0.03 mg/kg/dose IV q 6-8h prn. Usual dose 0.05-0.06 mg/kg/dose; maximum of 0.1 mg/kg.

UNAPPROVED ADULT - Chemo-induced nausea: 2.5-5 mg IV/IM q 3-4h prn.

UNAPPROVED PEDS - Chemo-induced nausea: 0.05-0.06 mg/kg/dose IV/IM q 4-6h prn.

NOTES - Has no analgesic or amnestic effects. Consider lower doses in geriatric, debilitated, or high-risk patients such as those receiving other CNS depressants. May cause hypotension or tachycardia, EPS, drowsiness.

metoclopramide (Reglan, ✦Maxeran) ▶K ♀B ▶? $

ADULT - Gastroesophageal reflux: 10-15 mg PO qid 30 min before meals and qhs. Diabetic gastroparesis: 10 mg PO/IV/IM 30 min before meals and bedtime. Prevention of chemo-induced emesis: 1-2 mg/kg 30 min before chemo and then q2h for 2 doses then q3h for 3 doses prn. Prevention of post-op nausea: 10-20 mg IM/IV near end of surgical procedure, may repeat q3-4 h prn. Intubation of small intestine, radiographic exam of upper GI tract: 10 mg IV.

PEDS - Intubation of small intestine: Age <6 yo: 0.1 mg/kg IV. 6-14 yo: 2.5-5 mg IV. Radiographic exam of upper GI tract: Age <6 yo: 0.1 mg/kg IV; 6-14 yo: 2.5-5 mg IV.

UNAPPROVED ADULT - Prevention/treatment of chemo-induced emesis: 3 mg/kg over 1h followed by continuous IV infusion of 0.5 mg/kg/h for 12h. Migraine treatment: 10 mg IV. Migraine adjunct: 10 mg PO 5-10 min before ergotamine/analgesic/sedative.

UNAPPROVED PEDS - Gastroesophageal reflux: 0.4-0.8 mg/kg/day in 4 divided doses. Prevention of chemo-induced emesis: 1-2 mg/kg 30 min before chemo and then q3h prn, maximum of 5 doses/day or 5-10 mg/kg/day.

FORMS - Generic/Trade: tabs 5,10 mg, Generic only: soln 5 mg/5 mL.

NOTES - To reduce incidence and severity of akathisia, consider giving IV doses over 15 minutes. If EPS reactions occur (especially with high IV doses) give diphenhydramine IM/IV. Adjust dose in renal dysfunction. May cause drowsiness, agitation, seizures, hallucinations, galactorrhea, hyperprolactinemia, constipation, diarrhea. Increases cyclosporine and ethanol absorption. Do not use if bowel perforation or mechanical obstruction present. Levodopa decreases metoclopramide effects. Tardive dyskinesia in <1% with long-term use.

nabilone (*Cesamet*) ▶L ♀C ▶- ©II $$$$
ADULT - Nausea/vomiting in cancer chemotherapy with poor response to other agents: 1 to 2 mg PO bid, 1 to 3 hours before chemo. Max dose 6 mg/day in 3 divided doses.

PEDS - Not approved in children.

FORMS - Trade only: cap 1 mg.

NOTES - Contraindicated in known sensitivity to marijuana or other cannabinoids, current or past psychiatric reactions. Additive CNS effects with alcohol, sedatives, hypnotics, psychomimetics. Additive cardiac effects with amphetamines, antihistamines, anticholinergics.

phosphorated carbohydrates (*Emetrol*) ▶L ♀A ▶+ $
ADULT - Nausea: 15-30 mL PO q15 min until nausea subsides or up to 5 doses.

PEDS - Nausea: 2-12 yo: 5-10 mL q15 min until nausea subsides or up to 5 doses.

UNAPPROVED ADULT - Morning sickness: 15-30 mL PO upon rising, repeat q3h prn. Motion sickness or nausea due to drug therapy or anesthesia: 15 mL/dose.

UNAPPROVED PEDS - Regurgitation in infants: 5-10 mL PO 10-15 min prior to each feeding. Motion sickness or nausea due to drug therapy or anesthesia: 5 mL/dose.

FORMS - OTC Generic/Trade: Solution containing dextrose, fructose, and phosphoric acid.

NOTES - Do not dilute. Do not ingest fluids before or for 15 min after dose. Monitor blood glucose in diabetic patients.

prochlorperazine (*Compazine*, ✦*Stemetil*) ▶LK ♀C ▶? $
ADULT - Nausea/vomiting: 5-10 mg PO/IM tid-qid max 40 mg/day; 15-30 mg PO daily or 10 mg PO q12h of sustained release or 15 mg PO qam of sustained release; 25 mg PR q12h; 5-10 mg IV over at least 2 min q3-4h prn max 40 mg/day; 5-10 mg IM q3-4h prn max 40 mg/day.

PEDS - Nausea and vomiting: Age <2 yo or <10 kg: not recommended. >2 yo: 0.4 mg/kg/day PO/PR in 3-4 divided doses; 0.1-0.15 mg/kg/dose IM; IV not recommended.

UNAPPROVED ADULT - Migraine: 10 mg IV/IM or 25 mg PR single dose for acute headache.

UNAPPROVED PEDS - N/V during surgery: 5-10 mg IM 1-2 hr before anesthesia induction, may repeat in 30 min; 5-10 mg IV 15-30 min before anesthesia induction, may repeat once.

FORMS - Generic/Trade: tabs 5,10,25 mg, supp 25 mg. Trade only: extended-release caps (Compazine Spansules) 10,15,30 mg, supp 2.5,5 mg, liquid 5 mg/5 mL.

NOTES - May cause extrapyramidal reactions (especially in elderly), hypotension (with IV), arrhythmias, sedation, seizures, hyperprolactinemia, gynecomastia, dry mouth, constipation, urinary retention, leukopenia, thrombocytopenia. Elderly more prone to adverse effects.

promethazine (*Phenergan*) ▶LK ♀C ▶- $
WARNING - Contraindicated if <2 yo due to risk of fatal respiratory depression; caution if older.

ADULT - Nausea / vomiting: 12.5-25 mg q4-6h PO/IM/PR prn. Motion sickness: 25 mg PO/PR 30-60 min prior to departure and q12h prn. Hypersensitivity reactions: 25 mg IM/IV, may repeat in 2 hours. Allergic conditions: 12.5 mg PO/PR/IM/IV qid or 25 mg PO/PR qhs.

PEDS - N/V, ≥2 yo: 0.25-1 mg/kg/dose PO/IM/PR q4-6h prn. Motion sickness: 0.5 mg/kg PO 30-60 min prior to departure and q12h prn. Max 25 mg/dose. Hypersensitivity reactions, >2 yo: 6.25-12.5 mg PO/PR/IM/IV q6h prn.

UNAPPROVED ADULT - Nausea / vomiting: 12.5-25 mg IV q4h prn.

UNAPPROVED PEDS - Nausea / vomiting, ≥2 yo: 0.25-0.5 mg/kg/dose IV q4h prn.

FORMS - Generic/Trade: tab/supp 12.5, 25, 50 mg. Generic only: syrup 6.25 mg/5ml

NOTES - May cause sedation, extrapyramidal reactions (esp. with high IV doses), hypotension with rapid IV administration, anticholinergic side effects, eg, dry mouth, blurred vision.

scopolamine (*Transderm-Scop, Scopace, ♥Transderm-V*) ▶L ♀C ▶+ $

ADULT - Motion sickness: 1 disc behind ear at least 4h before travel and q3 days prn or 0.4-0.8 mg PO 1 hour before travel and q8h prn. Prevention of post-op N/V: Apply patch behind ear 4 h before surgery, remove 24 h after surgery. Spastic states, postencephalitic parkinsonism: 0.4-0.8 mg PO q8h prn.

PEDS - Not approved in children <12 yo.

UNAPPROVED PEDS - Pre-op and antiemetic: 6 mcg/kg/dose IM/IV/SC (max dose 0.3 mg/dose). May repeat q6-8h. Has been used in severe drooling.

FORMS - Trade only: topical disc 1.5 mg/72h, box of 4. Oral tablet 0.4 mg.

NOTES - Dry mouth common. Also causes drowsiness, blurred vision.

thiethylperazine (*Torecan*) ▶L ♀? ▶? $

ADULT - N/V: 10 mg PO/IM 1-3 times/day.

PEDS - Not approved in children.

FORMS - Trade only: tab 10 mg.

trimethobenzamide (*Tigan*) ▶LK ♀C but + ▶? $

ADULT - Nausea and vomiting: 250 mg PO q6-8h, 200 mg PR/IM q6-8h.

PEDS - N/V: Children <13.6kg (except neonates): 100 mg PR q6-8h. Children 13.6-40.9 kg: 100-200 mg PO/IM q6-8h.

FORMS - Generic/Trade: Caps 300 mg. Generic only: Caps 250 mg.

NOTES - Not for IV use. May cause sedation.

GASTROENTEROLOGY: Antiulcer – Antacids

***Alka-Seltzer* (aspirin + citrate + bicarbonate)** ▶LK ♀? (- 3rd trimester) ▶? $

ADULT - Relief of upset stomach: 2 regular strength tablets in 4 oz. water q4h PO prn, maximum 8 tablets (<60 yo) or 4 tablets (>60 yo) in 24h or 2 extra-strength tablets in 4 oz. water q6h PO prn, maximum 7 tablets (<60 yo) or 4 tablets (>60 yo) in 24h.

PEDS - Not approved in children.

FORMS - OTC Trade only: regular strength, original: ASA 325 mg + citric acid 1000 mg + sodium bicarbonate 1916 mg. Regular strength lemon lime and cherry: 325 mg + 1000 mg + 1700 mg. Extra-strength: 500 mg + 1000 mg + 1985 mg. Not all forms of Alka Seltzer contain aspirin (eg, Alka Seltzer Heartburn Relief).

NOTES - Avoid ASA-containing forms in children/teenagers due to Reye's syndrome risk.

aluminum hydroxide (*Alternagel, Amphojel, Alu-Tab, Alu-Cap, ♥Basalgel, Mucaine*) ▶K ♀+ (? 1st trimester) ▶? $

ADULT - Hyperphosphatemia in chronic renal failure (short term treatment only to avoid aluminum accumulation): 30-60 mL PO with meals. Upset stomach, indigestion: 5-10 mL or 1-2 tabs PO 6 times/day, between meals and qhs and prn.

PEDS - Not approved in children.

UNAPPROVED ADULT - Hyperphosphatemia in chronic renal failure (short term treatment only to avoid aluminum accumulation): 30-60 mL PO with meals. Symptomatic reflux: 15-30 mL PO q30-60 min. For long-term management of reflux disease: 15-30 mL PO 1 and 3 h after meals and qhs prn. Peptic ulcer disease: 15-45 mL or 1-3 tab PO 1 and 3h after meals and qhs. Prophylaxis against GI bleeding (titrate dose to maintain gastric pH >3.5): 30-60 mL or 2-4 tab PO q1-2h.

UNAPPROVED PEDS - Peptic ulcer disease: 5-15 mL PO 1 and 3h after meals and qhs. Prophylaxis against GI bleeding (titrate dose to maintain gastric pH >3.5): Neonates 0.5-1 mL/kg/dose PO q4h. Infants 2-5 mL PO q1-2h. Child: 5-15 mL PO q1-2h.

FORMS - OTC Generic/Trade: cap 475 mg, susp 320 & 600 mg/5 mL. Trade only: cap 400 mg (Alu-Cap)

NOTES - For concentrated suspensions, use ½ the recommended dose. May cause constipation. Avoid administration with tetracyclines, digoxin, iron, isoniazid, buffered/enteric aspirin, diazepam, fluoroquinolones.

***Citrocarbonate* (bicarbonate + citrate)** ▶K ♀? ▶? $

ADULT - 1-2 teaspoonfuls in cold water PO 15 minutes to 2 hours after meals prn.

PEDS - 6-12 yo: ¼-1/2 teaspoonful in cold water

PO after meals prn.
FORMS - OTC Trade only: sodium bicarbonate 0.78 g + sodium citrate anhydrous 1.82 g in each 1 teaspoonful dissolved in water, 150, 300g.
NOTES - Chronic use may cause metabolic alkalosis. Contains sodium.

***Gaviscon* (aluminum hydroxide + magnesium carbonate)** ▶K ♀? ▶? $
ADULT - 2-4 tabs or 15-30 mL (regular strength) or 10 mL (extra strength) PO qid prn.
PEDS - Not approved in children.
UNAPPROVED PEDS - Peptic ulcer disease: 5-15 mL PO after meals and prn.
FORMS - OTC Trade only: Tab: regular strength (Al hydroxide 80 mg + Mg trisilicate 20 mg), extra strength (Al hydroxide 160 mg + Mg carbonate 105 mg). Liquid: regular strength (Al hydroxide 95 mg + Mg carbonate 358 mg per 15 mL), extra strength (Al hydroxide 508 mg + Mg carbonate 475 mg per 30 mL)
NOTES - Contains alginic acid or sodium alginate which is considered an "inactive" ingredient. Alginic acid forms foam barrier which floats in stomach to minimize esophageal contact with acid. Chronic use may cause metabolic alkalosis. Contains sodium.

***Maalox* (aluminum hydroxide + magnesium hydroxide)** ▶K ♀+ (? 1st trimester) ▶? $
ADULT - Heartburn/indigestion: 10-20 mL or 1-4 tab PO qid, after meals and qhs and prn.
PEDS - Not approved in children.
UNAPPROVED PEDS - Peptic ulcer disease: 15-45 mL PO 1 & 3h after meals & qhs. Symptomatic reflux: 15-30 mL PO q30-60 min prn. For long-term management of reflux disease: 15-30 mL PO 1 and 3 h after meals & qhs prn. Prophylaxis against GI bleeding (titrate dose to maintain gastric pH >3.5): 30-60 mL PO q1-2h.
UNAPPROVED PEDS - Peptic ulcer disease: 5-15 mL PO 1 and 3h after meals and qhs. Prophylaxis against GI bleeding (titrate dose to maintain gastric pH >3.5): Neonates 1 mL/kg/dose PO q4h. Infants 2-5 mL PO q1-2h. Child: 5-15 mL PO q1-2h.
FORMS - OTC Generic/Trade: regular strength chew tab (Al hydroxide + Mg hydroxide 200/200 mg), susp (225/200 mg per 5 mL).
NOTES - Maalox Extra Strength and Maalox TC are more concentrated than Maalox. Maalox Plus has added simethicone. May cause constipation or diarrhea. Avoid concomitant administration with tetracyclines, digoxin, iron, isoniazid, buffered/enteric aspirin, diazepam, fluoroquinolones. Avoid chronic use in patients with renal dysfunction due to potential for magnesium accumulation.

magaldrate (Riopan) ▶K ♀+ (? 1st trimester) ▶? $
ADULT - Relief of upset stomach: 5-10 mL between meals and qhs and prn.
PEDS - Not approved in children.
UNAPPROVED PEDS - Peptic ulcer disease: 5-10 mL PO 1 and 3h after meals and qhs.
FORMS - OTC Trade only: susp 540 mg/5 mL. Riopan Plus (with simethicone) available as susp 540/20 mg/5 mL, chew tab 540/20 mg.
NOTES - Riopan Plus has added simethicone. Avoid concomitant administration with tetracyclines, fluoroquinolones, digoxin, iron, isoniazid, buffered/enteric aspirin, diazepam. Avoid chronic use in patients with renal failure.

***Mylanta* (aluminum hydroxide + magnesium hydroxide + simethicone)** ▶K ♀+ (? 1st trimester) ▶? $
ADULT - Heartburn/indigestion: 10-45 mL or 2-4 tab PO qid, after meals and qhs and prn.
PEDS - Safe dosing has not been established.
UNAPPROVED ADULT - Peptic ulcer disease: 15-45 mL PO 1 and 3h after meals and qhs. Symptomatic reflux: 15-30 mL PO q30-60 min. For long-term management of reflux: 15-30 mL PO 1 and 3 h postprandially and qhs prn.
UNAPPROVED PEDS - Peptic ulcer disease: 5-15 mL PO 1 and 3h after meals and qhs.
FORMS - OTC Generic/Trade: Liquid, double strength liquid, tab, double strength tab. Trade only: tab sodium + sugar + dye free.
NOTES - Mylanta Gelcaps contain calcium carbonate and magnesium hydroxide. May cause constipation or diarrhea. Avoid concomitant administration with tetracyclines, fluoroquinolones, digoxin, iron, isoniazid, buffered/enteric aspirin, diazepam. Avoid chronic use in renal dysfunction.

***Rolaids* (calcium carbonate + magnesium hydroxide)** ▶K ♀? ▶? $
ADULT - 2-4 tabs PO q1h prn, max 12 tabs/day (regular strength) or 10 tabs/day (extra-strength).
PEDS - Not approved in children.
FORMS - OTC Trade only: Tab: regular strength (Ca carbonate 550 mg, Mg hydroxide 110 mg), extra-strength (Ca carbonate 675 mg, Mg hydroxide 135 mg).
NOTES - Chronic use may cause metabolic alkalosis.

GASTROENTEROLOGY: Antiulcer – H2 Antagonists

cimetidine (*Tagamet, Tagamet HB*) ▶LK ♀B ▶+ $$$

ADULT - Treatment of duodenal or gastric ulcer: 800 mg PO qhs or 300 mg PO qid with meals and qhs or 400 mg PO bid. Prevention of duodenal ulcer: 400 mg PO qhs. Erosive esophagitis: 800 mg PO bid or 400 mg PO qid. Prevention or treatment of heartburn (OTC product only approved for this indication): 200 mg PO prn max 400 mg/day for up to 14 days. Hypersecretory conditions: 300 mg PO qid with meals and qhs. Patients unable to take oral medications: 300 mg IV/IM q6-8h or 37.5 mg/h continuous IV infusion. Prevention of upper GI bleeding in critically ill patients: 50 mg/h continuous infusion.

PEDS - Not approved in children.

UNAPPROVED ADULT - Prevention of aspiration pneumonitis during surgery: 400-600 mg PO or 300 mg IV 60-90 min prior to anesthesia. Has been used as adjunctive therapy with H1 antagonist for severe allergic reactions.

UNAPPROVED PEDS - Treatment of duodenal or gastric ulcers, erosive esophagitis, hypersecretory conditions: Neonates: 5-10 mg/kg/day PO/IV/IM q 8-12h. Infants: 10-20 mg/kg/day PO/IV/IM divided q6h. Children: 20-40 mg/kg/day PO/IV/IM divided q6h. Chronic viral warts in children: 25-40 mg/kg/day PO in divided doses.

FORMS - Rx Generic/Trade: tab 200, 300, 400, 800 mg. Rx Generic liquid 300 mg/5 mL. OTC Generic/Trade: tab 200 mg.

NOTES - May cause dizziness, drowsiness, headache, diarrhea, nausea. Decreased absorption of ketoconazole, itraconazole. Increased levels of carbamazepine, cyclosporine, diazepam, labetalol, lidocaine, theophylline, phenytoin, procainamide, quinidine, propranolol, tricyclic antidepressants, valproic acid, warfarin. Stagger doses of cimetidine and antacids. Decrease dose with CrCl <30 mL/min.

famotidine (*Pepcid, Pepcid AC, Maximum Strength Pepcid AC*) ▶LK ♀B ▶? $$

ADULT - Treatment of duodenal ulcer: 40 mg PO qhs or 20 mg PO bid. Maintenance of duodenal ulcer: 20 mg PO qhs. Treatment of gastric ulcer: 40 mg PO qhs. GERD: 20 mg PO bid. Treatment or prevention of heartburn: (OTC product only approved for this indication) 10-20 mg PO prn. Hypersecretory conditions:

20 mg PO q6h. Patients unable to take oral medications: 20 mg IV q12h.

PEDS - Not approved in children.

UNAPPROVED ADULT - Prevention of aspiration pneumonitis during surgery: 40 mg PO/IM prior to anesthesia. Upper GI bleeding: 20 mg IV q12h. Has been used as adjunct to H1 antagonist for severe allergic reactions.

UNAPPROVED PEDS - Treatment of duodenal or gastric ulcers, GERD, hypersecretory conditions: 0.6-0.8 mg/kg/day IV in 2-3 divided doses or 1-1.2 mg/kg/day PO in 2-3 divided doses, maximum 40 mg/day. GERD: <3 mo: 0.5 mg/kg PO daily; 3-12 months: 0.5 mg/kg PO bid; 1-16 yo:1 mg/kg/day PO divided bid.

FORMS - Generic/Trade: tab 10 mg (OTC, Pepcid AC Acid Controller), 20 (Rx and OTC, Maximum Strength Pepcid AC), 30, 40 mg. Rx Trade only: susp.40 mg/5 mL.

NOTES - May cause dizziness, headache, constipation, diarrhea. Decreased absorption of ketoconazole, itraconazole. Adjust dose in patients with CrCl <60 mL/min.

nizatidine (*Axid, Axid AR*) ▶K ♀B ▶? $$$$

ADULT - Treatment of duodenal or gastric ulcer: 300 mg PO qhs or 150 mg PO bid. Maintenance of duodenal ulcer: 150 mg PO qhs. GERD: 150 mg PO bid. Treatment or prevention of heartburn: (OTC product only approved for this) 75 mg PO prn, max 150 mg/day.

PEDS - Age ≥12 yo: Esophagitis, GERD: 150 mg PO bid.

UNAPPROVED ADULT - Has been used as adjunctive therapy with H1 antagonist for severe allergic reactions.

UNAPPROVED PEDS - 6 mos-11 yo (limited data): 6-10 mg/kg/day PO in 2 divided doses.

FORMS - OTC Trade only (Axid AR): tabs 75 mg Rx Trade: oral solution 15 mg/mL (120, 480 mL). Rx Generic/Trade: cap 150, 300 mg.

NOTES - May cause dizziness, headache, constipation, diarrhea. Decrease absorption of ketoconazole, itraconazole. Adjust dose if CrCl <80 mL/min.

Pepcid Complete (famotidine + calcium carbonate + magnesium hydroxide) ▶LK ♀B ▶? $

ADULT - Treatment of heartburn: 1 tab PO prn. Max 2 tabs/day.

PEDS - Not approved in children.

FORMS - OTC: Trade only: chew tab famotidine

10 mg with calcium carbonate 800 mg & magnesium hydroxide 165 mg.

ranitidine (Zantac, Zantac 25, Zantac 75, Zantac 150, Peptic Relief) ▶K ♀B ▶? $$$
ADULT - Treatment of duodenal ulcer: 150 mg PO bid or 300 mg qhs. Treatment of gastric ulcer or GERD: 150 mg PO bid. Maintenance of duodenal or gastric ulcer: 150 mg PO qhs. Treatment of erosive esophagitis: 150 mg PO qid. Maintenance of erosive esophagitis: 150 mg PO bid. Prevention/treatment of heartburn: (OTC product only approved for this indication) 75-150 mg PO prn, max 300 mg/day. Hypersecretory conditions: 150 mg PO bid. Patients unable to take oral meds: 50 mg IV/IM q6-8h or 6.25 mg/h continuous IV infusion.
PEDS - Children 1 month - 16 years: Treatment of duodenal or gastric ulcers: 2-4 mg/kg/24h PO divided bid (max 300 mg) or 2-4 mg/kg/day IV divided q6-8h. GERD, erosive esophagitis: 5-10 mg/kg/24h PO divided bid or 2-4 mg/kg/day IV divided q6-8h. Maintenance of duodenal or gastric ulcers: 2-4 mg/kg/24h PO daily (max 150 mg).
UNAPPROVED ADULT - Prevention of upper GI bleeding in critically ill patients: 6.25 mg/h continuous IV infusion (150 mg/d). Has been used as adjunctive therapy with H1 antagonist for severe allergic reactions.
UNAPPROVED PEDS - Treatment of duodenal or gastric ulcers, GERD, hypersecretory conditions: Neonates: 2-4 mg/kg/24h PO divided q12h or 2 mg/kg/24h IV divided q12h. Infants and children: 2-4 mg/kg/24h IV/IM divided q12h or 0.1-0.2 mg/kg/h continuous IV infusion. Premature and term infants <2 weeks of age: 2 mg/kg/day PO divided q12h. 1.5 mg/kg IV x1 then 12 h later 1.5-2 mg/kg/day IV divided q12h. Continuous infusion 1.5 mg/kg x1 then 0.04-0.08 mg/kg/h infusion.
FORMS - Generic/Trade: tabs 75 mg (OTC, Zantac 75, Zantac 150), 150,300 mg, syrup 75 mg/5 mL. Rx Trade only: effervescent tab 25,150 mg. Rx Generic only: caps 150,300 mg.
NOTES - May cause dizziness, sedation, headache, drowsiness, rash, nausea, constipation, diarrhea. Variable effects on warfarin, decreased absorption of ketoconazole, itraconazole. Dissolve granules and effervescent tablets in water. Stagger doses of ranitidine and antacids. Adjust dose if CrCl <50 mL/min.

HELICOBACTER PYLORI THERAPY

- Triple therapy PO x 7-14 days: clarithromycin 500 mg bid + amoxicillin 1 g bid (or metronidazole 500 mg bid) + a proton pump inhibitor*
- Quadruple therapy PO x 14 days: bismuth subsalicylate 525 mg (or 30 mL) tid-qid + metronidazole 500 mg tid-qid + tetracycline 500 mg tid-qid + a proton pump inhibitor* or a H2 blocker†

*PPI's esomeprazole 40 mg qd, lansoprazole 30 mg bid, omeprazole 20 mg bid, pantoprazole 40 mg bid, rabeprazole 20 mg bid. †H2 blockers cimetidine 400 mg bid, famotidine 20 mg bid, nizatidine 150 mg bid, ranitidine 150 mg bid. Adapted from *Medical Letter Treatment Guidelines* 2004.

GASTROENTEROLOGY: Antiulcer – Helicobacter pylori Treatment

NOTE: For "notes", see components.

Helidac **(bismuth subsalicylate + metronidazole + tetracycline)** ▶LK ♀D ▶- $$$$
ADULT - Active duodenal ulcer associated with Helicobacter pylori: 1 dose PO qid, at meals and qhs for 2 weeks with an H2 antagonist.
PEDS - Not approved in children.
UNAPPROVED ADULT - Active duodenal ulcer associated with H pylori: Same as "adult", but substitute proton inhibitor for H2 antagonist.
FORMS - Trade: Each dose: bismuth subsalicylate 524 (2x262 mg) chewable tab + metronidazole 250 mg tab + tetracycline 500 mg cap.

PrevPac **(lansoprazole + amoxicillin + clarithromycin, ✦HP-Pac)** ▶LK ♀C ▶? $$$$$
ADULT - Active duodenal ulcer associated with H pylori: 1 dose PO bid x 10-14 days.
PEDS - Not approved in children.
FORMS - Trade only: lansoprazole 30 mg x 2 + amoxicillin 1 g (2x500 mg) x 2, clarithromycin 500 mg x 2.

Pylera **(biskalcitrate + metronidazole + tetracycline)** ▶LK ♀D ▶- $$$$$
ADULT - Duodenal ulcer associated with H. pylori: 3 capsules PO qid (after meals and at bedtime) x 10 days. To be given with omeprazole 20 mg PO bid.
PEDS - Not approved in children.
FORMS - Trade: Capsule: biskalcitrate 140 mg + metronidazole 125 mg + tetracycline 125 mg.

GASTROENTEROLOGY: Antiulcer – Proton Pump Inhibitors

esomeprazole (Nexium) ▶L ♀B ▶? $$$$
ADULT - Erosive esophagitis: 20-40 mg PO daily x 4-8 weeks. Maintenance of erosive esophagitis: 20 mg PO daily. Zollinger-Ellison: 40 mg PO bid x 4-8 weeks, may repeat for additional 4-8 weeks. GERD: 20 mg PO daily x 4 weeks. GERD with esophagitis: 20-40 mg IV daily x 10 days until taking PO. Prevention of NSAID-associated gastric ulcer: 20-40 mg PO daily x up to 6 months. H pylori eradication: 40 mg PO daily with amoxicillin 1000 mg PO bid & clarithromycin 500 mg PO bid x 10 days.
PEDS - 12-17 yo: GERD: 20-40 mg daily for up to 8 weeks. Not approved in children <12 yo.
FORMS - Trade only: delayed release cap 20, 40 mg. Suspension powder 20, 40 mg.
NOTES - May decrease absorption of ketoconazole, itraconazole, digoxin, iron, and ampicillin. Concomitant voriconazole may lead to a more than doubling of esomeprazole exposure.

lansoprazole (Prevacid, Prevacid Napra-Pac) ▶L ♀B ▶? $$$$
ADULT - Erosive esophagitis: 30 mg PO daily or 30 mg IV daily x 7 days or until taking PO. Maintenance therapy following healing of erosive esophagitis: 15 mg PO daily. NSAID-induced gastric ulcer: 30 mg PO daily x 8 weeks (treatment), 15 mg PO daily for up to 12 weeks (prevention). GERD: 15 mg PO daily. Duodenal ulcer treatment and maintenance: 15 mg PO daily. Gastric ulcer: 30 mg PO daily. Part of a multidrug regimen for H. pylori eradication: 30 mg PO bid with amoxicillin 1000 mg PO bid & clarithromycin 500 mg PO bid x 10-14 days (see table) or 30 mg PO tid with amoxicillin 1000 mg PO tid x 14 days. Hypersecretory conditions: 60 mg PO daily.
PEDS - Erosive esophagitis and GERD (1-11 yo) ≤30 kg: 15 mg PO daily x up to 12 weeks. >30 kg: 30 mg PO daily x up to 12 weeks. Non-erosive GERD (12-17 yo): 15 mg PO daily x up to 8 weeks. GERD with erosive esophagitis (12-17 yo): 30 mg PO daily x up to 8 weeks.
FORMS - Trade only: cap 15,30 mg. Susp 15,30 mg packets. Orally disintegrating tab 15,30 mg. Prevacid NapraPac: 7 lansoprazole 15 mg caps packaged with 14 naproxen tabs 375 mg or 500 mg.
NOTES - Take before meals. Avoid concomitant sucralfate. May decrease absorption of atazanavir, ketoconazole, itraconazole, ampicillin, digoxin and iron. Orally disintegrating tablets can be dissolved water (15 mg tab in 4 mL, 30 mg tab in 10 mL) and administered via an oral syringe or nasogastric tube ≥8 French.

omeprazole (Prilosec, ✦Losec) ▶L ♀C ▶? $$$$
ADULT - GERD, duodenal ulcer, erosive esophagitis: 20 mg PO daily. Heartburn (OTC): 20 mg PO daily x 14 days. Gastric ulcer: 40 mg PO daily. Hypersecretory conditions: 60 mg PO daily. Part of a multidrug regimen for H pylori: 20 mg PO bid with amoxicillin 1000 mg PO bid & clarithromycin 500 mg PO bid x 10 days, with additional 18 days of omeprazole 20 mg PO daily if ulcer present (see table). Or 40 mg PO daily with clarithromycin 500 mg PO tid x 14 days, with additional 14 days of omeprazole 20 mg PO daily if ulcer present.
PEDS - GERD (2-16 yo) <20 kg: 10 mg PO daily. ≥20 kg: 20 mg PO daily.
UNAPPROVED ADULT - Upper gastrointestinal bleeding: 80 mg IV, then infusion 8 mg/hour until endoscopy.
UNAPPROVED PEDS – Gastric/duodenal hypersecretory states/ulcers: 0.7-3.3 mg/kg/dose PO daily. GERD: 1 mg/kg/day PO daily or bid.
FORMS - Rx Generic/Trade: Cap 10, 20 mg. Trade only: Cap 40 mg. OTC: 20 mg.
NOTES - Take before meals. Caps contain enteric-coated granules; do not chew. Caps may be opened and administered in acidic liquid (eg, apple juice). May increase levels of diazepam, warfarin, and phenytoin. May decrease absorption of ketoconazole, itraconazole, iron, ampicillin, and digoxin. Reduces plasma levels of atazanavir. Concomitant administration with voriconazole may more than double omeprazole exposure. Avoid with sucralfate.

pantoprazole (Protonix, ✦Pantoloc) ▶L ♀B ▶? $$$$
ADULT - 40 mg PO daily for 8-16 weeks. Maintenance therapy following healing of erosive esophagitis: 40 mg PO daily. Zollinger-Ellison syndrome: 80 mg IV q8-12h x 6 days until taking PO. GERD associated with a history of erosive esophagitis: 40 mg IV daily x 7-10 days until taking PO.
PEDS - Not approved in children.
UNAPPROVED ADULT - Has been studied as part of various multidrug regimens for H. pylori eradication. Decreases peptic ulcer rebleeding

after hemostasis: 80 mg IV bolus, then 8 mg/h continuous IV infusion x 3 days, followed by oral therapy (or 40 mg IV q12h for 4-7 days if unable to tolerate PO).

UNAPPROVED PEDS - GERD associated with a history of erosive esophagitis: 0.5-1 mg/kg/day (max 40 mg/day).

FORMS - Trade only: Tabs 20, 40 mg.

NOTES - May decrease absorption of ketoconazole, itraconazole, digoxin, iron, and ampicillin. Can increase INR when used with warfarin.

rabeprazole (*Aciphex*, ♥*Pariet*) ▶L ♀B ▶? $$$$

ADULT - GERD: 20 mg PO daily x 4-16 weeks. Duodenal ulcers: 20 mg PO daily x 4 weeks. Zollinger-Ellison syndrome: 60 mg PO daily, may increase up to 100 mg daily or 60 mg bid. Part of a multidrug regimen for H. pylori: 20 mg PO bid, with amoxicillin 1000 mg PO bid & clarithromycin 500 mg PO bid x 7 days.

PEDS - Not approved in children.

FORMS - Generic/Trade: Tab 20 mg.

NOTES - May decrease absorption of ketoconazole, itraconazole, digoxin, iron, and ampicillin.

***Zegerid* (omeprazole + bicarbonate)** ▶L ♀C ▶? $$$$

ADULT - Duodenal ulcer, GERD, erosive esophagitis: 20 mg PO daily x 4-8 weeks. Gastric ulcer: 40 mg PO once daily x 4-8 weeks. Reduction of risk of upper GI bleed in critically ill (susp only): 40 mg PO, then 40 mg 6-8h later, then 40 mg once daily thereafter x 14 days.

PEDS - Not approved in children.

FORMS - Trade: Caps 20/1,100 & 40/1,100 mg omeprazole/sodium bicarbonate, powder packets for suspension 20/1,680 & 40/1,680 mg.

NOTES - Do not combine two 20 mg doses for a 40 mg dose, since the dose of sodium bicarbonate is the same in both dose strengths. May increase levels of diazepam, warfarin, and phenytoin. May decrease absorption of ketoconazole, itraconazole, iron, ampicillin, and digoxin. Reduces plasma levels of atazanavir. Avoid administration with sucralfate.

GASTROENTEROLOGY: Antiulcer – Other

***Bellergal-S* (phenobarbital + belladonna + ergotamine, ♥*Bellergal Spacetabs*)** ▶LK ♀X ▶- $

WARNING - Serious or life-threatening peripheral ischemia has been noted with ergotamine when used with P450 3A4 inhibitors such as ritonavir, nelfinavir, indinavir, erythromycin, clarithromycin, ketoconazole, and itraconazole.

ADULT - Hypermotility/hypersecretion: 1 tab PO bid.

PEDS - Not approved in children.

FORMS - Generic/Trade: Tab phenobarbital 40 mg, ergotamine 0.6 mg, belladonna 0.2 mg.

NOTES - May decrease INR in patients receiving warfarin. Variable effect on phenytoin levels. May cause sedation especially with alcohol, phenothiazines, opioids, or tricyclic antidepressants. Additive anticholinergic effects with tricyclic antidepressants.

dicyclomine (*Bentyl, Bentylol, Antispas*, ♥*Formulex, Protylol, Lomine*) ▶LK ♀B ▶- $$

ADULT - Treatment of functional bowel/irritable bowel syndrome (irritable colon, spastic colon, mucous colon): Initiate with 20 mg PO qid and increase to 40 mg PO qid, if tolerated. If unable to take oral medications: 20 mg IM q6h.

PEDS - Not approved in children.

UNAPPROVED PEDS - Treatment of functional / irritable bowel syndrome: Infants >6 months: 5 mg PO tid-qid. Children: 10 mg PO tid-qid.

FORMS - Generic/Trade: Tab 20 mg, cap 10 mg, syrup 10 mg/5 mL. Generic: cap 20 mg.

NOTES - Although some use lower doses (i.e., 10-20 mg PO qid), the only adult oral dose proven to be effective is 160 mg/day.

***Donnatal* (phenobarbital + atropine + hyoscyamine + scopolamine)** ▶LK ♀C ▶- $

ADULT - Adjunctive therapy of irritable bowel syndrome or adjunctive treatment of duodenal ulcers: 1-2 tabs/caps or 5-10 mL PO tid-qid or 1 extended release tab PO q8-12h.

PEDS - Adjunctive therapy of irritable bowel syndrome: 0.1 mL/kg/dose PO q4h, maximum dose 5 mL. Adjunctive treatment of duodenal ulcers: 0.1 mL/kg/dose q4h. Alternative dosing regimen: Weight 4.5kg: 0.5 mL PO q4h or 0.75 mL PO q6h; 9.1kg: 1 mL PO q4h or 1.5 mL PO q6h; 13.6kg: 1.5 mL PO q4h or 2 mL PO q6h; 22.7kg: 2.5 mL PO q4h or 3.75 mL PO q6h; 34kg: 3.75 mL PO q4h or 5 mL PO q6h; ≥45.5kg: 5 mL PO q4h or 7.5 mL PO q6h.

FORMS - Generic/Trade: Phenobarbital 16.2 mg + hyoscyamine 0.1 mg + atropine 0.02 mg + scopolamine 6.5 mcg in each tab, cap or 5 mL. Extended-release tab 48.6 + 0.3111 +

0.0582 + 0.0195 mg.

NOTES - The FDA has classified Donnatal as "possibly effective" for treatment of irritable bowel syndrome and duodenal ulcer. Heat stroke may occur in hot weather. Can cause anticholinergic side effects; use caution in narrow-angle glaucoma, BPH, etc.

"GI cocktail" ("green goddess") ▶LK ♀See individual ▶See individual $

ADULT - See components

PEDS - Not approved in children.

UNAPPROVED ADULT - Acute GI upset: mixture of Maalox/Mylanta 30 mL + viscous lidocaine (2%) 10 mL + Donnatal 10 mL administered PO in a single dose.

NOTES - Avoid repeat dosing due to risk of lidocaine toxicity.

hyoscyamine (*Anaspaz, A-spaz, Cystospaz, ED Spaz, Hyosol, Hyospaz, Levbid, Levsin, Levsinex, Medispaz, NuLev, Spacol, Spasdel, Symax*) ▶LK ♀C ▶- $

ADULT - Bladder spasm, control gastric secretion, GI hypermotility, irritable bowel syndrome: 0.125-0.25 mg PO q4h or prn. 0.375-0.75 mg PO q12h (extended release). Max 1.5 mg/day.

PEDS - Bladder spasm >12 yo: Adult dosing. Control gastric secretion, GI hypermotility, irritable bowel syndrome, and others: If <2 yo, dose by weight: <2 yo: 12.5 mcg (2.3 kg), 16.7 mcg (3.4 kg), 20.8 mcg (5 kg), 25 mcg (7 kg), 31.3-33.3 mcg (10 kg), and 45.8 mcg (15 kg). Alternatively, if <2 yo: 3 drops (2.3 kg), 4 drops (3.4 kg), 5 drops (5 kg), 6 drops (7 kg), 8 drops (10 kg), 11 drops (15 kg). Doses can be repeated q4h prn, but maximum daily dose is six times initial dose. If 2-12 yo, dose by weight: 31.3-33.3 mcg (10kg), 62.5 mcg (20kg), 93.8 mcg (40kg), and 125 mcg (50kg). Doses may be repeated q4h, but maximum daily dose should not exceed 750 mcg.

FORMS - Generic/Trade: Tab 0.125. Sublingual Tab 0.125 mg. Extended release Tab 0.375 mg. Extended release Cap 0.375 mg. Elixir 0.125 mg/ 5 mL. Drops 0.125 mg/1 mL. Trade: Tab 0.15 mg (Hyospaz, Cystospaz). Tab, orally disintegrating 0.125 (NuLev).

NOTES - May cause dizziness, drowsiness, blurred vision, dry mouth, N/V, urinary retention. Contraindicated in glaucoma, obstructive conditions (eg, pyloric, duodenal or other intestinal obstructive lesions, ileus, achalasia, GI hemorrhage, obstructive uropathies), unstable cardiovascular status, myasthenia gravis.

mepenzolate (*Cantil*) ▶LK ♀B ▶? $$$$$

ADULT - Adjunctive therapy in peptic ulcer: 25-50 mg PO tid-qid, with meals and qhs.

PEDS - Not approved in children.

FORMS - Trade only: tab: 25 mg.

NOTES - Contraindicated in glaucoma, obstructive uropathy, paralytic ileus, toxic megacolon, myasthenia gravis.

methscopolamine (*Pamine, Pamine Forte*) ▶LK ♀C ▶? $$$$

ADULT - Adjunctive therapy in peptic ulcer disease: 2.5-5 mg PO 30 min ac & qhs.

PEDS - Not approved in children.

FORMS - Generic/Trade: tab 2.5 mg (Pamine), 5 mg (Pamine Forte).

NOTES - Has not been shown to be effective in treating peptic ulcer disease.

misoprostol (*PGE1, Cytotec*) ▶LK ♀X ▶- $

WARNING - Contraindicated in desired early or preterm pregnancy due to abortifacient property. Pregnant women should avoid contact/exposure to the tabs. Uterine rupture reported with use for labor induction & medical abortion.

ADULT - Prevention of NSAID-induced gastric ulcers: 200 mcg PO qid. If not tolerated, use 100 mcg PO qid.

PEDS - Not approved in children.

UNAPPROVED ADULT - Cervical ripening and labor induction: 25 mcg intravaginally q3-6h (or 50 mcg q6h). First-trimester pregnancy failure: 800 mcg intravaginally, repeat on day 3 if expulsion incomplete. Medical abortion ≤49 days gestation: w/ mifepristone, see mifepristone; w/ methotrexate: 800 mcg intravaginally 5-7 days after 50 mg/m² PO or IM methotrexate. Preop cervical ripening: 400 mcg intravaginally 3-4h before mechanical cervical dilation. Postpartum hemorrhage: 800 mcg PR x 1. Oral dosing has been used but is controversial. Treatment of duodenal ulcers: 100 mcg PO qid.

UNAPPROVED PEDS - Improvement in fat absorption in cystic fibrosis in children 8 - 16 yo: 100 mcg PO qid.

FORMS - Generic/Trade: Oral tabs 100 & 200 mcg.

NOTES - Contraindicated with prior C-section. Oral tabs can be inserted into the vagina for labor induction/cervical ripening. Monitor for uterine hyperstimulation & abnormal fetal heart rate. Risk factors for uterine rupture: prior uterine surgery & ≥5 previous pregnancies.

propantheline (*Pro-Banthine,* ✚*Propanthel*) ▶LK ♀C ▶- $$$

ADULT - Adjunctive therapy in peptic ulcer: 7.5-15 mg PO 30 min before meals and qhs.

PEDS - Not approved in children.

UNAPPROVED ADULT - Irritable bowel, pancreatitis, urinary bladder spasms: 7.5-15 mg PO qid.

UNAPPROVED PEDS - Antisecretory effects: 1.5 mg/kg/day PO in 3-4 divided doses. Antispasmodic effects: 2-3 mg/kg/day PO divided q4-6h and qhs.

FORMS - Generic/Trade: tab 15 mg. Trade only: tab 7.5 mg.

NOTES - For elderly adults and those with small stature use 7.5 mg dose. May cause constipation, dry mucous membranes.

simethicone (*Mylicon, Gas-X, Phazyme, ❖Ovol*) ▶Not absorbed ♀C but + ▶? $

ADULT - Excessive gas in GI tract: 40-160 mg PO after meals and qhs prn, max 500 mg/day.

PEDS - Excessive gas in GI tract: <2 yo: 20 mg PO qid prn, maximum of 240 mg/d. Children 2-12 yo: 40 mg PO qid prn.

UNAPPROVED PEDS - Although used to treat infant colic (in approved dose for gas), several studies suggest no benefit.

FORMS - OTC: Generic/Trade: tab 60,95 mg, chew tab 40,80,125 mg, cap 125 mg, drops 40 mg/0.6 mL.

NOTES - For administration to infants, may mix dose in 30 mL of liquid. Chew tabs should be chewed thoroughly.

sucralfate (*Carafate*, ❖*Sulcrate*) ▶Not absorbed ♀B ▶? $$$

ADULT - Duodenal ulcer: 1g PO qid, 1h before meals and qhs. Maintenance therapy of duodenal ulcer: 1g PO bid.

PEDS - Not approved in children.

UNAPPROVED ADULT - Gastric ulcer, reflux esophagitis, NSAID-induced GI symptoms, stress ulcer prophylaxis: 1g PO qid 1h before meals & qhs. Oral and esophageal ulcers due to radiation/chemo/sclerotherapy: (suspension only) 5-10 mL swish and spit /swallow qid.

UNAPPROVED PEDS - Reflux esophagitis, gastric or duodenal ulcer, stress ulcer prophylaxis: 40-80 mg/kg/day PO divided q6h. Alternative dosing: children <6 yo: 500 mg PO qid, children >6 yo: 1g PO qid.

FORMS - Generic/Trade: tab 1 g, susp 1g/10 mL.

NOTES - May cause constipation. May reduce absorption of cimetidine, ciprofloxacin, digoxin, ketoconazole, itraconazole, norfloxacin, phenytoin, ranitidine, tetracycline, theophylline, warfarin; separate doses by ≥2 hours. Antacids should be separated by ≥30 minutes.

GASTROENTEROLOGY: Laxatives – Bulk-Forming

methylcellulose (*Citrucel*) ▶Not absorbed ♀+ ▶? $

ADULT - Laxative: 1 heaping tablespoon in 8 ounces cold water PO daily-tid.

PEDS - Laxative: Age 6-12 yo: 1½ heaping teaspoons in 4 ounces cold water daily-tid PO prn.

FORMS - OTC Trade only: regular & sugar-free packets and multiple use canisters, clear-mix solution, caplets 500 mg.

NOTES - Must be taken with water to avoid esophageal obstruction or choking.

polycarbophil (*FiberCon, Fiberall, Konsyl Fiber, Equalactin*) ▶Not absorbed ♀+ ▶? $

ADULT - Laxative: 1 g PO qid prn.

PEDS - Laxative: Children 3-5 yo: 500 mg PO daily-bid prn. ≥6 yo: 500 mg PO daily-tid prn.

UNAPPROVED ADULT - Diarrhea: 1 g PO q30min prn. Max daily dose 6 g.

UNAPPROVED PEDS - Diarrhea: Children 3-5 yo: 500 mg PO q30min prn. Max daily dose 1.5 g. >6 yo: 500 mg PO daily-tid or prn. Max daily dose 3 g.

FORMS - OTC Generic/Trade: tab 500,625 mg, chew tab 500,1000 mg.

NOTES - When used as a laxative, take with ≥8 ounces of fluid. Do not administer concomitantly with tetracycline; separate by ≥2 hours.

psyllium (*Metamucil, Fiberall, Konsyl, Hydrocil*, ❖*Prodium Plain*) ▶Not absorbed ♀+ ▶? $

ADULT - Laxative: 1 rounded tsp or 1 packet in liquid, or 1 wafer with liquid PO daily-tid.

PEDS - Laxative (children 6-11yo): ½-1 rounded tsp in liquid, ½-1 packet in liquid or 1 wafer with liquid PO daily-tid.

UNAPPROVED ADULT - Reduction in cholesterol: 1 rounded tsp in liquid, 1 packet in liquid or 1-2 wafers with liquid PO tid. Prevention of GI side effects with orlistat: 6 g in liquid with each orlistat dose or 12 g in liquid qhs.

FORMS - OTC: Generic/Trade: regular and sugar-free powder, granules, capsules, wafers, including various flavors and various amounts of psyllium.

NOTES - Powders and granules must be mixed with liquid prior to ingestion. Start with 1 dose/

day and gradually increase to minimize gas and bloating. Can bind with warfarin, digoxin, potassium-sparing diuretics, salicylates, tetracycline and nitrofurantoin; space ≥3 h apart.

GASTROENTEROLOGY: Laxatives – Osmotic

glycerin (Fleet) ▶Not absorbed ♀C ▶? $
ADULT - Constipation: 1 adult supp PR prn.
PEDS - Constipation: Neonates: 0.5 mL/kg/dose PR prn. Children <6 yo: 1 infant supp or 2-5 mL rectal solution as an enema PR prn. Children ≥6 yo: 1 adult supp or 5-15 mL of rectal solution as enema PR prn.
FORMS - OTC Generic/Trade: supp infant & adult, solution (Fleet Babylax) 4 mL/applicator.

lactulose (Chronulac, Cephulac, Kristalose) ▶Not absorbed ♀B ▶? $$
ADULT - Constipation: 15-30 mL (syrup) or 10-20 g (powder for oral solution) PO daily. Evacuation of barium following barium procedures: 5-10 mL (syrup) PO bid. Acute hepatic encephalopathy: 30-45 mL syrup/dose PO q1h until laxative effect observed or 300 mL in 700 mL water or saline PR as a retention enema q4-6h. Prevention of encephalopathy: 30-45 mL syrup PO tid-qid.
PEDS - Prevention or treatment of encephalopathy: Infants: 2.5-10 mL/day (syrup) PO in 3-4 divided doses. Children/adolescents: 40-90 mL/day (syrup) PO in 3-4 divided doses.
UNAPPROVED ADULT - Restoration of bowel movements in hemorrhoidectomy patients: 15 mL syrup PO bid on day before surgery and for 5 days following surgery.
UNAPPROVED PEDS - Constipation: 7.5 mL syrup PO daily, after breakfast.
FORMS - Generic/Trade: syrup 10 g/15 mL. Trade only (Kristalose): 10, 20 g packets for oral solution.
NOTES - May be mixed in water, juice or milk to improve palatability. Packets for oral solution should be mixed in 4 oz of water. Titrate dose to produce 2-3 soft stools/day.

magnesium citrate (✿Citro-Mag) ▶K♀+▶? $
ADULT - Evacuate bowel prior to procedure: 150-300 mL PO divided daily-bid.
PEDS - Evacuate bowel prior to procedure, <6 yo: 2-4 mL/kg/24h PO divided daily-bid. 6-12 yo: 100-150 mL/24h PO divided daily-bid.
FORMS - OTC Generic only: solution 300 mL/bottle. Low sodium & sugar-free available.
NOTES - Use caution with impaired renal function. May decrease absorption of phenytoin, ciprofloxacin, benzodiazepines, and glyburide.

May cause additive CNS depression with CNS depressants. Chill to improve palatability.

magnesium hydroxide (Milk of Magnesia) ▶K ♀+ ▶? $
ADULT - Laxative: 30-60 mL PO as a single dose or divided doses. Antacid: 5-15 mL/dose PO qid prn or 622-1244 mg PO qid prn.
PEDS - Age <2 yo: 0.5 mL/kg PO as a single dose. 2-5 yo: 5-15 mL/day PO as a single dose or in divided doses. 6-11 yo: 15-30 mL PO in a single dose or in divided doses. Antacid (children >12yo): 2.5-5 mL/dose PO qid prn.
FORMS - OTC Generic/Trade: susp 400 mg/5ml. Trade only: chew tab 311 mg. Generic only: susp (concentrated) 1200 mg/5 mL, sugar-free 400 mg/5 mL.
NOTES - Milk of magnesia concentrated liquid contains 800 mg/5 mL, so use half of the dose. Use caution with impaired renal function.

polyethylene glycol (MiraLax, GlycoLax) ▶Not absorbed ♀C ▶? $
ADULT - Constipation: 17 g (1 heaping tablespoon) in 4-8 oz water, juice, soda, coffee, or tea PO daily.
PEDS - Not approved in children.
UNAPPROVED PEDS - Constipation: 0.8 g/kg/day PO in 2 divided doses.
FORMS - OTC Generic/Trade: powder for oral solution 17g/scoop. Rx Trade only: 17 g packets for oral solution.
NOTES - Takes 2-4 days to produce bowel movement. Indicated for up to 14 days.

polyethylene glycol with electrolytes (GoLytely, Colyte, TriLyte, NuLytely, Moviprep, HalfLytely and Bisacodyl Tablet Kit, ✿Klean-Prep, Electropeg, Peg-Lyte) ▶Not absorbed ♀C ▶? $
ADULT - Bowel cleansing prior to GI examination: 240 mL PO every 10 min or 20-30 mL/min NG until 4L are consumed or rectal effluent is clear. Movieprep: 240 mL q15 min x 4 (over 1 hr) the night before plus 16 additional ounces of clear liquid and 240 mL q15 min x (over 1 hr) plus 16 additional ounces of clear liquid on the morning of the colonoscopy. Alternatively, 240 mL q15 min x 4 (over 1 hr) at 6pm on the evening before the colonoscopy and then 1.5 hours later, 240 mL q15 min x 4 (over 1hr) plus

32 additional ounces of clear liquid on the evening before the colonoscopy (Moviprep only).

PEDS - Bowel prep, >6 months (NuLYTELY, TriLyte): 25 mL/kg/hour PO/NG, until rectal effluent is clear, maximum 4L.

UNAPPROVED ADULT - Chronic constipation: 125-500 mL/day PO daily-bid.

UNAPPROVED PEDS - Bowel cleansing prior to GI examination: 25-40 mL/kg/h PO/NG for 4-10 h or until rectal effluent is clear or 20-30 mL/min NG until 4L are consumed or rectal effluent is clear. Acute iron overdoses: children <3 yo: 0.5 L/h.

FORMS - Generic/Trade: powder for oral soln in disposable jug 4L or 2L (Moviprep). Also, as a kit of 2L bottle of polyethylene glycol with electrolytes and 4 bisacodyl tabs 5 mg (HalfLytely and Bisacodyl Tablet Kit). Trade only (GoLytely): packet for oral solution to make 3.785 L.

NOTES - Solid food should not be given within 2 h of solution. Effects should occur within 1-2 hours. Chilling improves palatability.

sodium phosphate (*Fleet enema, Fleet Phospho-Soda, Accu-Prep, Visicol, ♣Enemol, Phoslax*) ▶Not absorbed ♀C▶? $

WARNING - Phosphate-containing bowel regimens have been rarely reported to cause acute phosphate nephropathy. Risk factors include advanced age, kidney disease or decreased intravascular volume, and medications that affect renal perfusion or function such as diuretics, ACE inhibitors, ARBs, and maybe NSAIDs.

ADULT - 1 adult or pediatric enema PR or 20-30 mL of oral soln PO prn (max 45 mL/24 h). Visicol: Evening before colonoscopy: 3 tabs with 8 oz clear liquid q15 min until 20 tabs are consumed. Day of colonoscopy: starting 3-5 h before procedure, 3 tabs with 8 oz clear liquid q15 min until 20 tabs are consumed.

PEDS - Laxative: 1 pediatric enema (67.5 mL) PR prn or 5-9 yo: 5 mL of oral solution PO prn. 10-12 yo: 10 mL of oral solution PO prn.

UNAPPROVED ADULT - Visicol: Evening before colonoscopy: 3 tabs with 8 oz clear liquid q15 min until 20 tabs are consumed. Day of colonoscopy: starting 3-5 h before procedure, 3 tabs with 8 oz clear liquid q15 min until 8-12 tabs are consumed.

FORMS - OTC Trade only: pediatric & adult enema, oral solution. Rx Trade only: Visicol tab (trade $$$): 1.5 g.

NOTES - Taking the last 2 doses of Visicol with ginger ale appears to minimize residue. Excessive doses (>45 mL/24 h) of oral products may lead to serious electrolyte disturbances. Use with caution in severe renal impairment.

sorbitol ▶Not absorbed ♀+ ▶? $

ADULT - Laxative: 30-150 mL (of 70% solution) PO or 120 mL (of 25-30% solution) PR. Cathartic: 1-2 mL/kg PO.

PEDS - Laxative: Children 2-11 yo: 2 mL/kg (of 70% solution) PO or 30-60 mL (of 25-30% solution) PR.

UNAPPROVED PEDS - Cathartic: 4.3 mL/kg of 35% soln (diluted from 70% soln) PO x 1.

FORMS - Generic only: solution 70%.

NOTES - When used as a cathartic, can be given with activated charcoal to improve taste and decrease gastric transit time of charcoal. May precipitate electrolyte changes.

GASTROENTEROLOGY: Laxatives – Stimulant

bisacodyl (*Correctol, Dulcolax, Feen-a-Mint*) ▶L ♀+ ▶? $

ADULT - Constipation/colonic evacuation prior to a procedure: 10-15 mg PO daily prn, 10 mg PR daily prn.

PEDS - Constipation/colonic evacuation prior to a procedure: 0.3 mg/kg/d PO daily prn. Children <2 yo: 5 mg PR prn. 2-11 yo: 5-10 mg PR prn. >11 yo: 10 mg PR prn.

FORMS - OTC Generic/Trade: tab 5 mg, supp 10 mg.

NOTES - Oral tab has onset of 6-10 h. Suppository onset approximately 15-60 min. Do not chew tabs, swallow whole. Do not give within 1h of antacids or dairy products. Chronic use of stimulant laxatives may be habit forming.

cascara ▶L ♀C ▶+ $

ADULT - Constipation: 325 mg PO qhs prn or 5 mL/day of aromatic fluid extract PO qhs prn.

PEDS - Constipation: Infants: 1.25 mL/day of aromatic fluid extract PO daily prn. 2-11 yo: 2.5 mL/day of aromatic fluid extract PO daily prn.

FORMS - OTC Generic only: tab 325 mg, liquid aromatic fluid extract.

NOTES - Cascara sagrada fluid extract is 5 times more potent than cascara sagrada aromatic fluid extract. Chronic use of stimulant laxatives may be habit forming.

castor oil (*Purge, Fleet Flavored Castor Oil*) ▶Not absorbed ♀- ▶? $

ADULT - Constipation: 15 mL PO daily prn. Colonic evacuation prior to procedure: 15-30 mL of castor oil or 30-60 mL emulsified castor oil PO as a single dose 16h prior to procedure.

PEDS - Colonic evacuation prior to procedure: Children <2 yo: 1-5 mL of castor oil or 5-15 mL emulsified castor oil PO as a single dose 16h prior to procedure. 2-11 yo: 5-15 mL of castor oil or 7.5-30 mL of emulsified castor oil PO as a single dose 16h prior to procedure.

FORMS - OTC Generic/Trade: liquid 30,60,120, 480 mL, emulsified susp 45,60,90,120 mL.

NOTES - Emulsions somewhat mask the bad taste. Onset of action approximately 2-6h. Do not give at bedtime. Chill or administer with juice to improve taste.

lubiprostone (*Amitiza*) ▶Gut ♀C ▶? $$$$
WARNING - Avoid if symptoms or history of mechanical gastrointestinal obstruction.
ADULT - Chronic idiopathic constipation: 24 mcg PO bid with meals.
PEDS - Not approved in children.

FORMS - Trade only: 24 mcg caps.

senna (*Senokot, SenokotXTRA, Ex-Lax, Fletcher's Castoria*, ✦*Glysennid*) ▶L ♀C ▶+ $

ADULT - Laxative or evacuation of the colon for bowel exams: 1 tsp granules in water or 10-15 mL or 2 tabs PO qhs. Max daily dose 4 tsp of granules, 30 mL of syrup, 8 tabs or 2 supp.

PEDS - Laxative: 10-20 mg/kg/dose PO qhs. Alternative regimen: 1 mo-2 yo: 1.25-2.5 mL syrup PO qhs, max 5 mL/day; 2-5yo: 2.5-3.75 mL syrup PO qhs, max 7.5 mL/day; 6-12 yo: 5-7.5 mL syrup PO qhs, max 15 mL/day.

FORMS - OTC Generic/Trade (All dosing is based on sennosides content; 1 mg sennosides = 21.7 mg standardized senna concentrate): granules 15 mg/tsp, syrup 8.8 mg/5 mL, liquid 3 mg/mL (Fletcher's Castoria), tab 8.6, 15, 17, 25 mg , chewable tab 15 mg.

NOTES - Onset 6-24 h after oral administration. Caution in renal dysfunction. Chronic use of stimulant laxatives may be habit forming.

GASTROENTEROLOGY: Laxatives – Stool Softener

docusate (*Colace, Kaopectate Stool Softener, Surfak*) ▶L ♀+ ▶? $
ADULT - Constipation. Docusate calcium: 240 mg PO daily. Docusate sodium: 50-500 mg/day PO in 1-4 divided doses.
PEDS - Constipation, docusate sodium: Children <3 yo: 10-40 mg/day PO in 1-4 divided doses. 3-6 yo: 20-60 mg/day PO in 1-4 divided doses. 6-12 yo: 40-150 mg/day PO in 1-4 divided doses.

UNAPPROVED ADULT - Docusate sodium, constipation: Can be given as a retention enema: Mix 50-100 mg docusate liquid with saline or oil retention enema for rectal use.
FORMS - Docusate calcium OTC Generic/Trade: cap 240 mg. Docusate sodium OTC Generic/Trade: cap 50,100, 250 mg, tab 50, 100 mg, liquid 10 & 50 mg/5 mL, syrup 16.75 & 20 mg/5 mL.
NOTES - 1-3 days to notably soften stools.

GASTROENTEROLOGY: Laxatives – Other or Combinations

mineral oil (*Kondremul, Fleet Mineral Oil Enema*, ✦*Lansoyl*) ▶Not absorbed ♀C ▶? $
ADULT - Laxative: 15-45 mL PO in a single dose or in divided doses, 60-150 mL PR.
PEDS - Laxative: Children 6-11 yo: 5-15 mL PO in a single dose or in divided doses. Children 2-11 yo: 30-60 mL PR.
FORMS - OTC Generic/Trade: plain mineral oil, mineral oil emulsion (Kondremul).
NOTES - Use with caution in young children due to concerns for aspiration pneumonitis. Although usual directions for plain mineral oil are to administer at bedtime, this increases risk of lipid pneumonitis. Mineral oil emulsions may be administered with meals.

Peri-Colace (docusate + sennosides) ▶L ♀C ▶? $
ADULT - Constipation: 2-4 tabs PO once daily or in divided doses prn.
PEDS - Constipation 6-12 yo: 1-2 tabs PO daily prn. 2-6 yo: up to 1 tab PO daily prn.
FORMS - OTC Generic/Trade: tab 50 mg docusate + 8.6 mg sennosides
NOTES - Dilute syrup in 6-8 oz. of juice, milk or infant formula to prevent throat irritation. Chronic use of stimulant laxatives (casanthranol) may be habit forming.

***Senokot-S* (senna + docusate)** ▶L ♀C ▶+ $
ADULT - 2 tabs PO daily, maximum 4 tabs bid.
PEDS - 6-12 yo: 1 tab PO daily, max 2 tabs bid.

2-6 yo: ½ tab PO daily, max 1 tab bid.
FORMS - OTC Generic/Trade: tab 8.6 mg
senna concentrate/50 mg docusate.

NOTES - Effects occur 6-24 h after taking. Use
caution in renal dysfunction. Chronic use of
stimulant laxatives may be habit forming.

GASTROENTEROLOGY: Ulcerative Colitis

balsalazide (*Colazal*) ▶Minimal absorption ♀B
▶? $$$$$
ADULT - Ulcerative colitis: 2.25 g PO tid x 8-12
weeks.
PEDS - 5-17 yo: Mild to moderately active ul-
cerative colitis: 2.25 g PO tid x 8 weeks. Alter-
natively, 750 mg PO tid x 8 weeks.
FORMS - Trade only: cap 750 mg.
NOTES - Contraindicated in salicylate allergy.
Caution with renal insufficiency.

**mesalamine (5-ASA, 5-aminosalicylic ac-
id, *Asacol, Lialda, Pentasa, Canasa, Rowasa, ✦Mesasal, Salofalk*)** ▶Gut ♀B ▶?
$$$$$
ADULT - Ulcerative colitis: Tab: 800-1600 mg
PO tid. Pentasa: 1 g PO qid. Lialda: 2.4-4.8 g
PO daily with a meal x 8 weeks. Susp: 4 g (60
mL) PR retained for 8h qhs. Maintenance of ulcerative colitis: 1600 mg/day PO in divided
doses. Ulcerative proctitis: Canasa supp: 500
mg PR bid-tid or 1000 mg PR qhs.
PEDS - Not approved in children.
UNAPPROVED ADULT - Active Crohn's: 0.4-
4.8 g/day PO in divided doses. Maintenance of
Crohn's remission: 2.4 g/day in divided doses.
UNAPPROVED PEDS - Tab: 50 mg/kg/day PO
divided q6-12h. Cap: 50 mg/kg/day PO divided
q8-12h.
FORMS - Trade only: delayed-release tab 400
mg (Asacol), controlled-release cap 250 & 500
mg (Pentasa), delayed-release tablet 1200 mg
(Lialda), rectal supp 1000 mg (Canasa). Ge-
neric/Trade: rectal susp 4 g/60 mL (Rowasa).
NOTES - Avoid in salicylate sensitivity or hepatic dysfunction. May decrease digoxin levels.
May discolor urine yellow-brown. Most common adverse effects include headache, abdominal pain, fever, rash.

olsalazine (*Dipentum*) ▶L ♀C ▶- $$$$
ADULT - Maintenance of remission of ulcerative
colitis in patients intolerant to sulfasalazine:
500 mg PO bid.
PEDS - Not approved in children.
UNAPPROVED ADULT - Crohn's: 1.5-3 g/day
PO in divided doses.
FORMS - Trade only: cap 250 mg.
NOTES - Diarrhea in up to 17%. Avoid in salicy-
late sensitivity.

**sulfasalazine (*Azulfidine, Azulfidine EN-
tabs, ✦Salazopyrin En-tabs, S.A.S.*)** ▶L
♀B ▶- $$
WARNING - Beware of hypersensitivity, marrow
suppression, renal & liver damage, irreversible
neuromuscular and CNS changes, fibrosing al-
veolitis.
ADULT - Colitis: Initially 500-1000 mg PO qid.
Maintenance: 500 mg PO qid. RA: 500 mg PO
daily-bid after meals to start. Increase to 1g PO
bid.
PEDS - JRA: ≥6 yo: 30-50 mg/kg/day (EN-
Tabs) PO divided bid to max of 2 g/day. Colitis,
>2 yo: Initially 30-60 mg/kg/day PO divided into
3-6 doses. Maximum 75 mg/kg/day. Mainte-
nance: 30 mg/kg/day PO divided qid.
UNAPPROVED ADULT - Ankylosing spondyli-
tis: 1-1.5 g PO bid. Psoriasis: 1.5-2g PO bid.
Psoriatic arthritis: 1g PO bid.
FORMS - Generic/Trade: Tabs 500 mg, scored.
Enteric coated, delayed-release (EN-Tabs) 500
mg.
NOTES - Contraindicated if <2 yo. Avoid with
hepatic or renal dysfunction, intestinal or uri-
nary obstruction, porphyria, sulfonamide or
salicylate sensitivity. Monitor CBC q 2-4 weeks
for 3 months, then q 3 months. Monitor LFTs &
renal function. Oligospermia & infertility, and
photosensitivity may occur. May decrease folic
acid, digoxin, cyclosporine & iron levels. May
turn body fluids, contact lenses, or skin orange-
yellow. Enteric coated (Azulfidine EN, Sala-
zopyrin EN) tabs may cause fewer GI adverse
effects.

GASTROENTEROLOGY: Other

alosetron (*Lotronex*) ▶L ♀B ▶? $$$$$
WARNING - Can cause severe constipation &
ischemic colitis. Concomitant use with fluvox-
amine, a potent CYP1A2 inhibitor, is contrain-
dicated. Use caution with moderate CYP1A2
inhibitors such as quinolone antibiotics and ci-

metidine. Use caution with strong inhibitors of CYP3A4 such as ketoconazole, clarithromycin, telithromycin, protease inhibitors, voriconazole and itraconazole. Can be prescribed only by drug company authorized clinicians using special sticker and written informed consent.
ADULT - Diarrhea-predominant irritable bowel syndrome in women who have failed conventional therapy: 1 mg PO daily for 4 weeks; may increase to 1 mg PO bid. Discontinue if symptoms not controlled in 4 weeks on 1 mg PO bid.
PEDS - Not approved in children.
FORMS - Trade only: tab 0.5, 1 mg.
NOTES - Specific medication guide must be distributed with prescriptions.

alpha-galactosidase (*Beano*) ▶Minimal absorption ♀? ▶? $
ADULT - 5 drops per ½ cup gassy food, 3 tabs PO (chew, swallow or crumble) or 15 drops per typical meal.
PEDS - Not approved in children <12 yo.
FORMS - OTC Trade only: drops 150 GalU/5 drops, tab 150 GalU.
NOTES - Beano produces 2-6 grams of carbohydrates for every 100 grams of food treated by Beano; may increase glucose levels.

budesonide (*Entocort EC*) ▶L ♀C ▶? $$$$$
ADULT - Mild-moderate Crohn's, induction of remission 9 mg PO daily x 8 weeks. May repeat 8 week course for recurring episodes. Maintenance: 6 mg PO daily x 3 months.
PEDS - Not approved in children.
UNAPPROVED PEDS - Mild-moderate Crohn's and ≥9 yo: 0.45 mg/kg up to 9 mg PO daily x 8-12 weeks.
FORMS - Trade only: cap 3 mg.
NOTES - May taper dose to 6 mg for 2 weeks prior to discontinuation.

chlordiazepoxide-clidinium ▶K ♀D ▶- $
ADULT - Irritable bowel syndrome: 1 cap PO tid-qid.
PEDS - Not approved in children.
FORMS - Generic only: cap clidinium 2.5 mg + chlordiazepoxide 5 mg.
NOTES - May cause drowsiness. After prolonged use, gradually taper to avoid withdrawal symptoms. Contains ingredients formerly contained in Librax.

cisapride (*Propulsid*) ▶LK ♀C ▶? from manufacturer only
WARNING - Available only through limited-access protocol through manufacturer. Can cause potentially fatal cardiac arrhythmias. Many drug and disease interactions.

ADULT - 10 mg PO qid, at least 15 min before meals and qhs. Some patients may require 20 mg PO qid. Max 80 mg/day.
PEDS - Not approved in children.
UNAPPROVED PEDS - Gastroesophageal reflux disease: 0.2-0.3 mg/kg/dose PO tid-qid.
FORMS - Trade only: Tab 10,20 mg, susp 1 mg/1 mL.

glycopyrrolate (*Robinul, Robinul Forte*) ▶K ♀B ▶? $$$$
ADULT - Drooling: 0.1 mg/kg PO bid-tid, max 8 mg/day. Pre-op/intraoperative respiratory antisecretory: 0.1 mg IV/IM prn.
PEDS - Not approved in children <16 yo.
UNAPPROVED PEDS - Drooling: 0.04-0.1 mg/kg PO tid-qid, max 8 mg/day. Pre-op/intraoperative respiratory antisecretory: 0.004-0.01 mg/kg IV/IM prn, max 0.2 mg/dose or 0.8 mg/24h.
FORMS - Trade only: tab 1, 2 mg.
NOTES - Contraindicated in glaucoma, obstructive uropathy, paralytic ileus or GI obstruction, myasthenia gravis, severe ulcerative colitis, toxic megacolon and unstable cardiovascular status in acute hemorrhage.

lactase (*Lactaid*) ▶Not absorbed ♀+ ▶+ $
ADULT - Swallow or chew 3 caplets (Original strength), 2 caplets (Extra strength), 1 caplet (Ultra) with first bite of dairy foods. Adjust dose based on response.
PEDS - Titrate dose based on response.
FORMS - OTC Generic/Trade: caplets, chew tab.

Librax (chlordiazepoxide + methscopolamine) ▶K ♀D ▶- $$$$$
ADULT - Irritable bowel syndrome: 1 cap PO tid-qid.
PEDS - Not approved in children.
FORMS - Trade only: cap methscopolamine 2.5 mg + chlordiazepoxide 5 mg.
NOTES - May cause drowsiness. After prolonged use, taper to avoid withdrawal symptoms.

neomycin (*Mycifradin, Neo-Fradin*) ▶Minimally absorbed ♀D ▶? $$$
ADULT - Suppression of intestinal bacteria (given with erythromycin): 1 g PO at 19h, 18h and 9h prior to procedure (i.e. 1 pm, 2 pm, 11 pm on prior day). Alternative regimen 1 g PO q1h for 4 doses then 1 g PO q4h for 5 doses. Hepatic encephalopathy: 4-12 g/day PO divided q6h. Diarrhea caused by enteropathogenic E. coli: 3 g/day PO divided q6h.
PEDS - Suppression of intestinal bacteria (given with erythromycin): 25 mg/kg PO at 19h, 18h and 9h prior to procedure (i.e. 1 pm, 2 pm, 11

pm on prior day). Alternative regimen 90 mg/kg/day PO divided q4h for 2-3 days. Hepatic encephalopathy: 50-100 mg/kg/day PO divided q6-8h. Diarrhea caused by enteropathogenic E. coli: 50 mg/kg/day PO divided q6h.

FORMS - Generic only: tab 350, 500 mg. Trade only (Neo-Fradin): solution 125 mg/5 mL.

NOTES - Increased INR with warfarin, decreased levels of digoxin, methotrexate.

octreotide (*Sandostatin, Sandostatin LAR*) ▶LK ♀B ▶? $$$$$

ADULT - Diarrhea associated with carcinoid tumors: 100-600 mcg/day SC/IV in 2-4 divided doses or 20 mg IM (Sandostatin LAR) q4 weeks x 2 months. Adjust dose based on response. Diarrhea associated with vasoactive intestinal peptide-secreting tumors: 200-300 mcg/day SC/IV in 2-4 divided doses or 20 mg IM (Sandostatin LAR) q4 weeks x 2 months. Adjust dose based on response.

PEDS - Not approved in children.

UNAPPROVED ADULT - Variceal bleeding: Bolus 50-100 mcg IV followed by 25-50 mcg/h continuous IV infusion. AIDS diarrhea: 100-500 mcg SC tid. Irritable bowel syndrome: 100 mcg as a single dose to 125 mcg SC bid. GI and pancreatic fistulas: 50-200 mcg SC/IV q8h.

UNAPPROVED PEDS - Diarrhea: initially 1-10 mcg/kg SC/IV q12h. Congenital hyperinsulinism 1 to 40 mcg/kg SC daily. Hypothalamic obesity, 6-17 yo: 40 mg IM every 4 weeks (Sandostatin LAR) or 5-15 mcg/ kg SC daily.

FORMS - Generic/Trade: injection vials 0.05, 0.1, 0.2, 0.5, 1 mg. Trade only: long-acting injectable susp (Sandostatin LAR) 10,20,30 mg.

NOTES - For the treatment of variceal bleeding, most studies treat for 3-5 days. Individualize dose based on response. Dosage reduction often necessary in elderly. May cause hypoglycemia, hyperglycemia; caution especially in diabetes. May cause hypothyroidism, cardiac arrhythmias. Increases bioavailability of bromocriptine. Sandostatin LAR only indicated for patients who are stabilized on Sandostatin.

orlistat (*Alli, Xenical*) ▶Gut ♀B ▶? $$$$$

ADULT - Weight loss/weight management: 120 mg PO tid with meals or up to 1 h after meals.

PEDS - Children 12-16 yo: 120 mg PO tid with meals. Not approved in children <12 yo.

FORMS - Trade: Caps 60 (OTC), 120 (Rx) mg.

NOTES - May cause fatty stools, fecal urgency, flatus with discharge and oily spotting in >20% of patients. GI adverse effects greater when taken with high fat diet.

pancreatin (*Creon, Donnazyme, Ku-Zyme, ✿Entozyme*) ▶Gut ♀C ▶? $$$

ADULT - Enzyme replacement (initial dose): 8,000-24,000 units lipase (1-2 cap/tab) PO with meals and snacks.

PEDS - Enzyme replacement (initial dose): <1 yo: 2,000 units lipase PO with meals. 1-6 yo: 4,000-8,000 units lipase PO with meals, 4,000 units lipase with snacks. 7-12 yo: 4,000-12,000 units lipase PO with meals and snacks.

FORMS - Tab, cap with varying amounts of pancreatin, lipase, amylase and protease.

NOTES - Titrate dose to stool fat content. Products are not interchangeable. Avoid concomitant calcium carbonate & magnesium hydroxide since these may affect the enteric coating. Do not crush/chew microspheres or tabs. Possible association of colonic strictures and high doses of lipase (>16,000 units/kg/meal) in pediatric patients.

pancrelipase (*Viokase, Pancrease, Pancrecarb, Cotazym, Ku-Zyme HP*) ▶Gut ♀C ▶? $$$

ADULT - Enzyme replacement (initial dose): 4,000-33,000 units lipase (1-3 cap/tab) PO with meals and snacks.

PEDS - Enzyme replacement (initial dose): 6 mo -1 yo: 2,000 units lipase or 1/8 tsp PO with feedings. 1-6 yo: 4,000-8,000 units lipase PO with meals, 4,000 units lipase with snacks. 7-12 yo: 4,000-12,000 units lipase PO w/ meals/snacks.

FORMS - Tab, cap, powder with varying amounts of lipase, amylase and protease.

NOTES - Titrate dose to stool fat content. Products are not interchangeable. Avoid concomitant calcium carbonate and magnesium hydroxide since these may affect the enteric coating. Do not crush/chew microspheres or tabs. Possible association of colonic strictures and high doses of lipase (>16,000 units/kg/meal) in pediatric patients.

pinaverium (✿*Dicetel*) ▶? ♀C ▶- $$$

ADULT - Canada only. Irritable bowel syndrome: 50 mg PO tid, may increase to maximum of 100 mg tid.

PEDS - Not for children.

FORMS - Trade only: tabs 50, 100 mg.

NOTES - Take with a full glass of water during meal or snack.

secretin (*SecreMax*) ▶Serum ♀C ▶? $$$$$

ADULT - Stimulation of pancreatic secretions, to aid in diagnosis of exocrine pancreas dysfunction: Test dose 0.2 mcg IV. If tolerated, 0.2 mcg/kg IV over 1 minute. Stimulation of gastrin to aid in diagnosis of gastrinoma: Test dose 0.2 mcg IV. If tolerated, 0.4 mcg/kg IV over 1 minute. Identification of ampulla of Vater and accessory papilla during ERCP: 0.2 mcg/kg IV over 1 minute.

PEDS - Not approved in children.

NOTES - Previously known as Secreflo. Contraindicated in acute pancreatitis.

tegaserod (*Zelnorm*) ▶stomach/L ♀B ▶? free (investigational)

WARNING - Restricted (investigational) use; contact manufacturer to obtain. Severe diarrhea leading to hypovolemia, hypotension and syncope has been reported, as has ischemic colitis and other forms of intestinal ischemia; discontinue immediately if symptoms occur.

ADULT - Constipation-predominant irritable bowel syndrome in women <55 yo: 6 mg PO bid before meals for 4-6 weeks. May repeat for an additional 4-6 weeks.

PEDS - Not approved in children.

FORMS - Restricted use only: tab 2, 6 mg.

ursodiol (*Actigall, Ursofalk, URSO, URSO Forte*) ▶Bile ♀B ▶? $$$$

ADULT - Radiolucent gallstone dissolution (Actigall): 8-10 mg/kg/day PO divided in 2-3 doses. Prevention of gallstones associated with rapid weight loss (Actigall): 300 mg PO bid. Primary biliary cirrhosis (URSO): 13-15 mg/kg/day PO divided in 2-4 doses.

PEDS - Not approved in children.

UNAPPROVED ADULT - Cholestasis of pregnancy: 300-600 mg PO bid.

UNAPPROVED PEDS - Biliary atresia: 10-15 mg/kg/day PO divided tid. Cystic fibrosis with liver disease: 30 mg/kg/day PO divided bid. TPN-induced cholestasis: 30 mg/kg/day PO divided tid.

FORMS - Generic/Trade: cap 300 mg. Trade only: tab 250 (URSO), 500 mg (URSO Forte).

NOTES - Gallstone dissolution requires months of therapy. Complete dissolution does not occur in all patients and 5-year recurrence up to 50%. Does not dissolve calcified cholesterol stones, radiopaque stones or radiolucent bile pigment stones. Avoid concomitant antacids, cholestyramine, colestipol, estrogen, oral contraceptives.

HEMATOLOGY: Anticoagulants – Heparin, LMW Heparins, & Fondaparinux

NOTE: See cardiovascular section for antiplatelet drugs & thrombolytics. Contraindicated in active major bleeding. High risk of spinal/epidural hematoma if spinal puncture or neuraxial anesthesia before/during treatment. Risk of bleeding increased by oral anticoagulants, ASA, dipyridamole, dextran, glycoprotein IIb/IIIA inhibitors, NSAIDs (including ketorolac), ticlopidine, clopidogrel, and thrombolytics. Monitor platelets, Hb, stool for occult blood.

dalteparin (*Fragmin*) ▶KL ♀B ▶+ $$$$

ADULT - DVT prophylaxis, acute medical illness with restricted mobility: 5,000 units SC daily x 12-14 days. DVT prophylaxis, abdominal surgery: 2,500 units SC 1-2 h preop and daily postop x 5-10 days. DVT prophylaxis, abdominal surgery in patients with malignancy: 5,000 units SC evening before surgery and daily postop x 5-10 days. Alternatively, 2,500 units SC 1-2 h preop and 12 h later, then 5,000 units SC daily x 5-10 days. DVT prophylaxis, hip replacement: Give SC for up to 14 days. Preop start regimens: 2,500 units 2 h preop and 4-8h postop, then 5,000 units daily starting ≥6h after second dose. Alternatively, 5,000 units 10-14 h preop, 4-8h postop, then daily (approximately 24h between doses). Postop start regimen: 2,500 units 4-8h postop, then 5,000 units daily starting ≥6h after first dose. Treatment of DVT/PE in cancer: 200 units/kg SC daily x 1 month, then 150 units/kg SC daily x 5 months. Max 18,000 units/day, round to nearest commercially available syringe dose. Unstable angina or non-Q-wave MI: 120 units/kg up to 10,000 units SC q12h with aspirin (75-165 mg/day PO) until clinically stable.

PEDS - Not approved in children.

UNAPPROVED ADULT - Therapeutic anticoagulation: 200 units/kg SC daily or 100-120 units/kg SC bid. Venous thromboembolism in pregnancy. Prevention: 5,000 units SC daily. Treatment: 100 units/kg SC q12h or 200 units/kg SC daily. To avoid unwanted anticoagulation during delivery, stop LMWH 24 h before elective induction of labor.

FORMS - Trade only: Single-dose syringes 2,500 & 5,000 anti-Xa units/0.2 mL, 7500 anti-Xa/0.3 mL, 10,000 anti-Xa units/1 mL, 12,500 anti-Xa units/0.5 mL, 15,000 anti-Xa units/0.6 mL, 18,000 anti-Xa units/0.72 mL; multi-dose vial 10,000 units/mL, 9.5 mL and 25,000 units/mL, 3.8 mL.

NOTES - Longer prophylaxis may be warranted based on individual thromboembolic risk. ACCP recommendations suggest that patients with total hip or knee replacement or hip fracture surgery receive prophylaxis for ≥10 days; consider extended prophylaxis (28-35 days) in hip replacement or hip fracture surgery. Contraindicated in heparin or pork allergy, history of heparin-induced thrombocytopenia. Use caution and consider monitoring anti-Xa levels if morbidly obese, underweight, pregnant, or renal/liver failure.

enoxaparin (*Lovenox*) ▶KL ♀B ▶+ $$$$$

ADULT - DVT prophylaxis, acute medical illness with restricted mobility: 40 mg SC daily for ≤14 days (CrCl <30 ml/min): 30 mg SC daily). DVT prophylaxis, hip/knee replacement: 30 mg SC q12h starting 12-24 h postop for ≤14 days (CrCl <30 ml/min: 30 mg SC daily). Alternative for hip replacement: 40 mg SC daily starting 12 h preop. After hip replacement may continue 40 mg SC daily x 3 weeks. DVT prophylaxis, abdominal surgery: 40 mg SC daily starting 2 h preop for ≤12 days (CrCl <30 ml/min: 30 mg SC daily). Outpatient treatment of DVT without pulmonary embolus: 1 mg/kg SC q12h. Inpatient treatment of DVT with/without pulmonary embolus: 1 mg/kg SC q12h or 1.5 mg/kg SC q24h (CrCl <30 ml/min: 1 mg/kg SC daily). Give at the same time each day. Continue enoxaparin for ≥5 days and until therapeutic oral anticoagulation established. Unstable angina or non-Q-wave MI: 1 mg/kg SC q12h with aspirin (100-325 mg PO daily) for ≥2 days and until clinically stable (CrCl <30 ml/min: 1 mg/kg SC daily). Acute ST-elevation MI: if ≤75 yo: 30 mg IV bolus plus 1 mg/kg SC dose then 1 mg/kg (max 100 mg for the first two doses) SC q12 hours (CrCl <30 ml/min: 30 mg IV bolus plus 1 mg/kg SC dose then 1 mg/kg SC daily); if >75 yo: 0.75 mg/kg (max 75 mg for the first two doses, no bolus) SC q12 hours (CrCl <30 ml/min: 1 mg/kg SC daily, no bolus). Given with aspirin (75-325 mg PO daily) until hospital discharge or for ≥8 days.

PEDS - Not approved in children.

UNAPPROVED ADULT - Prevention of venous thromboembolism. After major trauma: 30 mg SC q12h starting 12-36 h postinjury if hemostasis achieved. Acute spinal cord injury: 30 mg SC q12h. Venous thromboembolism in pregnancy: Prevention: 40 mg SC daily. Treatment: 1 mg/kg SC q12h. To avoid unwanted anticoagulation during delivery, stop LMWH 24 h before elective induction of labor.

UNAPPROVED PEDS - Therapeutic anticoagulation: Age <2 mo: 1.5 mg/kg/dose SC q12h titrated to anti-Xa level of 0.5-1 units/mL. Age >2 mo: 1 mg/kg/dose SC q12h titrated to anti-Xa level of 0.5-1.0 units/mL. DVT prophylaxis: Age <2 mo: 0.75 mg/kg/dose q12h. Age >2 mo: 0.5 mg/kg/dose q12h.

FORMS - Trade only: Multi-dose vial 300 mg; Syringes 30,40 mg; graduated syringes 60,80,100,120,150 mg. Concentration is 100 mg/mL except for 120,150 mg which are 150 mg/mL.

NOTES - Longer prophylaxis may be warranted based on individual thromboembolic risk. ACCP recommendations suggest that patients with total hip or knee replacement or hip fracture surgery receive prophylaxis for ≥10 days; consider extended prophylaxis (28-35 days) in hip replacement or hip fracture surgery. Dosage adjustments for CrCl <30 mL/min. Use caution and consider monitoring anti-Xa levels if renal dysfunction, pregnancy, morbidly obese, underweight, or abnormal coagulation/bleeding. In unstable angina, can give 30 mg IV bolus before first SC dose. In acute ST-elevation MI, if administered with thrombolytic give between 15 minutes before or 30 minutes after start of thrombolytic therapy. In acute ST-elevation MI in patients with PCI, if last enoxaparin administration was >8h before balloon inflation, give 0.3 mg/kg IV bolus. Contraindicated in patients with heparin or pork allergy, history of heparin-induced thrombocytopenia. Use caution in mechanical heart valves, especially in pregnancy; reports of valve thrombosis (maternal & fetal deaths reported). Congenital anomalies linked to enoxaparin use during pregnancy; causality unclear. Multidose formulation contains benzyl alcohol, which can cause hypersensitivity and cross placenta in pregnancy.

fondaparinux (*Arixtra*) ▶K ♀B ▶? $$$$$

ADULT - DVT prophylaxis, hip/knee replacement or hip fracture surgery, abdominal surgery: 2.5 mg SC daily starting 6-8 h postop (giving earlier increases risk of bleeding). Usual duration is 5-9 days; extend prophylaxis up to 24 additional days (max 32 days) in hip fracture surgery. DVT / PE treatment based on weight: 5 mg (if <50 kg), 7.5 mg (if 50-100 kg), 10 mg (if >100 kg) SC daily for ≥5 days & therapeutic oral anticoagulation.

PEDS - Not approved in children.

UNAPPROVED ADULT - Unstable angina or non-ST elevation MI: 2.5 mg SC daily until hospital discharge or for up to 8 days. ST-elevation MI: 2.5 mg SC daily until hospital discharge or for up to 8 days.

FORMS - Trade only: Pre-filled syringes 2.5 mg/0.5 mL, 5 mg/0.4 mL, 7.5 mg/0.6 mL, 10 mg/0.8 mL.

NOTES - May cause thrombocytopenia, however, lacks in vitro cross-reactivity with heparin-induced thrombocytopenia antibodies. Risk of major bleeding increased in elderly. Contraindicated if CrCl <30 mL/minute due to increased bleeding risk. Caution advised if CrCl 30-50 mL/minute. Monitor renal function in all patients; discontinue if severely impaired or labile. In DVT prophylaxis, contraindicated if body weight <50 kg. Protamine ineffective for reversing anticoagulant effect. Factor VIIa partially reverses anticoagulant effect in small studies. Store at room temperature.

heparin (♥Hepalean) ▶Reticuloendothelial system ♀C but + ▶+ $

ADULT - Venous thrombosis/pulmonary embolus treatment: Load 80 units/kg IV, then initiate infusion at 18 units/kg/h. Adjust based on coagulation testing (PTT). DVT prophylaxis: 5000 units SC q8-12h. Low-dose for prevention of thromboembolism in pregnancy: 5,000-10,000 units SC q12h. Treatment of thromboembolism in pregnancy: 80 units/kg IV load, then infuse 18 units/kg/h with dose titrated to achieve full anticoagulation for ≥5 days. Then continue via SC route with ≥10,000 units SC q8-12h adjusted to achieve PTT of 1.5-2.5 x control. To avoid unwanted anticoagulation during delivery, stop SC heparin 24 h before elective induction of labor.

PEDS - Venous thrombosis/pulmonary embolus treatment: Load 50 units/kg IV, then 25 units/kg/h infusion.

UNAPPROVED ADULT - Venous thrombosis/pulmonary embolus treatment: Load 333 units/kg SC, then 250 units/kg SC q12h based on max 100 kg weight. Adjust to achieve goal PTT 1.5-2 x control (approximately 50-70 seconds). Anticoagulation for acute MI not treated with thrombolytics: 75 units/kg IV load, then initiate infusion at 1,000-1,200 units/h adjusted to achieve PTT of 1.5-2.5 x control. Unstable angina/MI ST-elevation MI: 60-70 units/kg IV load (max 5000 units), then initiate infusion at 12-15 units/kg/h (max 1000 units) and adjust to achieve goal PTT 1.5-2.5 x control. Adjunct to

thrombolytics for acute MI. For use with alteplase, reteplase, or tenecteplase: 60 units/kg IV load (max 4,000 units), then initial infusion 12 units/kg/h (max 1,000 units/h) adjusted to achieve goal PTT 1.5-2 x control (approximately 50-70 seconds). Maintain for ≥48 h, duration based on concomitant therapy and patient thromboembolic risk. For use with streptokinase: start ≥4 h after start of streptokinase and PTT <70 seconds; 12,500 units SC q12h. IV heparin only for patients receiving streptokinase who are at high risk for systemic/venous thromboembolism, duration based on concomitant therapy and patient thromboembolic risk.

UNAPPROVED PEDS - Venous thrombosis/pulmonary embolus treatment: Load 75 units/kg IV over 10 minutes, then 28 units/kg/h if age <1 yo, 20 units/kg/h if age >1 yo.

FORMS - Generic only: 1000, 2500, 5000, 7500, 10,000, 20,000 units/mL in various vial and syringe sizes.

NOTES - Beware of heparin-induced thrombocytopenia (HIT; immune-mediated thrombocytopenia associated with thrombotic events), elevated LFTs, hyperkalemia/ hypoaldosteronism. HIT can occur up to several weeks after heparin discontinued. Osteoporosis with long-term use. Bleeding risk increased by high dose; concomitant thrombolytic or platelet GPIIb/IIIa receptor inhibitor; recent surgery, trauma, or invasive procedure; concomitant hemostatic defect. Monitor platelets, hemoglobin, stool for occult blood. Anti-Xa is an alternative to PTT for monitoring.

tinzaparin (Innohep) ▶K ♀B ▶+ $$$$$

ADULT - DVT with/without pulmonary embolus: 175 units/kg SC daily for ≥6 days & until adequate anticoagulation with warfarin.

PEDS - Not approved in children.

UNAPPROVED ADULT - Treatment of venous thromboembolism in pregnancy: 175 units/kg SC daily.

FORMS - Trade only: 20,000 anti-Xa units/mL, 2 mL multi-dose vial.

NOTES - Contraindicated if history of heparin-induced thrombocytopenia, or allergy to heparin, pork, sulfites, or benzyl alcohol. Can cause thrombocytopenia, priapism (rare), increased AST/ALT. Tinzaparin may slightly prolong PT; draw blood for INR just before giving tinzaparin. Use caution and consider monitoring anti-Xa levels if morbidly obese, underweight, pregnant, or renal dysfunction.

WEIGHT-BASED HEPARIN DOSING FOR DVT/PE*

Initial dose: 80 units/kg IV bolus, then 18 units/kg/h. Check PTT in 6 h.
PTT <35 secs (<1.2 x control): 80 units/kg IV bolus, then ↑ infusion rate by 4 units/kg/h.
PTT 35-45 secs (1.2-1.5 x control): 40 units/kg IV bolus, then ↑ infusion by 2 units/kg/h.
PTT 46-70 seconds (1.5-2.3 x control): No change.
PTT 71-90 seconds (2.3-3 x control): ↓ infusion rate by 2 units/kg/h.
PTT >90 seconds (>3 x control): Hold infusion for 1 h, then ↓ infusion rate by 3 units/kg/h.

* PTT = Activated partial thromboplastin time. Reagent-specific target PTT may differ; use institutional nomogram when appropriate. Adjusted dosing may be appropriate in obesity. Consider establishing a max bolus dose / max initial infusion rate or use an adjusted body weight in obesity. Monitor PTT 6h after heparin initiation and 6h after each dosage adjustment. When PTT is stable within therapeutic range, monitor every morning. Therapeutic PTT range corresponds to anti-factor Xa activity of 0.3-0.7 units/mL. Check platelets between days 3-5. Can begin warfarin on 1st day of heparin; continue heparin for ≥4 to 5 days of combined therapy. Adapted from *Ann Intern Med* 1993;119:874; *Chest* 2004:126:191S-192S, *Circulation* 2001; 103:2994.

HEMATOLOGY: Anticoagulants – Other

argatroban ►L ♀B ▶- $$$$$
ADULT - Prevention/treatment of thrombosis in heparin-induced thrombocytopenia: Start 2 mcg/kg/min IV infusion. Get PTT at baseline and 2 h after starting infusion. Adjust dose (up to 10 mcg/kg/min) until PTT is 1.5-3 times baseline (but not >100 seconds). Percutaneous coronary intervention in those with or at risk for heparin-induced thrombocytopenia: Bolus 350 mcg/kg IV over 3 to 5 minutes then 25 mcg/kg/min infusion. Adjust to therapeutic activated clotting time (ACT: 300-450 seconds) using guidelines in package insert.
PEDS - Not approved in children.
NOTES - Argatroban prolongs INR with warfarin; discontinue when INR >4 on combined therapy. Dosage reduction recommended in liver dysfunction.

bivalirudin (*Angiomax*) ►proteolysis/K ♀B ▶? $$$$$
ADULT - Anticoagulation in PCI (including patients with or at risk of heparin-induced thrombocytopenia or heparin-induced thrombocytopenia and thrombosis syndrome): 0.75 mg/kg IV bolus prior to intervention, then 1.75 mg/kg/hr for duration of procedure (with provisional Gp IIb/IIIa inhibition) and optionally up to 4 hours post-procedure. For CrCl <30 mL/min, reduce infusion dose to 1mg/kg/hr after bolus. For patients on dialysis, reduce infusion dose to 0.25 mg/kg/hr. Use with aspirin 300-325 mg PO daily. Additional bolus of 0.3 mg/kg if activated clotting time <225 sec. Can additionally infuse 0.2 mg/kg/h for up to 20 h more.
PEDS - Not approved in children.

UNAPPROVED ADULT - Anticoagulation with streptokinase thrombolysis in ST elevation MI & known heparin-induced thrombocytopenia, start 3 min before streptokinase: 0.25 mg/kg bolus followed by 0.5 mg/kg/hr for first 12 hours, then 0.25 mg/kg/hr for subsequent 36 hours (consider dose reduction if PTT >75 seconds within first 12 hours). Acute coronary syndrome (with or without Gp IIb/IIIa inhibition): 0.1 mg/kg bolus followed by 0.25 mg/kg/hr. If PCI, then additional bolus 0.5 mg/kg then 1.75 mg/kg/hr. Use with aspirin.
NOTES - Contraindicated in active major bleeding. Monitor activated clotting time. Former trade name Hirulog.

lepirudin (*Refludan*) ►K ♀B ▶? $$$$$
ADULT - Anticoagulation in heparin-induced thrombocytopenia (HIT) and associated thromboembolic disease: Bolus 0.4 mg/kg up to 44 mg IV over 15-20 seconds, then infuse 0.15 mg/kg/h up to 16.5 mg/h x 2-10 days. Adjust dose to maintain APTT ratio of 1.5-2.5.
PEDS - Not approved in children.
UNAPPROVED ADULT - Adjunct to thrombolytics for acute MI in patients with HIT: 0.1 mg/kg IV bolus, then infuse 0.15 mg/h.
NOTES - May increase INR. Dosage adjustment for renal impairment: Bolus 0.2 mg/kg IV followed by 0.075 mg/kg/h for CrCl 45-60 mL/min, 0.045 mg/kg/h for CrCl 30-44 mL/min, 0.0225 mg/kg/h for CrCl 15-29 mL/min. Hemodialysis/CrCl <15 mL/min: Bolus 0.1 mg/kg IV qod if APTT ratio <1.5. Severe anaphylactic reactions resulting in death have been reported upon initial or re-exposure.

THERAPEUTIC GOALS FOR ANTICOAGULATION

INR Range*	Indication
2.0-3.0	Atrial fibrillation, deep venous thrombosis, pulmonary embolism, bioprosthetic heart valve, mechanical prosthetic heart valve (aortic position, bileaflet or tilting disk with normal sinus rhythm and normal left atrium)
2.5-3.5	Mechanical prosthetic heart valve: (1) mitral position, (2) aortic position with atrial fibrillation, (3) caged ball or caged disk

*Aim for an INR in the middle of the INR range (e.g. 2.5 for range of 2-3 and 3.0 for range of 2.5-3.5).
Adapted from: *Chest suppl 2004*; 126: 416S, 450S, 474S; see for additional info and other indications.

WARFARIN – SELECTED DRUG INTERACTIONS

Assume possible interactions with any new medication. When starting/stopping a medication, the INR should be checked at least weekly for ≥2-3 weeks and dose adjusted accordingly. For further information regarding mechanism or management, refer to the *Tarascon Pocket Pharmacopoeia* drug interactions database (PDA edition).Similarly monitor if significant change in diet (including supplements) or illness resulting in decreased oral intake.

Increased anticoagulant effect of warfarin / Increased risk of bleeding

Monitor INR when agents below started, stopped, or dosage changed. Consider alternative agent.
acetaminophen ≥2 g/day for ≥3-4 days, allopurinol, amiodarone*, amprenavir, **anabolic steroids**, aspirin¶, cefixime, cefoperazone, celecoxib, chloramphenicol, cimetidine†, **corticosteroids**, danazol, danshen, delavirdine, disulfiram, dong quai , erlotinib, **fibrates**, fish oil, fluconazole, **fluoroquinolones**, fluorouracil, fluvoxamine, fosphenytoin (acute), garlic supplements, gemcitabine, gemfibrozil, ginkgo, ifosfamide, imatinib, isoniazid, itraconazole, ketoconazole, leflunomide, lepirudin, levothyroxine#, **macrolides**‡, metronidazole, miconazole(intravaginal), neomycin (PO for >1-2 days), **NSAIDs**¶, olsalazine, omeprazole, paroxetine, penicillin (high-dose IV), pentoxifylline, phenytoin (acute), propafenone, propoxyphene, quinidine, quinine, **statins**§, sulfinpyrazone (with later inhibition), **sulfonamides**, tamoxifen, **testosterones**, **tetracyclines**, tramadol, tigecycline, **tricyclic antidepressants**, valproate, voriconazole, vitamin A (high-dose), vitamin E, zafirlukast, zileuton

Decreased anticoagulant effect of warfarin / Increased risk of thrombosis

Monitor INR when agents below started, stopped, or dosage changed. Consider alternative agent.
Aminoglutethimide, aprepitant, azathioprine, barbiturates, bosentan, carbamazepine, coenzyme Q-10, dicloxacillin, fosphenytoin (chronic), ginseng (American), griseofulvin, mercaptopurine, mesalamine, methimazole#, mitotane, nafcillin, oral contraceptives**, phenytoin (chronic), primidone, propylthiouracil#, raloxifene, ribavirin, rifabutin, rifampin, rifapentine, ritonavir, St John's wort, vitamin C (high-dose).
Use alternative to agents below. Or give at different times of day and monitor INR when agent started, stopped, or dose/dosing schedule changed
cholestyramine, colestipol††, sucralfate

*Interaction may be delayed; monitor INR for several weeks after starting & several months after stopping amiodarone. May need to decrease warfarin dose by 33% to 50%.
† Famotidine, nizatidine or ranitidine are alternatives.
‡ Azithromycin appears to have lower risk of interaction than clarithromycin or erythromycin.
§ Pravastatin appears to have lower risk of interaction.
# Hyperthyroidism/thyroid replacement increases metabolism of clotting factors, increasing response to warfarin therapy and increased bleed risk (typically requires lowering warfarin dose).
¶ Does not necessarily increase INR, but increases bleeding risk. Check INR frequently and monitor for GI bleeding.
**Do not necessarily ↓INR, but may induce hypercoagulability.
†† Likely lower risk than cholestyramine

Table adapted from: Coumadin® product information; *Am Fam Phys* 1999;59:635; *Chest* 2004; 126: 204S; *Hansten and Horn's Drug Interactions Analysis and Management*; *Ann Intern Med* 2004;141:23; *Arch Intern Med* 2005;165:1095. *Tarascon Pocket Pharmacopoeia* drug interactions database (PDA edition).

warfarin (Coumadin, Jantoven) ▶L ♀X ▶+ $

WARNING - Many important drug interactions that increase/decrease INR, see table.

ADULT - Oral anticoagulation for prophylaxis/ treatment of DVT/PE, thromboembolic complications associated with A-fib, mechanical and bioprosthetic heart valves: Start 2-5 mg PO daily x 3-4 days, then adjust dose to maintain therapeutic PT/INR. Consider initial dose <5 mg/day if elderly, malnourished, liver disease, or high bleeding risk. Target INR of 2-3 for most indications, 2.5-3.5 for mechanical heart valves. See table for specific target INR and duration of anticoagulation.

PEDS - Not approved in children.

UNAPPROVED ADULT - Oral anticoagulation treatment of acute DVT/PE: Start 5-10 mg PO daily (with ≥5 days of LMWH/heparin) until target INR (2.0 to 3.0) reached. See table for target INR and duration of anticoagulation for specific indications.

FORMS - Generic/Trade: Tabs 1, 2, 2.5, 3, 4, 5, 6, 7.5, 10 mg.

NOTES - ACCP guidelines suggest initial dose of 2-10 mg, with lower doses if high risk of bleeding, elderly, malnourished or congestive heart failure. Consider lower initial dose if genetic variation in CYP2C9 and VKORC1 enzymes. Tissue necrosis in protein C or S deficiency. Many important drug interactions that increase/decrease INR, see table. Warfarin onset of action is within 24 hours, peak effect delayed by 3-4 days. Most patients can begin warfarin at the same time as heparin/LMWH. Continue heparin/LMWH treatment for thrombosis until the INR has been in the therapeutic range for ≥2 days. See phytonadione (vitamin K) entry for management of high INR.

HEMATOLOGY: Antihemophilic Agents

anti-inhibitor coagulant complex (Feiba VH, ✤Feiba VH Immuno) ▶L ♀C ▶? $$$$$

ADULT - Hemophilia A or B with factor VIII inhibitors, XI and XII (if surgery or active bleeding): 50-100 units/kg IV; specific dose and frequency based on site of bleeding, max 200 units/kg/day.

PEDS - Not approved in children.

NOTES - Contraindicated if normal coagulation. Human plasma product, thus risk of infectious agent transmission. Avoid in active or impending disseminated intravascular coagulation (DIC).

factor VIIa (NovoSeven, ✤Niastase) ▶L ♀C ▶? $$$$$

ADULT, PEDS - Hemophilia A or B: individualize factor VIIa dose.

UNAPPROVED ADULT - Reversal of excessive warfarin anticoagulation (INR >10): 15-20 mcg/kg IV over 3-5 min. Intracerebral hemorrhage (within 4 hours of symptom onset): 40-160 mcg/kg IV over 1 to 2 min. Perioperative blood loss in retropubic prostatectomy: 20 or 40 mcg/kg IV bolus.

FORMS - Trade: 1200, 2400, 4800 mcg/vial.

NOTES - Contraindicated with hypersensitivity to mouse, hamster or bovine proteins. Patients with DIC, advanced atherosclerotic disease, crush injury or septicemia may be at increase thrombotic risk. If DIC or thrombosis confirmed, reduce dose or stop treatment depending on symptoms.

factor VIII (Advate, Alphanate, Hemofil M, Humate P, Monoclate P, Monarc-M, ReFacto, ✤Kogenate, Recombinate) ▶L ♀C ▶? $$$$$

ADULT - Hemophilia A: individualize factor VIII dose. Surgical procedures in patients with von Willebrand disease (Alphanate, Humate P): individualized dosing.

PEDS - Hemophilia A: individualize factor VIII dose.

FORMS - Specific formulation usually chosen by specialist in Hemophilia Treatment Center. Advate is only current recombinant formulation of factor VIII.

NOTES - Risk of HIV/hepatitis transmission varies by product; no such risk with recombinant product. Reduced response with development of factor VIII inhibitors. Hemolysis with large/repeated doses in patients with A, B, AB blood type.

factor IX (Benefix, Mononine, ✤Immunine VH) ▶L ♀C ▶? $$$$$

ADULT, PEDS - Hemophilia B: individualize factor IX dose.

FORMS - Specific formulation usually chosen by specialist in Hemophilia Treatment Center.

NOTES - Risk of HIV/hepatitis transmission varies by product. Products that contain factors II, VII, & X may cause thrombosis in at-risk patients. Stop infusion if signs of DIC.

HEMATOLOGY: Colony Stimulating Factors

darbepoetin (Aranesp, NESP) ▶cellular sialidases, L ♀C ▶? $$$$$

WARNING - Use lowest dose for gradual rise in Hb to minimum level to avoid blood transfusion. When administered to target Hb of >12 mg/dL, increased risk of death and serious cardiovascular events, including arterial and venous thrombotic events. Consider antithrombotic DVT prophylaxis. Not approved for use in cancer patients with anemia not due to concurrent chemotherapy; may not provide benefit and may increase risk of death. May shorten time to tumor progression in cancer patients and increase risk of death.

ADULT - Anemia of chronic renal failure: 0.45 mcg/kg IV/SC q weekly, or SC q 2 weeks for some patients. Maintenance dose may be lower in predialysis patients than dialysis patients. Anemia in cancer chemo patients: initially 2.25 mcg/kg SC q week, or 500 mcg SC every 3 weeks. For weekly administration, max 4.5 mcg/kg/dose. Weekly dose conversion to darbepoetin (D) from erythropoietin (E): 6.25 mcg D for <2,500 units E; 12.5 mcg D for 2,500-4,999 units E; 25 mcg D for 5,000-10,999 units E; 40 mcg D for 11,000-17,999 units E; 60 mcg D for 18,000-33,999 units E; 100 mcg D for 34,000-89,999 units E; 200 mcg D for ≥90,000 units E. Give D once weekly for patients taking E 2-3 times weekly; give D once every 2 weeks for patients taking E once weekly. Monitor Hb weekly until stable, then at least monthly. Target Hb not to exceed 12 g/dL. Reduce dose by 25% if Hb is increasing and approaches 12 g/dL or if Hb increases by 1 g/dL per 2 week time period; hold if >12 g/dL. Increase dose by 25% if Hb increases by <1 g/dL over 1 month. Increase dose at intervals of 1 month or more.

PEDS - Not approved in children.

UNAPPROVED ADULT - Chemotherapy-induced anemia: 3 mcg/kg or 200 mcg SC q2 wks.

FORMS - Trade: All available with or without albumin. Single-dose vials 25, 40, 60, 100, 200, 300, 500 mcg/1 mL, and 150 mcg/0.75 mL. Single-dose prefilled syringes or autoinjectors - 25 mcg/0.42 mL, 40 mcg/0.4 mL, 60 mcg/0.3 mL, 100 mcg/0.5 mL, 150 mcg/0.3 mL, 200 mcg/0.4 mL, 300 mcg/0.6 mL, 500 mcg/1 mL.

NOTES - May exacerbate HTN; contraindicated if uncontrolled HTN. Not for immediate correction of anemia. Evaluate iron stores before and during treatment; most patients eventually require iron supplements. Consider other causes of anemia if no response. Use only one dose per vial/syringe; discard any unused portion. Do not shake. Protect from light.

erythropoietin (Epogen, Procrit, epoetin, ♥Eprex) ▶L ♀C ▶? $$$$$

WARNING - Use lowest dose for gradual rise in Hb to minimum level to avoid blood transfusion. When administered to target Hb of >12 mg/dL, increased risk of death and serious cardiovascular events, including arterial and venous thrombotic events. Consider antithrombotic DVT prophylaxis. Not approved for use in cancer patients with anemia not due to concurrent chemotherapy; may not provide benefit and may increase risk of death. May shorten time to tumor progression in cancer patients and increase risk of death.

ADULT - Anemia of chronic renal failure: Initial dose 50-100 units/kg IV/SC 3 times/week. Zidovudine-induced anemia in HIV-infected patients: 100-300 units/kg IV/SC 3 times/week. Anemia in cancer chemo patients: 150-300 units/kg SC 3 times/week or 40,000 units SC once/week. Monitor Hb weekly until stable, then at least monthly. Target Hb not to exceed 12 g/dL. Reduce dose by 25% if Hb is increasing and approaches 12 g/dL or if Hb increases by 1 g/dL per 2 week time period; hold if >12 g/dL. Increase dose by 25% if Hb increases by <1 g/dL over 1 month. Increase dose at intervals of 1 month or more. Reduction of allogeneic blood transfusion in surgical patients: 300 units/kg/day SC x 10 days preop, on the day of surgery, and 4 days postop. Or 600 units/kg SC once weekly starting 21 days preop and ending on day of surgery (4 doses).

PEDS - Not approved in children.

UNAPPROVED PEDS - Anemia of chronic renal failure: Initial dose 50-100 units/kg IV/SC 3 times/week. Zidovudine-induced anemia in HIV-infected patients: 100 units/kg SC 3 times/week; max of 300 units/kg/dose.

FORMS - Trade only: Single-dose 1 mL vials 2,000, 3,000, 4,000, 10,000, 40,000 units/mL. Multi-dose vials 10,000 units/mL 2 mL & 20,000 units/mL 1 mL.

NOTES - May exacerbate HTN; contraindicated if uncontrolled HTN. Not for immediate correction of anemia. Evaluate iron stores before and during treatment; most patients eventually require iron supplements. Consider other causes of anemia if no response. Single-dose vials contain no preservatives. Use 1 dose per vial; do not re-enter vial. Discard unused portion.

filgrastim (G-CSF, Neupogen) ▶L ♀C ▶?
$$$$$
ADULT - Reduction of febrile neutropenia after chemo for non-myeloid malignancies: 5 mcg/kg/day SC/IV for ≤2 weeks until post-nadir ANC is ≥10,000/mm3. Can increase by 5 mcg/kg/day with each cycle prn.
PEDS - Reduction of febrile neutropenia after chemo for non-myeloid malignancies: 5 mcg/kg/day SC/IV.
UNAPPROVED ADULT - AIDS: 0.3-3.6 mcg/kg/day.
FORMS - Trade only: Single-dose vials 300 mcg/1 mL, 480 mcg/1.6 mL. Single-dose syringes 300 mcg/0.5 mL, 480 mcg/0.8 mL.
NOTES - Allergic-type reactions, bone pain, cutaneous vasculitis. Do not give <24h before/after cytotoxic chemotherapy. Store in refrigerator; use <24 h when kept at room temperature.

oprelvekin (Neumega) ▶K ♀C ▶? $$$$$
ADULT - Prevention of severe thrombocytopenia after chemo for nonmyeloid malignancies: 50 mcg/kg SC daily starting 6-24 h after chemo and continuing until post-nadir platelet count is ≥50,000 cells/mcL.
PEDS - Not approved in children. Safe and effective dose not established. Papilledema with 100 mcg/kg; 50 mcg/kg ineffective.
FORMS - Trade only: 5 mg single-dose vials with diluent.
NOTES - Fluid retention - monitor fluid and electrolyte balance. Transient atrial arrhythmias, visual blurring, papilledema.

pegfilgrastim (Neulasta) ▶Plasma ♀C ▶?
$$$$$
WARNING - Do not use if <45 kg.
ADULT - To reduce febrile neutropenia after chemo for non-myeloid malignancies: 6 mg SC once each chemo cycle.
PEDS - Not approved in children.
FORMS - Trade only: Single-dose syringes 6 mg/0.6 mL.
NOTES - Bone pain common. Do not give <14 days before or 24 h after cytotoxic chemo. Store in refrigerator. Stable at room temperature for ≤48 h. Protect from light

sargramostim (GM-CSF, Leukine) ▶L ♀C ▶?
$$$$$
ADULT - Specialized dosing for leukemia, bone marrow transplantation.
PEDS - Not approved in children.

HEMATOLOGY: Other (See endocrine section for vitamins and minerals.)

---

aminocaproic acid (Amicar) ▶K ♀D ▶? $$
ADULT - Hemostasis when fibrinolysis contributes to bleeding: 4-5 g IV/PO over 1h, then 1 g/h for 8h or until bleeding controlled.
PEDS - Not approved in children.
UNAPPROVED ADULT - Prevention of recurrent subarachnoid hemorrhage: 6 g IV/PO q4h (6 doses/day). Reduction of postop bleeding after cardiopulmonary bypass: 5 g IV, then 1 g/h x 6-8 h.
UNAPPROVED PEDS - To improve hemostasis when fibrinolysis contributes to bleeding: 100 mg/kg or 3 g/m2 IV infusion during first h, then continuous infusion of 33.3 mg/kg/h or 1 g/m2/h. Max dose of 18 g/m2/day. IV prep contains benzyl alcohol - do not use in newborns.
FORMS - Generic/Trade: Syrup or oral soln 250 mg/mL, tabs 500 mg.
NOTES - Contraindicated in active intravascular clotting. Do not use in DIC without heparin. Can cause intrarenal thrombosis, hyperkalemia. Skeletal muscle weakness, necrosis with prolonged use - monitor CPK. Use with estrogen/oral contraceptives can cause hypercoagulability. Rapid IV administration can cause hypotension, bradycardia, arrhythmia.

anagrelide (Agrylin) ▶LK ♀C ▶? $$$$$
ADULT - Thrombocythemia due to myeloproliferative disorders (including essential thrombocythemia): Start 0.5 mg PO qid or 1 mg PO bid, then after 1 week adjust to lowest effective dose that maintains platelets <600,000/mcL. Max 10 mg/day or 2.5 mg as a single dose. Usual dose 1.5 to 3 mg/day.
PEDS - Limited data. Thrombocythemia due to myeloproliferative disorders (including essential thrombocythemia): Start 0.5 mg PO daily, then after 1 week adjust to lowest effective dose that maintains platelets <600,000/mcL. Max 10 mg/day or 2.5 mg as a single dose. Usual dose 1.5 to 3 mg/day.
FORMS - Generic/Trade: Caps, 0.5, 1 mg.
NOTES - Caution with heart disease -- may cause vasodilation, tachycardia, palpitations,

heart failure. Contraindicated in severe hepatic impairment; caution in mild to moderate hepatic impairment. Dosage should be increased by not more than 0.5 mg/day in any one week.

aprotinin (Trasylol) ▶lysosomal enzymes, K ♀B ▶? $$$$$
WARNING - May increase the risk of death, serious renal damage, CHF, MI, and stroke; use only when reduced blood loss is essential and outweighs these risks. Anaphylaxis can occur even with test dose and when test dose was tolerated. Risk low in previously unexposed patients. Risk high with reexposure ≤12 months after previous dose; use special precautions.
ADULT - To reduce blood loss during CABG: 1 mL IV test dose ≥10 min before loading dose. Regimen A: 200 mL loading dose, then 200 mL pump prime dose, then 50 mL/h. Regimen B: 100 mL loading dose, then 100 mL pump prime dose, then 25 mL/h. Pick regimen based on bleeding risk.
PEDS - Safety and efficacy not established.
NOTES - Hypotension with rapid administration. Prolongation of activated clotting time (ACT) by aprotinin may overestimate heparin anticoagulation. Effect of aprotinin on ACT may vary by ACT formulation. Determine dose of protamine to reverse heparin based on heparin dose rather than ACT value.

protamine ▶Plasma ♀C ▶? $
ADULT - Heparin overdose: 1 mg antagonizes ~100 units heparin. Give IV over 10 minutes in doses of not >50 mg.
PEDS - Not approved in children.
UNAPPROVED ADULT - Reversal of low molecular weight heparin: 1 mg protamine per 100 anti-Xa units of dalteparin or tinzaparin. Give additional 0.5 mg protamine per 100 anti-Xa

units of tinzaparin if PTT remains prolonged 2-4 h after first infusion of protamine. 1 mg protamine per 1 mg enoxaparin.
UNAPPROVED PEDS - Heparin overdose: <30 min since last heparin dose, give 1 mg protamine per 100 units of heparin received; 30-60 min since last heparin dose, give 0.5-0.75 mg protamine per 100 units of heparin received; 60-120 min since last heparin dose, give 0.375-0.5 mg protamine per 100 units of heparin; >120 min since last heparin dose, give 0.25-0.375 mg protamine/100 units of heparin.
NOTES - Severe hypotension/anaphylactoid reaction with too rapid administration. Allergic reactions in patients with fish allergy, previous exposure to protamine (including insulin). Risk of allergy unclear in infertile/vasectomized men with anti-protamine antibodies. Additional doses of protamine may be required in some situations (neutralization of SC heparin, heparin rebound after cardiac surgery). Monitor APTT to confirm heparin neutralization.

tranexamic acid (Cyklokapron) ▶K ♀B ▶- $$$
ADULT - Prophylaxis/reduction of tooth extraction bleeding in hemophilia: 10 mg/kg IV immediately prior, then 25 mg/kg PO 3-4 times/day for 2-8 days following surgery. Additional regimens include: 10 mg/kg IV 3-4 times/day if intolerant of oral therapies or 25 mg/kg PO 3-4 times/day beginning 1 day before surgery.
PEDS - Not approved in children.
NOTES – Adjust dose in renal impairment-Creat 1.36-2.83 mg/dL: 10 mg/kg IV bid or 15 mg/kg PO bid. Creat 2.83-5.66 mg/dL: 10 mg/kg IV daily or 15 mg/kg PO daily. Creat >5.66 mg/dL: 10 mg/kg IV q48h or 5 mg/kg IV q24h; 15 mg/kg PO q48h or 7.5 mg/kg PO q24h.

HERBAL & ALTERNATIVE THERAPIES

NOTE: For all, FORMS are not by prescription. In the US, herbal and alternative therapy products are regulated as dietary supplements, not drugs. Premarketing evaluation and FDA approval are not required unless specific therapeutic claims are made. Since these products are not required to demonstrate efficacy, it is unclear whether many of them have health benefits. In addition, there may be considerable variability in content from lot to lot or between products. See www.tarascon.com/herbals for the evidence-based efficacy ratings used by Tarascon editorial staff.

aloe vera (acemannan, burn plant) ▶LK ♀oral- topical +? ▶oral- topical +? $
UNAPPROVED ADULT - Topical: Efficacy unclear for seborrheic dermatitis, psoriasis, genital herpes, partial-thickness skin burns. Does not appear effective for radiation-induced skin injury. Do not apply to surgical incisions; impaired healing reported. Oral: Mild to moderate active ulcerative colitis (possibly effective): 100 mL PO bid. Efficacy unclear for type 2 DM.
UNAPPROVED PEDS - Not for use in children.
NOTES - OTC laxatives containing aloe were

removed from the US market in 2002 due to concerns about increased risk of colon cancer. International Aloe Science Council seal may help ensure aloe content.

androstenedione (*andro*) ▶L, peripheral conversion to estrogens & androgens ♀- ▶- $

UNAPPROVED ADULT - Marketed as anabolic steroid to enhance athletic performance. Advise patients against use because of potential for androgenic and estrogenic side effects.

UNAPPROVED PEDS - Not for use in children.

NOTES - In 2004 FDA warned manufacturers to stop marketing. Also banned by many athletic associations. In theory, chronic use may increase risk of hormone-related cancers (prostate, breast, ovarian). Increase in androgen levels could exacerbate hyperlipidemia.

aristolochic acid (*Aristolochia, Asarum, Bragantia*) ▶? ♀- ▶- $

UNAPPROVED ADULT - Do not use. Was promoted for weight loss.

UNAPPROVED PEDS - Do not use.

NOTES - Banned by FDA due to risk of nephrotoxicity and cancer. May be present as an adulterant in other Chinese herbal products like Akebia, Clematis, Stephania, and others. Rule out aristolochic acid nephrotoxicity in cases of unexplained renal failure. List of Internet products that may contain aristolochic acid available at http://potency.berkeley.edu/text/FDA AristolochicAcidLetter.pdf

arnica (*Arnica montana, leopard's bane, wolf's bane*) ▶? ♀- ▶- $

UNAPPROVED ADULT - Toxic if taken by mouth. Topical preparations promoted for treatment of skin wounds, bruises, aches, and sprains; but insufficient data to assess efficacy. Do not use on open wounds.

UNAPPROVED PEDS - Not for use in children.

NOTES - Repeated topical application can cause skin reactions.

artichoke leaf extract (*Cynara-SL, Cynara scolymus*) ▶? ♀? ▶? $

UNAPPROVED ADULT - May reduce total cholesterol, but clinical significance is unclear. Cynara-SL is promoted as digestive aid (possibly effective for dyspepsia) at a dose of 1-2 caps PO daily. Does not appear to prevent alcohol-induced hangover.

UNAPPROVED PEDS - Not for use in children.

NOTES - Advise against for bile duct obstruction or gallstones. Artichoke leaf is an ingredient in CholesTame and Digestive Formula.

astragalus (*Astragalus membranaceus, huang qi, vetch*) ▶? ♀? ▶? $

UNAPPROVED ADULT - Used in combination with other herbs in traditional Chinese medicine, but efficacy unclear for CHD, CHF, chronic kidney disease, viral infections, upper respiratory tract infections. Astragalus-based Chinese herbal medicine may improve survival, tumor response, and performance status of patients receiving platinum-based chemotherapy for non-small cell lung cancer.

UNAPPROVED PEDS - Not for use in children.

NOTES - Not used for >3 weeks without close follow-up in traditional Chinese medicine. In theory, may enhance activity of drugs for diabetes, hypertension, and anticoagulation.

bilberry (*Vaccinium myrtillus, huckleberry, Tegens, VMA extract*) ▶Bile, K ♀- ▶- $

UNAPPROVED ADULT - Cataracts (efficacy unclear): 80-160 mg PO bid-tid of 25% anthocyanosides extract. Insufficient data to evaluate efficacy for macular degeneration. Does not appear effective for improving night vision.

UNAPPROVED PEDS - Not for use in children.

NOTES - High doses may impair platelet aggregation, affect clotting time, cause GI distress.

bitter melon (*Momordica charantia, karela*) ▶? ♀- ▶- $$

UNAPPROVED ADULT - Possibly effective for type 2 diabetes. Dose unclear; juice may be more potent than dried fruit powder.

UNAPPROVED PEDS - Not for use in children. Two cases of hypoglycemic coma in children ingesting bitter melon tea.

bitter orange (*Citrus aurantium, Seville orange, Acutrim Natural AM, Dexatrim Natural Ephedrine Free*) ▶K ♀- ▶- $

UNAPPROVED ADULT - Marketed as substitute for ephedra in weight-loss dietary supplements; safety and efficacy not established.

UNAPPROVED PEDS - Not for use in children.

NOTES - Contains sympathomimetics including synephrine and octopamine. Case reports of stroke and MI in patients taking bitter orange with caffeine. Do not use within 14 days of an MAOI. Juice may inhibit CYP 3A4 metabolism of felodipine and midazolam.

black cohosh (*Cimicifuga racemosa, Remifemin, Menofem*) ▶? ♀- ▶- $

UNAPPROVED ADULT - Ineffective for relief of menopausal symptoms.

UNAPPROVED PEDS - Not for use in children.

NOTES - Unclear if estrogenic effects. Potential for endometrial stimulation unclear; some experts recommend monitoring with vaginal ultrasound if long-term use.

butterbur (*Petesites hybridus, Petadolex, Petaforce, Tesalin, ZE 339*) ▶? ♀- ▶- $

UNAPPROVED ADULT - Migraine prophylaxis (possibly effective): Petadolex 50-75 mg PO bid. Allergic rhinitis prophylaxis (possibly effective): Petadolex 50 mg PO bid or Tesalin (ZE 339; 8 mg petasin/tab) 1 tab PO qid or 2 tabs tid. Efficacy unclear for asthma.

UNAPPROVED PEDS - Not for children.

Standardized pyrrolizidine-free extracts: Petadolex (7.5 mg of petasin & isopetasin/50 mg tab). Tesalin (ZE 339; 8 mg petasin/tab).

NOTES - Do not use raw butterbur; it may contain hepatotoxic pyrrolizidine alkaloids which are removed by processing. Butterbur is related to Asteraceae and Compositae; consider the potential for cross-allergenicity between plants in these families.

chamomile (*Matricaria recutita* - German chamomile, *Anthemis nobilis* - Roman chamomile) ▶? ♀- ▶? $

UNAPPROVED ADULT - Promoted as a sedative or anxiolytic, to relieve GI distress, for skin infections or inflammation, many other indications. Efficacy unclear for any indication. Does not appear to reduce mucositis caused by 5-fluorouracil or radiation.

UNAPPROVED PEDS - Supplements not for children. Efficacy/safety unclear for treatment of infant colic with multi-ingredient teas/extracts of chamomile, fennel, and lemon balm.

NOTES - Theoretical concern (no clinical evidence) for interactions due to increased sedation, increased risk of bleeding (contains coumarin derivatives), delayed GI absorption of other drugs (due to antispasmodic effect). Increased INR with warfarin attributed to chamomile in single case report.

chaparral (*Larrea divaricata, creosote bush*) ▶? ♀- ▶- $

UNAPPROVED ADULT - Do not use. Promoted as cancer cure.

UNAPPROVED PEDS - Not for use in children.

NOTES - Reports of irreversible liver damage.

chasteberry (*Vitex agnus castus fruit extract, Femaprin*) ▶? ♀- ▶- $

UNAPPROVED ADULT - Premenstrual syndrome (possibly effective): 20 mg PO daily of extract ZE 440 (ratio 6-12:1; standardized for casticin).

UNAPPROVED PEDS - Not for use in children.

NOTES - Liquid formulations may contain alcohol. Avoid concomitant dopamine antagonists

such as haloperidol or metoclopramide.

chondroitin ▶K ♀? ▶? $

UNAPPROVED ADULT - Does not appear effective for relief of knee osteoarthritis pain, but possibly reduces joint space narrowing. Glucosamine/ Chondroitin Arthritis Intervention Trial (GAIT) did not find improvement in pain of knee OA with chondroitin 400 mg PO tid +/- glucosamine. Glucosamine + chondroitin improved pain in subgroup of patients with moderate to severe knee OA.

UNAPPROVED PEDS - Not for use in children.

NOTES - Chondroitin content not standardized and known to vary. Cosamin DS contains 3 mg manganese/cap; tolerable upper limit of manganese is 11 mg/day. Some products made from bovine cartilage. Case report of increased INR with warfarin/chondroitin/glucosamine.

coenzyme Q10 (*CoQ-10, ubiquinone*) ▶Bile ♀- ▶- $

UNAPPROVED ADULT - Heart failure: 100 mg/day PO divided bid-tid (conflicting clinical trials; may reduce hospitalization, dyspnea, edema, but Am Heart Assoc does not recommend). Statin-induced muscle pain: 100-200 mg PO daily (conflicting clinical trials). Parkinson's disease: 1200 mg/day PO divided qid at meals and hs ($$$$; efficacy unclear; might slow progression slightly, but Am Acad Neurol does not recommend). Study for progression of Huntington's disease was inconclusive. Prevention of migraine: 100 mg PO tid (possibly effective). Efficacy unclear for improving athletic performance. Appears ineffective for diabetes.

UNAPPROVED PEDS - Not for use in children.

NOTES - Case reports of increased INR with warfarin; but a crossover study did not find an interaction.

comfrey (*Symphytum officinale*) ▶? ♀- ▶- $

UNAPPROVED ADULT - Do not use, even externally (application on broken skin could lead to systemic absorption). Topical use promoted for bruises, burns and sprains.

UNAPPROVED PEDS - Do not use, even externally (application on broken skin could lead to systemic absorption). Topical use promoted for bruises, burns and sprains.

NOTES - Reports of fatal hepatic veno-occlusive disease in humans. Contains pyrrolizidine alkaloids. FDA banned comfrey products from US market in 2001.

cranberry (*Cranactin, Vaccinium macrocarpon*) ▶? ♀? ▶? $

UNAPPROVED ADULT - Prevention of UTI

(possibly effective): 300 mL/day PO cranberry juice cocktail. Usual dose of cranberry juice extract caps/tabs is 300-400 mg PO bid. Insufficient data to assess efficacy for treatment of UTI. Not a substitute for antibiotics in UTI.

UNAPPROVED PEDS - Insufficient data to assess efficacy for prevention/treatment of UTI. Does not appear to treat or prevent UTI in children with neurogenic bladder. Should not be a substitute for antibiotics in acute UTI.

NOTES - Warfarin product labeling advises patients to avoid ingestion of cranberry products based on case reports of increased INRs and bleeding. However, new clinical trials did not find an increase in the INR with cranberry. ~100 calories/6 oz of cranberry juice cocktail. Advise diabetics that some products have high sugar content. Not a substitute for antibiotics to treat UTI. Increases urinary oxalate excretion; may increase risk of oxalate kidney stones.

creatine ▶LK ♀- ▶- $

UNAPPROVED ADULT - Promoted to enhance athletic performance. No benefit for endurance exercise, but modest benefit for intense anaerobic tasks lasting <30 seconds. Usually taken as loading dose of 20 g/day PO x 5 days, then 2-5 g/day. A 5-year phase III NIH trial is evaluating for neuroprotection in Parkinson's disease (http://www.parkinsontrial.ninds.nih.gov). Possibly effective for increasing muscle strength in Duchenne muscular dystrophy. Does not appear effective for myotonic dystrophy Type 1, amyotrophic lateral sclerosis. Research ongoing in Huntington's disease.

UNAPPROVED PEDS - Not for use in children.

NOTES - Caffeine may antagonize the ergogenic effects of creatine. Creatine is metabolized to creatinine. In young healthy adults, large doses can increase serum creatinine slightly without affecting CrCl. The effect in elderly is unknown.

danshen (Salvia miltiorrhiza) ▶? ♀? ▶? $

UNAPPROVED ADULT - Used for treatment of cardiovascular diseases in traditional Chinese medicine.

UNAPPROVED PEDS - Not for use in children.

NOTES - Case reports of increased INR with warfarin.

dehydroepiandrosterone (DHEA, Aslera, Fidelin, Prasterone) ▶Peripheral conversion to estrogens and androgens ♀- ▶- $

UNAPPROVED ADULT - No convincing evidence that DHEA slows aging or improves cognition in elderly. To improve well-being in wom-

en with adrenal insufficiency: 50 mg PO daily (possibly effective; conflicting clinical trials). Used by athletes as a substitute for anabolic steroids; but no convincing evidence of enhanced athletic performance or increased muscle mass. Banned by many sports organizations.

UNAPPROVED PEDS - Not for use in children.

NOTES - In theory, chronic use may increase risk of hormone-related cancers (prostate, breast, ovarian).

devil's claw (Harpagophytum procumbens, Phyto Joint, Doloteffin, Harpadol) ▶? ♀- ▶- $

UNAPPROVED ADULT - Osteoarthritis, acute exacerbation of chronic low back pain (possibly effective): 2400 mg extract/day (50-100 mg harpagoside/day) PO divided bid-tid.

UNAPPROVED PEDS - Not for children.

Extracts standardized to harpagoside (iridoid glycoside) content.

dong quai (Angelica sinensis) ▶? ♀- ▶- $

UNAPPROVED ADULT - Appears ineffective for postmenopausal symptoms; North American Menopause Society recommends against use. Used with other herbs for treatment and prevention of dysmenorrhea, TIA, stroke, PVD, and cardiovascular conditions in traditional Chinese medicine.

UNAPPROVED PEDS - Not for use in children.

NOTES - Increased risk of bleeding with warfarin with/without increase in INR; avoid concurrent use.

echinacea (E. purpurea, E. angustifolia, E. pallida, cone flower, EchinaGuard, Echinacin Madaus) ▶? ♀- ▶- $

UNAPPROVED ADULT - Promoted as immune stimulant. Conflicting clinical trials for prevention/treatment of upper respiratory infections.

UNAPPROVED PEDS - Not for use in children. Appears ineffective for treatment of upper respiratory tract infections in children. A formulation combining echinacea, vitamin C, and propolis (Chizukit; not available in US) appears effective for preventing respiratory infections.

NOTES - Single case reports of precipitation of thrombotic thrombocytopenic purpura and exacerbation of pemphigus vulgaris; causality unclear. Rare allergic reactions including anaphylaxis. Cross-hypersensitivity possible with other plants in Compositae family (arnica, chamomile, chrysanthemum, feverfew, ragweed, Artemisia). Photosensitivity possible. Could interact with immunosuppressants due to immunomodulating effects. Some experts limit use to

≤8 weeks and recommend against use with autoimmune disorders. May inhibit P450 1A2.

elderberry (*Sambucus nigra, Rubini, Sambucol, Sinupret*) ▶? ♀- ▶- $

UNAPPROVED ADULT - Efficacy unclear for influenza, sinusitis, and bronchitis.

UNAPPROVED PEDS - Not for use in children.

NOTES - Sinupret and Sanbucol also contain other ingredients. Eating uncooked elderberries may cause nausea or cyanide toxicity.

ephedra (*Ephedra sinica, ma huang, Metabolife 356, Biolean, Ripped Fuel, Xenadrine*) ▶K ♀- ▶- $

UNAPPROVED ADULT - Little evidence of efficacy for obesity, other than modest short-term weight loss. Traditional use as bronchodilator. FDA banned ephedra supplements in 2004.

UNAPPROVED PEDS - Not for use in children.

NOTES - Linked to CVA, MI, sudden death, HTN, palpitations, tachycardia, seizures. Risk of serious reactions may increase with dose, strenuous exercise, or concomitant use of other stimulants like caffeine (as in Biolean & Dexatrim Results). Metabolife 356 can prolong QT interval and increase systolic BP. Country mallow (Sida cordifolia) contains ephedrine.

evening primrose oil (*Oenothera biennis*) ▶? ♀? ▶? $

UNAPPROVED ADULT - Appears ineffective for premenstrual syndrome, postmenopausal symptoms, atopic dermatitis.

UNAPPROVED PEDS - Not for use in children.

fenugreek (*Trigonelle foenum-graecum*) ▶? ♀- ▶? $$

UNAPPROVED ADULT - Efficacy unclear for diabetes or hyperlipidemia. Insufficient data to evaluate efficacy as galactagogue.

UNAPPROVED PEDS - Not for use in children.

NOTES - Case report of increased INR with warfarin possibly related to fenugreek. Can cause maple syrup-like body odor. Fiber content could decrease absorption of some drugs.

feverfew (*Chrysanthemum parthenium, Migra-Lief, MigraSpray, Tanacetum parthenium L.*) ▶? ♀- ▶- $

UNAPPROVED ADULT - Prevention of migraine (possibly effective): 50-100 mg extract PO daily; 2-3 fresh leaves PO daily; 50-125 mg freeze-dried leaf PO daily. Take either leaf form with or after meals. Benefit of alcoholic extract questioned. May take 1-2 months to be effective. Inadequate data to evaluate efficacy for acute migraine.

UNAPPROVED PEDS - Not for use in children.

NOTES - May cause uterine contractions; avoid with pregnancy. Migra-Lief contains feverfew, riboflavin and magnesium. MigraSpray and Gelstat are homeopathic products that are unlikely to be beneficial.

flavocoxid (*Limbrel*) ▶? ♀- ▶- $$$

UNAPPROVED ADULT - Osteoarthritis (efficacy unclear): 250-500 mg PO bid. Max 2000 mg/day short-term. Taking 1 h before or after meals may increase absorption.

UNAPPROVED PEDS - Not for use in children.

FORMS - Caps 250,500 mg. Marketed as medical food by prescription only (not all medical foods require a prescription). Medical foods are intended to be given under physician supervision to meet distinctive nutritional needs of a disease, but they do not undergo an approval process to establish safety and efficacy.

NOTES - Be alert for confusion between the brand names, Limbrel and Enbrel, as well misidentification of flavocoxid as a COX-2 inhibitor.

garcinia (*Garcinia cambogia, Citri Lean*) ▶? ♀- ▶- $

UNAPPROVED ADULT - Appears ineffective for weight loss.

UNAPPROVED PEDS - Not for use in children.

garlic supplements (*Allium sativum, Kwai, Kyolic*) ▶LK ♀- ▶- $

UNAPPROVED ADULT - Ineffective for hyperlipidemia, and Am College of Cardiology does not recommend for this indication. Small reduction in BP, but efficacy in HTN unclear. Does not appear effective for diabetes.

UNAPPROVED PEDS - Not for use in children.

NOTES - Significantly decreases saquinavir levels; may also interact with other protease inhibitors. May increase warfarin bleeding risk with/ without increase in INR. Kyolic (aged garlic extract) did not affect the INR in a clinical study.

ginger (*Zingiber officinale*) ▶? ♀? ▶? $

UNAPPROVED ADULT - Prevention of motion sickness (efficacy unclear): 500-1000 mg powdered rhizome PO single dose 1 h before exposure. American College of Obstetrics and Gynecology considers ginger 250 mg PO qid a nonpharmacologic option for N/V of pregnancy. Some experts advise pregnant women to limit dose to usual dietary amount (≤1 g/day). Conflicting clinical trials for postop N/V. Efficacy unclear for relief of osteoarthritis pain.

UNAPPROVED PEDS - Not for use in children.

NOTES - Increased INR >10 attributed to ginger in a phenprocoumon-treated patient, but study in healthy volunteers found no effect of ginger on INR or pharmacokinetics of warfarin.

ginkgo biloba (*EGb 761, Ginkgold, Ginkoba, Quanterra Mental Sharpness*) ▶K ♀- ▶- $

UNAPPROVED ADULT - Dementia (modest benefit for mild to moderate disease): 40 mg PO tid of standardized extract containing 24% ginkgo flavone glycosides and 6% terpene lactones. It may take up to 4 weeks to be effective. Does not appear to improve memory in elderly with normal cognitive function. Does not appear effective for prevention of acute altitude sickness. Limited benefit in intermittent claudication. Am College of Cardiology found insufficient evidence for treatment of peripheral vascular disease. ArginMax (also contains L-arginine and other ingredients) promoted for SSRI-induced sexual dysfunction.

UNAPPROVED PEDS - Not for use in children.

NOTES - Case reports of intracerebral, subdural, and ocular bleeding. Does not appear to increase INR with warfarin, but monitoring for bleeding is advised. Ginkgo seeds contain a neurotoxin. A few reports attributing exacerbation or precipitation of seizures to ginkgo supplements has raised concern about possible contamination with the neurotoxin. Some experts advise caution or avoidance of ginkgo by those with seizures or taking drugs that lower the seizure threshold.

ginseng - American (*Panax quinquefolius L.*) ▶K ♀- ▶- $

UNAPPROVED ADULT - Reduction of postprandial glucose in type 2 diabetes (possibly effective): 3 g ground root caps PO taken with or up to 2h before meal.

UNAPPROVED PEDS - Not for use in children.

NOTES - Ginseng content varies widely and some products are mislabeled or adulterated with caffeine. American, Asian, and Siberian ginseng are often misidentified. Decreased INR with warfarin.

ginseng - Asian (*Panax ginseng, Ginsana, Ginsai, G115, Korean red ginseng*) ▶? ♀- ▶- $

UNAPPROVED ADULT - Promoted to improve vitality and well-being: 200 mg PO daily. Ginsana: 2 caps PO daily or 1 cap PO bid. Ginsana Sport: 1 cap PO daily. Efficacy unclear for improving physical or psychomotor performance, diabetes, herpes simplex infections, cognitive or immune function. American College of Obstetrics and Gynecologists and North American Menopause Society recommend against use

for postmenopausal hot flashes .

UNAPPROVED PEDS - Not for use in children.

NOTES - Some formulations may contain up to 34% alcohol. Ginsana Gold also contains vitamins and minerals. Reports of an interaction with the MAOI, phenelzine. Decreased INR with warfarin. Ginseng content varies widely and some products are mislabeled or adulterated with caffeine. American, Asian, and Siberian ginseng are often misidentified. May interfere with FPIA and MEIA digoxin assays.

ginseng - Siberian (*Eleutherococcus senticosus, Ci-wu-jia*) ▶? ♀- ▶- $

UNAPPROVED ADULT - Does not appear to improve athletic endurance. Did not appear effective in single clinical trial for chronic fatigue syndrome.

UNAPPROVED PEDS - Not for use in children.

NOTES - May interfere with FPIA and MEIA digoxin assays. A case report of thalamic stroke attributed to Siberian ginseng plus caffeine.

glucosamine (*Aflexa, Cosamin DS, Dona, Flextend, Promotion*) ▶? ♀- ▶- $

UNAPPROVED ADULT - Osteoarthritis: Glucosamine HCl 500 mg PO tid. Glucosamine sulfate (Dona) 1500 mg PO once daily (a packet dissolved in glass of water or caplet). Efficacy for OA is unclear (conflicting data). GAIT (glucosamine/chondroitin arthritis intervention trial) did not find improvement in knee OA pain with glucosamine HCl 500 mg +/- chondroitin 400 mg both PO tid, although it did improve pain in the subgroup with moderate to severe OA. Some earlier studies reported improved pain with a different salt [glucosamine sulfate (Dona) 1500 mg PO once daily].

UNAPPROVED PEDS - Not for use in children.

NOTES - Avoid or caution in shellfish allergy. Case report of increased INR with warfarin in patient taking chondroitin + glucosamine.

goldenseal (*Hydrastis canadensis*) ▶? ♀- ▶- $

UNAPPROVED ADULT - Often used in attempts to achieve false-negative urine test for illicit drug use (efficacy unclear). Often combined with echinacea in cold remedies; but insufficient data to assess efficacy of goldenseal for the common cold or URIs.

UNAPPROVED PEDS - Not for use in children.

NOTES - Alkaloids in goldenseal with antibacterial activity not well-absorbed orally. Oral use contraindicated in pregnancy (may cause uterine contractions), newborns (may cause kernicterus), and HTN (high doses may cause peripheral vasoconstriction). Adding goldenseal directly to urine turns it brown. May inhibit CYP 2D6 and 3A4. Berberine, a component of goldenseal, may increase cyclosporine levels.

grape seed extract (*Vitis vinifera L.*, *procyanidolic oligomers, PCO*) ▶? ♀? ▶? $

UNAPPROVED ADULT - Small trials suggest benefit in chronic venous insufficiency. No benefit in single study of seasonal allergic rhinitis.

UNAPPROVED PEDS - Not for use in children.

NOTES - Pine bark (pycnogenol) and grape seed extract are often confused; they both contain oligomeric proanthocyanidins.

green tea (*Camellia sinensis*) ▶? ♀+ in moderate amount in food, - in supplements ▶+ in moderate amount in food, - in supplements $

PEDS - Not for children.

UNAPPROVED ADULT - Some population studies suggest a reduction in adenomatous polyps and chronic atrophic gastritis in green tea drinkers. Efficacy unclear for cancer prevention, weight loss, hypercholesterolemia. Phase I studies of green tea extract in advanced lung and prostate cancer did not suggest antineoplastic activity. Under evaluation for prevention of prostate cancer in men with high-grade prostate intraepithelial neoplasia.

Green tea extract available in caps standardized to polyphenol content.

NOTES - Case report of decreased INR with warfarin attributed to drinking large amounts of green tea (due to vitamin K content). The vitamin K content of green tea is low with usual consumption.

guarana (*Paullinia cupana*) ▶? ♀+ in food, - in supplements ▶+ in food, - in supplements $

UNAPPROVED ADULT - Marketed as an ingredient in weight-loss supplements. Seeds contain caffeine. Guarana in weight loss supplements may provide high doses of caffeine.

UNAPPROVED PEDS - Not for children.

guggulipid (*Commiphora mukul extract, guggul*) ▶? ♀- ▶- $$

UNAPPROVED ADULT - Does not appear effective for hyperlipidemia. A USA randomized controlled trial with 1000 mg or 2000 mg PO tid reported no change in total cholesterol, triglycerides, or HDL, and a small increase in LDL. Earlier studies of weaker design reported reductions in total cholesterol of up to 27%.

UNAPPROVED PEDS - Not for use in children.

NOTES - May decrease levels of propranolol and diltiazem.

hawthorn (*Crataegus laevigata, monogyna, oxyacantha, standardized extract WS 1442 - Crataegutt novo, HeartCare*) ▶? ♀- ▶- $

UNAPPROVED ADULT - Symptomatic improvement of mild CHF (NYHA I-II; possibly effective): 80 mg PO bid to 160 mg PO tid of standardized extract (19% oligomeric procyanidins; WS 1442; HeartCare 80 mg tabs); doses as high as 900-1800 mg/day have been studied. Am College of Cardiology found evidence insufficient to recommend for mild heart failure. Does not appear effective for hypertension.

UNAPPROVED PEDS - Not for use in children.

NOTES - Unclear whether hawthorn and digoxin should be used together; mechanisms of action may be similar.

horse chestnut seed extract (*Aesculus hippocastanum, HCE50, Venastat*) ▶? ♀- ▶- $

UNAPPROVED ADULT - Chronic venous insufficiency (effective): 1 cap Venastat PO bid with water before meals. Response within 1 month. Venastat is 16% aescin in standardized extract. Am College of Cardiology found evidence insufficient to recommend for peripheral vascular disease.

UNAPPROVED PEDS - Not for use in children.

NOTES - Venastat does not contain aesculin, a toxin in horse chestnuts.

kava (*Piper methysticum, One-a-day Bedtime & Rest, Sleep-Tite*) ▶K ♀- ▶- $

UNAPPROVED ADULT - Promoted as anxiolytic (possibly effective) or sedative; recommend against use due to hepatotoxicity.

UNAPPROVED PEDS - Not for use in children.

NOTES - Reports of severe hepatotoxicity leading to liver transplantation. May potentiate CNS effects of benzodiazepines and other sedatives, including alcohol. Reversible yellow skin discoloration with long-term use.

kombucha tea (*Manchurian or Kargasok tea*) ▶? ♀- ▶- $

UNAPPROVED ADULT - Promoted for many indications, but no scientific evidence to support benefit for any condition. FDA advises caution due to a case of fatal acidosis.

UNAPPROVED PEDS - Not for use in children.

NOTES - Culture of bacteria and yeast that is very acidic after preparation. Tea is made by steeping mushroom culture in tea and sugar for ~1 week. Tea may contain alcohol, ethyl acetate, acetic acid, and lactate.

licorice (*Glycyrrhiza glabra, Glycyrrhiza uralensis*) ▶Bile ♀- ▶- $

UNAPPROVED ADULT - Insufficient data to assess efficacy for postmenopausal vasomotor symptoms.

UNAPPROVED PEDS - Not for use in children.

NOTES - Diuretics or stimulant laxatives could potentiate licorice-induced hypokalemia. In the US, "licorice" candy usually does not contain licorice. Deglycyrrhizinated licorice does not have mineralocorticoid effects.

melatonin (N-acetyl-5-methoxytryptamine)
▶L ♀- ▶- $

UNAPPROVED ADULT - To reduce jet lag after flights across >5 time zones (possibly effective; especially traveling East; may also help for 2-4 times zones): 0.5-5 mg PO qhs (10 pm to midnight) x 3-6 nights starting on day of arrival. Faster onset and better sleep quality with 5 mg over 0.5 mg, but no greater benefit with >5 mg. No benefit with use before departure or slow-release forms. Do not take earlier in day (may cause drowsiness and delay adaptation to local time). Orphan drug for circadian rhythm-related sleep disorders in blind patients with no light perception. Possibly effective for difficulty falling asleep, but not for staying asleep.

UNAPPROVED PEDS - Not usually for use in children. Sleep-onset insomnia in ADHD, ≥6 yo (possibly effective): 3-6 mg PO qhs. Orphan drug for circadian rhythm-related sleep disorders in blind patients with no light perception.

NOTES - High melatonin levels linked to nocturnal asthma; some experts advise patients with nocturnal asthma to avoid melatonin supplements until more data available.

methylsulfonylmethane (MSM, dimethyl sulfone, crystalline DMSO2) ▶? ♀- ▶- $

UNAPPROVED ADULT - Insufficient data to assess efficacy of oral and topical MSM for arthritis pain.

UNAPPROVED PEDS - Not for use in children.

NOTES - Can cause nausea, diarrhea, headache. DMSO metabolite promoted as a source of sulfur without odor.

milk thistle (Silybum marianum, Legalon, silymarin, Thisylin) ▶LK ♀- ▶- $

UNAPPROVED ADULT - Hepatic cirrhosis (possibly effective): 100-200 mg PO tid of standardized extract with 70-80% silymarin. Hepatitis C: May decrease serum transaminase levels, but does not appear to improve viral load or liver histology; Am Gastroenterol Assoc recommends against use. Used in Europe to treat Amanita mushroom poisoning.

UNAPPROVED PEDS - Not for use in children.

NOTES - May inhibit cytochrome P450 2C9 and 3A4; but no effect on pharmacokinetics of indinavir in human studies. May decrease blood glucose in patients with cirrhosis and diabetes.

nettle root (stinging nettle, Urtica dioica radix) ▶? ♀- ▶- $

UNAPPROVED ADULT - Efficacy unclear for treatment of BPH.

UNAPPROVED PEDS - Not for use in children.

NOTES - Lead contamination led to recall of some lots of Nature's Way nettle caps.

noni (Morinda citrifolia) ▶? ♀- ▶- $$$

UNAPPROVED ADULT - Promoted for many medical disorders; but insufficient data to assess efficacy.

UNAPPROVED PEDS - Not for use in children.

NOTES - Potassium concentration comparable to orange juice. Hyperkalemia reported in a patient with chronic renal failure. Case reports of hepatotoxicity.

policosanol (One-A-Day Cholesterol Plus, CholeRx, Cholest Response, Cholesstor, Cholestin) ▶? ♀- ▶- $

UNAPPROVED ADULT - Ineffective for hyperlipidemia. A Cuban formulation (unavailable in US) reduced LDL cholesterol in studies by a single group of researchers, but studies by other groups found no benefit. Study of a US formulation (Cholesstor) also found no benefit.

UNAPPROVED PEDS - Not for use in children.

NOTES - An old formulation of Cholestin contained red yeast rice; the current formulation contains policosanol.

probiotics (Acidophilus, Bifidobacteria, Lactobacillus, Bacid, Culturelle, Florastor, IntestiFlora, Lactinex, LiveBac, Power-Dophilus, Primadophilus, Probiotica, Saccharomyces boulardii, VSL#3) ▶? ♀+ ▶+ $

ADULT - VSL#3 approved as medical food for ulcerative colitis (possibly effective) or pouchitis (effective): 4 packets/day for >8 bowel movements/day; 2-4 packets for 5-8 bowel movements; 1-2 packets for <5 bowel movements. Mix powder with ≥4 oz of cold water before taking.

PEDS - VSL#3 approved as medical food for ulcerative colitis (possibly effective) or pouchitis (effective), age ≥3 months: Dose based on weight and number of bowel movements/day. Use adult dose for ≥15 yo. Mix powder with ≥4 oz of cold water before taking.

UNAPPROVED ADULT - Antibiotic-associated diarrhea (effective): Saccharomyces boulardii

500 mg PO bid (Florastor 2 caps PO bid). Give 2 h before/after antibiotic so culture isn't killed. Prevention of recurrent C difficile diarrhea (possibly effective): S boulardii 500 mg PO bid (Florastor 2 caps PO bid) x 4 weeks. Efficacy of probiotics unclear for travelers' diarrhea (conflicting evidence), Crohn's disease, H pylori, radiation enteritis, irritable bowel syndrome. Lactobacillus GG appears ineffective for prevention of post-antibiotic vulvovaginitis.

UNAPPROVED PEDS - Prevention of antibiotic-associated diarrhea (effective): Lactobacillus GG 10-20 billion cells/day PO (Culturelle 1 cap PO once daily or bid) or S boulardii 250 mg PO bid (Floraster 1 cap PO bid). Rotavirus gastroenteritis: Lactobacillus GG ≥10 billion cells/day PO started early in illness. Efficacy of probiotics unclear for travelers' diarrhea (conflicting evidence), radiation enteritis, irritable bowel syndrome. Lactobacillus GG does not appear effective for Crohn's disease in children. Research ongoing for prevention and treatment of atopic dermatitis.

FORMS - Culturelle contains Lactobacillus GG 10 billion cells/cap. Florastor contains Saccharomyces boulardii 5 billion cells/250 mg cap. Probiotica contains Lactobacillus reuteri 100 million cells/chew tab. VSL#3 contains 450 billion cells/packet (Bifidobacterium breve, longum, infantis; Lactobacillus acidophilus, plantarum, casei, bulgaricus; Streptococcus thermophilus). VSL#3 is marketed as non-prescription medical food. Medical foods are intended to be given under physician supervision to meet distinctive nutritional needs of a disease, but they do not undergo an approval process to establish safety and efficacy.

NOTES - Use cautiously in immunosuppressed patients; acquired infection possible. Lactobacillus sepsis and Saccharomyces fungemia reported rarely in probiotic-treated patients; possible central venous access port contamination in some cases. Microbial type and content varies by product. Pick yogurt products labeled "Live and active cultures". Refrigerate packets of VSL#3; can store at room temp for 1 week.

pycnogenol (*French maritime pine tree bark*) ▶L ♀? ▶? $

UNAPPROVED ADULT - Promoted for many medical disorders, but insufficient data to assess efficacy. Data is limited to small studies in chronic venous insufficiency, sperm dysfunction, melasma, and ADHD.

UNAPPROVED PEDS - Not for use in children.

NOTES - Pine bark (pycnogenol) and grape seed extract are often confused; they both contain oligomeric proanthocyanidins.

pygeum africanum (*African plum tree, Prostata, Prostatonin, Provol*) ▶? ♀- ▶- $

UNAPPROVED ADULT - Benign prostatic hypertrophy (may have modest efficacy): 50-100 mg PO bid or 100 mg PO daily of standardized extract containing 14% triterpenes. Prostatonin (also contains Urtica dioica): 1 cap PO bid with meals; up to 6 weeks for full response. Prostata also contains saw palmetto and other ingredients.

UNAPPROVED PEDS - Not for use in children.

NOTES - Appears well-tolerated. Self-treatment could delay diagnosis of prostate cancer.

red clover isoflavone extract (*Trifolium pratense, trefoil, Promensil, Rimostil, Supplifem, Trinovin*) ▶Gut, L, K ♀- ▶- $$

UNAPPROVED ADULT - Promensil (1 tab PO daily-bid with meals) marketed for menopausal symptoms; Rimostil (1 tab PO daily) for bone & cholesterol health, and to promote health & well-being after menopause; Trinovin (1 tab PO daily) for maintaining prostate health & urinary function in men. Conflicting evidence of efficacy for postmenopausal vasomotor symptoms. Does not appear effective overall, but may have modest benefit for severe symptoms. Efficacy unclear for prevention of osteoporosis & treatment of hyperlipidemia in postmenopausal women, and for BPH sx in men.

UNAPPROVED PEDS - Not for use in children.

FORMS - Isoflavone content (genistein, daidzein, biochanin, formononetin) is 40 mg/tab in Promensil and Trinovin, 57 mg/tab in Rimostil.

NOTES - Does not appear to stimulate endometrium. Effect on breast cancer risk is unclear; some experts recommend against use by women with breast cancer. No effect on breast density in women with Wolfe P2 or DY mammographic breast density patterns. H2 blockers, proton pump inhibitors, and antibiotics may decrease metabolic activation of isoflavones in GI tract. Ingesting large amounts of red clover can cause bleeding in cattle; bleeding risk of supplements in humans is theoretical. Supplifem contains soy and red clover extract (51 mg isoflavones/caplet).

red yeast rice (*Monascus purpureus, Xuezhikang, Zhibituo, Hypocol, Lipolysar*) ▶L ♀- ▶- $$

UNAPPROVED ADULT - Efficacy of currently available US products for hyperlipidemia is unclear. A formulation of Cholestin that is no longer marketed did lower cholesterol; it contained lovastatin and other statins formed in the fermentation process. Xuezhikang (reduces LDL by 10-33%) was effective for secondary prevention of CHD events in Chinese trial. Xuezihang 2 caps PO bid or Zhibituo 3 tabs PO tid provides ~ 10 mg lovastatin/day.

UNAPPROVED PEDS - Not for use in children. Xuezhikang marketed in Asia, Norway (Hypo-Col), Italy (Lipolysar).

NOTES - In 1997, a red yeast rice product called Cholestin was marketed in the US as a cholesterol-lowering supplement. It was removed from the market in 2001 because it contained lovastatin (5-7 mg/day at usual doses). Current products may have statin activity. Cholestin later returned to the market; it now contains policosanol (ineffective for hyperlipidemia).

s-adenosylmethionine (*SAM-e, sammy*) ▶L ♀? ▶? $$$

UNAPPROVED ADULT - Depression (possibly effective): 400-1600 mg/day PO. Osteoarthritis (possibly effective): 400-1200 mg/day PO. Onset of response in OA in 2-4 weeks. Efficacy unclear for alcoholic liver disease.

UNAPPROVED PEDS - Not for use in children.

NOTES - Serotonin syndrome possible with SSRIs. Do not use within 2 weeks of an MAOI or in bipolar disorder.

Saint John's wort (*Alterra, Hypericum perforatum, Kira, Movana, One-a-day Tension & Mood, LI-160, St John's wort*) ▶L ♀- ▶- $

UNAPPROVED ADULT - Short-term treatment of mild depression (effective): 300 mg PO tid of standardized extract (0.3% hypericin). Conflicting trials for moderate major depression.

UNAPPROVED PEDS - Not for use in children.

NOTES - Photosensitivity possible with >1800 mg/day. Inducer of hepatic cytochrome P450 3A4, 2C9, 2C19, and P-glycoprotein. May decrease efficacy of drugs with hepatic metabolism including alprazolam, cyclosporine, methadone, non-nucleoside reverse transcriptase inhibitors, omeprazole, oral contraceptives, protease inhibitors, statins, voriconazole. May need increased dose of digoxin, theophylline, tricyclic antidepressants. Decreased INR with warfarin. Administration with SSRIs, nefazodone, triptans may cause serotonin syndrome. Do not use within 14 days of MAO inhibitors.

saw palmetto (*Serenoa repens, One-a-day Prostate Health, Quanterra*) ▶? ♀- ▶- $

UNAPPROVED ADULT - BPH (possibly effective for mild to moderate; appears ineffective for moderate to severe): 160 mg PO bid or 320 mg PO daily of standardized liposterolic extract. Take with food. Brewed teas may not be effective.

UNAPPROVED PEDS - Not for use in children.

NOTES - Not for use by women of child-bearing potential. Does not interfere with PSA test. Self-treatment could delay diagnosis of prostate cancer.

shark cartilage (*BeneFin, Cancenex, Cartilade*) ▶? ♀- ▶- $$$$$

UNAPPROVED ADULT - Appears ineffective for palliative care of advanced cancer. Neovastat (AE-941), a derivative of shark cartilage, is in clinical trials for non-small cell lung cancer.

UNAPPROVED PEDS - Not for use in children.

silver - colloidal (*mild & strong silver protein, silver ion*) ▶? ♀- ▶- $

UNAPPROVED ADULT - The FDA does not recognize OTC colloidal silver products as safe or effective for any use.

UNAPPROVED PEDS - Not for use in children.

May come as silver chloride, cyanide, iodide, oxide, or phosphate.

NOTES - Silver accumulates in skin (leads to grey tint), conjunctiva, and internal organs with chronic use.

soy (*Genisoy, Healthy Woman, Novasoy, Phytosoya, Supro*) ▶Gut, L, K ♀+ for food, ? for supplements ▶+ for food, ? for supplements $

UNAPPROVED ADULT - Cardiovascular risk reduction: ≥25 g/day soy protein (50 mg/day isoflavones) PO. Hypercholesterolemia: ~50 g/day soy protein PO reduces LDL cholesterol by ~3%; effects on HDL, triglycerides, BP appear insignificant. No apparent benefit for isoflavone supplements. Postmenopausal vasomotor symptoms (modest benefit if any): 20-60 g/day soy protein PO (40-80 mg/day isoflavones). Conflicting clinical trials for postmenopausal bone loss. Am Heart Assn recommends against isoflavone supplements for treatment or prevention of hyperlipidemia, or breast, endometrial, or prostate cancer.

UNAPPROVED PEDS - Soy foods are regarded as safe for children.

NOTES - Effect on breast cancer risk is unclear; some experts recommend against use of isoflavone or phytoestrogen supplements by women with endometrial or breast cancer (esp. estrogen receptor-positive tumor or receiving tamoxifen). Case report of decreased INR with ingestion of soy milk by patient taking warfarin. Report of decreased levothyroxine absorption with soy protein.

stevia (*Stevia rebaudiana*) ▶L ♀? ▶? $

UNAPPROVED ADULT - Leaves traditionally used as a sweetener, but not enough safety data for FDA approval as such. Efficacy unclear for treatment of type 2 diabetes or HTN.

UNAPPROVED PEDS - Not for use in children.

NOTES - Stevia available as dietary supplement, but not approved by the FDA as sweetener in the US.

tea tree oil (*melaleuca oil, Melaleuca alternifolia*) ▶? ♀- ▶- $

UNAPPROVED ADULT - Not for oral use; CNS toxicity reported. Efficacy unclear for onychomycosis, tinea pedis, acne vulgaris, dandruff, pediculosis.

UNAPPROVED PEDS - Not for use in children.

valerian (*Valeriana officinalis, Alluna, One-a-day Bedtime & Rest, Sleep-Tite*) ▶? ♀- ▶- $

UNAPPROVED ADULT - Insomnia (possibly effective): 400-900 mg of standardized extract PO 30 minutes before bedtime. Response reported in 2-4 weeks. Alluna (valerian + hops): 2 tabs PO 1 h before bedtime. Some products have unpleasant smell.

UNAPPROVED PEDS - Not for use in children.

NOTES - Do not combine with CNS depressants. Withdrawal symptoms reported after long-term use. Valerian does not appear to inhibit CYP 1A2, 2D6, 2E1, or 3A4.

wild yam (*Dioscorea villosa*) ▶L ♀? ▶? $

UNAPPROVED ADULT - Ineffective as topical "natural progestin".

UNAPPROVED PEDS - Not for use in children.

willow bark extract (*Salix alba, Salicis cortex, Assalix, salicin*) ▶K ♀- ▶- $

UNAPPROVED ADULT - Osteoarthritis, low back pain (possibly effective): 60 to 240 mg/day salicin PO divided bid-tid. Onset of pain relief is about 2 h. Often included in multi-ingredient weight-loss supplements based on preliminary research suggesting that aspirin increases thermogenesis.

UNAPPROVED PEDS - Not for use in children. Do not give to febrile children who could develop Reye's syndrome.

FORMS - Some products standardized to 15% salicin content.

NOTES - Contraindicated in third trimester of pregnancy, and in intolerance or allergy to aspirin or other NSAIDs. Consider contraindications and precautions that apply to other salicylates. Avoid concomitant use of NSAIDs.

yohimbe (*Corynanthe yohimbe, Pausinystalia yohimbe, Potent V*) ▶L ♀- ▶- $

UNAPPROVED ADULT - Nonprescription yohimbe promoted for impotence and as aphrodisiac, but these products rarely contain much yohimbine (active constituent). FDA considers yohimbe bark in herbal remedies an unsafe herb. Yohimbine HCl is available in US as a prescription drug.

UNAPPROVED PEDS - Not for use in children.

FORMS - Yohimbine is the primary alkaloid in the bark of the yohimbe tree. Yohimbine HCl is a prescription drug in the US; yohimbe bark is available without prescription. Yohimbe bark (not by prescription) and prescription yohimbine HCl are not interchangeable.

NOTES - Can cause CNS stimulation. High doses have MAOI activity and can increase BP. Avoid in hypotension, diabetes, heart, liver or kidney disease. Reports of renal failure, seizures, death in patients taking yohimbe.

IMMUNOLOGY: Immunizations

NOTE: For vaccine info see CDC (www.cdc.gov).

avian influenza vaccine H5N1 - inactivated injection ♀C ▶? ?

ADULT - 18-64 yo: 1 mL IM x 2 doses, separated by 21-35 days.

PEDS - Not approved for use in children.

NOTES - Caution if hypersensitivity to chicken or egg proteins. The immunocompromised may have a blunted immune response.

BCG vaccine (*Tice BCG, ♥Oncotice, Immucyst*) ♀C ▶? $$$$

ADULT - 0.2-0.3 mL percutaneously (using 1 mL sterile water for reconstitution).

PEDS - Age >1 month: use adult dose. Age <1 month: Decrease concentration by 50% using 2 mL sterile water for reconstitution, then 0.2-0.3 mL percutaneously. May revaccinate with full dose (adult dose) after 1 yo if necessary.

Comvax (*haemophilus b + hepatitis B vaccine*) ♀C ▶? $$$

ADULT - Do not use in adults.

PEDS - Infants born of HBsAg (-) mothers: 0.5

mL IM x 3 doses at 2, 4, and 12-15 mo.

NOTES - Combination of PedvaxHIB (haemophilus b vaccine) + Recombivax HB (hepatitis B vaccine). For infants >8 weeks of age.

diphtheria tetanus and acellular pertussis vaccine (*DTaP, Tdap, Tripedia, Infanrix, Daptacel, Boostrix, Adacel, ♥Tripacel*) ♀C ▶- $$

ADULT - 0.5 mL IM in deltoid as a single dose, 2 to 5 years since last tetanus dose (Adacel).

PEDS - Check immunization history: DTaP is preferred for all DTP doses. Give first dose of 0.5 mL IM at approximately 2 months, second dose at 4 months, third dose at 6 months, fourth dose at 15-18 months, and fifth dose (booster) at 4-6 yo. Use Boostrix only if adolescents 10-18 yo, and ≥2-5 years after last childhood dose of DTP. Use Adacel only in adolescents ≥11 yo and at least 2 to 5 years after last childhood dose of DTP or Td.

NOTES - When feasible, use same brand for first 3 doses. Do not give if prior DTP vaccination caused anaphylaxis/encephalopathy within 7 days. Avoid Tripedia if thimerosal allergy. Do not use Boostrix or Adacel for primary childhood vaccination series, if prior DTP vaccination caused anaphylaxis/encephalopathy, or if progressive neurologic disorders (eg, encephalopathy) or uncontrolled epilepsy. Adacel is only DTaP vaccine approved for adults up to 64 yo. For adolescents and adults, only one dose should be given, at least 2-5 years after last tetanus dose. No information available on repeat doses in adolescents or adults.

diphtheria-tetanus toxoid (*Td, DT, ♥D2T5*) ♀C ▶? $

ADULT - Age ≥7 yo: 0.5 mL IM, second dose 4-8 weeks later, and third dose 6-12 months later. Give 0.5 mL booster dose at 10 year intervals. Use adult formulation (Td) for adults and children ≥7 years of age.

PEDS - Age 6 weeks- 6 yo: 0.5 mL IM , second dose 4-8 weeks later, and third dose 6-12 months later using DT for pediatric use. If immunization of infants begins in the first year of life using DT rather than DTP (i.e. pertussis is contraindicated), give three 0.5 mL doses 4- 8 weeks apart, followed by a fourth dose 6- 12 months later.

FORMS - Injection DT (pediatric: 6 weeks- 6 yo). Td (adult children: ≥7years).

NOTES - DTaP is preferred for most children <7 years of age. Td is preferred for adults and children ≥7 yo. Avoid in thimerosal allergy.

haemophilus b vaccine (*ActHIB, HibTITER, PedvaxHIB*) ♀C ▶? $

PEDS - Doses vary depending on formulation used and age at first dose. ActHIB/ OmniHIB/ HibTITER: 2- 6 months- 0.5 mL IM x 3 doses at two month intervals. 7- 11 months- 0.5 mL IM x 2 doses at two month intervals. 12- 14 months- 0.5 mL IM x 1 dose. A single 0.5 mL IM (booster) dose is given to children ≥15 months old, and at least 2 months after the previous injection. 15- 60 months: 0.5 mL IM x 1 dose (no booster). PedvaxHIB: 2- 14 months- 0.5 mL IM x 2 doses at two month intervals. If the 2 doses are given before 12 months of age, a third 0.5 mL IM (booster) dose is given at least 2 months after the second dose. 15- 60 months- 0.5 mL IM x 1 dose (no booster).

UNAPPROVED ADULT - Asplenia, ≥14 days prior to elective splenectomy, or immunodeficiency: 0.5 mL IM x 1 dose of any Hib conjugate vaccine.

UNAPPROVED PEDS - Asplenia, ≥14 days prior to elective splenectomy, or immunodeficiency age ≥5 yo: 0.5 mL IM x 1 dose of any Hib vaccine.

NOTES - Not for IV use. No data on interchangeability between brands; AAP & ACIP recommend use of any product in children >12-15 months of age.

hepatitis A vaccine (*Havrix, Vaqta, ♥Avaxim, Epaxal*) ♀C ▶+ $$$

ADULT - Havrix ≥18 yo: 1 mL (1440 ELU) IM, then 1 mL (1440 ELU) IM booster dose 6- 12 months later. Vaqta ≥18 yo: 1 mL (50 U) IM, then 1 mL (50 U) IM booster 6 months later.

PEDS - Havrix 1-18 yo: 0.5 mL (720 ELU) IM x 1 dose, then 0.5 mL (720 ELU) IM booster 6-12 months after first dose. Vaqta 1-18 yo: 0.5 mL (25 U) IM x 1 dose, then 0.5 mL (25 U) IM booster 6-18 months later.

FORMS - Single dose vial (specify peds, adult).

NOTES - Do not inject IV, SC, ID. Brands may be used interchangeably. Need for boosters unclear. Post-exposure prophylaxis with vaccine alone not recommended. Should be given 4 weeks prior to travel to endemic area. May be given at the same time as immune globulin, but preferably at different site.

hepatitis B vaccine (*Engerix-B, Recombivax HB*) ♀C ▶+ $$$

ADULT - Engerix-B ≥20 yo: 1 mL (20 mcg) IM, repeat in 1 and 6 months. Hemodialysis: Give 2.0 mL (40 mcg) IM, repeat in 1, 2, & 6 months. Give 2.0 mL (40 mcg) IM booster when antibody levels <10 mIU/mL. Recombivax HB: 1 mL (10 mcg) IM, repeat in 1 and 6 months. Hemodialysis: 1 mL (40 mcg) IM, repeat in 1 & 6 months. Give 1 mL (40 mcg) IM booster when antibody levels <10 mIU/mL.

PEDS - Specialized dosing based on age and maternal HBsAg status. Infants of hepatitis B negative and positive mothers, children, adolescents <20 years: Engerix-B 10 mcg (0.5 mL) IM 0, 1, 6 months. Recombivax 5 mcg (0.5 mL) IM 0, 1, 6 months. In adolescents 11-15 year, a 2-dose schedule can be used (Recombivax HB 10 mcg (1.0 mL) IM 0, 4-6 months).

NOTES - Infants born to hepatitis B positive mothers should also receive hepatitis B immune globulin and hepatitis B vaccine within 12 hours of birth. Not for IV or ID use. May interchange products. Recombivax HB Dialysis Formulation is intended for adults only. Avoid if yeast allergy. Adult formulations contain thimerosal; avoid if allergy.

human papillomavirus recombinant vaccine (*Gardasil*) ♀B ♪? $$$$$

ADULT - Females up to age 26 years: 0.5 mL IM at time 0, 2 and 6 months.

PEDS - Females 9 years or older: 0.5 mL IM at time 0, 2 and 6 months.

NOTES - Includes types 6, 11, 16, 18. Counsel to continue to use condoms. Immunosuppression may reduce response.

influenza vaccine - inactivated injection (*Fluarix, FluLaval, Fluzone, Fluvirin, ♣Fluviral, Vaxigrip*) ♀C ♪+ $

ADULT - 0.5 mL IM single dose once yearly.

PEDS - Fluarix and FluLaval are not indicated in children. All others: Age 6- 35 months: 0.25 mL IM, repeat dose ≥4 weeks. Age 3- 8 yo: 0.5 mL IM, repeat dose ≥4 weeks. Age 9- 12 yo: 0.5 mL IM once yearly. Healthy children 5-17 yo: 1 dose (0.2 mL) intranasally (FluMist), repeat dose in 2 months in children 5-8 yo receiving for first time. When using the intramuscular formulations, use only the split virus vaccine (i.e. subvirion or purified surface antigen) in children 6 months- 8 yo. Give repeat dose only in previously unvaccinated children.

NOTES - Avoid in Guillain-Barre Syndrome, chicken egg allergy, ASA therapy, thimerosal allergy. Optimal administration Oct to Nov.

influenza vaccine - live intranasal (*FluMist*) ♀C ♪+ $

ADULT - Healthy adults ages 18-49 yo: 1 dose (0.2 mL) intranasally once yearly (FluMist).

PEDS - Healthy children 5-17 yo: 1 dose (0.2 mL) intranasally (FluMist), repeat in 2 months in children 5-8 yo receiving for first time.

NOTES - Avoid in Guillain-Barre Syndrome, chicken egg allergy, ASA therapy. Optimal administration October to November. Since FluMist is a live vaccine, do not use in immune deficiencies (e.g., HIV, malignancy) or altered immune status (e.g., taking systemic corticosteroids, chemotherapy, radiation).

Japanese encephalitis vaccine (*JE-Vax*) ♀C ♪? $$$$

ADULT - 1 mL SC x 3 doses on days 0, 7, 30.

PEDS - Age ≥3 yo: 1.0 mL SC x 3 doses on days 0, 7, and 30. Age 1-3 yo: 0.5 mL SC x 3 doses on days 0, 7, and 30.

NOTES - Give at least 10 days before travel to endemic areas. An abbreviated schedule on days 0, 7, and 14 can be given if time limits. A booster dose may be given after 2 years. Avoid in thimerosal allergy.

measles mumps & rubella vaccine (*M-M-R II, ♣Priorix*) ♀C ♪+ $$$

ADULT - 0.5 mL (1 vial) SC.

PEDS - 12-15 months of age: 0.5 mL (1 vial) SC. Revaccinate prior to elementary and/or middle school according to local health guidelines. If measles outbreak, may immunize infants 6-12 mo with 0.5 mL SC; then start 2 dose regimen between 12-15 mo.

NOTES - Do not inject IV. Contraindicated in pregnancy. Advise women to avoid pregnancy for 4 weeks following vaccination. Live virus, contraindicated in immunocompromised patients. Avoid if allergic to neomycin or gelatin; caution in egg allergy.

meningococcal polysaccharide vaccine (*Menomune-A/C/Y/W-135, Menactra, ♣Menjugate*) ♀C ♪? $$$$

WARNING - Reports of associated Guillain-Barre Syndrome; avoid if prior history of such.

ADULT - 0.5 mL SC (Menomune) or IM (Menactra).

PEDS - Age ≥2 yo: 0.5 mL SC.

UNAPPROVED PEDS - Age 3-18 months: 0.5 mL SC x 2 doses separated by 3 months

NOTES - Give 2 weeks before elective splenectomy or travel to endemic areas. May consider revaccination q3-5 yrs in high risk patients. Do not inject IV. Contraindicated in pregnancy. Consider vaccinating 11-12 year olds and first-year college students living in dormitories. Avoid in thimerosal allergy.

Pediarix (diphtheria tetanus and acellular pertussis vaccine + hepatitis B vaccine

+ polio vaccine ♀C ▶? $$$
PEDS - 0.5 mL at 2, 4, 6 months IM.
NOTES - Do not administer before 6 weeks old.

plague vaccine ♀C ▶+ $
ADULT - Age 18-61 yo: 1 mL IM x 1 dose, then 0.2 mL IM 1-3 months after the 1st dose, then 0.2 mL IM 5-6 months after the 2nd dose.
PEDS - Not approved in children.
NOTES - Up to 3 booster doses (0.2 mL) may be administered at 6 month intervals in high risk patients. Jet injector gun may be used for IM administration.

pneumococcal 23-valent vaccine (*Pneumovax*, ✿ *Pneumo 23*) ♀C ▶+ $$
ADULT - 0.5 mL IM/SC. Routine revaccination not recommended if immunocompetent. Consider revaccination once in patients ≥65 yo (if <65 yo at initial vaccination) or patients at high risk of developing serious pneumococcal infection if >5 years from initial vaccine.
PEDS - ≥2 yo: 0.5 mL IM/SC. Consider revaccination once in patients at high risk of developing serious pneumococcal infection after 3-5 yr from initial vaccine in patients that would be ≤10 yo at revaccination.
NOTES - Do not give IV or ID. May be co-administered with influenza virus vaccine at different site. OK for high risk children ≥2 yo who received Prevnar already to provide additional serotype coverage. Avoid in thimerosal allergy.

pneumococcal 7-valent conjugate vaccine (*Prevnar*) ♀C ▶? $$$
ADULT - Not approved in adults.
PEDS - 0.5 mL IM x 3 doses 6-8 weeks apart starting at 2-6 months of age, followed by a 4th dose of 0.5 mL IM at 12-15 months. For previously unvaccinated older infants and children age 7-11 months: 0.5 mL x 2 doses 6-8 weeks apart, followed by a 3rd dose of 0.5 mL at 12-15 months. Age 12-23 months: 0.5 mL x 2 doses 6-8 weeks apart. Age 2-9 yo: 0.5 mL x 1 dose; give 2nd dose 4 weeks later in immunocompromised or chronically ill children.
NOTES - For IM use only; do not inject IV. Shake susp vigorously prior to administration.

polio vaccine (*IPOL*) ♀C ▶? $$
ADULT - Not generally recommended. Previously unvaccinated adults at increased risk of exposure should receive a complete primary immunization series of 3 doses (two doses at intervals of 4-8 weeks; a third dose at 6-12 months after the second dose). Accelerated schedules are available. Travelers to endemic areas who have received primary immunization

should receive a single booster in adulthood.
PEDS - 0.5 mL IM or SC at 2 months of age, with 2nd dose at 4 months, 3rd dose at 6-18 months, and 4th dose at 4-6 yo.
NOTES - Oral polio vaccine no longer available.

***ProQuad* (measles mumps & rubella vaccine + varicella vaccine)** ♀C ▶? $$$$
ADULT - Not indicated in adults.
PEDS - 12 months - 12 yo: 0.5 mL (1 vial) SC.
NOTES - Give ≥1 month after a MMR-containing vaccine and ≥3 months after a varicella-containing vaccine. Do not inject IV. Contraindicated in pregnancy. Following vaccination avoid pregnancy for 3 months and ASA / salicylates for 6 weeks. Live virus, contraindicated in immunocompromise or untreated TB. Avoid if neomycin allergic; caution with egg allergies.

rabies vaccine (*RabAvert, Imovax Rabies, BioRab, Rabies Vaccine Adsorbed*) ♀C ▶? $$$$$
ADULT - Post-exposure prophylaxis: Give rabies immune globulin (20 IU/ kg) immediately after exposure, then give rabies vaccine 1 mL IM in deltoid region on days 0, 3, 7, 14, and 28. If pre-exposure immunization, give 1 mL IM rabies vaccine on days 0 and 3 only without rabies immune globulin. Pre-exposure immunization: 1 mL IM rabies vaccine on days 0, 7, and between days 21-28. Or 0.1 mL ID on days 0, 7, and between days 21-28. (Imovax Rabies I.D. vaccine formula only). Repeat q2-5 years based on antibody titer.
PEDS - Same as adults.
NOTES - Do not use ID preparation for post-exposure prophylaxis.

rotavirus vaccine (*RotaTeq*) ♀ ▶? $$$$$
ADULT - Not recommended.
PEDS - Give the first dose (2 mL PO) between 6-12 weeks of age, and then the 2nd & 3rd doses at 4-10 weeks intervals thereafter (last dose no later than 32 weeks).
FORMS - Trade only: Oral suspension 2 mL.
NOTES - Live vaccine so potential for transmission, especially to immunodeficient close contacts. Safety unclear in immunocompromised infants.

smallpox vaccine (*Dryvax, vaccinia vaccine*) ♀C ▶- Not available to civilians.
ADULT - Prevention of smallpox or monkeypox: Specialized administration using a bifurcated needle SC x 1.
PEDS - >1 yo: Specialized administration using a bifurcated needle SC x 1.
NOTES - Contraindicated in polymyxin, neomy-

cin, tetracycline, or streptomycin allergy. Avoid in those (or household contacts of those) with eczema or a history of eczema, those with a rash due to other causes (eg, burns, zoster, impetigo, psoriasis), immunocompromise, or pregnancy. Persons with known cardiac disease (or 3+ risk factors) should not be vaccinated as response team members in the pre-event smallpox vaccination program.

tetanus toxoid ♀C ▶+ $

WARNING - Td is preferred in adults and children ≥7 yo. DTP is preferred in children <7 yo. Use fluid tetanus toxoid in assessing cell-mediated immunity only.

ADULT - 0.5 mL IM (adsorbed) x 2 doses 4-8 wks apart. Give third dose 6-12 months after 2nd injection. Give booster q10 yrs. Assess cell-mediated immunity: 0.1 mL of 1:100 diluted skin-test reagent or 0.02 mL of 1: 10 diluted skin-test reagent injected intradermally.

PEDS - 0.5 mL IM (adsorbed) x 2 doses 4-8 wks apart. Give third dose 6-12 months after 2nd injection. Give booster q10 years.

NOTES - May use tetanus toxoid fluid for active immunization in patients hypersensitive to the aluminum adjuvant of the adsorbed formulation: 0.5 mL IM or SC x 3 doses at 4- 8 week intervals. Give fourth dose 6- 12 months after third injection. Give booster dose q10 years. Avoid in thimerosal allergy

TriHibit **(haemophilus b + diphtheria tetanus and acellular pertussis vaccine)** ♀C ▶- $$$

PEDS - For 4th dose only, 15-18 mos: 0.5 mL IM.

NOTES - Tripedia (DTaP) is used to reconstitute ActHIB (Haemophilus b) to make TriHIBit and will appear whitish in color. Use within 30 min. Avoid in thimerosal allergy.

Twinrix **(hepatitis A vaccine + hepatitis B vaccine)** ♀C ▶? $$$

ADULT - ≥18 yo: 1 mL IM in deltoid only, repeat in 1 & 6 months. Accelerated dosing schedule: 0, 7, 21-30 days; booster dose at 12 months.

PEDS - Not approved in children.

NOTES - Not for IV or ID use. 1 mL = 720 ELU inactivated hepatitis A + 20 mcg hepatitis B surface antigen.

typhoid vaccine - inactivated injection (*Typhim Vi*, ✤*Typherix*) ♀C ▶? $$

ADULT - 0.5 mL IM x 1 dose given at least 2 weeks prior to potential exposure. May consider revaccination q2 yrs in high risk patients.

PEDS - Age ≥2 yo: same as adult dose.

NOTES - Recommended for travel to endemic areas.

typhoid vaccine - live oral (*Vivotif Berna*) ♀C ▶? $$

ADULT - 1 cap 1 hr before a meal with cold or lukewarm drink qod x 4 doses to be completed ≥1 week prior to potential exposure. May consider revaccination q5 yrs in high risk patients.

PEDS - Age ≥6 yo: same as adult dose.

FORMS - Trade only: Caps

NOTES - Recommended for travel to endemic areas. Oral vaccine may be inactivated by antibiotics, including antimalarials.

varicella vaccine (*Varivax*, ✤*Varilrix*) ♀C ▶+ $$$

ADULT - 0.5 mL SC. Repeat 4- 8 weeks later.

PEDS - age 1- 12 yo: 0.5 mL SC x 1 dose. Age ≥13 yo: same as adult dose. Not recommended for infants <1 yo.

UNAPPROVED PEDS - Postexposure prophylaxis: 0.5 mL SC within 3-5 days of exposure.

NOTES - Do not inject IV. Following vaccination avoid pregnancy for 3 months and ASA / salicylates for 6 weeks. The need for booster doses is not defined. This live vaccine is contraindicated in immunocompromised. Vaccine is stored in freezer; thawed vaccine must be used within 30 minutes.

yellow fever vaccine (*YF-Vax*) ♀C ▶+ $$$

ADULT - 0.5 mL SC.

PEDS - 0.5 mL SC into the thigh (6 mo - 3 yo) or deltoid region (≥3 yo).

NOTES - Approval by state and/or federal authorities required to obtain vaccine. A booster dose (0.5 mL) may be administered q10 years.

zoster vaccine - live (*Zostavax*) ♀C ▶? $$$$

ADULT - Adults ≥60 years: 0.65 mL SC x 1.

PEDS - Not approved in children.

NOTES - Avoid if history of anaphylactic/anaphylactoid reaction to gelatin or neomycin, if primary or acquired immunodeficiency states, or if taking immunosuppressives. Do not administer if active untreated tuberculosis or in possible pregnancy. Theoretically possible to transmit to pregnant household contact who has not had varicella infection or immunocompromised contact. Do not substitute for Varivax in children.

CHILDHOOD IMMUNIZATION SCHEDULE*

Age	Birth	1	2	4	6	12	15	18	2	4-6	11-12
						Months				Years	
Hepatitis B	HB	HB			HB						
Rotavirus			Rota	Rota	Rota						
DTP			DTaP	DTaP	DTaP		DTaP			DTaP	TDaP
H influenza b			Hib	Hib	Hib	Hib					
Pneumococci			PCV	PCV	PCV	PCV					
Polio			IPV	IPV		IPV				IPV	
Influenza†					Influenza (yearly)†						
MMR						MMR				MMR	
Varicella						Varicella				Vari	
Hepatitis A¶						Hep A x 2¶					
Papillomavirus§											HPV x 3§
Meningococcal											MCV

*2007 schedule from the CDC, ACIP, AAP, & AAFP, see CDC website (www.cdc.gov). †If ≥5 yo and healthy can use intranasal form. If <9 yo receiving for first time, should get 2 doses ≥4 weeks apart for injected form and ≥6 weeks apart for intranasal. ¶Two doses at least 6 months apart. §Second and third doses 2 and 6 months after first dose.

ADULT IMMUNIZATION SCHEDULE*

Tetanus, diphtheria (Td): For all ages, 1 dose booster every 10 years. *Pertussis*: Consider single dose of pertussis in adults <65 years old (as part of Tdap (*Adacel*), at least 10 years since last tetanus dose. *Influenza*: 1 yearly dose if ≥50 years old. If <50 years, then 1 yearly dose if healthcare worker, pregnant, chronic underlying illness, household contact of person with chronic underlying illness or household contact with children <5 years old, or those who request vaccination. Intranasal vaccine indicated for healthy adults <50 years. *Pneumococcal* (polysaccharide): 1 dose if ≥65 years old. If <65 years, consider immunizing if chronic underlying illness, nursing home resident, or Native American. Consider revaccination 5 years later if high risk or if ≥65 years and received primary dose before age 65. *Hepatitis A*: For all ages with clotting factor disorders, chronic liver disease, or exposure risk (travel to endemic areas, illegal drug use, men having sex with men), 2 doses (0, 6-12 months). *Hepatitis B*: For all ages with medical (hemodialysis, clotting factor recipients, chronic liver disease), occupational (healthcare or public safety workers with blood exposure), behavioral (illegal drug use, multiple sex partners, those seeking evaluation or treatment of sexually transmitted disease, men having sex with men) or other (household/sex contacts of those with chronic HBV or HIV infections, clients/staff of developmentally disabled, >6 month travel to high risk areas, inmates of correctional facilities) indications , 3 doses (0, 1-2, 4-6 months). *Measles, mumps, rubella (MMR)*: If <50 years old and immunity in doubt, see cdc.gov. *Varicella*: For all ages if immunity in doubt, if ≥13 years, 2 doses separated by 4-8 weeks. *Meningococcal* (conjugate vaccine is preferred for ≤ 55 years): For all ages if medical (complement deficiency, anatomic or functional asplenia) or other (travel to endemic regions, college dormitory residents, military recruits) indications, 1 dose. Consider revaccination in 3-5 years if high-risk. *Human papillomavirus*: Consider HPV vaccine in women 9 to 26 years at 0, 2 and 6 months. *Herpes zoster*: Consider single dose of HZ vaccine in individuals 60 years of age or older.

*2007 schedule from the CDC, ACIP, & AAFP, see: www.cdc.gov/vaccines/recs/schedules/default.htm

TETANUS WOUND CARE

TETANUS WOUND CARE (www.cdc.gov)	Uncertain or <3 prior tetanus immunizations	≥3 prior tetanus immunizations
Non tetanus prone wound (e.g., clean and minor)	Td (DT if <7 yo)	Td if >10 years since last dose
Tetanus prone wound (e.g., dirt, contamination, punctures, crush components)	Td (DT if <7 yo), tetanus immune globulin 250 units IM at site other than Td.	Td if >5 years since last dose

When immunizing adults or adolescents ≥10 yo consider DTaP (*Adacel* if 11-64 yo, *Boostrix* if 10-18 yo) if patient has never received a pertussis booster.

IMMUNOLOGY: Immunoglobulins

NOTE: Adult IM injections should be given in the deltoid region; injection in the gluteal region may result in suboptimal response.

antivenin - crotalidae immune Fab ovine polyvalent (CroFab) ▶? ♀C ▶? $$$$$

ADULT - Rattlesnake envenomation: Give 4-6 vials IV infusion over 60 minutes, <6 h of bite if possible. Administer 4-6 additional vials if no initial control of envenomation syndrome, then 2 vials q6h for up to 18 h (3 doses) after initial control has been established.

PEDS - Same as adults, although specific studies in children have not been conducted.

NOTES - Contraindicated in allergy to papaya or papain. Start IV infusion slowly over the first 10 minutes at 25-50 mL/hr and observe for allergic reaction, then increase to full rate of 250 mL/hr.

antivenin - crotalidae polyvalent ▶L ♀C ▶? $$$$$

ADULT - Pit viper envenomation: minimal envenomation: 20-40 mL (2-4 vials) IV infusion; moderate envenomation: 50-90 mL (5-9 vials) IV infusion; severe envenomation: ≥100-150 mL (10-15 vials) IV infusion. Administer within 4h of bite, less effective after 8h, and of questionable value after 12h. May give additional 10-50 mL (1-5 vials) IV infusion based on clinical assessment and response to initial dose.

PEDS - Larger relative doses of antivenin are needed in children and small adults because of small volume of body fluid to dilute the venom. The dose is not based on weight.

NOTES - Test first for sensitivity to horse serum. Serum sickness may occur 5-24 days after dose. IV route is preferred. May give IM.

antivenin - latrodectus mactans ▶L♀C▶? $$$

ADULT, PEDS - Specialized dosing for black widow spider toxicity; consult poison center.

NOTES – Pre-test for horse serum sensitivity. Serum sickness may occur after 5-24 days.

botulism immune globulin (BabyBIG) ▶L ♀? ▶? $$$$$

ADULT - Not approved in >1 yo.

PEDS - Infant botulism <1 yo: 1 mL (50 mg)/kg IV.

cytomegalovirus immune globulin human (Cytogam) ▶L ♀C ▶? $$$$$

ADULT, PEDS - Specialized dosing based on indication and time since transplant.

hepatitis B immune globulin (H-BIG, Bay-Hep B, HepaGam B, NABI-HB) ▶L ♀C ▶? $$$

ADULT - Post-exposure prophylaxis for needle-stick, ocular, mucosal exposure: 0.06 mL/kg IM (usual dose 3- 5 mL) within 24 h of exposure. Initiate hepatitis B vaccine series within 7 days. Consider a second dose of hepatitis B immune globulin (HBIG) one month later if patient refuses hepatitis B vaccine series. Post-exposure prophylaxis for sexual exposure: 0.06 mL/kg IM within 14d of sexual contact. Initiate hepatitis B vaccine series. Prevention of hepatitis B recurrence following liver transplantation in HBsAg-positive (HepaGam B): first dose given during transplantation surgery. Subsequent doses daily for 7 days, then biweekly up to 3 months and monthly thereafter. Doses adjusted based on regular monitoring of HBsAg, HBV-DNA, HBeAg and anti-HBs antibody levels.

PEDS - Prophylaxis of infants born to HBsAg (+) mothers: 0.5 mL IM within 12 h of birth. Initiate hepatitis B vaccine series within 7 days. If hepatitis B vaccine series is refused, repeat HBIG dose at 3 and 6 months. Household exposure <12 months of age: 0.5 mL IM within 14d of exposure. Initiate hep B vaccine series.

NOTES - HBIG may be administered at the same time or up to 1 month prior to hepatitis B vaccine without impairing the active immune response from hepatitis B vaccine.

immune globulin - intramuscular (Baygam, ✳Gamastan) ▶L ♀C ▶? $$$$

ADULT - Hepatitis A post-exposure prophylaxis for household or institutional contacts): 0.02 mL/kg IM within 2 weeks of exposure. Hepatitis A pre-exposure prophylaxis (ie, travel to endemic area): <3 months length of stay = 0.02 mL/kg IM. >3 months length of stay = 0.06 mL/kg IM and repeat q4-6 months. Measles: 0.2-0.25 mL/ kg IM within 6 days of exposure, max 15 mL. Varicella zoster (if VariZIG unavailable): 0.6-1.2 mL/kg IM. Rubella exposure in pregnant, susceptible women: 0.55 mL/kg IM. Immunoglobulin deficiency: 0.66 mL/kg IM every 3-4 weeks.

PEDS - Not approved in children.

UNAPPROVED PEDS - Measles: 0.2-0.25 mL/ kg IM within 6 days of exposure. In susceptible immunocompromised children use 0.5 mL/kg IM (max 15 mL) immediately after exposure. Varicella zoster (if VariZIG unavailable): 0.6-1.2 mL/kg IM.

NOTES - Human derived product, increased infection risk. Hepatitis A vaccine preferred over immune globulin for persons >2 years old who plan to travel to high risk areas repeatedly or for long periods of time.

immune globulin - intravenous (Carimune, Polygam, Panglobulin, Octagam, Flebogamma, Gammagard, Gamunex, Iveegam, Venoglobulin) ▶L ♀C ▶? $$$$$

ADULT - Idiopathic thrombocytopenic purpura (induction): 400 mg/kg IV daily x 5 days (or 1 g/kg IV daily for 1-2 days). Bone marrow transplant (>20 yo): 500 mg/kg IV daily, given 7 and 2 days before transplant, and then weekly until 90 days post transplant. Primary humoral immunodeficiency: 200-300 mg/kg IV each month; increase as needed to max 400-800 mg/kg/month. B-cell chronic lymphocytic leukemia: specialized dosing.

PEDS - Pediatric HIV: 400 mg/kg IV q28 days. Idiopathic thrombocytopenic purpura (induction): 400 mg/kg IV daily x 5 days (or 1 g/kg IV daily for 1-2 days). Kawasaki Syndrome (acute): 400 mg/kg IV daily x 4 days (or 2 g/kg IV x 1 over 10 hours). Primary humoral immunodeficiency: 200-300 mg/kg IV each month; increase prn to max 400-800 mg/kg/month.

UNAPPROVED ADULT - First-line therapy in severe Guillain-Barré syndrome, chronic inflammatory demyelinating polyneuropathy, multifocal motor neuropathy, severe post-transfusion purpura, inclusion body myositis, fetomaternal alloimmune thrombocytopenia; second-line therapy in stiff-person syndrome, dermatomyositis, myasthenia gravis, and Lambert-Eaton myasthenic syndrome: Various dosing regimens have been used; a common one is myasthenia gravis (induction): 400 mg/kg IV daily x 5 days (total 2 g/kg). Has been used in multiple sclerosis and inflammatory myositis (polymyositis & dermatomyositis), renal transplant rejection, systemic lupus erythematosus, toxic epidermal necrolysis and Stevens-Johnson syndrome, Clostridium difficile colitis, Graves' ophthalmopathy, pemphigus.

UNAPPROVED PEDS - Myasthenia gravis (induction): 400 mg/kg IV daily x 5 days. Other dosing regimens have been used.

NOTES - Indications and doses vary by product. Follow LFTs, renal function, vital signs, and urine output closely. Contraindicated in IgA deficiency. Use caution (and lower infusion rates) if risk factors for thrombosis, heart failure, or renal insufficiency. Use slower infusion rates for initial doses. Consider pretreatment with acetaminophen and/or diphenhydramine to minimize some infusion-related adverse effects. Human-derived product; although donors are carefully screened there is risk of transmission of infectious agents.

immune globulin - subcutaneous (Vivaglobulin) ▶L ♀C ▶? $$$$$

ADULT - Primary immune deficiency: 100-200 mg/kg SC weekly. In patients already receiving IV immune globulin: SC dose = (previous IV dose x 1.37) divided by frequency of IV regimen in weeks.

PEDS - Limited information. Dosing appears to be same as in adults.

NOTES - Do not administer IV. Contraindicated in IgA deficiency. Human-derived product, increased infection risk.

lymphocyte immune globulin (Atgam) ▶L ♀C ▶? $$$$$

ADULT - Renal allograft recipients: 10-30 mg/kg IV daily. Delaying onset of allograft rejection: 15 mg/kg IV daily x 14 days, then qod x 14 days. Treatment of renal transplant rejection: 10-15 mg/kg IV x 14 days. Aplastic anemia: 10-20 mg/kg IV daily x 8-14 days, then qod, as needed, up to 21 total doses.

PEDS - Limited experience. Has been safely administered to a limited number of children with renal transplant and aplastic anemia at doses comparable to adults.

NOTES - Equine product. Doses should be administered over ≥4 hours.

rabies immune globulin human (Imogam Rabies-HT, HyperRAB S/D) ▶L ♀C ▶? $$$$$

ADULT - Post-exposure prophylaxis: 20 units/kg (0.133 mL/kg), with as much as possible infiltrated around the bite and the rest given IM. Give as soon as possible after exposure. Administer with the first dose of vaccine, but in a different extremity.

PEDS - Not approved in children.

UNAPPROVED PEDS - Use adult dosing.

NOTES - Do not repeat dose once rabies vaccine series begins. Do not give to patients who have been completely immunized with rabies vaccine. Do not administer IV.

RSV immune globulin (RespiGam) ▶Plasma ♀C ▶? $$$$$

PEDS - RSV prophylaxis in children <24 months: 1.5 mL/kg/hr x 15 minutes. Increase rate as clinical condition permits to 3 mL/kg/hr x 15 minutes, then to a maximum rate of 6 mL/kg/hr. Max total dose/ month is 750 mg/kg.

NOTES - May cause fluid overload; monitor vital signs frequently during IV infusion. RSV season is typically November-April.

tetanus immune globulin (*BayTet*, ✚*Hypertet*) ▶L ♀C ▶? $$$$
ADULT - See tetanus wound management table. Post-exposure prophylaxis in tetanus prone wounds in patients ≥7 years of age: if <3 doses of tetanus vaccine have been administered or if history is uncertain, give 250 units IM x 1 dose along with dT. If ≥3 doses of tetanus vaccine have been administered in the past, do not give tetanus immune globulin. Tetanus treatment: 3000-6000 units IM in combination with other therapies.

PEDS - <7 yo: 4 units/ kg IM or 250 units IM. Initiate tetanus toxoid vaccine (DTP or DT).

NOTES - Do not give tetanus immune globulin for clean, minor wounds. May be given at the same time as tetanus toxoid active immunization. Do not inject IV.

varicella-zoster immune globulin (*VariZIG*) ▶L ♀C ▶? $$$$$
ADULT, PEDS - Specialized dosing for post-exposure prophylaxis.

IMMUNOLOGY: Immunosuppression

basiliximab (*Simulect*) ▶Plasma ♀B ▶? $$$$$
ADULT, PEDS - Specialized dosing for organ transplantation.

cyclosporine (*Sandimmune, Neoral, Gengraf*) ▶L ♀C ▶- $$$$$
ADULT - Specialized dosing for organ transplantation, rheumatoid arthritis, and psoriasis.

PEDS - Not approved in children.

UNAPPROVED ADULT - Specialized dosing for autoimmune eye disorders, vasculitis, inflammatory myopathies, Behcet's disease, psoriatic arthritis, chronic refractory idiopathic thrombocytopenia.

UNAPPROVED PEDS - Specialized dosing for organ transplantation, chronic refractory idiopathic thrombocytopenia.

FORMS - Generic/Trade: microemulsion Caps 25, 100 mg. Generic/Trade: Caps (Sandimmune) 25, 100 mg, solution (Sandimmune) 100 mg/mL, microemulsion solution (Neoral, Gengraf) 100 mg/mL.

NOTES - Monitor blood levels closely. Many drug interactions including atorvastatin, azithromycin, lovastatin, oral contraceptives, rosuvastatin, simvastatin, sirolimus, terbinafine, voriconazole. Caution when combining with methotrexate or potassium sparing drugs such as ACE inhibitors. Reduce dose in renal dysfunction. Monitor blood pressure and renal function closely. Avoid excess UV light exposure. Monitor patients closely when switching from Sandimmune to microemulsion formulations.

daclizumab (*Zenapax*) ▶L ♀C ▶? $$$$$
ADULT - Specialized dosing for organ transplantation.

PEDS - Not approved in children.

UNAPPROVED PEDS - Specialized dosing for organ transplantation.

mycophenolate mofetil (*Cellcept, Myfortic*) ▶? ♀C ▶? $$$$$
ADULT - Specialized dosing for organ transplantation.

PEDS - Not approved in children.

UNAPPROVED ADULT - Lupus nephritis: 1000 mg PO bid. Has been used in pemphigus and bullous pemphigoid.

UNAPPROVED PEDS - Specialized dosing for organ transplantation.

FORMS - Trade only (CellCept): caps 250 mg, tabs 500 mg, oral suspension 200 mg/mL. Trade (Myfortic): tablet, extended-release: 180, 360 mg.

sirolimus (*Rapamune*) ▶L ♀C ▶- $$$$$
WARNING - Increased risk of infection and lymphoma. Combination of sirolimus plus cyclosporine or tacrolimus is associated with hepatic artery thrombosis in liver transplant patients. Combination with tacrolimus and corticosteroids in lung transplant patients may cause bronchial anastomotic dehiscence. Can cause hypersensitivity reactions including anaphylactic and/or anaphylactoid reactions, angioedema, vasculitis. Avoid with strong inhibitors of CYP3A4 and/or P-glycoprotein (ketoconazole, voriconazole, itraconazole, erythromycin, telithromycin, clarithromycin) or strong inducers CYP3A4 and/or P-glycoprotein (rifampin, rifabutin). Monitor level if cyclosporine is discontinued or has dose markedly changed.

ADULT - Specialized dosing for organ transplantation.

PEDS - Not approved in children.

UNAPPROVED PEDS - Specialized dosing for organ transplantation.

FORMS - Trade only: oral solution 1 mg/mL (60 mL). Tab 1, 2 mg.
NOTES - Wear protective clothing and sunscreen when exposed to sunlight to reduce the risk of skin cancer. Adjust dose by 1/3 in liver dysfunction.

tacrolimus (*Prograf, FK 506*) ▶L ♀C ▶- $$$$$
ADULT, PEDS - Specialized dosing for organ transplantation.
UNAPPROVED ADULT - Rheumatoid arthritis (approved in Canada), active vasculitis, systemic lupus erythematosus nephritis & vasculitis.
FORMS - Trade only: Caps 1,5 mg.
NOTES - Reduce dose in renal dysfunction. Monitor blood pressure and renal function closely. Many drug interactions.

IMMUNOLOGY: Other

hymenoptera venom ▶Serum ♀C ▶? $$$$
ADULT, PEDS - Specialized desensitization dosing protocol. Products available: honey bee (Apis mellifera) and yellow jacket (Vespula sp.), yellow hornet (Dolichovespula arenaria), white-faced hornet (Dolichovespula maculata) and wasp (Polistes sp.). Mixed vespid venom protein (yellow jacket, yellow hornet and white-faced hornet) is also available.

tuberculin PPD (*Aplisol, Tubersol, Mantoux, PPD*) ▶L ♀C ▶+ $
ADULT - 5 TU (0.1 mL) intradermally.
PEDS - Same as adult dose. AAP recommends screening at 12 months, 4- 6 yo, and 14- 16 yo.
NOTES - Avoid SC injection. Read 48- 72 h after intradermal injection. Repeat testing in patients with known prior positive PPD may cause scarring at injection site.

NEUROLOGY: Alzheimer's Disease – Cholinesterase Inhibitors

NOTE: Avoid concurrent use of anticholinergic agents. Use caution in asthma/COPD. May be co-administered with memantine.

donepezil (*Aricept*) ▶LK ♀C ▶? $$$$
ADULT - Alzheimer's disease: Start 5 mg PO qhs. May increase to 10 mg PO qhs in 4-6 weeks. For severe disease (MMSE ≤10), the recommended dose is 10 mg/day.
PEDS - Not approved in children.
UNAPPROVED ADULT - Dementia in Parkinson's disease: 5-10 mg/day.
FORMS - Trade only: Tabs 5,10 mg. Orally disintegrating tabs 5,10 mg.
NOTES - Some clinicians start with 5 mg PO qod to minimize GI side effects.

galantamine (*Razadyne, Razadyne ER, ✦Reminyl*) ▶LK ♀B ▶? $$$$
ADULT - Alzheimer's disease: Extended release: Start 8 mg PO q am with food; increase to 16 mg q am after 4 weeks. May increase to 24 mg q am after another 4 weeks. Immediate release: Start 4 mg PO bid with food; increase to 8 mg bid after 4 weeks. May increase to 12 mg PO bid after another 4 weeks.
PEDS - Not approved in children.
UNAPPROVED ADULT - Dementia in Parkinson's disease: 4-8 mg PO bid (immediate release).

FORMS - Trade only: Tabs (Razadyne) 4, 8, 12 mg; oral solution 4 mg/mL. Extended release caps (Razadyne ER) 8, 16, 24 mg. Prior to April 2005 was called Reminyl.
NOTES - Do not exceed 16 mg/day with renal or hepatic impairment. Use caution with CYP3A4 and CYP2D6 inhibitors (eg, cimetidine, ranitidine, ketoconazole, erythromycin, paroxetine). Avoid abrupt discontinuation. If therapy has been interrupted for several days or more, then restart at the lowest dose.

rivastigmine (*Exelon, Exelon Patch*) ▶K ♀B ▶? $$$$
ADULT - Alzheimer's disease: Start 1.5 mg PO bid with food. Increase to 3 mg bid after 2 wks. Usual effective dose is 6-12 mg/day. Max 12 mg/day. Patch: Start 4.6 mg/24h once daily; may increase after ≥1 month to max 9.5 mg/24h. Dementia associated with Parkinson's disease: Start 1.5 mg bid with food. Increase by 3 mg/day at intervals >4 weeks to max 12 mg/day. Patch: Start 4.6 mg/24h once daily; may increase after ≥1 month to max 9.5 mg/24h.
PEDS - Not approved in children.
FORMS - Trade: Caps 1.5, 3, 4.5, 6 mg. Oral soln 2 mg/mL (120 mL). Transdermal: 4.6 mg/24h (9 mg/patch), 9.5 mg/24h (18 mg/patch).
NOTES - Restart treatment with the lowest daily dose (ie, 1.5 mg PO bid) if discontinued for

several days to reduce the risk of severe vomiting. When changing from PO to patch, patients taking <6 mg/day can be placed on 4.6 mg/24h patch.

For those taking 6-12 mg/day, start with 9.5 mg/24h patch. Have patient start the day after stopping oral dosing. Rotate application sites and do not apply to same spot for 14 days.

NEUROLOGY: Alzheimer's Disease – NMDA Receptor Antagonists

memantine (Namenda, ✹Ebixa) ▶KL ♀B ▶?
$$$$
ADULT - Alzheimer's disease (moderate to severe): Start 5 mg PO daily. Increase by 5 mg/day at weekly intervals to max 20 mg/day. Doses >5 mg/day should be divided bid.
PEDS - Not approved in children.

FORMS - Trade only: Tabs 5, 10 mg. Oral soln 2 mg/mL.
NOTES - May be used in combination with acetylcholinesterase inhibitors. Reduce target dose to 5 mg PO bid in severe renal impairment (CrCl 5-29 mL/min). No adjustment needed for mild-moderate renal impairment.

NEUROLOGY: Anticonvulsants

NOTE: Avoid rapid discontinuation of anticonvulsants, since this can precipitate seizures or other withdrawal symptoms.

carbamazepine (Tegretol, Tegretol XR, Carbatrol, Epitol, Equetro) ▶LK ♀D ▶+ $$
WARNING - Risk of aplastic anemia and agranulocytosis; contraindicated if prior marrow depression. Monitor CBC at baseline and periodically.
ADULT - Epilepsy: Start 200 mg PO bid. Increase by 200 mg/day at weekly intervals divided tid-qid (regular release), bid (extended-release), or qid (suspension) to max 1,600 mg/day. Trigeminal neuralgia: Start 100 mg PO bid or 50 mg PO qid (suspension); increase by 200 mg/day until pain relief. Max 1,200 mg/day. Bipolar disorder, acute manic/mixed episodes (Equetro): Start 200 mg PO bid; increase by 200 mg/day to max 1,600 mg/day. See "unapproved adult" section for alternative bipolar dosing.
PEDS - Epilepsy, age >12 yo: Start 200 mg PO bid or 100 mg PO qid (suspension); increase by 200 mg/day at weekly intervals divided tid-qid (regular release), bid (extended-release), or qid (suspension) to max 1,000 mg/day (age 12-15 yo) or 1,200 mg/day (age >15 yo). Epilepsy, age 6-12 yo: Start 100 mg PO bid or 50 mg PO qid (suspension); increase by 100 mg/day at weekly intervals divided tid-qid (regular release), bid (extended-release), or qid (suspension) to max 1,000 mg/day. Epilepsy, age <6 yo: Start 10-20 mg/kg/day PO divided bid-tid or qid (suspension). Increase weekly prn. Max 35 mg/kg/day.

UNAPPROVED ADULT - Neuropathic pain: Start 100 mg PO bid; usual effective dose is 200 mg PO bid-qid. Max 1,200 mg/day. Mania (American Psychiatric Association guidelines): Start 200-600 mg/day divided tid-qid (standard release) or bid (extended-release), then increase by 200 mg/day q2-4 days. Mean effective dose is 1,000 mg/day. Max 1,600 mg/day.
UNAPPROVED PEDS - Bipolar disorder (manic or mixed phase): Start 100-200 mg PO daily or bid; titrate to usual therapeutic level of 4-12 mcg/mL. Usual effective dose is 200-600 mg/day for children and up to 1,200 mg/day for adolescents.
FORMS - Generic/Trade: Tabs 200 mg, chew tabs 100 mg, susp 100 mg/5 ml. Generic Only: Tabs 100,300,400 mg, chew tabs 200 mg. Trade only: Extended-release tabs (Tegretol XR): 100, 200, 400 mg. Extended-release caps (Carbatrol & Equetro): 100, 200, 300 mg.
NOTES - Usual therapeutic range = 4-12 mcg/mL. Stevens-Johnson Syndrome, hepatitis, aplastic anemia, and hyponatremia may occur. Monitor CBC and LFTs. Many drug interactions. Should not be used for absence or atypical absence seizures.

clobazam (✹Frisium) ▶L ♀X (first trimester) D (2nd/3rd trimesters) ▶- $
WARNING - Caution in the elderly; may accumulate and cause side effects such as psychomotor impairment.
ADULT - Canada only. Epilepsy, adjunctive: Start 5-15 mg PO daily. Gradually increase prn to max 80 mg/day.
PEDS - Canada only. Epilepsy, adjunctive, <2 yo: Start 0.5-1 mg/kg PO daily. 2-16 yo: Start 5

mg daily; may increase prn to max 40 mg/day.

FORMS - Generic/Trade: Tabs 10 mg.

NOTES - Reduce dose in hepatic or renal dysfunction. Drug interactions with enzyme-inducing anticonvulsants such as carbamazepine and phenytoin; may need to adjust dose.

ethosuximide (Zarontin) ▶LK ♀C ▶+ $$$$

ADULT - Absence seizures: Start 500 mg PO given once daily or divided bid. Increase by 250 mg/day q4-7 days prn. Max 1.5 g/day.

PEDS - Absence seizures, 3-6 yo: Start 250 mg PO daily or divided bid. Max 500 mg/day. Age >6 yo: use adult dosing.

UNAPPROVED PEDS - Absence seizures, age <3 yo: start 15 mg/kg/day PO divided bid. Increase q4-7 days prn. Usual effective dose is 15-40 mg/kg/day divided bid. Max 500 mg/day.

FORMS - Generic/Trade: Caps 250 mg. Syrup 250 mg/5 mL.

NOTES - Usual therapeutic range = 40-100 mcg/mL. Monitor CBC for blood dyscrasias. Caution in hepatic and renal impairment. May increase the risk of grand mal seizures in some.

felbamate (Felbatol) ▶KL ♀C ▶- $$$$$

WARNING - Aplastic anemia and fatal hepatic failure have occurred.

ADULT - Severe, refractory epilepsy: Start 400 mg PO tid. Increase by 600 mg/day q2 weeks to max 3,600 mg/day.

PEDS - Lennox-Gastaut syndrome, adjunctive therapy, age 2-14 yo: Start 15 mg/kg/day PO in 3-4 divided doses. Increase by 15 mg/kg/day at weekly intervals to max 45 mg/kg/day.

FORMS - Trade only: Tabs 400, 600 mg. Susp 600 mg/5 mL.

NOTES - Use only after discussing the risks and obtaining written informed consent. Many drug interactions.

fosphenytoin (Cerebyx) ▶L ♀D ▶+ $$$$$

ADULT - Status epilepticus: Load 15-20 mg "phenytoin equivalents" (PE) per kg IV no faster than 100-150 mg PE/minute. Non-emergent loading dose: 10-20 mg PE/kg IM/IV at rate ≤150 mg/minute. Maintenance: 4-6 mg PE/kg/day.

PEDS - Not approved in children.

UNAPPROVED PEDS - Status epilepticus: 15-20 mg PE/kg IV at a rate <2 mg PE/kg/min. Nonemergent use >7 yo: 4-6 mg PE/kg/24 hr IV/IM no faster than 100-150 mg PE/minute.

NOTES - Fosphenytoin is dosed in "phenytoin equivalents" (PE). Use beyond 5 days has not been systematically studied. Monitor ECG & vital signs continuously during and after infusion.

Contraindicated in cardiac conduction block. Many drug interactions. Usual therapeutic level = 10-20 mcg/mL if normal hepatorenal function. Renal/hepatic disease may change protein binding and levels. Low albumin levels may increase free fraction.

gabapentin (Neurontin) ▶K ♀C ▶? $$$$

ADULT - Partial seizures, adjunctive therapy: Start 300 mg PO qhs. Increase gradually to usual effective dose of 300-600 mg PO tid. Max 3,600 mg/day. Postherpetic neuralgia: Start 300 mg PO on day 1. Increase to 300 mg bid on day 2, and to 300 mg tid on day 3. Max 1,800 mg/day divided tid.

PEDS - Partial seizures, adjunctive therapy, 3-12 yo: Start 10-15 mg/kg/day PO divided tid. Titrate over 3 days to usual effective dose of 25-40 mg/kg/day divided tid. Max 50 mg/kg/day. Age >12 yo: Use adult dosing.

UNAPPROVED ADULT - Partial seizures, initial monotherapy: Titrate as above. Usual effective dose is 900-1,800 mg/day. Neuropathic pain: 300 mg PO tid, max 3,600 mg/day in 3-4 divided doses. Migraine prophylaxis: Start 300 mg daily, then gradually increase to 1,200-2,400 mg/day in 3-4 divided doses. Restless legs syndrome: Start 300 mg PO qhs. Max 3,600 mg/day divided tid. Hot flashes: 300 mg PO tid.

UNAPPROVED PEDS - Neuropathic pain: Start 5 mg/kg PO at bedtime. Increase to 5 mg/kg bid on day 2 and 5 mg/kg tid on day 3. Titrate to usual effective range of 8-35 mg/kg/24 hr.

FORMS - Generic only: Tabs 100, 300, 400 mg. Generic/Trade: Caps 100, 300, 400 mg. Tabs 600, 800 mg (scored). Soln 50 mg/mL.

NOTES - Decrease dose in renal impairment (CrCl <60 mL/min); table in package insert. Discontinue gradually over ≥1 week.

lamotrigine (Lamictal, Lamictal CD) ▶LK ♀C (see notes) ▶- $$$$

WARNING - Potentially life-threatening rashes (eg, Stevens-Johnson Syndrome) reported in 0.3% of adults and 0.8% of children, usually within 2-8 weeks of initiation; discontinue at first sign of rash. Drug interaction with valproate – see adjusted dosing guidelines.

ADULT - Partial seizures, Lennox Gastaut syndrome, or generalized tonic-clonic seizures, adjunctive therapy with an enzyme-inducing anticonvulsant (age >12 yo): Start 50 mg PO daily x 2 weeks, then 50 mg PO bid x 2 weeks. Increase by 100 mg/day q1-2 weeks to usual maintenance dose of 150-250 mg PO bid. Partial seizures, conversion to monotherapy from adjunctive therapy with a single enzyme-inducing anticonvulsant (age ≥16 yo): Use above guidelines to gradually increase the dose to 250 mg PO bid; then taper the enzyme-inducing anticonvulsant by 20% a week over 4 wks. Partial seizures, Lennox-Gastaut syndrome, or generalized tonic-clonic seizures, adjunctive therapy with valproate (age >12 yo): Start 25 mg PO qod x 2 weeks, then 25 mg PO daily x 2 weeks. Increase by 25-50 mg/day q1-2 weeks to usual maintenance dose of 100-400 mg/day (lamotrigine + valproate and other anticonvulsants) or 100-200 mg/day if used with valproate alone given once daily or divided bid. Partial seizures, conversion to monotherapy from adjunctive therapy with valproate (age ≥16 yo): Use above guidelines to gradually increase the dose to 200 mg/day PO given daily or divided bid; then decrease valproate weekly by ≤500 mg/day to an initial goal of 500 mg/day. After 1 week at these doses, increase lamotrigine to 300 mg/day and decrease valproate to 250 mg/day divided bid. A week later, discontinue valproate; then increase lamotrigine weekly by 100 mg/day to usual maintenance dose of 500 mg/day. Partial seizures, Lennox-Gastaut syndrome, or generalized tonic-clonic seizures, adjunctive therapy with other anticonvulsants (not valproate or enzyme inducers) (>12 yo): Start 25 mg PO daily x 2 weeks, the 50 mg PO daily x 2 weeks. Increase by 50 mg/day q1-2 weeks to usual maintenance dose of 225-375 mg/day divided bid. See psychiatry section for bipolar disorder dosing.

PEDS - Partial seizures, Lennox-Gastaut syndrome or generalized tonic-clonic seizures, adjunctive therapy with an enzyme-inducing anticonvulsant, age 2-12 yo: Start 0.6 mg/kg/day PO divided bid x 2 weeks, then 1.2 mg/kg/day PO divided bid x 2 weeks. Increase q1-2 weeks by 1.2 mg/kg/day (rounded down to the nearest whole tablet) to usual maintenance dose of 5-15 mg/kg/day. Max 400 mg/day. Partial seizures, Lennox-Gastaut syndrome, or generalized tonic-clonic seizures, adjunctive therapy with valproate, age 2-12 yo: Start 0.15 mg/kg/day PO (given daily or divided bid) x 2 weeks, then 0.3 mg/kg/day PO (given daily or divided bid) x 2 weeks. Increase q1-2 weeks by 0.3 mg/kg/day (rounded down to nearest whole tablet) to usual maintenance dose of 1-5 mg/kg/day (lamotrigine + valproate and other anticonvulsants) or 1-3 mg/kg/day if used with valproate alone. Max 200 mg/day. Partial seizur-

es, Lennox-Gastaut syndrome, or generalized tonic-clonic seizures, adjunctive therapy with other anticonvulsants (not valproate or enzyme inducers), age 2-12 yo: Start 0.3 mg/kg/day (given daily or divided bid) x 2 weeks, then 0.6 mg/kg/day x 2 weeks. Increase q1-2 weeks by 0.6 mg/kg/day (rounded down to nearest whole tablet) to usual maintenance dose of 4.5-7.5 mg/kg/day. Max 300 mg/day. Age >12 yo: use adult dosing for all of the above indications.

UNAPPROVED ADULT - Initial monotherapy for partial seizures: Start 25 mg PO daily. Usual maintenance dose is 100-300 mg/day divided bid. Max 500 mg/day.

UNAPPROVED PEDS - Initial monotherapy for partial seizures: Start 0.5 mg/kg/day given daily or divided bid. Max 10 mg/kg/day. Newly-diagnosed absence seizures: Titrate as above. Usual effective dose is 2-15 mg/kg/day.

FORMS - Generic/Trade: Chewable dispersible tabs 5, 25 mg. Trade only: Tabs 25, 100, 150, 200 mg. Chewable dispersible tabs (Lamictal CD) 2 mg not available in pharmacies; obtain through manufacturer representative, or by calling 1-888-825-5249.

NOTES - Drug interactions with valproate and enzyme-inducing antiepileptic drugs (ie, carbamazepine, phenobarbital, phenytoin, primidone); may need to adjust dose. May increase carbamazepine toxicity. Women taking estrogen-containing oral contraceptives without an enzyme-inducing anticonvulsant will generally require an increase of the lamotrigine maintenance dose by up to 2-fold. Consider increasing the lamotrigine dose when the contraceptive is started. Taper lamotrigine by ≤25% of daily dose q week over a 2-week period if the contraceptive is stopped. Preliminary evidence suggests that exposure during the first trimester of pregnancy is associated with a risk of cleft palate and/or cleft lip. Please report all fetal exposure to the Lamotrigine Pregnancy Registry (800-336-2176) and the North American Antiepileptic Drug Pregnancy Registry (888-233-2334).

levetiracetam (*Keppra*) ▶K ♀C ▶? $$$$$
ADULT - Partial seizures, juvenile myoclonic epilepsy (JME), or primary generalized tonic-clonic seizures (GTC), adjunctive therapy: Start 500 mg PO/IV bid; increase by 1,000 mg/day q2 weeks prn to max 3,000 mg/day (partial seizures) or to target dose of 3,000 mg/day (JME or GTC).

PEDS - Partial seizures, adjunctive therapy, age

>4 yo: Start 20 mg/kg/day PO/IV divided bid. Increase q2 weeks as tolerated to target dose of 60 mg/kg/day. Juvenile myoclonic epilepsy, adjunctive therapy, age ≥12 yo: Use adult dosing. Primary generalized tonic-clonic seizures (GTC), adjunctive therapy, 6-15 yo: Start 20 mg/kg/day PO divided bid. Increase by 20 mg/kg/day q2 weeks to target dose of 60 mg/day. GTC, adjunctive therapy, age >16 yo: Use adult dosing.

UNAPPROVED ADULT - Myoclonus: Start 500-1,000 mg/day in divided doses. May increase to max 1,500-3,000 mg/day or 50 mg/kg/day.

FORMS - Trade only: Tabs 250, 500, 750, 1,000 mg. Oral solution 100 mg/mL.

NOTES - Drug interactions unlikely. Decrease dose in renal dysfunction (CrCl <80 mL/min). Emotional lability, hostility, and depression may occur. Use same dose when switching between IV and PO forms.

oxcarbazepine (*Trileptal*) ▶LK ♀C ▶- $$$$$
WARNING - Serious multi-organ hypersensitivity reactions and life-threatening rashes (eg, Stevens-Johnson Syndrome, toxic epidermal necrolysis) have occurred, with some fatalities. Consider discontinuation if skin reactions.

ADULT - Partial seizures, monotherapy: Start 300 mg PO bid. Increase by 300 mg/day q3 days to usual effective dose of 1,200 mg/day. Max 2,400 mg/day. Partial seizures, adjunctive: Start 300 mg PO bid. Increase by ≤600 mg/day at weekly intervals to usual effective dose of 1,200 mg/day. Max 2,400 mg/day.

PEDS - Partial seizures, adjunctive, age 2-16 yo: Start 8-10 mg/kg/day PO divided bid (max starting dose 600 mg/day). Titrate to max 60 mg/kg/day (age 2 to <4 yo), or to target dose of 900 mg/day (20-29 kg), 1,200 mg/day (29.1-39 kg), or 1,800 mg/day (>39 kg). May consider using a starting dose of 16-20 mg/kg for children aged 2 to <4 yo who weigh <20 kg to account for higher clearance. Partial seizures, initial monotherapy, 4-16 yo: Start 8-10 mg/kg/day divided bid. Increase by 5 mg/kg/day q3 days to recommended dose (in mg/day) of: 600-900 if ~20 kg, 900-1,200 if ~25-30 kg, 900-1,500 if ~35-40 kg, 1,200-1,500 if ~45 kg, 1,200-1,800 if ~50-55 kg, 1,200-2,100 if ~60-65 kg, 1,500-2,100 if ~70 kg. Partial seizures, conversion to monotherapy, age 4-16 yo: Start 8-10 mg/kg/day divided bid. Increase at weekly intervals by ≤10 mg/kg/day to target dose listed for initial monotherapy.

FORMS - Trade only: Tabs (scored) 150, 300, 600 mg. Oral suspension 300 mg/5 mL.

NOTES - Monitor serum sodium. Decrease initial dose by one-half in renal dysfunction (CrCl <30 mL/min). Inhibits CYP 2C19 and induces CYP 3A4/5. Interactions with other antiepileptic drugs, oral contraceptives, and dihydropyridine calcium channel blockers.

phenobarbital (*Luminal*) ▶L ♀D ▶- ©IV $
ADULT - Epilepsy: 100-300 mg/day PO divided daily-tid. Status epilepticus: 20 mg/kg IV at rate ≤60 mg/min.

PEDS - Epilepsy: 3-5 mg/kg/day PO divided bid-tid. Status epilepticus: 20 mg/kg IV at rate ≤60 mg/min.

UNAPPROVED ADULT - Status epilepticus: may give up to a total dose of 30 mg/kg IV.

UNAPPROVED PEDS - Status epilepticus: 15-20 mg/kg IV load; may give additional 5 mg/kg doses q15-30 minutes to max total dose of 30 mg/kg. Epilepsy: 3-5 mg/kg/day given once daily or divided bid (neonates), 5-6 mg/kg/day given once daily or divided bid (infants), 6-8 mg/kg/day given once daily or divided bid (age 1-5 yo), 4-6 mg/kg/day given once daily or divided bid (age 6-12 yo), or 1-3 mg/kg/day given once daily or divided bid (age >12 yo).

FORMS - Generic only: Tabs 15, 16.2, 30, 32.4, 60, 100 mg. Elixir 20 mg/5 mL.

NOTES - Usual therapeutic range = 15- 40 mcg/mL. Monitor cardiopulmonary function closely when administering IV. Decrease dose in renal or hepatic dysfunction. Many drug interactions.

phenytoin (*Dilantin, Phenytek*) ▶L ♀D ▶+ $$
ADULT - Status epilepticus: 10-15 mg/kg IV at rate ≤50 mg/ min, then 100 mg IV/PO q6-8h. Epilepsy, oral loading dose: 400 mg PO initially, then 300 mg in 2h and 4h. Epilepsy, maintenance dose: 300 mg/day PO given once daily (extended release) or divided tid (standard release) and titrated to a therapeutic level.

PEDS - Epilepsy, >6 yo: 5 mg/kg/day PO divided bid-tid, to max 300 mg/day. Status epilepticus: 15-20 mg/kg IV at a rate ≤1 mg/kg/min.

FORMS - Generic/Trade: Extended-release caps 100 mg (Dilantin). Suspension 125 mg/5 mL. Trade only: Extended-release caps 30 mg (Dilantin), 200, 300 mg (Phenytek). Chew tabs 50 mg (Dilantin Infatabs).

NOTES - Usual therapeutic range is 10-20 mcg/mL. Monitor ECG and vital signs when administering IV. Many drug interactions. Monitor levels closely when switching between forms (free acid vs. sodium salt). The free fraction may be increased in patients with low albumin levels. IV loading doses of 15-20 mg/kg have also been recommended. May need to reduce loading dose if patient is already on phenytoin.

pregabalin (*Lyrica*) ▶K ♀C ▶? ©V $$$$
ADULT - Painful diabetic peripheral neuropathy: Start 50 mg PO tid; may increase within 1 week to max 100 mg PO tid. Postherpetic neuralgia: Start 150 mg/day PO divided bid-tid; may increase within 1 week to 300 mg/day divided bid-tid; max 600 mg/day. Partial seizures (adjunctive): Start 150 mg/day PO divided bid-tid; may increase prn to max 600 mg/day divided bid-tid. Fibromyalgia: Start 75 mg PO bid; may increase to 150 mg bid within 1 week; max dose 225 mg bid.
PEDS - Not approved in children.
FORMS - Trade only: Caps 25, 50, 75, 100, 150, 200, 225, 300 mg.
NOTES - Adjust dose if CrCl <60 mL/min; refer to package insert. Warn patients to report changes in visual acuity, muscle pain. May increase creatine kinase. Must taper if discontinuing to avoid withdrawal symptoms. Increased risk of peripheral edema when used in conjunction with thiazolidinedione antidiabetic agents.

primidone (*Mysoline*) ▶LK ♀D ▶- $$$$
ADULT - Epilepsy: Start 100-125 mg PO qhs. Increase over 10 days to usual maintenance dose of 250 mg PO tid-qid. Max 2 g/day.
PEDS - Epilepsy <8 yo: Start 50 mg PO qhs. Increase over 10 days to usual maintenance dose of 125-250 mg tid or 10-25 mg/kg/day.
UNAPPROVED ADULT - Essential tremor: Start 12.5-25 mg PO qhs. May increase weekly prn by 50 mg/day to 250 mg/day given once daily or in divided doses. Max 750 mg/day.
FORMS - Generic/Trade: Tabs 50, 250 mg.
NOTES - Usual therapeutic level = 5-12 mcg/mL. Metabolized to phenobarbital.

tiagabine (*Gabitril*) ▶L ♀C ▶? $$$$$
WARNING - New onset-seizures and status epilepticus may occur when used in patients without epilepsy, particularly when combined with other medications that lower the seizure threshold. Avoid off-label use.
ADULT - Partial seizures, adjunct with an enzyme-inducing anticonvulsant: Start 4 mg PO daily. Increase by 4-8 mg/day at weekly intervals prn to max 56 mg/day divided bid-qid.
PEDS - Partial seizures, adjunctive therapy with an enzyme-inducing anticonvulsant, 12-18 yo: Start 4 mg PO daily. Increase by 4 mg/day q1-2 weeks prn to max 32 mg/day divided bid-qid.
FORMS - Trade only: Tabs 2, 4, 12, 16 mg.

NOTES - Take with food. Dosing is for patients on enzyme-inducing anticonvulsants such as carbamazepine, phenobarbital, phenytoin, or primidone. Reduce dosage in patients who are not taking enzyme-inducing medications, and in those with liver dysfunction.

topiramate (*Topamax*) ▶K ♀C ▶? $$$$$
ADULT - Partial seizures or primary generalized tonic-clonic seizures, monotherapy: Start 25 mg PO bid (week 1), 50 mg bid (week 2), 75 mg bid (week 3), 100 mg bid (week 4), 150 mg bid (week 5), then 200 mg bid as tolerated. Partial seizures, primary generalized tonic-clonic seizures, or Lennox Gastaut Syndrome, adjunctive therapy: Start 25-50 mg PO qhs. Increase weekly by 25-50 mg/day to usual effective dose of 200 mg PO bid. Doses >400 mg/day not shown to be more effective. Migraine prophylaxis: Start 25 mg qhs (week 1), then 25 mg bid (week 2), 25 mg q am and 50 mg q pm (week 3), then 50 mg bid (week 4 and thereafter).
PEDS - Partial seizures or primary generalized tonic-clonic seizures, monotherapy (age >10 yo): Use adult dosing. Partial seizures, primary generalized tonic-clonic seizures, or Lennox-Gastaut Syndrome, adjunctive therapy, 2-16 yo: Start 1-3 mg/kg (max 25 mg) PO qhs. Increase by 1-3 mg/kg/day q 1-2 weeks to usual effective dose of 5-9 mg/kg/day divided bid.
UNAPPROVED ADULT - Essential tremor: Start 25 mg PO daily. Increase by 25 mg/day at weekly intervals to 100 mg/day; max 400 mg/day. Bipolar disorder: Start 25-50 mg PO daily. Titrate prn to max 400 mg/day.
FORMS - Trade only: Tabs 25, 50, 100, 200 mg. Sprinkle Caps 15, 25 mg.
NOTES - Give ½ usual adult dose in renal impairment (CrCl <70 mL/min). Confusion, nephrolithiasis, glaucoma, and weight loss may occur. Risk of oligohidrosis and hyperthermia, particularly in children; use caution in warm ambient temperatures and/or with vigorous physical activity. Hyperchloremic, non-anion gap metabolic acidosis may occur; monitor serum bicarbonate and either reduce dose or taper off entirely if this occurs. Max dose tested was 1,600 mg/day.

valproic acid (*Depakene, Depakote, Depakote ER, Depacon, divalproex, sodium valproate, ✚Epival, Deproic*) ▶L ♀D ▶+ $$$$
WARNING - Fatal hepatic failure has occurred; monitor LFTs during first 6 months of treat-

ment. Life-threatening pancreatitis has been reported after initial or prolonged use. Evaluate for abdominal pain, N/V, and/or anorexia. Discontinue if pancreatitis occurs. May be more teratogenic than other anticonvulsants (eg, carbamazepine, lamotrigine, and phenytoin). Hepatic failure and clotting disorders have occurred when used during pregnancy.

ADULT - Epilepsy: 10-15 mg/kg/day PO or IV infusion over 60 min (≤20 mg/min) divided bid to qid (standard release, delayed release, or IV) or given once daily (Depakote ER). Increase dose by 5-10 mg/kg/day at weekly intervals to max 60 mg/kg/day. Migraine prophylaxis: Start 250 mg PO bid (Depakote) or 500 mg PO daily (Depakote ER) x 1 week, then increase to max 1,000 mg/day PO divided bid (Depakote) or given once daily (Depakote ER).

PEDS - Seizures >2 yo: 10-15 mg/kg/day PO or IV infusion over 60 min (rate ≤20 mg/min). Increase dose by 5-10 mg/kg/day at weekly intervals to max 60 mg/kg/day. Divide doses >250 mg/day into bid-qid; may give once daily (Depakote ER) if >10 yo.

UNAPPROVED ADULT - Status epilepticus (not first-line): Load 20-40 mg/kg IV (rate ≤ 6 mg/kg/min), then continue 4-8 mg/kg IV tid to achieve therapeutic level. May use lower loading dose if already on valproate.

UNAPPROVED PEDS - Status epilepticus, age >2 yo (not first-line): Load 20-40 mg/kg IV over 1-5 min, then 5 mg/kg/hr adjusted to achieve therapeutic level. May use lower loading dose if already on valproate.

FORMS - Generic/Trade: Immediate release caps 250 mg (Depakene), syrup (Depakene, valproic acid) 250 mg/5 mL. Trade (Depakote): Delayed release sprinkle caps 125 mg, delayed release tabs 125, 250, 500 mg; extended release tabs (Depakote ER) 250, 500mg.

DERMATOMES

MOTOR NERVE ROOTS

Level	Motor function
C4	Spontaneous breathing
C5	Shoulder shrug / deltoid
C6	Biceps / wrist extension
C7	Triceps / wrist flexion
C8/T1	finger flexion
T1-T12	Intercostal/abd muscles
T12	cremasteric reflex
L1/L2	hip flexion
L2/L3/L4	hip adduction / quads
L5	great toe dorsiflexion
S1/S2	foot plantarflexion
S2-S4	rectal tone

LUMBOSACRAL NERVE ROOT COMPRESSION	Root	Motor	Sensory	Reflex
	L4	quadriceps	medial foot	knee-jerk
	L5	dorsiflexors	dorsum of foot	medial hamstring
	S1	plantarflexors	lateral foot	ankle-jerk

GLASGOW COMA SCALE

Eye Opening	Verbal Activity	Motor Activity
4. Spontaneous	5. Oriented	6. Obeys commands
3. To command	4. Confused	5. Localizes pain
2. To pain	3. Inappropriate	4. Withdraws to pain
1. None	2. Incomprehensible	3. Flexion to pain
	1. None	2. Extension to pain
		1. None

NOTES - Contraindicated in urea cycle disorders or hepatic dysfunction. Usual therapeutic trough level is 50-100 mcg/mL. Depakote and Depakote ER are not interchangeable. Depakote ER is ~10% less bioavailable than Depakote. Depakote releases divalproex sodium over 8-12h (daily-qid dosing); Depakote ER releases divalproex sodium over 18-24h (daily dosing). Many drug interactions. Patients receiving other anticonvulsants may require higher doses of valproic acid. Reduce dose in the elderly. Hyperammonemia, GI irritation, or thrombocytopenia may occur.

vigabatrin (✿Sabril) ▶K ♀C ▶- $$$$

WARNING - Ophthalmologic abnormalities have been reported. Visual field testing should be performed prior to treatment and q3 months thereafter. In view of difficulties in testing in children <9 yo, use only if clearly indicated. Do not use with other retinotoxic drugs.

ADULT - Canada only. Epilepsy (adjunct treatment): Start: 1 g/day in divided doses, maintenance: 2-3 g/day in divided doses.

PEDS - Canada only. Epilepsy (adjunct treatment), infantile spasms (monotherapy): Start: 40 mg/kg/day, maintenance: 50-100 mg/kg/day in divided doses.

FORMS - Trade only: Tabs 500 mg. Oral powder 500 mg/sachet.

zonisamide (Zonegran) ▶LK ♀C ▶? $$$$

ADULT - Partial seizures, adjunctive: Start 100 mg PO daily x 2 weeks, then increase to 200 mg daily. May increase prn q2 weeks to 300-400 mg daily (or divided bid). Max 600 mg/day.

PEDS - Not approved in children.

FORMS - Generic/Trade: Caps 25, 50, 100 mg.

NOTES - This is a sulfonamide; contraindicated in sulfa allergy. Fatalities and severe reactions including Stevens-Johnson syndrome, toxic epidermal necrolysis, fulminant hepatic necrosis, and blood dyscrasias have occurred with sulfonamides. Clearance is affected by CYP 3A4 inhibitors or inducers such as phenytoin, carbamazepine, phenobarbital, and valproic acid. Nephrolithiasis may occur. Oligohidrosis and hyperthermia may occur, and are more common in children. Patients with renal disease may require slower dose titration.

NEUROLOGY: Migraine Therapy – Triptans (5-HT1 Receptor Agonists)

NOTE: None are FDA-approved in children. May cause vasospasm. Avoid in ischemic or vasospastic heart disease, cerebrovascular syndromes, peripheral arterial disease, uncontrolled HTN, and hemiplegic or basilar migraine. Do not use within 24 hours of ergots or other triptans. Risk of serotonin syndrome with SSRIs, MAOIs.

almotriptan (Axert) ▶LK ♀C ▶? $$

ADULT - Migraine treatment: 6.25-12.5 mg PO. May repeat in 2 hours prn. Max 25 mg/day.

FORMS - Trade only: Tabs 6.25, 12.5 mg.

NOTES - MAOIs inhibit metabolism; use together only with extreme caution. Use lower doses (6.25 mg) in renal and/or hepatic dysfunction.

eletriptan (Relpax) ▶LK ♀C ▶? $$

ADULT - Migraine treatment: 20-40 mg PO at onset. May repeat in >2 hours prn. Max 40 mg/dose or 80 mg/day.

FORMS - Trade only: Tabs 20, 40 mg.

NOTES - Do not use within 72 hours of potent CYP3A4 inhibitors such as ketoconazole, itraconazole, nefazodone, troleandomycin, clarithromycin, ritonavir, or nelfinavir.

frovatriptan (Frova) ▶LK ♀C ▶? $

ADULT - Migraine treatment: 2.5 mg PO. May repeat in 2 hours prn. Max 7.5 mg/24 hours.

FORMS - Trade only: Tabs 2.5 mg.

naratriptan (Amerge) ▶KL ♀C ▶? $$

ADULT - Migraine treatment: 1-2.5 mg PO. May repeat in 4 hours prn. Max 5 mg/24 hours.

FORMS - Trade only: Tabs 1, 2.5 mg.

NOTES - Contraindicated in severe renal or hepatic impairment.

rizatriptan (Maxalt, Maxalt MLT) ▶LK ♀C ▶? $$

ADULT - Migraine treatment: 5-10 mg PO; May repeat in 2 hours prn. Max 30 mg/24 hours.

FORMS - Trade only: Tabs 5, 10 mg. Orally disintegrating tabs (MLT) 5, 10 mg.

NOTES - Should not be combined with MAOIs. MLT form dissolves on tongue without liquids.

sumatriptan (Imitrex) ▶K ♀C ▶+ $$

ADULT - Migraine treatment: 4-6 mg SC. May repeat in 1 hour prn. Max 12 mg/24 hours. Tablets: 25-100 mg PO (50 mg most common). May repeat q2h prn with 25-100 mg doses. Max 200 mg/24 hours. Intranasal spray: 5-20 mg. May repeat q2h prn. Max 40 mg/24 hours. Cluster headache dose: 6 mg SC. May repeat in >1h prn. Max 12 mg/24 hours. Initial oral dose of 50 mg appears to be more effective than 25 mg. If HA returns after initial SC injection, then tablets may be used q2h prn, max 100 mg/24 hours.

UNAPPROVED PEDS - Acute migraine, 8-17 yo: 20 mg intranasal spray (if ≥40 kg) or 10 mg (if 20-39 kg) at headache onset. May repeat after 2 hours prn.

FORMS - Trade only: Tabs 25, 50, 100 mg. Nasal spray 5, 20 mg/ spray. Injection 6 mg/0.5 mL, 4 & 6 mg cartridges (STATdose System).

NOTES - Should not be combined with MAOIs. Avoid IM/IV route.

zolmitriptan (*Zomig, Zomig ZMT*) ▶L ♀C ▶? $$

ADULT - Migraine treatment: Tabs: 1.25-2.5 mg PO q2h. Max 10 mg/24 hours. Orally disintegrating tabs (ZMT): 2.5 mg PO. May repeat in 2 hours prn. Max 10 mg/24 hours. Nasal spray: 5 mg (1 spray) in one nostril. May repeat in 2 hours prn. Max 10 mg/24 hours.

FORMS - Trade only: Tabs 2.5, 5 mg. Orally disintegrating tabs $$$ (ZMT) 2.5, 5 mg. Nasal spray 5 mg/spray.

NOTES - Risk of vasospastic complications. Should not be combined with MAOIs. Use lower doses (<2.5 mg) in hepatic dysfunction. May break 2.5 mg tabs in half.

NEUROLOGY: Migraine Therapy – Other

***Cafergot* (ergotamine + caffeine)** ▶L♀X ▶- $

WARNING - Contraindicated with concomitant use of potent CYP 3A4 inhibitors (e.g., macrolides, protease inhibitors) due to risk of serious / life-threatening peripheral ischemia. Ergots have been associated with potentially life-threatening fibrotic complications.

ADULT – Migraine, cluster headache treatment: 2 tabs PO at onset, then 1 tab q30 minutes prn to max 6 tabs/attack or 10 tabs/week. Suppositories: 1 suppository PR at onset; may repeat in 1h prn. Max 2 suppositories/attack or 5/wk.

PEDS - Not approved in children.

UNAPPROVED PEDS - Migraine treatment: 1 tab PO at onset, then 1 tab q 30 minutes prn to max 3 tabs/attack.

FORMS - Trade only: Tabs 1/100 mg ergotamine/caffeine.

NOTES - Contraindicated in sepsis, CAD, peripheral arterial disease, HTN, impaired hepatic or renal function, malnutrition, severe pruritus.

dihydroergotamine (*D.H.E. 45, Migranal*) ▶L ♀X ▶- $$

WARNING - Contraindicated with concomitant use of potent CYP 3A4 inhibitors (e.g., macrolides, protease inhibitors) due to risk of serious / life-threatening peripheral ischemia. Ergots have been associated with potentially life-threatening fibrotic complications.

ADULT - Migraine treatment: Solution (DHE 45): 1 mg IV/IM/SC; may repeat q1h prn to max 2 mg (IV) or 3 mg (IM/SC) per 24 hours. Nasal spray (Migranal): 1 spray (0.5 mg) in each nostril; may repeat in 15 min prn to max 6 sprays (3 mg)/ 24 hours or 8 sprays (4 mg)/week.

PEDS - Not approved in children.

FORMS - Trade only: Nasal spray 0.5 mg/spray (Migranal). Self-injecting solution (D.H.E. 45): 1 mg/mL.

NOTES - Contraindicated in basilar or hemiplegic migraine, sepsis, ischemic or vasospastic cardiac disease, peripheral vascular disease, vascular surgery, impaired hepatic or renal function, or uncontrolled HTN. Avoid concurrent ergotamine, methysergide, or triptan use.

flunarizine (❋*Sibelium*) ▶L ♀C ▶- $$

ADULT - Canada only. Migraine prophylaxis: 10 mg PO qhs. If side effects, then 5 mg qhs. Safety of long-term use (>4 months) has not been established.

PEDS - Not approved in children.

FORMS - Generic/Trade: Caps 5 mg

NOTES - Gradual benefit over 6-8 weeks. Not for acute therapy. Contraindicated if history of depression or extrapyramidal disorders.

***Midrin* (isometheptene + dichloralphenazone + acetaminophen, *Amidrine, Durdrin, Migquin, Migratine, Migrazone, VaZone*)** ▶L ♀? ▶? ©IV $

ADULT - Tension and vascular headache treatment: 1-2 caps PO q4h, to max of 8 caps/day. Migraine treatment: 2 caps PO x 1, then 1 cap q1h prn to max 5 caps/12 hours.

PEDS - Not approved in children.

FORMS - Generic only: Caps 65/100/325 mg of isometheptene / dichloralphenazone / acetaminophen.

NOTES - Midrin brand no longer available; generics only. FDA has classified as "possibly effective" for migraine treatment. Contraindicated in glaucoma, severe renal disease, heart disease, hepatic disease, or concurrent MAOI use. Use caution in HTN, peripheral arterial disease, or recent MI.

NEUROLOGY: Multiple Sclerosis

glatiramer (*Copaxone*) ▶Serum ♀B ▶? $$$$$
ADULT - Multiple sclerosis (relapsing-remitting): 20 mg SC daily.
PEDS - Not approved in children.
FORMS - Trade only: Injection 20 mg single dose vial.
NOTES - Do not inject IV.

interferon beta-1A (*Avonex, Rebif*) ▶L ♀C ▶? $$$$$
WARNING - Risk of severe hepatic injury and failure, possibly greater when used with other hepatotoxic drugs. Monitor LFTs. Suicidality risk; use caution in depression.
ADULT - Multiple sclerosis (relapsing forms): Avonex- 30 mcg (6 million units) IM q week. Rebif- start 8.8 mcg SC three times weekly; titrate over 4 weeks to maintenance dose of 44 mcg three times weekly.
PEDS - Not approved in children.
FORMS - Trade only: Avonex: Injection 33 mcg (6.6 million units) single dose vial. Rebif: Starter kit 20 mcg pre-filled syringe, 22 & 44 mcg prefilled syringes.
NOTES - Caution with depression, seizure disorders, or cardiac disease. Follow LFTs and CBC. Avonex: indicated for the first attack of MS. Rebif: give same dose 3 days each week, with at least 48 hours between doses.

interferon beta-1B (*Betaseron*) ▶L ♀C ▶? $$$$$
ADULT - Multiple sclerosis (relapsing-remitting): Start 0.0625 mg SC qod; titrate over six weeks to 0.25 mg (8 million units) SC qod.
PEDS - Not approved in children.
FORMS - Trade only: Injection 0.3 mg (9.6 million units) single dose vial.
NOTES - Suicidality risk; use caution in depression. Check LFTs after 1, 3, and 6 months and then periodically. Product can be stored at room temp until reconstituted; then refrigerate and use within 3 hours.

natalizumab (*Tysabri*) ▶Serum ♀C ▶? $$$$$
WARNING - May cause progressive multifocal leukoencephalopathy. Avoid concomitant use of other immunomodulators.
ADULT - Relapsing multiple sclerosis (monotherapy): 300 mg IV infusion over 1 hour q4 wks.
PEDS - Not approved in children.
UNAPPROVED ADULT - Crohn's disease: Two doses of 3 mg/kg IV given 4 weeks apart. Alternative "ENCORE" dose: 300 mg IV at weeks 0, 4, and 8.
NOTES - Not first line - recommended only when there has been an inadequate response or failure to tolerate other therapies. Available only through the TOUCH prescribing program at 1-800-456-2255. Observe closely for infusion reactions & signs of leukoencephalopathy.

NEUROLOGY: Myasthenia Gravis

edrophonium (*Tensilon, Enlon*) ▶Plasma ♀C ▶? $
ADULT - Evaluation for myasthenia gravis: 2 mg IV over 15-30 seconds (test dose) while on cardiac monitor, then 8 mg IV after 45 seconds. Reversal of neuromuscular blockade: 10 mg IV over 30-45 seconds; repeat prn to max 40 mg.
PEDS - Evaluation for myasthenia gravis, weight ≤34 kg: 1 mg IV (test dose), then 1 mg IV q30-45 seconds to max 5 mg. Weight >34 kg: 2 mg IV (test dose), then 2 mg IV q30- 45 seconds to max 10 mg.
UNAPPROVED ADULT - Reversal of non-depolarizing neuromuscular blocking agents: 0.5-1.0 mg/kg IV together with atropine 0.007-0.014 mg/kg.
NOTES - Not for maintenance therapy of myasthenia gravis because of short action (5-10 minutes). May give IM. Monitor cardiac function. Atropine should be readily available in case of cholinergic reaction. Contraindicated in mechanical urinary or intestinal obstruction.

neostigmine (*Prostigmin*) ▶L ♀C ▶? $$$
ADULT - Myasthenia gravis: 15-375 mg/day PO in divided doses, or 0.5 mg IM/SC when oral therapy is not possible. Reversal of non-depolarizing neuromuscular blocking agents: 0.5-2.0 mg slow IV (preceded by atropine 0.6-1.2 mg or glycopyrrolate 0.2-0.6 mg); repeat prn to max 5 mg.
PEDS - Not approved in children.
UNAPPROVED PEDS - Myasthenia gravis: 7.5-15 mg PO tid-qid; or 0.03 mg/kg IM q2-4h. Reversal of non-depolarizing neuromuscular blocking agents: 0.025-0.08 mg/kg/dose slow IV, preceded by either atropine (0.4 mg for each mg of neostigmine) or glycopyrrolate (0.2 mg for each mg of neostigmine).

FORMS - Trade only: Tabs 15 mg.
NOTES - Oral route preferred when possible.
pyridostigmine (Mestinon, Mestinon Timespan, Regonal) ▶Plasma, K ♀C ▶+ $$
ADULT - Myasthenia gravis, standard release tabs: Start 60 mg PO tid; gradually increase to usual therapeutic dose of 200 mg PO tid. Extended release tabs: Start 180 mg PO daily or divided bid. Max 1,500 mg/day. May give 2 mg IM or slow IV injection q2-3h.
PEDS - Not approved in children.

UNAPPROVED PEDS - Myasthenia gravis, neonates: 5 mg PO q4-6h or 0.05- 0.15 mg/kg IM/IV q4-6h. Myasthenia gravis, children: 7 mg/kg/day PO in 5-6 divided doses, or 0.05-0.15 mg/kg/dose IM/IV q4-6h. Max 10 mg IM/IV single dose.
FORMS - Generic/Trade: Tabs 60 mg. Trade only: Extended release tabs 180 mg. Syrup 60 mg/5 mL.
NOTES - Give injection at 1/30th of oral dose when oral therapy is not possible.

NEUROLOGY: Parkinsonian Agents – Anticholinergics

benztropine mesylate (Cogentin) ▶LK ♀C ▶? $
ADULT - Parkinsonism: Start 0.5-2 mg/day PO/IM/IV. Increase in 0.5 mg increments at weekly intervals to max 6 mg/day. May divide doses daily-qid. Drug-induced extrapyramidal disorders: 1-4 mg PO/IM/IV given once daily or divided bid.
PEDS - Not approved in children.
UNAPPROVED PEDS - Parkinsonism (>3 yo): 0.02-0.05 mg/kg/dose given once daily or divided bid. Use caution; potential for undesired anticholinergic effects.
FORMS - Generic only: Tabs 0.5, 1, 2 mg.
NOTES - Contraindicated in narrow-angle glaucoma. Anticholinergic side effects are enhanced in the elderly, and may worsen cognition or cause delirium. Avoid concomitant donepezil, rivastigmine, galantamine, or tacrine.
biperiden (Akineton) ▶LK ♀C ▶? $$$
ADULT - Parkinsonism: 2 mg PO tid-qid. Titrate to max 16 mg/day. Drug-induced extrapyramidal disorders: 2 mg PO daily-tid to max 8 mg/24 hours.
PEDS - Not approved in children.
FORMS - Trade only: Tabs 2 mg
NOTES - Contraindicated in narrow-angle glaucoma, bowel obstruction, and megacolon.
procyclidine (Kemadrin, ♣Procyclid) ▶LK ♀C ▶? $$$
ADULT - Parkinsonism: Start 2.5-5 mg PO tid; may add qhs dose. Usual max 20 mg/day. Drug-induced extrapyramidal side effects: 2.5-5 mg PO tid.
PEDS - Not approved in children.
FORMS - Trade only: Tabs 5 mg.
NOTES - Contraindicated in narrow-angle glaucoma.
trihexyphenidyl (Artane) ▶LK ♀C ▶? $
ADULT - Parkinsonism: 1 mg PO daily. Increase by 2 mg/day at 3-5 day intervals to usual therapeutic dose of 6-10 mg/day divided tid with meals. Max 15 mg/day.
PEDS - Not approved in children.
FORMS - Generic only: Tabs 2, 5 mg. Elixir 2 mg/5 mL.

NEUROLOGY: Parkinsonian Agents – COMT Inhibitors

entacapone (Comtan) ▶L ♀C ▶? $$$$$
ADULT - Parkinson's disease, adjunctive: Start 200 mg PO with each dose of carbidopa/levodopa. Max 8 tabs (1,600 mg)/day.
PEDS - Not approved in children.
FORMS - Trade only: Tabs 200 mg.

NOTES - Adjunct to end-of-dose "wearing off" with carbidopa/levodopa; has no antiparkinsonian effect on its own. Avoid concomitant non-selective MAOIs. Use caution in hepatobiliary dysfunction. Avoid rapid withdrawal, which may precipitate neuroleptic malignant syndrome.

NEUROLOGY: Parkinsonian Agents – Dopaminergic Agents & Combinations

NOTE: May cause hallucinations, particularly when used in combination. They have also been associated with the development of impulse control disorders such as compulsive gambling, hypersexuality, and hyperphagia. Avoid rapid discontinuation, which may precipitate neuroleptic malignant syndrome.

apomorphine (Apokyn) ▶L ♀C ▶? $$$$$
WARNING - Never administer IV due to risk of severe adverse effects including pulmonary embolism.
ADULT - Acute, intermittent treatment of hypomobility ("off episodes") in Parkinson's disease: Start 0.2 mL SC test dose in the presence of medical personnel. May increase dose by 0.1 mL every few days as tolerated. Max 0.6 mL/dose or 2 mL/day. Monitor for orthostatic hypotension after initial dose and with dose escalation. Potent emetic - pretreat with trimethobenzamide 300 mg PO tid (or domperidone 20 mg PO tid) starting three days prior to use, and continue for ≥2 months before weaning.
PEDS - Not approved in children.
FORMS - Trade: Cartridges (for injector pen, 10 mg/mL) 3 mL. Ampules (10 mg/mL) 2 mL.
NOTES - Write doses exclusively in mL rather than mg to avoid errors. Most effective when administered at (or just prior to) the onset of an "off" episode. Avoid concomitant use of 5HT3 antagonists (eg, ondansetron, granisetron, dolasetron, palonosetron, alosetron), which can precipitate severe hypotension and loss of consciousness. Inform patients that the dosing pen is labeled in mL (not mg), and that it is possible to dial in a dose of medication even if the cartridge does not contain sufficient drug. Rotate injection sites. Restart at 0.2 mL/day if treatment is interrupted for ≥1 week. Adjust dosing in hepatic impairment. Reduce starting dose to 0.1 mL in patients with mild or moderate renal failure. Contains sulfites.

carbidopa (Lodosyn) ▶LK ♀C ▶? $$$
ADULT - Parkinson's Disease, adjunct to carbidopa/levodopa: start 25 mg PO daily with first daily dose of carbidopa/levodopa. May give an additional 12.5-25 mg with each dose of carbidopa/levodopa as needed. Max 200 mg/day.
PEDS - Not approved in children.
FORMS - Trade only: Tabs 25 mg.
NOTES - Adjunct to carbidopa/levodopa to reduce peripheral side-effects such as nausea. Also increases the CNS availability of levodopa. Monitor for CNS side-effects such as dyskinesias and hallucinations when initiating therapy, and reduce levodopa dose as necessary.

carbidopa-levodopa (Sinemet, Sinemet CR, Parcopa) ▶L ♀C ▶- $$$$
ADULT - Parkinsonism: Standard release and orally disintegrating tablet: start 1 tab (25/100 mg) PO tid. Increase by 1 tab/day q 1-2 days prn. Use 1 tab (25/250 mg) PO tid-qid when higher levodopa doses are needed. Sustained release: Start 1 tab (50/200 mg) PO bid; separate doses by ≥4 hrs. Increase as needed at intervals ≥3 days. Typical max dose is 1,600-2,000 mg/day of levodopa, but higher doses have been used.
PEDS - Not approved in children.
UNAPPROVED ADULT - Restless legs syndrome: start 1/2 tab (25/100 mg) PO qhs; increase q3-4d to max 50/200 mg (two 25/100 tabs) qhs. If symptoms recur during the night, then a combination of standard release (25/100 mg, 1-2 tabs qhs) and sustained release (25/100 or 50/200 mg qhs) tablets may be used.
FORMS - Generic/Trade: Tabs (carbidopa/levodopa) 10/100, 25/100, 25/250 mg. Tabs, sustained release (Sinemet CR, carbidopa-levodopa ER) 25/100, 50/200 mg. Trade only: orally disintegrating tablet (Parcopa) 10/100, 25/100, 25/250.
NOTES - Motor fluctuations and dyskinesias may occur. The 25/100 mg tablets are preferred as initial therapy, since most patients require at least 70-100 mg/day of carbidopa to reduce the risk of N/V. The 10/100 mg tabs have limited clinical utility. Extended-release formulations have a lower bioavailability than conventional preparations. Do not use within two weeks of a nonselective MAOI. When used for restless legs syndrome, may precipitate rebound (recurrence of symptoms during the night) or augmentation (earlier daily onset of symptoms). Orally disintegrating tablet is placed on top of the tongue and does not require water or swallowing, but is absorbed through the GI tract (not sublingually). Use caution in patients with undiagnosed skin lesions or a history of melanoma.

pramipexole (Mirapex) ▶K ♀C ▶? $$$$$
ADULT - Parkinson's disease: Start 0.125 mg PO tid x 1 week, then 0.25 mg x 1 week; after that, increase by 0.75 mg/week divided tid. Usual effective dose is 0.5-1.5 mg PO tid. Restless legs syndrome: Start 0.125 mg PO 2-3 hrs prior to bedtime. May increase q4-7 days to 0.25 mg then 0.5 mg if needed.
PEDS - Not approved in children.
FORMS - Trade only: Tabs 0.125, 0.25, 0.5, 1, 1.5 mg.
NOTES - Decrease dose in renal impairment. Sleep attacks, syncope, and/or orthostatic hypotension may occur. Titrate slowly.

ropinirole (Requip) ▶L ♀C ▶? $$$$
ADULT - Parkinson's disease: Start 0.25 mg PO

tid. Increase by 0.25 mg/dose at weekly intervals to 1 mg PO tid. Max 24 mg/day. Restless legs syndrome: Start 0.25 mg PO 1-3 hr before sleep for 2 days, then increase to 0.5 mg/day on days 3-7. Increase by 0.5 mg/d at weekly intervals prn to max 4 mg/d given 1-3 hours before sleep.

PEDS - Not approved in children.

FORMS - Trade only: Tabs 0.25, 0.5, 1, 2, 3, 4, 5 mg.

NOTES - Sleep attacks, impulse control disorders, syncope, and/or orthostatic hypotension may occur. Titrate slowly.

rotigotine (Neupro) ▶L ♀C ▶? $$$$$
ADULT - Parkinson's disease: Start 2 mg/24 hours patch daily x 1 week, then increase to lowest effective dose of 4 mg/24 hours. May increase prn in ≥1 week to max 6 mg/24 hours.

PEDS - Not approved in children.

FORMS - Trade only: Transdermal patch 2, 4, 6 mg/24 hours.

NOTES - Contains sulfites. Remove prior to MRI or cardioversion to avoid burns. Apply to clean, dry, intact skin of the abdomen, thigh, flank, shoulder, or upper arm, and hold in place for 20-30 seconds. Rotate application sites daily, and wash skin after removal. Taper by 2 mg/24 hours every other day when discontinuing.

***Stalevo* (carbidopa + levodopa + entacapone)** ▶L ♀C ▶- $$$$$
ADULT - Parkinson's disease (conversion from carbidopa-levodopa +/- entacapone): Start Stalevo tablet that contains the same amount of carbidopa-levodopa as the patient was previously taking, and titrate to desired response. May need to lower the dose of levodopa in patients not already taking entacapone. Max 1,600 mg/day of entacapone or 1,600-2,000 mg/day of levodopa.

PEDS - Not approved in children.

FORMS - Trade only: Tabs (carbidopa/levodopa /entacapone): Stalevo 50 (12.5/50/200 mg), Stalevo 100 (25/100/200 mg), Stalevo 150 (37.5/150/200 mg).

NOTES – If not currently taking entacapone, consider titrating individual components before conversion to this fixed-dose preparation. Avoid concomitant use of non-selective MAOIs. Use caution in hepatobiliary dysfunction. Motor fluctuations and dyskinesias may occur. Should not be used in patients with undiagnosed skin lesions or a history of melanoma.

NEUROLOGY: Parkinsonian Agents – Monoamine Oxidase Inhibitors (MAOIs)

rasagiline (Azilect) ▶L ♀C ▶? $$$$$
ADULT - Parkinson's disease, monotherapy: 1 mg PO qam. Parkinson's disease, adjunctive: 0.5 mg PO qam. Max 1 mg/day.

PEDS - Not approved in children.

FORMS - Trade only: Tabs 0.5, 1 mg.

NOTES - Requires an MAOI diet. Contraindicated (risk of hypertensive crisis) with meperidine, methadone, tramadol, propoxyphene, dextromethorphan, sympathomimetic amines (eg, pseudoephedrine, phenylephrine, ephedrine), antidepressants, other MAOIs, cyclobenzaprine, and general anesthesia. Discontinue ≥14 days before liberalizing diet, starting one of these medications, or proceeding with elective surgery that requires general anesthesia. May need to reduce levodopa dose when used in combination. Reduce dose to 0.5 mg when used with CYP1A2 inhibitors (eg, ciprofloxacin) and in mild hepatic impairment. Do not use in moderate or severe liver disease.

selegiline (Eldepryl, Zelapar) ▶LK ♀C ▶? $$$$
ADULT - Parkinsonism (adjunct to levodopa): 5 mg PO q am and q noon; max 10 mg/day. Zelapar ODT: Start 1.25 mg SL q am for >6 weeks, then increase prn to max 2.5 mg q am.

PEDS - Not approved in children.

UNAPPROVED ADULT - Parkinsonism (monotherapy): 5 mg PO q am and q noon; max 10 mg/day.

FORMS - Generic/Trade: Caps 5 mg. Tabs 5 mg. Trade only (Zelapar): Oral disintegrating tabs (ODT) 1.25 mg.

NOTES – Don't use with meperidine or other opioids. Risk of non-selective MAO inhibition at high doses. Zelapar should be taken in the morning before food and without water.

NEUROLOGY: Other

betahistine (✤Serc) ▶LK ♀? ▶? $
ADULT - Canada only. Vertigo of Meniere's disease: 8-16 mg PO tid.

PEDS - Not approved in children.

FORMS - Trade only: Tabs 8, 16 mg.

NOTES - Contraindicated in peptic ulcer disease and pheochromocytoma; use caution in asthmatics.

botulinum toxin type A (Botox, Botox Cosmetic) ▶Not absorbed ♀C ▶? $$$$$

ADULT - Moderate to severe glabellar lines, ≤65 yo: inject 0.1 mL into each of 5 sites. Blepharospasm: 1.25-5 units IM into each of several sites in the orbicularis oculi of upper and lower lids q 3 months; use lower doses at initial visit. Strabismus: 1.25-5.0 units depending on diagnosis, injected into extraocular muscles. Cervical dystonia: 15-100 units IM (with or without EMG guidance) into affected muscles q 3 months (e.g., splenius capitis/cervicis, sternocleidomastoid, levator scapulae, trapezius, semispinalis, scalene, longissimus); usual total dose is 200-300 units/treatment. Primary axillary hyperhidrosis: 50 units/axilla intradermally, divided over 10-15 sites.

PEDS - Not approved in children <12 yo (for blepharospasm), <16 yo (for cervical dystonia), or <18 yo (for hyperhidrosis).

UNAPPROVED ADULT - Hemifacial spasm: 1.25-2.5 units IM into affected muscles q 3-4 months (e.g., corrugator, orbicularis oculi, zygomaticus major, buccinator, depressor anguli oris, platysma); usual total dose is 10-34 units/treatment.

FORMS - Trade only: 100 unit single-use vials.

NOTES - Clinical benefit occurs in ≤2 weeks (2-3 days for facial injections), peaks at 1-6 weeks, and wears off in about 3 months. Contraindicated in peripheral motor neuropathic disease (e.g., ALS, motor neuropathy) or neuromuscular junction disease (e.g., myasthenia gravis, Lambert-Eaton syndrome). The use of lower doses and longer dosing intervals may decrease the risk of neutralizing antibodies. Increased risk of dysphagia when >100 units are injected into the sternocleidomastoid or with bilateral sternocleidomastoid injections.

botulinum toxin type B (Myobloc) ▶Not significantly absorbed ♀+ ▶? $$$$$

ADULT - Cervical dystonia: Start 2,500-5,000 units IM in affected muscles. Use lower initial dose if no prior history of botulinum toxin therapy. Benefits usually last for 12-16 weeks when a total dose of 5,000-10,000 units has been administered. Titrate to effective dose. Give treatments ≥3 months apart to decrease the risk of producing neutralizing antibodies.

PEDS - Not approved in children.

NOTES - Low systemic concentrations are expected with IM injection; monitor closely for dysphagia. Caution in peripheral motor neuropathic disease (eg, ALS, motor neuropathy) or neuromuscular junction disease (eg, myasthenia gravis, Lambert-Eaton syndrome due to an increased risk of systemic effects) and with other drugs that block neuromuscular function (eg, aminoglycosides, curare-like compounds).

mannitol (Osmitrol, Resectisol) ▶K ♀C ▶? $$

ADULT - Intracranial HTN: 0.25-2 g/kg IV over 30-60 minutes as a 15, 20, or 25% solution.

PEDS - Not approved in children.

UNAPPROVED ADULT - Increased ICP/Head trauma: 0.25-1 g/kg IV push over 20 minutes. Repeat q4-6h prn.

UNAPPROVED PEDS - Increased ICP/Cerebral edema: 0.25-1 g/kg/dose IV push over 20-30 minutes, then 0.25-0.5 g/kg/dose IV q4-6h prn.

NOTES - Monitor fluid and electrolyte balance and cardiac function. Filter IV solutions with concentrations ≥20%; crystals may be present.

nimodipine (Nimotop) ▶L ♀C ▶- $$$$$

ADULT - Subarachnoid hemorrhage: 60 mg PO q4h for 21 days.

PEDS - Not approved in children.

FORMS - Generic/Trade: Caps 30 mg.

NOTES - Begin therapy within 96 hours. Give 1 hour before or 2 hours after meals. May give cap contents SL or via NG tube. Reduce dose in hepatic dysfunction.

oxybate (Xyrem, GHB, gamma hydroxybutyrate) ▶L ♀B ▶? ©III $$$$$

WARNING - CNS depressant with abuse potential; avoid concurrent alcohol or sedative use.

ADULT - Narcolepsy-associated cataplexy or excessive daytime sleepiness: 2.25 g PO qhs. Repeat in 2.5-4 hours. May increase by 1.5 g/day at >2 week intervals to max 9 g/day. Dilute each dose in 60 mL water.

PEDS - Not approved in children.

FORMS - Trade only: Solution 180 mL (500 mg/mL) supplied with measuring device and child-proof dosing cups.

NOTES - Available only through the Xyrem Success Program centralized pharmacy (1-866-997-3688). Adjust dose in hepatic dysfunction. Prepare doses just prior to bedtime, and use within 24 hours. May need an alarm to signal second dose.

riluzole (Rilutek) ▶LK ♀C ▶- $$$$$

ADULT - Amyotrophic lateral sclerosis: 50 mg PO q12h.

PEDS - Not approved in children.
FORMS - Trade only: Tabs 50 mg.
NOTES - Take 1 hour before or 2 hours after meals. Monitor LFTs.

tetrabenazine (✸*Nitoman*) ▶L ♀? ▶- $$$$
WARNING - Contraindicated if history of depression or suicidality; monitor closely and discontinue at the first signs thereof.
ADULT - Hyperkinetic movement disorders (Canada only): Start 12.5 mg PO bid-tid. May increase by 12.5 mg/day q3-5 days to usual dose of 25 mg PO tid. Max 200 mg/day, but most patients do not tolerate more than 75 mg/day. Discontinue if there is no benefit after 7 days of treatment at max tolerated dose.

PEDS - Not approved in children.
UNAPPROVED PEDS - Limited data suggest that ½ of the adult dose may be used and titrated as tolerated.
FORMS - Trade only: Tabs 25 mg.
NOTES - Used for the treatment of Huntington's chorea, hemiballismus, senile chorea, tic disorders (including Tourette's syndrome), and tardive dyskinesia. May cause or exacerbate parkinsonism, depression, and/or suicidality. Contraindicated in Parkinson's disease or depression. Don't use with MAOIs; use caution when used with antipsychotics and other dopamine receptor blocking agents. May attenuate the effects of levodopa and antidepressants.

OB/GYN: Contraceptives – Other (Oral Contraceptives on page 252)

etonogestrel (*Implanon*) ▶L ♀X ▶+ $$$$$
WARNING - Increased risk of thromboembolism & stroke. Effectiveness may be reduced by hepatic enzyme-inducing drugs such as certain anticonvulsants, barbiturates, griseofulvin, rifampin. Additionally, products that contain St John's wort may decrease efficacy; an additional form of birth control may be advisable.
ADULT - Contraception: 1 subdermal implant every three years.
PEDS - Not approved in children.
FORMS - Trade only: Single rod implant, 68 mg.
NOTES - Not studied in women >130% of ideal body weight; may be less effective in them.

levonorgestrel (*Plan B*) ▶L ♀X ▶- $$
ADULT - Emergency contraception: 1 tab PO ASAP but within 72h of intercourse. 2nd tab 12h later.
PEDS - Not approved in children.
UNAPPROVED ADULT - 2 tabs (1.5 mg) PO ASAP but within 72h of intercourse (lesser efficacy at up to 120 hours).
FORMS - OTC: Trade only: Kit contains 2 tabs 0.75 mg.
NOTES - OTC if ≥ 18 yo; Rx if younger. Nausea uncommon, however, if vomiting occurs within 1h, initial dose must be given again. Consider adding an antiemetic. Patients should be instructed to then contact their healthcare providers. Can be used at any time during the menstrual cycle.

NuvaRing (ethyl estradiol vaginal ring + etonogestrel) ▶L ♀X ▶- $$
WARNING - Not recommended in women >35 yo who smoke. Increased risk of thromboem-

bolism, stroke, MI, hepatic neoplasia & gallbladder disease. Vaginitis, headache, nausea & weight gain are common side effects. Effectiveness is reduced by hepatic enzyme-inducing drugs such as certain anticonvulsants and barbiturates, rifampin, rifabutin, griseofulvin & protease inhibitors. Additionally, products that contain St John's wort may decrease efficacy; consider an additional form of birth control.
ADULT - Contraception: 1 ring intravaginally x 3 weeks each month.
PEDS - Not approved in children.
FORMS - Trade only: Flexible intravaginal ring, 15 mcg ethinyl estradiol/0.120 mg etonogestrel/day. 1 and 3 rings/box.
NOTES - Insert on day 5 of cycle or within 7 days of the last oral contraceptive pill. The ring must remain in place continuously for 3 weeks, including during intercourse. Remove for 1 week, then insert a new ring. May be used continuously for 4 weeks & replaced immediately to skip a withdrawal week. Store at room temperature. In case of accidental removal, reinsert ASAP after rinsing with cool to lukewarm water. If removal >3 hours, use back up method until ring in place for ≥7 days.

Ortho Evra (norelgestromin + ethyl estradiol transdermal, ✸*Evra*) ▶L ♀X ▶- $$$
WARNING - Average estrogen concentration 60% higher than common oral contraceptives (ie, 35 mcg ethinyl estradiol), which may further increase the risk of thromboembolism. Not recommended in women >35 yo who smoke. Increased risk of thromboembolism, stroke, MI, hepatic neoplasia & gallbladder disease. Nau-

ORAL CONTRACEPTIVES* ▶L ♀X **Monophasic**	Estrogen (mcg)	Progestin (mg)
Norinyl 1+50, Ortho-Novum 1/50, Necon 1/50	50 mestranol	1 norethindrone
Ovcon-50		
Demulen 1/50, Zovia 1/50E	50 ethinyl estradiol	1 ethynodiol
Ovral, Ogestrel		0.5 norgestrel
Norinyl 1+35, Ortho-Novum 1/35, Necon 1/35, Nortrel 1/35	35 ethinyl estradiol	1 norethindrone
Brevicon, Modicon, Necon 0.5/35, Nortrel 0.5/35		0.5 norethindrone
Ovcon-35, Femcon Fe		0.4 norethindrone
Previfem		0.18 norgestimate
Ortho-Cyclen, MonoNessa, Sprintec-28		0.25 norgestimate
Demulen 1/35, Zovia 1/35E, Kelnor 1/35		1 ethynodiol
Loestrin 21 1.5/30, Loestrin Fe 1.5/30, Junel 1.5/30, Junel 1.5/30 Fe, Microgestin Fe 1.5/30	30 ethinyl estradiol	1.5 norethindrone
Cryselle, Lo/Ovral, Low-Ogestrel		0.3 norgestrel
Apri, Desogen, Ortho-Cept, Reclipsen		0.15 desogestrel
Levlen, Levora, Nordette, Portia, Seasonale, Seasonique†, Quasense		0.15 levonorgestrel
Yasmin		3 drospirenone
Loestrin 21 1/20, Loestrin Fe 1/20, Loestin 24 Fe, Junel 1/20, Junel Fe 1/20, Microgestin Fe 1/20	20 ethinyl estradiol	1 norethindrone
Alesse, Aviane, Lessina, Levlite, Lutera		0.1 levonorgestrel
Lybrel		0.09 levonorgestrel
Yaz		3 drospirenone
Progestin-only		
Micronor, Nor-Q.D., Camila, Errin, Jolivette, Nora-BE	none	0.35 norethindrone
Ovrette		0.075 norgestrel
Biphasic (estrogen & progestin contents vary)		
Kariva, Mircette	20/10 eth estra	0.15/0 desogestrel
Ortho Novum 10/11, Necon 10/11	35 eth estradio	0.5/1 norethindrone
Triphasic (estrogen & progestin contents vary)		
Cyclessa, Velivet	25 ethinyl estradiol	0.100/0.125/0.150 desogestrel
Ortho-Novum 7/7/7, Necon 7/7/7, Nortrel 7/7/7	35 ethinyl estradiol	0.5/0.75/1 norethindr
Tri-Norinyl, Leena		0.5/1/0.5 norethindr
Enpresse, Tri-Levlen, Triphasil, Trivora-28	30/40/30 eth estradiol	0.5/0.75/0.125 levonorgestrel
Ortho Tri-Cyclen, Trinessa, Tri-Sprintec, Tri-Previfem	35 eth estrad	0.18/0.215/0.25 norgestimate
Ortho Tri-Cyclen Lo	25 eth estrad	
Estrostep Fe	20/30/35 e.e.	1 norethindrone

***All**: Not recommended in smokers. Increase risk of thromboembolism, stroke, MI, hepatic neoplasia & gallbladder disease. Nausea, breast tenderness, & breakthrough bleeding are common transient side effects. Effectiveness reduced by hepatic enzyme-inducing drugs such as certain anticonvulsants and barbiturates, rifampin, rifabutin, griseofulvin, & protease inhibitors. Coadministration with St. John's wort may decrease efficacy. Vomiting or diarrhea may also increase the risk of contraceptive failure. Consider an additional form of birth control in above circumstances. See product insert for instructions on missing doses. Most available in 21 and 28 day packs. **Progestin only**: Must be taken at the same time every day. Because much of the literature regarding OC adverse effects pertains mainly to estrogen/progestin combinations, the extent to which progestin-only contraceptives cause these effects is unclear. No significant interaction has been found with broad-spectrum antibiotics. The effect of St. John's wort is unclear. No placebo days, start new pack immediately after finishing current one. Available in 28 day packs. Readers may find the following website useful: www.managingcontraception.com. †84 light blue-green active pills followed by 7 yellow pills w/ 10 mcg ethinyl estradiol.

sea, breast tenderness, & breakthrough bleeding are common transient side effects. Effectiveness is reduced by hepatic enzyme-inducing drugs such as certain anticonvulsants and barbiturates, rifampin, rifabutin, griseofulvin & protease inhibitors. Additionally, products that contain St John's wort may decrease efficacy; consider additional birth control.
ADULT - Contraception: 1 patch q week x 3 weeks, then 1 week patch-free.

PEDS - Not approved in children.
FORMS - Trade only: Transdermal patch: 150 mcg norelgestromin + 20 mcg ethinyl estradiol/day. 1 and 3 patches/box.
NOTES - May be less effective in women ≥90 kg (198 lbs). Apply new patch on the same day each week. Do not exceed 7 days between patches. Rotate application sites, avoid the waistline. Do not use earlier than 4 weeks postpartum if not breastfeeding.

EMERGENCY CONTRACEPTION within 72 hours of unprotected sex: Take first dose ASAP, then identical dose 12h later. *Plan B* kit contains 2 levonorgestrel 0.75mg tabs. Each dose is 1 pill. The progestin-only method causes less nausea & may be more effective. Alternate regimens: Each dose is either 2 pills of *Ovral* or *Ogestrel*, 4 pills of *Cryselle, Levlen, Levora, Lo/Ovral, Nordette, Tri-Levlen*, Triphasil*, Trivora*,* or *Low Ogestrel,* or 5 pills of *Alesse, Aviane, Lessina,* or *Levlite.* If vomiting occurs within 1 hour of taking either dose of medication, consider whether or not to repeat that dose with an antiemetic 1h prior. More info at: www.not-2-late.com.

*Use 0.125 mg levonorgestrel/30 mcg ethinyl estradiol tabs.

OB/GYN: Estrogens (See also Hormone Combinations)

NOTE: Unopposed estrogens increase the risk of endometrial cancer in postmenopausal women. Malignancy should be ruled out in cases of persistent or recurrent abnormal vaginal bleeding. In women with an intact uterus, a progestin should be administered daily throughout the month or for the last 10-12 days of the month. Do not use during pregnancy. May increase the risk of DVT/ PE, gallbladder disease. Interactions with oral anticoagulants, certain anticonvulsants, rifampin, barbiturates, corticosteroids & St. John's wort. Estrogens should not be used in the prevention of cardiovascular disease. In the Women's Health Initiative, the use of conjugated estrogens (Premarin) caused an increase in the risk of CVA & PE. Additionally, the combination with medroxyprogesterone increased the risk of breast cancer and MI. Women >65 yo with 4 years of therapy had an increased risk of dementia. Estrogens should be prescribed at the lowest effective doses and for the shortest durations. Patients should be counseled regarding the risks/benefits.

esterified estrogens (*Menest*) ▸L ♀X ▸- $
ADULT - Moderate to severe menopausal vasomotor symptoms: 1.25 mg PO daily. Atrophic vaginitis: 0.3 to 1.25 mg PO daily. Female hypogonadism: 2.5 - 7.5 mg PO daily in divided doses for 20 days followed by a 10-day rest period. Repeat until bleeding occurs. Bilateral oophorectomy & ovarian failure: 1.25 mg PO daily. Prevention of postmenopausal osteoporosis: 0.3 - 1.25 mg PO daily.
PEDS - Not approved in children.
FORMS - Trade: Tabs 0.3, 0.625, 1.25, 2.5 mg.
NOTES - Typical hormone replacement regimen consists of a daily estrogen dose with a progestin added either daily or for the last 10-12 days of the cycle.

estradiol (*Estrace, Gynodiol*) ▸L ♀X ▸- $
ADULT - Moderate to severe menopausal vasomotor symptoms & atrophic vaginitis, female hypogonadism, bilateral oophorectomy & ovarian failure: 1-2 mg PO daily. Prevention of postmenopausal osteoporosis: 0.5 mg daily.
PEDS - Not approved in children.
FORMS - Generic/Trade: Tabs, micronized 0.5, 1, 2 mg, scored. Trade only: 1.5 mg (Gynodiol).
NOTES - Typical hormone replacement regimen consists of a daily estrogen dose with a progestin added either daily or for the last 10-12 days of the cycle.

estradiol acetate (*Femtrace*) ▸L ♀X ▸- $$
ADULT - Moderate to severe menopausal vasomotor symptoms: 0.45-1.8 mg PO daily.
PEDS - Not approved in children.
FORMS - Trade only: Tabs, 0.45, 0.9, 1.8 mg.
NOTES - Typical hormone replacement regimen consists of a daily estrogen dose with a progestin added either daily or for the last 10-12 days of the cycle.

estradiol acetate vaginal ring (*Femring*) ▸L ♀X ▸- $$

WARNING - A few cases of toxic shock syndrome have been reported.

ADULT - Menopausal atrophic vaginitis or vasomotor symptoms: insert ring into the vagina and replace after 90 days.

PEDS - Not approved in children.

FORMS - Trade: 0.05 mg/day and 0.1 mg/day.

NOTES - Should the ring fall out or be removed during the 90 day period, rinse in lukewarm water and re-insert.

estradiol cypionate (Depo-Estradiol) ▶L ♀X ▶- $

ADULT - Moderate to severe menopausal vasomotor symptoms: 1-5 mg IM q3-4 weeks. Female hypogonadism: 1.5-2 mg IM q month.

PEDS - Not approved in children.

estradiol gel (Divigel, Estrogel, Elestrin) ▶L ♀X ▶- $$$

ADULT - Moderate to severe menopausal vasomotor symptoms & atrophic vaginitis: Thinly apply contents of one complete pump depression to one entire arm, from wrist to shoulder (Estrogel) or upper arm (Elestrin) or contents of one foil packet to left or right upper thigh on alternating days. Allow to dry completely before dressing. Wash both hands after application.

PEDS - Not approved in children.

FORMS - Trade only: Gel 0.06% in non-aerosol, metered-dose pump with 64 1.25 g doses (Estrogel) & 100 0.87 g doses (Elestrin). Gel 0.1% in single dose foil packets of 0.25, 0.5 & 1.0 g, carton of 30.

NOTES - Depress the pump twice to prime. Concomitant sunscreen may increase absorption. Typical hormone replacement regimen consists of a daily estrogen dose with a progestin added either daily or for the last 10-12 days of the cycle.

estradiol topical emulsion (Estrasorb) ▶L ♀X ▶- $$

ADULT - Moderate to severe menopausal vasomotor symptoms: Apply entire contents of one pouch each to left and right legs (spread over thighs & calves) qam. Rub for 3 minutes until entirely absorbed. Allow to dry completely before dressing. Wash both hands after application. Daily dose = two 1.74 g pouches.

PEDS - Not approved in children.

FORMS - Trade only: Topical emulsion, 56 pouches/carton.

NOTES - Typical hormone replacement regimen consists of a daily estrogen dose with a progestin added either daily or for the last 10-12 days of the cycle. Concomitant sunscreen may

increase absorption.

estradiol transdermal patch (Alora, Climara, Esclim, Estraderm, FemPatch, Menostar, Vivelle, Vivelle Dot, ♥Estradot, Oesclim) ▶L ♀X ▶- $$

ADULT - Moderate to severe menopausal vasomotor symptoms & atrophic vaginitis, female hypogonadism, bilateral oophorectomy & ovarian failure: start with 0.025-0.05 mg/day patch once or twice weekly, depending on the product (see FORMS). Prevention of postmenopausal osteoporosis: 0.025-0.1 mg/day patch.

PEDS - Not approved in children.

FORMS - Generic/Trade: Transdermal patches doses in mg/day: Climara (q week) 0.025, 0.0375, 0.05, 0.06, 0.075, 0.1. Trade only: FemPatch (q week) 0.025. Esclim (twice/week) 0.025, 0.0375, 0.05, 0.075, 0.1. Vivelle, Vivelle Dot (twice/week) 0.025, 0.0375, 0.05, 0.075, 0.1. Estraderm (twice/week) 0.05, & 0.1. Alora (twice/week) 0.025, 0.05, 0.075, 0.1.

NOTES - Rotate application sites, avoid waistline. Transdermal may be preferable for women with high triglycerides/chronic liver disease.

estradiol transdermal spray (Evamist) ▶L ♀X ▶- ?

ADULT - Moderate to severe menopausal vasomotor symptoms: Initial: 1 spray daily to adjacent non-overlapping inner surface of the forearm. Allow to dry for 2 minutes and do not wash for 30 minutes. Adjust up to 3 sprays daily based on clinical response.

PEDS - Not approved in children.

FORMS - Trade: Spray: 1.53 mg estradiol/90 mcL spray, 56 sprays per metered-dose pump.

NOTES - Depress the pump three times with the cover on to prime each new applicator. Hold upright and vertical for spraying; rest the plastic cone against the skin. Typical hormone replacement regimen consists of a daily estrogen dose with a progestin added either daily or for the last 10-12 days of the cycle.

estradiol vaginal ring (Estring) ▶L ♀X ▶- $$

WARNING - Do not use during pregnancy.

ADULT - Menopausal atrophic vaginitis: insert ring into upper 1/3 of the vaginal vault and replace after 90 days.

PEDS - Not approved in children.

FORMS - Trade only: 2 mg ring single pack.

NOTES - Should the ring fall out or be removed during the 90 day period, rinse in lukewarm water and re-insert. Minimal systemic absorption, probable lower risk of adverse effects than systemic estrogens.

estradiol vaginal tab (Vagifem) ▶L ♀X ▶- $-
$$
WARNING - Do not use during pregnancy.
ADULT - Menopausal atrophic vaginitis: Begin
with 1 tab vaginally daily x 2 weeks, mainte-
nance 1 tab vaginally 2x/week.
PEDS - Not approved in children.
FORMS - Trade only: Vaginal tab: 25 mcg in
disposable single-use applicators, 8 & 18/pack.

estradiol valerate (Delestrogen) ▶L ♀X ▶- $
ADULT - Moderate to severe menopausal vaso-
motor symptoms & atrophic vaginitis: 10-20 mg
IM q4 weeks. Female hypogonadism, bilateral
oophorectomy & ovarian failure: 10-20 mg IM
q4 weeks.
PEDS - Not approved in children.

**estrogen vaginal cream (Premarin, Es-
trace)** ▶L ♀X ▶? $$$
ADULT - Menopausal atrophic vaginitis: Pre-
marin: 0.5-2 g intravaginally daily. Estrace: 2-4
g intravaginally daily for 1-2 weeks. Gradually
reduce to maintenance dose of 1 g 1-3 x/week.
PEDS - Not approved in children.
FORMS - Trade only: Vaginal cream. Premarin:
0.625 mg conjugated estrogens/g in 42.5 g
with or w/o calibrated applicator. Estrace: 0.1
mg estradiol/g in 42.5 g w/calibrated applicator.
NOTES - Possibility of absorption through the
vaginal mucosa. Uterine bleeding might be pro-
voked by excessive use in menopausal wom-
en. Breast tenderness & vaginal discharge due
to mucus hypersecretion may result from excessive estrogenic stimulation. Endometrial
bleeding may occur if use is discontinued.

**estrogens conjugated (Premarin, C.E.S.,
Congest)** ▶L ♀X ▶- $$
ADULT - Moderate to severe menopausal vaso-
motor symptoms, atrophic vaginitis, & urethri-
tis: 0.3-1.25 mg PO daily. Female hypogonad-
ism: 0.3-0.625 mg PO daily for 3 weeks with
one week off every month. Bilateral oophorec-
tomy & ovarian failure: 1.25 mg PO daily for 3
weeks with one week off every month. Preven-
tion of postmenopausal osteoporosis: 0.625
mg PO daily. Abnormal uterine bleeding: 25
mg IV/IM. Repeat in 6-12 hours if needed.
PEDS - Not approved in children.

UNAPPROVED ADULT - Prevention of post-
menopausal osteoporosis: 0.3 mg PO daily.
Normalizing bleeding time in patients with AV
malformations or underlying renal impairment:
30-70 mg IV/PO daily until bleeding time nor-
malized.
FORMS - Trade only: Tabs 0.3, 0.45, 0.625, 0.9,
1.25 mg.

**estrogens synthetic conjugated A (Cen-
estin)** ▶L ♀X ▶- $$
ADULT - Moderate to severe menopausal vaso-
motor symptoms: 0.3-1.25 mg PO daily.
PEDS - Not approved in children.
FORMS - Trade only: Tabs 0.3, 0.45, 0.625, 0.9,
1.25 mg.
NOTES - The difference between synthetic conjugated estrogens A and B is the additional
component of delta- 8,9-dehydroestrone sulfate in the B preparation. The clinical significance of this is unknown.

**estrogens synthetic conjugated B (Enju-
via)** ▶L ♀X ▶- $$
ADULT - Moderate to severe menopausal vaso-
motor symptoms: 0.3-1.25 mg PO daily.
PEDS - Not approved in children.
FORMS - Trade only: Tabs 0.3, 0.45, 0.625, 0.9,
1.25 mg.
NOTES - Typical hormone replacement regimen
consists of a daily estrogen dose with a pro-
gestin either daily or for the last 10-12 days of
the cycle. The difference between synthetic
conjugated estrogens A and B is the additional
component of delta- 8,9-dehydroestrone sul-
fate in the B preparation. The clinical signifi-
cance of this is unknown.

estropipate (Ogen, Ortho-Est) ▶L ♀X ▶- $
ADULT - Moderate to severe menopausal vaso-
motor symptoms, vulvar & vaginal atrophy:
0.75 to 6 mg PO daily. Female hypogonadism,
bilateral oophorectomy, or ovarian failure: 1.5-9
mg PO daily. Prevention of osteoporosis: 0.75
mg PO daily.
PEDS - Not approved in children.
FORMS - Generic/Trade: Tabs 0.75, 1.5, 3, 6
mg of estropipate.
NOTES - 6 mg estropipate = 5 mg sodium es-
trone sulfate.

OB/GYN: GnRH Agents

Anaphylaxis has occurred with GnRH agents.

cetrorelix acetate (Cetrotide) ▶Plasma ♀X ▶-
$$$$$

ADULT - Infertility: Multiple dose regimen: 0.25
mg SC daily during the early to mid follicular
phase. Continue treatment daily until the day of

hCG administration. Single dose regimen: 3 mg SC x 1 usually on stimulation day 7.

PEDS - Not approved in children.

FORMS - Trade only: Injection 0.25 mg in 1 & 7-dose kits. 3 mg in 1 dose kit.

NOTES - Best sites for SC self-injection are on the abdomen around the navel. Storage in original carton: 0.25 mg refrigerated (36-46F); 3 mg room temperature (77F). Contraindicated with severe renal impairment.

ganirelix (*Follistim-Antagon Kit*, ✚*Orgalutran*) ▶Plasma ♀X ▶? $$$$$

ADULT - Infertility: 250 mcg SC daily during the early to mid follicular phase. Continue treatment daily until the day of hCG administration.

PEDS - Not approved in children.

FORMS - Trade only: Injection 250 mcg/0.5 mL in pre-filled, disposable syringes with 3 vials follitropin beta.

NOTES - Best sites for SC self-injection are on the abdomen around the navel or upper thigh. Store at room temperature (77F) for up to 3 months. Protect from light. Packaging contains natural rubber latex which may cause allergic reactions.

nafarelin (*Synarel*) ▶L ♀X ▶- $$$$$

ADULT - Endometriosis: 200 mcg spray into one nostril q am & the other nostril q pm. May be increased to one 200 mcg spray into each nostril bid. Duration of treatment: 6 months.

PEDS - Central precocious puberty: 2 sprays into each nostril bid for a total of 1600 mcg/day. May be increased to 1800 mcg/day. Allow 30 seconds to elapse between sprays.

FORMS - Trade only: Nasal soln 2 mg/mL in 8 mL bottle (200 mcg per spray) about 80 sprays/bottle.

NOTES - Ovarian cysts have occurred in the first 2 months of therapy. Symptoms of hypoestrogenism may occur. Elevations of phosphorus & eosinophil counts, and decreases in calcium & WBC counts have been documented. Consider norethindrone as "addback" therapy to decrease bone loss (see norethindrone).

OB/GYN: Hormone Combinations

NOTE: See also estrogens. Unopposed estrogens increase the risk of endometrial cancer in postmenopausal women. Malignancy should be ruled out in cases of persistent or recurrent abnormal vaginal bleeding. Do not use during pregnancy. May increase the risk of DVT/PE, gallbladder disease. Interactions with oral anticoagulants, phenytoin, rifampin, barbiturates, corticosteroids and St. John's wort. For preparations containing testosterone derivatives, observe women for signs of virilization and lipid abnormalities. In the Women's Health Initiative, the combination of conjugated estrogens and medroxyprogesterone (PremPro) caused an increase in the risk of breast cancer, MI, CVA, & DVT/PE and did not improve overall quality of life. Women >65 yo with 4 years of therapy had an increased risk of dementia. Estrogen/progestin combinations should be prescribed at the lowest effective doses and for the shortest durations. Patients should be counseled regarding the risks/benefits of hormone replacement.

Activella (estradiol + norethindrone) ▶L ♀X ▶- $$

ADULT - Moderate to severe menopausal vasomotor symptoms, vulvar & vaginal atrophy, prevention of postmenopausal osteoporosis: 1 tab PO daily.

PEDS - Not approved in children.

FORMS - Trade only: Tab 1/0.5 mg and 0.5/0.1 mg estradiol/norethindrone acetate in calendar dial pack dispenser.

Angeliq (estradiol + drospirenone) ▶L ♀X ▶- $$$

ADULT - Moderate to severe menopausal vasomotor symptoms, vulvar & vaginal atrophy: 1 tab PO daily.

PEDS - Not approved in children.

FORMS - Trade only: Tabs 1 mg estradiol/0.5 mg drospirenone.

NOTES - May cause hyperkalemia in high-risk patients due to antimineralocorticoid activity of drospirenone. Monitor potassium in patients on ACEIs, ARBs, potassium-sparing diuretics, heparin, aldosterone antagonists, & NSAIDs. Should not be used if renal insufficiency, hepatic dysfunction or adrenal insufficiency.

Climara Pro (estradiol + levonorgestrel) ▶L ♀X ▶- $$

ADULT - Moderate to severe menopausal vasomotor symptoms, prevention of postmenopausal osteoporosis: 1 patch weekly.

PEDS - Not approved in children.

FORMS - Trade only: Transdermal 0.045/0.015 estradiol/levonorgestrel in mg/day, 4 patches/box.

NOTES - Rotate application sites; avoid the waistline.

CombiPatch (estradiol + norethindrone, ♥Estalis) ▶L ♀X ▶- $$

ADULT - Moderate to severe menopausal vasomotor symptoms, vulvar & vaginal atrophy, female hypogonadism, bilateral oophorectomy, & ovarian failure, prevention of postmenopausal osteoporosis: 1 patch twice weekly.

PEDS - Not approved in children.

FORMS - Trade only: Transdermal patch 0.05 estradiol/ 0.14 norethindrone & 0.05 estradiol/ 0.25 norethindrone in mg/day, 8 patches/box.

NOTES - Rotate application sites, avoid the waistline.

Estratest (esterified estrogens + methyltestosterone) ▶L ♀X ▶- $$$$

ADULT - Moderate to severe menopausal vasomotor symptoms: 1 tab PO daily.

PEDS - Not approved in children.

UNAPPROVED ADULT - Menopause-associated decrease in libido: 1 tab PO daily.

FORMS - Trade only: Tabs 1.25 mg esterified estrogens/2.5 mg methyltestosterone.

NOTES - Monitor LFTs and lipids.

Estratest H.S. (esterified estrogens + methyltestosterone) ▶L ♀X ▶- $$$

ADULT - Moderate to severe menopausal vasomotor symptoms: 1 tab PO daily.

PEDS - Not approved in children.

UNAPPROVED ADULT - Menopause-associated decrease in libido: 1 tab PO daily.

FORMS - Trade only: Tabs 0.625 mg esterified estrogens/1.25 mg methyltestosterone.

NOTES - HS = half-strength. Monitor LFTs and lipids.

FemHRT (ethinyl estradiol + norethindrone) ▶L ♀X ▶- $$

WARNING - Multiple strengths; see FORMS & write specific product on Rx.

ADULT - Moderate to severe menopausal vasomotor symptoms, prevention of postmenopausal osteoporosis: 1 tab PO daily.

PEDS - Not approved in children.

FORMS - Trade only: Tabs 5/1 and 2.5/0.5 mcg ethinyl estradiol/mg norethindrone, 28/blister card.

Prefest (estradiol + norgestimate) ▶L ♀X ▶- $$$

ADULT - Moderate to severe menopausal vasomotor symptoms, vulvar atrophy, atrophic vaginitis, prevention of postmenopausal osteoporosis: 1 pink tab PO daily x 3 days followed by 1 white tab PO daily x 3 days, sequentially

throughout the month.

PEDS - Not approved in children.

FORMS - Trade only: Tabs in 30-day blister packs 1 mg estradiol (15 pink) & 1 mg estadiol/0.09 mg norgestimate (15 white).

Premphase (estrogens conjugated + medroxyprogesterone) ▶L ♀X ▶- $$

ADULT - Moderate to severe menopausal vasomotor symptoms, vulvar/vaginal atrophy, & prevention of postmenopausal osteoporosis: 0.625 mg conjugated estrogens PO daily days 1-14 & 0.625 mg conjugated estrogens/5 mg medroxyprogesterone PO daily days 15-28.

PEDS - Not approved in children.

FORMS - Trade only: Tabs in 28-day EZ-Dial dispensers: 0.625 mg conjugated estrogens (14) & 0.625 mg/5 mg conjugated estrogens/ medroxyprogesterone (14).

Prempro (estrogens conjugated + medroxyprogesterone, ♥Premplus) ▶L ♀X ▶- $$

WARNING - Multiple strengths; see FORMS & write specific product on Rx.

ADULT - Moderate to severe menopausal vasomotor symptoms, vulvar/vaginal atrophy, & prevention of postmenopausal osteoporosis: 1 PO daily.

PEDS - Not approved in children.

FORMS - Trade only: Tabs in 28-day EZ-Dial dispensers: 0.625 mg/5 mg, 0.625 mg/2.5 mg, 0.45 mg/1.5 mg, or 0.3 mg/1.5 mg conjugated estrogens/medroxyprogesterone.

Syntest D.S. (esterified estrogens + methyltestosterone) ▶L ♀X ▶- $$

ADULT - Moderate to severe menopausal vasomotor symptoms: 1 tab PO daily.

PEDS - Not approved in children.

UNAPPROVED ADULT - Menopause-associated decrease in libido: 1 tab PO daily.

FORMS - Trade only: Tabs 1.25 mg esterified estrogens/2.5 mg methyltestosterone.

NOTES - Monitor LFTs and lipids. Same as Estratest.

Syntest H.S. (esterified estrogens + methyltestosterone) ▶L ♀X ▶- $$

ADULT - Moderate to severe menopausal vasomotor symptoms: 1 tab PO daily.

PEDS - Not approved in children.

UNAPPROVED ADULT - Menopause-associated decrease in libido: 1 tab PO daily.

FORMS - Trade only: Tabs 0.625 mg esterified estrogens/1.25 mg methyltestosterone.

NOTES - HS = half-strength. Monitor LFTs and lipids. Same as Estratest HS.

DRUGS GENERALLY ACCEPTED AS SAFE IN PREGNANCY (selected)

<u>Analgesics:</u> acetaminophen, codeine*, meperidine*, methadone*. <u>Antimicrobials:</u> penicillins, cephalosporins, erythromycins (not estolate), azithromycin, nystatin, clotrimazole, metronidazole**, nitrofurantoin***, *Nix*. Antivirals: acyclovir, valacyclovir, famciclovir. <u>CV:</u> labetalol, methyldopa, hydralazine. <u>Derm:</u> erythromycin, clindamycin, benzoyl peroxide. <u>Endo:</u> insulin, liothyronine, levothyroxine. <u>ENT:</u> chlorpheniramine, diphenhydramine, dimenhydrinate, dextromethorphan, guaifenesin, nasal steroids, nasal cromolyn. <u>GI:</u> trimethobenzamide, antacids*, simethicone, cimetidine, famotidine, ranitidine, nizatidine, psyllium, metoclopramide, bisacodyl, docusate, doxylamine, meclizine. <u>Heme:</u> Heparin, low molecular weight heparins. <u>Psych:</u> desipramine, doxepin. <u>Pulmonary:</u> short-acting inhaled beta-2 agonists, cromolyn, nedocromil, beclomethasone, budesonide, theophylline, prednisone**.
*Except if used long-term or in high does at term.   **Except 1st trimester.   ***Contraindicated at term and during labor and delivery.

APGAR SCORE				
	Heart rate	0. Absent	1. <100	2. >100
	Respirations	0. Absent	1. Slow/irreg	2. Good/crying
	Muscle tone	0. Limp	1. Some flexion	2. Active motion
	Reflex irritability	0. No response	1. Grimace	2. Cough/sneeze
	Color	0. Blue	1. Blue extremities	2. Pink

OB/GYN: Labor Induction / Cervical Ripening

NOTE: Fetal well-being should be documented prior to use.

dinoprostone *(PGE2, Prepidil, Cervidil, Prostin E2)* ▶Lung ♀C ▶? $$$$$
ADULT - Cervical ripening: Gel - one syringe via catheter placed into cervical canal below the internal os. May be repeated q6h to a max of 3 doses. Vaginal insert: place in posterior fornix. Evacuation of uterine contents after fetal death up to 28 weeks or termination of pregnancy 12-20th gestational week: 20 mg intravaginal suppository; repeat at 3-5 hour intervals until abortion occurs. Do not use for >2 days.
PEDS - Not approved in children.
FORMS - Trade only: Gel (Prepidil) 0.5 mg/3 g syringe. Vaginal insert (Cervidil) 10 mg. Vaginal suppository (Prostin E2) 20 mg.
NOTES - Patient should remain supine for 15-30 minutes after gel and 2 h after vaginal insert. For hospital use only. Monitor for uterine hyperstimulation & abnormal fetal heart rate. Caution with asthma or glaucoma. Contraindicated in prior C-section or major uterine surgery due to potential for uterine rupture.

oxytocin *(Pitocin)* ▶LK ♀? ▶- $
WARNING - Not approved for elective labor induction, although widely used.
ADULT - Induction/stimulation of labor: 10 units in 1000 mL NS, 1-2 milliunits/min IV as a continuous infusion (6-12 mL/hr). Increase in increments of 1-2 milliunits/min q30 minutes until a contraction pattern is established, up to a max of 20 milliunits/min. Postpartum bleeding: 10 units IM after delivery of the placenta. 10-40 units in 1000 mL NS IV infusion, infuse 20-40 milliunits/minute.
PEDS - Not approved in children.
UNAPPROVED ADULT - Augmentation of labor: 0.5-2 milliunits/min IV as a continuous infusion, increase by 1-2 milliunits/min q30 minutes until adequate pattern of labor to a max of 40 milliunits/min.
NOTES - Use a pump to accurately control the infusion and continuous fetal monitoring. Concurrent sympathomimetics may result in postpartum HTN. Anaphylaxis and severe water intoxication have occurred. Caution in patients undergoing a trial of labor after c-section.

OB/GYN: Ovulation Stimulants

NOTE: Potentially serious adverse effects include DVT/PE, ovarian hyperstimulation syndrome, adnexal torsion, ovarian enlargement & cysts, & febrile reactions.

choriogonadotropin alfa *(hCG, Ovidrel)* ▶L ♀X ▶? $$$
ADULT - Specialized dosing for ovulation induction.

PEDS - Not approved in children.

FORMS - Trade only: Powder for injection or, pre-filled syringe 250 mcg.

NOTES - Best site for SC self-injection is on the abdomen below the navel. Beware of multiple pregnancy & multiple adverse effects. Store in original package & protect from light. Use immediately after reconstitution.

chorionic gonadotropin (Clomid, Pregnyl, Profasi) ▶L ♀X ▶? $$

ADULT - Specialized dosing for ovulation induction.

PEDS - Not approved in children.

NOTES - Beware of multiple pregnancy & multiple adverse effects. For IM use only.

clomiphene (Clomid, Serophene) ▶L ♀D ▶? $$

ADULT - Specialized dosing for infertility.

PEDS - Not approved in children.

FORMS - Generic/Trade: Tabs 50 mg, scored.

NOTES - Beware of multiple pregnancy & multiple adverse effects.

follitropin alfa (FSH, Gonal-F, Gonal-F RFF Pen) ▶L ♀X ▶? $$$$$

ADULT - Specialized dosing for infertility.

PEDS - Not approved in children.

FORMS - Trade only: Powder for injection, 37.5 IU, 75 IU, & 150 IU FSH activity. 450 & 1200 IU multi-dose vial. Pre-filled, multiple-dose pen, 300 IU, 450 IU, & 900 IU FSH activity with single-use disposable needles.

NOTES - Best site for SC self-injection is on the abdomen below the navel. Beware of multiple gestation pregnancy & multiple adverse effects. Store in original package & protect from light. Use immediately after reconstitution. Pen may be stored at room temperature for up to 1 month or expiration, whichever is first.

follitropin beta (FSH, Follistim, Follistim AQ, ♣Puregon) ▶L ♀X ▶? $$$$$

ADULT - Specialized dosing for infertility.

PEDS - Not approved in children.

FORMS - Trade only: Powder for injection, 75 IU FSH activity. Cartridge, for use with the Follistim Pen, 150, 300, 600, 900 IU. Aqueous soln 75 & 150 IU FSH activity.

NOTES - Best site for SC self-injection is on the abdomen below the navel. Beware of multiple pregnancy & multiple adverse effects. Store in original package & protect from light. Use powder for injection immediately after reconstitution. Cartridge may be stored for up to 28 days. Store aqueous soln in refrigerator.

gonadotropins (menotropins, FSH and LH, Menopur, Pergonal, Repronex, ♣Propasi HP) ▶L ♀X ▶? $$$$$

ADULT - Specialized dosing for infertility.

PEDS - Not approved in children.

FORMS - Trade only: Powder or pellet for injection, 75 IU & 150 IU FSH/LH activity.

NOTES - Best site for SC self-injection is on the abdomen below the navel. Beware of multiple pregnancy & numerous adverse effects. Use immediately after reconstitution.

lutropin alfa (Luveris) ▶L ♀X ▶- $$$$$

ADULT - Specialized dosing for infertility.

PEDS - Not approved in children.

FORMS - Trade only: Powder for injection, 75 IU LH activity.

NOTES - For use with follitropin alfa. Best site for SC self-injection is on the abdomen below the navel. Protect from light. Use immediately after reconstitution.

urofollitropin (Bravelle, FSH, Fertinex) ▶L ♀X ▶? $$$$$

ADULT - Specialized dosing for infertility & polycystic ovary syndrome.

PEDS - Not approved in children.

FORMS - Trade: Powder or pellet for injection, 75 & 150 IU (FSH, Fertinex only) FSH activity.

NOTES - Best site for SC self-injection is on the abdomen below the navel. Beware of multiple pregnancy & numerous adverse effects. Use immediately after reconstitution.

OB/GYN: Progestins

NOTE: Do not use in pregnancy. DVT, PE, cerebrovascular disorders, & retinal thrombosis may occur. Effectiveness may be reduced by enzyme-inducing drugs such as certain anticonvulsants and barbiturates, rifampin, rifabutin, griseofulvin & protease inhibitors. The effects of St. John's wort on progestin only pills is currently unknown. In the Women's Health Initiative, the combination of conjugated estrogens and medroxyprogesterone caused a statistically significant increase in the risk of breast cancer, MI, CVA, & DVT/PE. Additionally, women >65 yo with 4 years of therapy had an increased risk of dementia. Estrogen/progestin combinations should be prescribed at the lowest effective doses and for the shortest durations. Patients should be counseled regarding the risks/benefits of hormones.

hydroxyprogesterone caproate ▶L ♀X ▶? $

ADULT - Amenorrhea, dysfunctional uterine bleeding, metrorrhagia: 375 mg IM. Production of secretory endometrium and desquamation: 125-250 mg IM on 10th day of the cycle, repeat q7days until suppression no longer desired.

PEDS - Not approved in children.

UNAPPROVED ADULT - Endometrial hyperplasia: 500 mg IM weekly. Prevention of preterm delivery in patients with a history of preterm birth: 250 mg IM weekly starting at 16-20 weeks gestation until 36 weeks or delivery.

medroxyprogesterone (Provera, Amen) ▶L ♀X ▶+ $

ADULT - Secondary amenorrhea: 5-10 mg PO daily x 5-10 days. Abnormal uterine bleeding: 5-10 mg PO daily x 5-10 days beginning on the 16th or 21st day of the cycle (after estrogen priming). Withdrawal bleeding usually occurs 3-7 days after therapy ends.

PEDS - Not approved in children.

UNAPPROVED ADULT - Add to estrogen therapy to prevent endometrial hyperplasia: 10 mg PO daily for 10-12 days of month, or 2.5-5 mg PO daily. Endometrial hyperplasia: 10-30 mg PO daily (long-term); 40-100 mg PO daily (short-term) or 500 mg IM twice/week.

FORMS - Generic/Trade: Tabs 2.5, 5, & 10 mg, scored.

NOTES - Breakthrough bleeding/spotting may occur. Amenorrhea usually after 6 months.

medroxyprogesterone (Depo-Provera, depo-subQ provera 104) ▶L ♀X ▶+ $$$

WARNING - Risk of significant bone loss (irreversible?) increases with duration of use. Use long-term use (>2 years) only if other methods of birth control are inadequate or symptoms of endometriosis return after discontinuation.

ADULT - Contraception/Endometriosis: 150 mg IM in deltoid or gluteus maximus or 104 mg SC in anterior thigh or abdomen q13 weeks. Also used for adjunctive therapy in endometrial & renal carcinoma.

PEDS - Not approved in children.

UNAPPROVED ADULT - Dysfunctional uterine bleeding: 150 mg IM in deltoid or gluteus maximus q13 weeks.

NOTES – May have breakthrough bleeding/spotting. Amenorrhea usually after 6 months. Weight gain common. To ensure non-pregnancy give injection only during the first 5 days after onset of a normal menstrual period or after a negative pregnancy test. May be given immediately post-pregnancy termination as well

as postpartum, including breastfeeding women. May be given as often as 11 weeks apart. If the time between injections is >14 weeks, exclude pregnancy before administering. Return to fertility can be variably delayed after last injection, with the median time to pregnancy being 10 months. Bone loss may occur with prolonged administration. Evaluate bone mineral density if considering retreatment for endometriosis.

megestrol (Megace, Megace ES) ▶L ♀D ▶? $$$$$

ADULT - AIDS anorexia: 800 mg (20 mL) suspension PO daily or 625 mg (5 mL) ES daily. Palliative treatment for advanced breast carcinoma: 40 mg (tabs) PO qid. Endometrial carcinoma: 40-320 mg/day (tabs) in divided doses.

PEDS - Not approved in children.

UNAPPROVED ADULT - Endometrial hyperplasia: 40-160 mg PO daily x 3-4 months. Cancer-associated anorexia/cachexia: 80-160 mg qid.

FORMS - Generic/Trade: Tabs 20 & 40 mg. Suspension 40 mg/mL in 240 mL. Trade only: Megace ES suspension 125 mg/mL (150 mL).

NOTES - In HIV-infected women, breakthrough bleeding/spotting may occur.

norethindrone (Aygestin, Micronor, Nor-Q.D., Camila, Errin, Jolivette, Nora-BE) ▶L ♀D/X ▶See notes $

ADULT - Contraception: 0.35 mg PO daily. Amenorrhea, abnormal uterine bleeding: 2.5-10 mg PO daily x 5-10 days during the second half of the menstrual cycle. Endometriosis: 5 mg PO daily x 2 weeks. Increase by 2.5 mg q 2 weeks to 15 mg/day.

PEDS - Not approved in children.

UNAPPROVED ADULT - "Addback" therapy with GnRH agonists (eg, leuprolide) to decrease bone loss: 5 mg PO daily.

FORMS - Generic/Trade: Tabs 5 mg, scored. Trade only: 0.35 mg tabs.

NOTES - Contraceptive doses felt compatible with breast feeding, but not higher doses.

progesterone gel (Crinone, Prochieve) ▶Plasma ♀- ▶? $$$

ADULT - Secondary amenorrhea: 45 mg (4%) intravaginally qod up to 6 doses. If no response, use 90 mg (8%) intravaginally qod up to 6 doses. Specialized dosing for infertility.

PEDS - Not approved in children.

FORMS - Trade only: 4%, 8% single-use, pre-filled applicators.

NOTES - An increase in dose from the 4% gel can only be accomplished using the 8% gel; doubling the volume of 4% does not increase absorption.

progesterone in oil ▶L ♀X ▶? $

WARNING - Contraindicated in peanut allergy since some products contain peanut oil.

ADULT - Amenorrhea, uterine bleeding: 5-10 mg IM daily for 6-8 days.

PEDS - Not approved in children.

NOTES - Discontinue with thrombotic disorders, sudden or partial loss of vision, proptosis, diplopia or migraine.

progesterone micronized (*Prometrium*) ▶L ♀B ▶+ $$

WARNING - Contraindicated in patients allergic to peanuts since caps contain peanut oil.

ADULT - Hormone therapy to prevent endome-trial hyperplasia: 200 mg PO qhs 10-12 days per month. Secondary amenorrhea: 400 mg PO qhs x 10 days.

PEDS - Not approved in children.

UNAPPROVED ADULT - Prevent endometrial hyperplasia: 100 mg qhs daily.

FORMS - Trade only: Caps 100 & 200 mg.

NOTES - Breast tenderness, dizziness, headache & abdominal cramping may occur.

progesterone vaginal insert (*Endometrin*) ▶Plasma ♀- ▶? ?

ADULT - Specialized dosing for infertility.

PEDS - Not approved in children.

FORMS - Trade only: 100 mg vaginal insert.

NOTES - Avoid with other vaginal products.

OB/GYN: Selective Estrogen Receptor Modulators

NOTE: Do not use during pregnancy.

raloxifene (*Evista*) ▶L ♀X ▶- $$$$

WARNING - May increase risk of stroke death.

ADULT - Postmenopausal osteoporosis prevention/treatment: 60 mg PO daily.

PEDS - Not approved in children.

UNAPPROVED ADULT - Breast cancer prevention: 60-120 mg PO daily.

FORMS - Trade only: Tabs 60 mg.

NOTES - Interactions with oral anticoagulants & cholestyramine. May increase risk of DVT/PE; stop 72h before and during prolonged immobilization. Does not decrease (and may increase) hot flashes. Leg cramps. Triglyceride levels may increase in women with prior estrogen-associated hypertriglyceridemia (>500 mg/dL).

tamoxifen (*Nolvadex, Soltamox, Tamone, ✿Tamofen*) ▶L ♀D ▶- $$$

WARNING - Uterine malignancies, stroke & pul-monary embolism, sometimes fatal. Visual disturbances, cataracts, hypercalcemia, increased LFTs, bone pain, fertility impairment, hot flashes, menstrual irregularities, endometrial hyperplasia & cancer, alopecia.

ADULT - Breast cancer prevention in high-risk women: 20 mg PO daily x 5 years. Breast cancer: 10-20 mg PO bid x 5 years.

PEDS - Not approved in children.

UNAPPROVED ADULT - Mastalgia: 10 mg PO daily x 4 months. Anovulation: 5-40 mg PO bid x 4 days.

FORMS - Generic/Trade: Tabs 10 & 20 mg, Trade only (Soltamox): sugar-free soln 10 mg/5mL (150 mL).

NOTES - Reliable contraception recommended. Monitor CBCs, LFTs. Regular gynecologic & ophthalmologic examinations. Interacts with warfarin. Does not decrease hot flashes.

OB/GYN: Uterotonics

carboprost (*Hemabate, 15-methyl-prosta-glandin F2 alpha*) ▶LK ♀C ▶? $$$

ADULT - Refractory postpartum uterine bleeding: 250 mcg deep IM. If necessary, may repeat at 15-90 minute intervals up to a total dose of 2 mg (8 doses).

PEDS - Not approved in children.

NOTES - Caution with asthma. Transient fever, HTN, nausea, bronchoconstriction & flushing. May augment oxytocics.

methylergonovine (*Methergine*) ▶LK ♀C ▶? $

ADULT - To increase uterine contractions & de-crease postpartum bleeding: 0.2 mg IM after delivery of the placenta, delivery of the anterior shoulder, or during the puerperium. Repeat q2-4h prn. 0.2 mg PO tid-qid in the puerperium for a max of 1 week.

PEDS - Not approved in children.

FORMS - Trade only: Tabs 0.2 mg.

NOTES - Contraindicated in pregnancy-induced hypertension/pre-eclampsia. Avoid IV route due to risk of sudden HTN and stroke. If IV absolutely necessary, give slowly over no less than 1 min, monitor BP.

OB/GYN: Vaginitis Preparations

NOTE: See also STD/vaginitis table in antimicrobial section. Many experts recommend 7 day antifungal therapy for pregnant women w/candida vaginitis. Many of these creams & suppositories are oil-based and may weaken latex condoms & diaphragms. Do not use latex products for 72 hrs after last dose.

boric acid ▶Not absorbed ♀? ▶- $

PEDS - Not approved in children.

UNAPPROVED ADULT - Resistant vulvovaginal candidiasis: 600 mg suppository intravaginally qhs x 2 weeks.

FORMS - No commercial preparation; must be compounded by pharmacist. Vaginal suppositories 600 mg in gelatin capsules.

NOTES - Reported use for azole-resistant non-albicans (C. glabrata) or recurrent albicans failing azole therapy. Do not use if abdominal pain, fever or foul-smelling vaginal discharge. Avoid vaginal intercourse during treatment.

butoconazole (Gynazole, Mycelex-3) ▶LK ♀C ▶? $(OTC), $$$(Rx)

ADULT - Local treatment of vulvovaginal candidiasis, nonpregnant patients: Mycelex 3: 1 applicatorful (~5g) intravaginally qhs x 3 days, up to 6 days, if necessary. Pregnant patients: (2nd & 3rd trimesters only) 1 applicatorful (~5g) intravaginally qhs x 6 days. Gynazole-1: 1 applicatorful (~5g) intravaginally daily x 1.

PEDS - Not approved in children.

FORMS - OTC: Trade only (Mycelex 3): 2% vaginal cream in 5 g pre-filled applicators (3s) & 20 g tube with applicators. Rx: Trade only (Gynazole-1): 2% vaginal cream in 5 g pre-filled applicator.

NOTES - Do not use if abdominal pain, fever or foul-smelling vaginal discharge. Since a small amount may be absorbed, use during the 1st trimester only when essential. During pregnancy, use of a vaginal applicator may be contraindicated & manual insertion may be preferred. Vulvar/vaginal burning may occur. Avoid vaginal intercourse during treatment.

clindamycin (Cleocin, Clindesse, ✿Dalacin) ▶L ♀- ▶+ $$

ADULT - Bacterial vaginosis: Cleocin: 1 applicatorful (~100 mg in 5g cream) intravaginally qhs x 7 days, or one supp qhs x 3 days. Clindesse: 1 applicatorful cream x 1.

PEDS - Not approved in children.

FORMS - Generic/Trade: 2% vaginal cream in 40 g tube with 7 disposable applicators (Cleocin). Vag supp (Cleocin Ovules) 100 mg (3) w/applicator. 2% vaginal cream in a single-dose prefilled applicator (Clindesse).

NOTES - Clindesse may degrade latex/rubber condoms & diaphragms for 5 days after the last dose (Cleocin up to 3 days). Not recommended during pregnancy despite B rating, as it does not prevent adverse effects of bacterial vaginosis (eg, pre-term birth, neonatal infection). Cervicitis, vaginitis, & vulvar irritation may occur. Avoid vaginal intercourse during treatment.

clotrimazole (Mycelex 7, Gyne-Lotrimin, ✿Canesten, Clotrimaderm) ▶LK ♀B ▶? $

ADULT - Local treatment of vulvovaginal candidiasis: 1 applicatorful 1% cream qhs x 7 days. 1 applicatorful 2% cream qhs x 3 days. 100 mg suppository intravaginally qhs x 7 days. 200 mg tablet qhs x 3 days. Topical cream for external symptoms bid x 7 days.

PEDS - Not approved in children.

FORMS - OTC: Generic/Trade: 1% vaginal cream with applicator (some pre-filled). 2% vaginal cream with applicator. Vaginal suppositories 100 mg (7) & 200 mg (3) with applicators. 1% topical cream in some combo packs.

NOTES - Do not use if abdominal pain, fever or foul-smelling vaginal discharge is present. Since small amounts of these drugs may be absorbed from the vagina, use during the 1st trimester only when essential. During pregnancy, use of a vaginal applicator may be contraindicated; manual insertion of tabs may be preferred. Skin rash, lower abdominal cramps, bloating, vulvar irritation may occur. Avoid vaginal intercourse during treatment.

metronidazole (MetroGel-Vaginal, Vandazole) ▶LK ♀B ▶? $$$

ADULT - Bacterial vaginosis: 1 applicatorful (~ 5 g containing ~ 37.5 mg metronidazole) intravaginally qhs or bid x 5 days.

PEDS - Not approved in children.

FORMS - Generic/Trade: 0.75% gel in 70 g tube with applicator.

NOTES - Cure rate same with qhs and bid dosing. Vaginally applied metronidazole could be absorbed in sufficient amounts to produce systemic effects. Caution in patients with CNS diseases due to rare reports of seizures, neuropathy & numbness. Do not administer to patients who have taken disulfiram within the last 2 weeks. Interaction with ethanol. Caution with warfarin. Candida cervicitis & vaginitis, & vaginal, perineal or vulvar itching may occur. Avoid vaginal intercourse during treatment.

miconazole (*Monistat, Femizol-M, M-Zole, Micozole, Monazole*) ▶LK ♀+ ▶? $

ADULT - Local treatment of vulvovaginal candidiasis: 1 applicatorful 2% cream intravaginally qhs x 7 days or 4% cream qhs x 3 days. 100 mg supp intravaginally qhs x 7 days, 400 mg qhs x 3 days, or 1200 mg x 1. Topical cream for external symptoms bid x 7 days.

PEDS - Not approved in children.

FORMS - OTC: Generic/Trade: 2% vaginal cream in 45 g with 1 applicator or 7 disposable applicators. Vaginal suppositories 100 mg (7) OTC: Trade only: 400 mg (3) & 1200 mg (1) with applicator. Generic/Trade: 4% vaginal cream in 25 g tubes or 3 prefilled applicators. Some in combination packs with 2% miconazole cream for external use.

NOTES - Do not use if abdominal pain, fever or foul-smelling vaginal discharge. Since a small amount may be absorbed, use during the 1st trimester only when essential. During pregnancy, use of a vaginal applicator may be contraindicated; manual insertion of suppositories may be preferred. Vulvovaginal burning, itching, irritation & pelvic cramps may occur. Avoid vaginal intercourse during treatment. May increase warfarin effect.

nystatin (*Mycostatin, ♥Nilstat, Nyaderm*) ▶Not metabolized ♀A ▶? $$

ADULT - Local treatment of vulvovaginal candidiasis: 100,000 units tab intravaginally qhs x 2 weeks.

PEDS - Not approved in children.

FORMS - Generic/Trade: Vaginal Tabs 100,000 units in 15s & 30s with or without applicator(s).

NOTES - Topical azole products more effective. Do not use if abdominal pain, fever or foul-

smelling vaginal discharge. During pregnancy use of a vaginal applicator may be contraindicated, manual insertion may be preferred. Avoid vaginal intercourse during treatment.

terconazole (*Terazol*) ▶LK ♀C ▶- $$

ADULT - Local treatment of vulvovaginal candidiasis: 1 applicatorful 0.4% cream intravaginally qhs x 7 days. 1 applicatorful 0.8% cream intravaginally qhs x 3 days. 80 mg supp intravaginally qhs x 3 days.

PEDS - Not approved in children.

FORMS - All forms supplied with applicators: Generic/Trade: Vag cream 0.4% (Terazol 7) in 45 g tube, 0.8% (Terazol 3) in 20 g tube. Vag supp (Terazol 3) 80 mg (#3).

NOTES - Do not use if abdominal pain, fever or foul-smelling vaginal discharge. Since a small amount may be absorbed, use during the 1st trimester only when essential. During pregnancy, use of a vaginal applicator may be contraindicated; manual insertion of suppositories may be preferred. Avoid vaginal intercourse during treatment. Vulvovaginal irritation, burning, & pruritus may occur.

tioconazole (*Monistat 1-Day, Vagistat-1*) ▶Not absorbed ♀C ▶- $

ADULT - Local treatment of vulvovaginal candidiasis: 1 applicatorful (~ 4.6 g) intravaginally qhs x 1.

PEDS - Not approved in children.

FORMS - OTC: Trade only: Vaginal ointment: 6.5% (300 mg) in 4.6 g prefilled single-dose applicator.

NOTES - Do not use if abdominal pain, fever or foul-smelling vaginal discharge. Since small amounts of these drugs may be absorbed from the vagina, use during the 1st trimester only when essential. During pregnancy, use of a vaginal applicator may be contraindicated. Avoid vaginal intercourse during treatment. Vulvovaginal burning & itching may occur.

OB/GYN: Other

danazol (*Danocrine, ♥Cyclomen*) ▶L ♀X ▶- $$$$$

ADULT - Endometriosis: Start 400 mg PO bid, then titrate downward to a dose sufficient to maintain amenorrhea x 3-6 months, up to 9 months. Fibrocystic breast disease: 100-200 mg PO bid x 4-6 months.

PEDS - Not approved in children.

UNAPPROVED ADULT - Menorrhagia: 100-400

mg PO daily x 3 months. Cyclical mastalgia: 100-200 mg PO bid x 4-6 months.

FORMS - Generic only: Caps 50, 100, 200 mg.

NOTES - Contraindications: impaired hepatic, renal or cardiac function. Androgenic effects may not be reversible even after the drug is discontinued. May alter voice. Hepatic dysfunction has occurred. Insulin requirements may increase in diabetics. Prolongation of PT/INR has been reported with concomitant warfarin.

mifepristone *(Mifeprex, RU-486)* ▶L ♀X ▶? $$$$$

WARNING - Rare cases of sepsis & death have occurred. Surgical intervention may be necessary with incomplete abortions. Patients need to be given info on where such services are available & what do in case of an emergency.

ADULT - Termination of pregnancy, up to 49 days: Day 1: 600 mg PO. Day 3: 400 mcg misoprostol (unless abortion confirmed). Day 14: confirmation of pregnancy termination.

PEDS - Not approved in children.

FORMS - Trade only: Tabs 200 mg.

NOTES - Bleeding/spotting & cramping most common side effects. Prolonged heavy bleeding may be a sign of incomplete abortion. Contraindications: ectopic pregnancy, IUD use, adrenal insufficiency & long-term steroid use, use of anticoagulants, hemorrhagic disorders & porphyrias. CYP3A4 inducers may increase metabolism & lower levels. Available through physician offices only.

***Premesis-Rx* (pyridoxine + folic acid + cyanocobalamin + calcium carbonate)** ▶L ♀A ▶+ $

ADULT - Treatment of pregnancy-induced nausea: 1 tab PO daily.

PEDS - Unapproved in children.

FORMS - Trade only: Tabs 75 mg vitamin B6 (pyridoxine), sustained-release, 12 mcg vitamin B12 (cyanocobalamin), 1 mg folic acid, and 200 mg calcium carbonate.

NOTES - May be taken in conjunction with prenatal vitamins.

RHO immune globulin *(HyperRHO S/D,*

MICRhoGAM, RhoGAM, Rhophylac, Win-Rho SDF) ▶L ♀C ▶? $$$$$

ADULT - Prevention of hemolytic disease of the newborn if mother Rh- and baby is or might be Rh+: 300 mcg vial IM to mother at 28 weeks gestation followed by a 2nd dose ≤72 hours of delivery. Doses >1 vial may be needed if large fetal-maternal hemorrhage occurs during delivery (see complete prescribing information to determine dose). Following amniocentesis, miscarriage, abortion, or ectopic pregnancy ≥13 weeks gestation: 1 vial (300 mcg) IM. <12 weeks gestation: 1 vial (50 mcg) microdose IM. Immune thrombocytopenic purpura (ITP), non-splenectomized (WinRho): 250 units/kg/dose (50 mcg/kg/dose) IV x 1 if hemoglobin >10 g/dL or 125-200 units/kg/dose (25-40 mcg/kg/dose) IV x 1 if hemoglobin <10 g/dL. Additional doses of 125-300 units/kg/dose (25-60 mcg/kg/dose) IV may be given based on patient's response.

PEDS - Immune thrombocytopenic purpura (ITP), nonsplenectomized (WinRho): 250 units/kg/dose (50 mcg/kg/dose) IV x 1 if hemoglobin >10g/dL or 125-200 units/kg/dose (25-40 mcg/kg/dose) IV x 1 if hemoglobin <10 g/dL. Additional doses of 125-300 units/kg/dose (25-60 mcg/kg/dose) IV may be given as determined by patient's response.

UNAPPROVED ADULT - Rh-incompatible transfusion: specialized dosing.

NOTES - One 300 mcg vial prevents maternal sensitization to the Rh factor if the fetomaternal hemorrhage is <15 mL fetal RBCs (30 mL of whole blood). When the fetomaternal hemorrhage exceeds this (as estimated by Kleihauer-Betke testing), administer >1 vial of 300 mcg.

ONCOLOGY

Alkylating agents: altretamine *(Hexalen)*, busulfan *(Myleran, Busulfex)*, carmustine *(BCNU, Bi-CNU, Gliadel)*, chlorambucil *(Leukeran)*, cyclophosphamide *(Cytoxan, Neosar)*, dacarbazine *(DTIC-Dome)*, ifosfamide *(Ifex)*, lomustine *(Cee-Nu, CCNU)*, mechlorethamine *(Mustargen)*, melphalan *(Alkeran)*, procarbazine *(Matulane)*, streptozocin *(Zanosar)*, temozolomide *(Temodar, ✦Temodal)*, thiotepa *(Thioplex)*. **Antibiotics**: bleomycin *(Blenoxane)*, dactinomycin *(Cosmegen)*, daunorubicin *(DaunoXome, Cerubicin)*, doxorubicin liposomal *(Doxil, ✦Caelyx, Myocet)*, doxorubicin non-liposomal *(Adriamycin, Rubex)*, epirubicin *(Ellence, ✦Pharmorubicin)*, idarubicin *(Idamycin)*, mitomycin *(Mutamycin, Mitomycin-C)*, mitoxantrone *(Novantrone)*, valrubicin *(Valstar, ✦Valtaxin)*. **Antimetabolites**: azacitidine *(Vidaza)*, capecitabine *(Xeloda)*, cladribine *(Leustatin, chlorodeoxyadenosine)*, clofarabine *(Clolar)*, cytarabine *(Cytosar-U, Tarabine, Depo-Cyt, Ara-C)*, decitabine *(Dacogen)*, floxuridine *(FUDR)*, fludarabine *(Fludara)*, fluorouracil *(Adrucil, 5-FU)*, gemcitabine *(Gemzar)*, hydroxyurea *(Hydrea, Droxia)*, mercaptopurine *(6-MP, Purinethol)*, nelarabine *(Arranon)*, pemetrexed *(Alimta)*, pentostatin *(Nipent)*, thioguanine *(Tabloid, ✦Lanvis)*. **Cytoprotective Agents**: amifostine *(Ethyol)*, dexrazoxane *(Zinecard)*, mesna *(Mesnex, ✦Uro-*

mitexan), palifermin (*Kepivance*). **Hormones**: abarelix (*Plenaxis*), anastrozole (*Arimidex*), bicalutamide (*Casodex*), cyproterone, ✤*Androcur, Androcur Depot*), estramustine (*Emcyt*), exemestane (*Aromasin*), flutamide (*Eulexin*, ✤*Euflex*), fulvestrant (*Faslodex*), goserelin (*Zoladex*), histrelin (*Vantas, Supprelin LA*), letrozole (*Femara*), leuprolide (*Eligard, Lupron, Lupron Depot, Oaklide, Viadur*), nilutamide (*Nilandron*), testolactone (*Teslac*), toremifene (*Fareston*), triptorelin (*Trelstar Depot*). **Immunomodulators**: aldesleukin (*Proleukin, interleukin-2*), alemtuzumab (*Campath*, ✤*MabCampath*), BCG (*Bacillus of Calmette & Guerin, Pacis, TheraCys, Tice BCG*, ✤*Oncotice, Immucyst*), bevacizumab (*Avastin*), cetuximab (*Erbitux*), dasatinib (*Sprycel*), denileukin (*Ontak*), erlotinib (*Tarceva*), gemtuzumab (*Mylotarg*), ibritumomab (*Zevalin*), imatinib (*Gleevec*), interferon alfa-2a (*Roferon-A*), lapatinib (*Tykerb*), panitumumab (*Vectibix*), rituximab (*Ritux-*

an), sunitinib (*Sutent*), temsirolimus (*Torisel*), tositumomab (*Bexxar*), trastuzumab (*Herceptin*). **Mitotic Inhibitors**: docetaxel (*Taxotere*), etoposide (*VP-16, Etopophos, Toposar, VePesid*), paclitaxel (*Taxol, Abraxane, Onxol*), teniposide (*Vumon, VM-26*), vinblastine (*Velban, VLB*), vincristine (*Oncovin, Vincasar, VCR*), vinorelbine (*Navelbine*). **Platinum-Containing Agents**: carboplatin (*Paraplatin*), cisplatin (*Platinol-AQ*), oxaliplatin (*Eloxatin*). **Radiopharmaceuticals**: samarium 153 (*Quadramet*), strontium-89 (*Metastron*). **Miscellaneous**: arsenic trioxide (*Trisenox*), asparaginase (*Elspar*, ✤*Kidrolase*), bexarotene (*Targretin*), bortezomib (*Velcade*), gefitinib (*Iressa*), irinotecan (*Camptosar*), lenalidomide (*Revlimid*), leucovorin (*Wellcovorin, folinic acid*), mitotane (*Lysodren*), pegaspargase (*Oncaspar*), porfimer (*Photofrin*), sorafenib (*Nexavar*), thalidomide (*Thalomid*), topotecan (*Hycamtin*), tretinoin (*Vesanoid*), vorinostat (*Zolinza*).

NOTE FOR ALL OPHTHALMOLOGY SECTIONS: Most eye medications can be administered 1 drop at a time despite common manufacturer recommendations of 1-2 drops concurrently. Even a single drop is typically more than the eye can hold and thus a second drop is both wasteful and increases the possibility of systemic toxicity. If twice the medication is desired separate single drops by ≥5 minutes.

OPHTHALMOLOGY: Antiallergy – Decongestants & Combinations

NOTE: Overuse can cause rebound dilation of blood vessels. Do not administer while wearing soft contact lenses. Wait 10 minutes after use before inserting contact lenses.

naphazoline (*Albalon, AK-Con, Vasocon, Naphcon, Allerest, Clear Eyes*) ▶? ♀C▶? $
ADULT - Ocular vasoconstrictor/decongestant: 1 gtt qid prn for up to 4 days.
PEDS - <6 yo: not approved. ≥6 yo: 1 gtt qid prn for up to 4 days.
FORMS - OTC Generic/Trade: solution 0.012, 0.02, 0.03% (15, 30 mL). Rx Generic/Trade: 0.1% (15 mL).

Naphcon-A (naphazoline + pheniramine,

***Visine-A*)** ▶L ♀C ▶? $
ADULT - Ocular decongestant: 1 gtt qid prn for up to 4 days.
PEDS - Age ≥6 yo: Use adult dose. <6 yo: Not approved.
FORMS - OTC Trade only: solution 0.025% + 0.3% (15 mL).

Vascon-A (naphazoline + antazoline) ▶L ♀C ▶? $
ADULT - Ocular decongestant: 1 gtt qid prn for up to 4 days.
PEDS - ≥6 yo: Adult dose. <6 yo: Not approved.
FORMS - OTC Trade only: solution 0.1% + 0.5% (15 mL).

OPHTHALMOLOGY: Antiallergy – Dual Antihistamine & Mast Cell Stabilizers

NOTE: Wait ≥10 minutes after use before inserting contact lenses.

azelastine (*Optivar*) ▶L ♀C ▶? $$
ADULT - Allergic conjunctivitis: 1 gtt bid.
PEDS - ≥3 yo: Adult dose. <3yo: Not approved.
FORMS - Trade only: solution 0.05% (3, 6 mL).

epinastine (*Elestat*) ▶K ♀C ▶? $$$

ADULT - Allergic conjunctivitis: 1 gtt bid.
PEDS - ≥3 yo: Adult dose. <3 yo: Not approved.
FORMS - Trade only: solution 0.05% (5,10 mL).

ketotifen (*Alaway, Zaditor*) ▶Minimal absorption ♀C ▶? $
ADULT - Allergic conjunctivitis: 1 gtt in each eye q8-12h.

PEDS - Allergic conjunctivitis children >3yo: 1 gtt in each eye q8-12h.
FORMS -OTC-Generic/Trade soln 0.025% 5 mL
olopatadine (*Pataday, Patanol*) ▶K♀C▶?$$$
ADULT - Allergic conjunctivitis: 1 gtt of 0.1% solution in each eye bid (Patanol) or 1 gtt of 0.2% solution in each eye daily (Pataday).
PEDS - ≥3 yo: Adult dose. <3 yo: Not approved.
FORMS - Trade only: solution 0.1% (5 mL, Patanol), 0.2% (2.5 mL, Pataday).
NOTES - Do not administer while wearing soft contact lenses.

OPHTHALMOLOGY: Antiallergy – Pure Antihistamines

NOTE - Wait 10 minutes after use before inserting contact lenses.
emedastine (*Emadine*) ▶L ♀B ▶? $$
ADULT - Allergic conjunctivitis: 1 gtt up to qid.
PEDS - ≥3 yo: Adult dose. <3yo: Not approved.
FORMS - Trade only: solution 0.05% (5 mL).

levocabastine (*Livostin*) ▶Minimal absorption ♀C ▶? $$$
ADULT - Allergic conjunctivitis: 1 gtt qid for up to 2 weeks.
PEDS - ≥12 yo: Adult dose.
FORMS - Trade: susp 0.05% (2.5, 5,10 mL).

Visual Acuity Screen

Hold card in good light 14 inches from eye. Record vision for each eye separately with and without glasses. Presbyopic patients should read through bifocal glasses. Myopic patients should wear glasses only.
Pupil Diameter (mm)

OPHTHALMOLOGY: Antiallergy – Pure Mast Cell Stabilizers

NOTE: Works best as preventative agent; use continually during at risk season. Wait 10 minutes after use before inserting contact lenses.

cromolyn (Crolom, Opticrom) ▶LK ♀B ▶? $$$
ADULT - Allergic conjunctivitis: 1-2 gtts 4-6 times/day.
PEDS - ≥4 yo: Adult dose. <4 yo: Not approved.
FORMS - Generic/Trade: solution 4% (10 mL).
NOTES - Response may take up to 6 weeks.

lodoxamide (Alomide) ▶K ♀B ▶? $$$
ADULT - Allergic conjunctivitis: 1-2 gtts in each eye qid for up to 3 months.
PEDS - ≥2 yo: Adult dose. <2 yo: Not approved.
FORMS - Trade only: solution 0.1% (10 mL).
NOTES - Do not administer while wearing soft contact lenses.

nedocromil (Alocril) ▶L ♀B ▶? $$$
ADULT - Allergic conjunctivitis: 1-2 gtts in each eye bid.
PEDS - Children >3 yo: Allergic conjunctivitis: 1-2 gtts bid. Not approved in children <3 yo.
FORMS - Trade only: solution 2% (5 mL).
NOTES - Soln normally appears slightly yellow.

pemirolast (Alamast) ▶? ♀C ▶? $$$
ADULT - Allergic conjunctivitis: 1-2 gtts in each eye qid.
PEDS - >3 yo: Adult dose. <3 yo: Not approved.
FORMS - Trade only: solution 0.1% (10 mL).
NOTES - Decreased itching may be seen within a few days, but full effect may require up to four weeks.

OPHTHALMOLOGY: Antibacterials – Aminoglycosides

gentamicin (Garamycin, Genoptic, Gentak, ✦Diogent) ▶K ♀C ▶? $
ADULT - Ocular infections: 1-2 gtts q2-4h or ½ inch ribbon of ointment bid- tid.
PEDS - Not approved in children.
UNAPPROVED PEDS - Ocular infections: 1-2 gtts q4h or ½ inch ribbon of ointment bid-tid.
FORMS - Generic/Trade: solution 0.3% (5 ,15 mL), ointment 0.3% (3.5 g tube).
NOTES - Severe infections up to 2 gtts q1h.

tobramycin (Tobrex) ▶K ♀B ▶- $
ADULT - Ocular infections, mild to moderate: 1-2 gtts q4h or ½ inch ribbon of ointment bid-tid. Ocular infections, severe: 2 gtts q1h, then taper to q4h or ½ inch ribbon of ointment q3-4h, then taper to bid-tid.
PEDS - ≥2 months: Ocular infections: 1-2 gtts q1-4h or ½ inch ribbon of ointment q3-4h or bid-tid.
UNAPPROVED PEDS - Ocular infections: 1-2 gtts q4h or ½ inch ribbon of ointment bid-tid.
FORMS - Generic/Trade: solution 0.3% (5 mL). Trade only: ointment 0.3% (3.5 g tube).

OPHTHALMOLOGY: Antibacterials – Fluoroquinolones

ciprofloxacin (Ciloxan) ▶LK ♀C ▶? $$
ADULT - Corneal ulcers/ keratitis: 2 gtts q15 minutes x 6 hours, then 2 gtts q30 minutes x 1 day; then, 2 gtts q1h x 1 day, and 2 gtts q4h x 3-14 days. Bacterial conjunctivitis: 1-2 gtts q2h while awake x 2 days, then 1-2 gtts q4h while awake x 5 days; or ½ inch ribbon ointment tid x 2 days, then ½ inch ribbon bid x 5 days.
PEDS - Bacterial conjunctivitis: use adult dose for age ≥1 yo (solution) and ≥2 yo (ointment). Not approved below these ages.
FORMS - Generic/Trade: solution 0.3% (2.5,5, 10 mL). Trade: ointment 0.3% (3.5 g tube).
NOTES - May cause white precipitate of drug at site of epithelial defect that may be confused with worsening infection. Resolves within 2 wks and does not necessitate discontinuation.

gatifloxacin (Zymar) ▶K ♀C ▶? $$$
ADULT - Bacterial conjunctivitis: 1-2 gtts q2h up to 8 times/day while awake on days 1&2, then 1-2 gtts q4h up to 4 times/day on days 3-7.
PEDS - >1 yo: Adult dose. <1 yo: Not approved.
FORMS - Trade only: solution 0.3%.

levofloxacin (Iquix, Quixin) ▶KL ♀C ▶? $$
ADULT - Bacterial conjunctivitis, Quixin: 1-2 gtts q2h while awake up to 8 times/day on days 1 & 2, then 1-2 gtts q4h up to 4 times/day on days 3-7. Bacterial conjunctivitis, Iquix: 1-2 gtts q30 min to 2h while awake and q4-6h overnight on days 1-3, then 1-2 gtts q1-4h while awake on days 4 to completion of therapy.
PEDS - Bacterial conjunctivitis, Quixin: ≤1 yo: Not approved. >1 yo: 1-2 gtts q2h while awake up to 8 times/day on days 1&2, then 1-2 gtts

q4h up to 4 times/day on days 3-7. Iquix: <6 yo: Not approved. ≥6 yo: 1-2 gtts q30 min to 2h while awake and q4-6h overnight on days 1-3, then 1-2 gtts q1-4h while awake on days 4 to completion of therapy.

FORMS - Trade only: solution 0.5% (Quixin, 5 mL), 1.5% (Iquix, 5 mL).

moxifloxacin (*Vigamox*) ▶LK ♀C ▶? $$$
ADULT - Bacterial conjunctivitis: 1 gtt tid x 7 days.
PEDS - >1 yo: Adult dose. <1 yo: Not approved.
FORMS - Trade only: solution 0.5% (3 mL).

norfloxacin (*Chibroxin*) ▶LK ♀C ▶? $
ADULT - Bacterial conjunctivitis: 1-2 gtts qid x 7

days. Severe infections may require 1-2 gtts q2h x 1-2 days, then qid.
PEDS - Bacterial conjunctivitis >1 year of age: 1-2 gtts qid x 7 days.
FORMS - Trade only: solution 0.3% (5 mL).

ofloxacin (*Ocuflox*) ▶LK ♀C ▶? $$
ADULT - Corneal ulcers/keratitis: 1-2 gtts q30 minutes while awake and 1-2 gtts 4-6 h after retiring x 2 days, then 1-2 gtts q1h while awake x 5 days, then 1-2 gtts qid x 3 days. Bacterial conjunctivitis: 1-2 gtts q2-4 h x 2 days, then 1-2 gtts qid x 5 days.
PEDS - ≥1 yo: Adult dose. <1 yo: Not approved.
FORMS - Generic/Trade: soln 0.3% (5, 10 mL).

OPHTHALMOLOGY: Antibacterials – Other

azithromycin (*Azasite*) ▶L ♀B ▶? ?
ADULT - Ocular infections: 1 gtt bid x 2 days, then 1 gtt daily x 5 more days.
PEDS - ≥1 yo: Adult dose.
FORMS - Trade only: solution 1% (2.5 mL).

bacitracin (*AK Tracin*) ▶Minimal absorption ♀C ▶? $
ADULT - Ocular infections: apply ¼-½ inch ribbon of ointment q3-4h or bid-qid.
PEDS - Not approved in children.
UNAPPROVED PEDS - Ocular infections: apply ½ inch ribbon of ointment q3-4h or bid-qid.
FORMS - Generic/Trade: ointment 500 units/g (3.5g tube)

erythromycin (*Ilotycin, AK-Mycin*) ▶L ♀B ▶+ $
ADULT - Ocular infections, corneal ulceration: ½ inch ribbon of ointment q3-4h or 2-8 times/day. For chlamydia infections: bid x 2 months or bid x 5 days/month for 6 months.
PEDS - Ophthalmia neonatorum prophylaxis: ½ inch ribbon to both eyes within 1 hour of birth.
FORMS - Generic: ointment 0.5% (1, 3.5 g tube).

fusidic acid (❉*Fucithalmic*) ▶L ♀? ▶? $
ADULT - Canada only. Eye infections: 1 gtt in both eyes q12h x 7 days.
PEDS - Canada only. ≥2 yo: Adult dose.
FORMS - Canada trade only: Drops 1%. Multidose tubes of 3, 5 g. Single dose preservative-free tubes of 0.2 g in a box of 12.

Neosporin ointment (neomycin + bacitracin + polymyxin) ▶K ♀C ▶? $
ADULT - Ocular infections: ½ inch ribbon of ointment q3-4 h x 7-10 days or ½ inch ribbon 2-3 times/day for mild-moderate infection.

PEDS - Not approved in children.
UNAPPROVED PEDS - ½ inch ribbon of ointment q3-4h x 7-10 days.
FORMS - Generic/Trade: ointment. (3.5 g tube).
NOTES - Contact dermatitis can occur after prolonged use.

Neosporin solution (neomycin + polymyxin + gramicidin) ▶KL ♀C ▶? $$
ADULT - Ocular infections:1-2 gtts q1-6h x 7-10 days.
PEDS - Not approved in children.
UNAPPROVED PEDS – Adult dose.
FORMS - Generic/Trade: solution (10 mL)
NOTES - Contact dermatitis can occur after prolonged use.

Polysporin (polymyxin + bacitracin) ▶K ♀C ▶? $
ADULT - Ocular infections: ½ inch ribbon of ointment q3-4h x 7-10 days or ½ inch ribbon bid-tid for mild-moderate infection.
PEDS - Not approved in children.
UNAPPROVED PEDS - Ocular infections: ½ inch ribbon of ointment q3-4h x 7-10 days.
FORMS - Generic/Trade: ointment (3.5 g tube).

Polytrim (polymyxin + trimethoprim) ▶KL ♀C ▶? $
ADULT - Ocular infections: 1-2 gtts q3-6h x 7-10 days. Max 6 gtts/day.
PEDS- ≥2 mo: Adult dose. <2 mo: Not approved
FORMS - Generic/Trade: solution (10 mL).

sulfacetamide (*Sulamyd, Bleph-10, Sulf-10, Isopto Cetamide, AK-Sulf*) ▶K ♀C ▶- $
ADULT - Ocular infections, corneal ulceration: 1-2 gtts q2-3h initially, then taper by decreasing frequency as condition allows x 7- 10 days or ½ inch ribbon of ointment q3-4h initially,

then taper x 7-10 days. Trachoma: 2 gtts q2h with systemic antibiotic such as doxycycline or azithromycin.

PEDS- ≥2 mo: Adult dose. <2 mo: Not approved

FORMS - Generic only: solution 10%, 30% (15 mL). Generic/Trade: ointment 10% (3.5g tube). Trade only: solution 10% (2.5,5,15 mL) 10, 15, 30% (15 mL)

NOTES - Ointment may be used as an adjunct to solution.

OPHTHALMOLOGY: Antiviral Agents

trifluridine (Viroptic) ▶Minimal absorption ♀C ▶- $$$

ADULT - HSV keratitis: 1 gtt q2h to maximum 9 gtts/day. After re-epithelialization, decrease dose to 1 gtt q4-6h while awake x 7-14 days. Maximum of 21 days of treatment.

PEDS - ≥6 yo: Adult dose. <6 yo: Not approved.

FORMS - Trade only: solution 1% (7.5 mL).

NOTES - Avoid continuous use >21 days; may cause keratitis and conjunctival scarring. Urge frequent use of topical lubricants (ie, tear substitutes) to minimize surface damage.

vidarabine (Vira-A) ▶Cornea ♀C ▶? $$$

ADULT - HSV keratitis: ½ inch ribbon of ointment 5 times daily x 5-7 days. After re-epithelialization, decrease dose to ½ inch ribbon bid x 5-7 days.

PEDS - Age ≥2 yo: Use adult dose. <2 yo: Not approved.

FORMS - Trade only: ointment 3% (3.5 g tube).

OPHTHALMOLOGY: Corticosteroid & Antibacterial Combinations

NOTE: Recommend that only ophthalmologists or optometrists prescribe due to infection, cataract, corneal/scleral perforation, glaucoma risk. Monitor IOP. Gradually taper when discontinuing.

Blephamide (prednisolone + sulfacetamide) ▶KL ♀C ▶? $

ADULT - Steroid-responsive inflammatory condition with bacterial infection or risk of bacterial infection: Start 1-2 gtts q1h during the day and q2h during the night, then 1 gtt q4-8h; or ½ inch ribbon (ointment) tid-qid initially, then daily-bid thereafter.

PEDS - Not approved in children.

FORMS - Generic/Trade: solution/suspension (5,10 mL), ointment (3.5 g tube).

Cortisporin (neomycin + polymyxin + hydrocortisone) ▶LK ♀C ▶? $

ADULT - Steroid-responsive inflammatory condition with bacterial infection or risk of bacterial infection: 1-2 gtts or ½ inch ribbon of ointment q3-4h or more frequently prn.

PEDS - Not approved in children.

UNAPPROVED PEDS - 1-2 gtts or ½ inch ribbon of ointment q3-4h.

FORMS - Generic/Trade: suspension (7.5 mL), ointment (3.5 g tube).

FML-S Liquifilm (prednisolone + Sulfacetamide) ▶KL ♀C ▶? $

ADULT - Steroid-responsive inflammatory condition with bacterial infection or risk of bacterial infection: Start 1-2 gtts q1h during the day and q2h during the night, then 1 gtt q4-8h; or ½ inch ribbon (ointment) tid-qid initially, then daily-bid thereafter.

PEDS - Not approved in children.

FORMS - Trade only: suspension (5,10 mL).

Maxitrol (dexamethasone + neomycin + polymyxin) ▶KL ♀C ▶? $

ADULT - Steroid-responsive inflammatory condition with bacterial infection or risk of bacterial infection: Start 1-2 gtts q1h during the day and q2h during the night, then 1 gtt q4-8h; or ½ -1 inch ribbon (ointment) tid-qid initially, then daily- bid thereafter.

PEDS - Not approved in children.

FORMS - Generic/Trade: suspension (5 mL), ointment (3.5 g tube).

Pred G (prednisolone + gentamicin) ▶KL ♀C ▶? $$

ADULT - Steroid-responsive inflammatory condition with bacterial infection or risk of bacterial infection: Start 1-2 gtts q1h during the day and q2h during the night, then 1 gtt q4-8h or ½ inch ribbon of ointment bid-qid.

PEDS - Not approved in children.

FORMS - Trade only: suspension (2,5,10 mL), ointment (3.5 g tube).

TobraDex (tobramycin + dexamethasone - ophthalmic) ▶L ♀C ▶? $$$

ADULT - Steroid-responsive inflammatory condition with bacterial infection or risk of bacterial infection: 1-2 gtts q2h x 1-2 days, then 1-2 gtts q4-6h; or ½ inch ribbon of ointment bid-qid.

PEDS - <2 yo: not approved. ≥2 yo: 1-2 gtts q2h x 1-2 days, then 1-2 gtts q4-6h; or ½ inch ribbon of ointment bid-qid.

FORMS - Trade only: suspension (2.5,5,10 mL), ointment (3.5 g tube).

Vasocidin (prednisolone + sulfacetamide) ▶KL ♀C ▶? $

ADULT - Steroid-responsive inflammatory condition with bacterial infection or risk of bacterial infection: Start 1-2 gtts q1h during the day and q2h during the night, then 1 gtt q4-8h; or ½ inch ribbon (ointment) tid-qid initially, then daily-bid thereafter.

PEDS - Not approved in children.

FORMS - Generic/Trade: solution (5,10 mL)

Zylet (loteprednol + tobramycin) ▶LK ♀C ▶? $$$

ADULT - 1-2 gtts q1-2h x 1-2 days then 1-2 gtts q4-6h.

PEDS - Not approved in children.

FORMS - Trade only: suspension 0.5% loteprednol + 0.3% tobramycin (2.5, 5, 10 mL)

OPHTHALMOLOGY: Corticosteroids

NOTE: Recommend that only ophthalmologists or optometrists prescribe due to infection, cataract, corneal/scleral perforation, glaucoma risk. Monitor IOP. Gradually taper when discontinuing.

fluorometholone (FML, FML Forte, Flarex, Fluor-Op) ▶L ♀C ▶? $$

ADULT - 1-2 gtts q1-2h or ½ inch ribbon of ointment q4h x 1-2 days, then 1-2 gtts bid-qid or ½ inch of ointment daily-tid.

PEDS - ≥2 yo: Adult dose. <2 yo: Not approved.

FORMS - Generic/Trade: suspension 0.1% (5, 10,15 mL). Trade only: suspension 0.25% (5,10,15 mL), ointment 0.1% (3.5 g tube)

NOTES - Fluorometholone acetate (Flarex) is more potent than fluorometholone (FML, FML Forte). Use caution in glaucoma.

loteprednol (Alrex, Lotemax) ▶L ♀C ▶? $$$

ADULT - 1-2 gtts qid, may increase to 1 gtt q1h during first week of therapy prn. Postoperative inflammation: 1-2 gtts qid.

PEDS - Not approved in children.

FORMS - Trade only: suspension 0.2% (Alrex 5,10 mL), 0.5% (Lotemax 2.5, 5,10,15 mL).

prednisolone (AK-Pred, Pred Forte, Pred Mild, Inflamase, Inflamase Forte, Econopred, Econopred Plus, ♣AK Tate, Diopred) ▶L ♀C ▶? $$

ADULT - Solution: 1-2 gtts up to q1h during day and q2h at night, when response observed, then 1 gtt q4h, then 1 gtt tid-qid. Suspension: 1-2 gtts bid-qid.

PEDS - Not approved in children.

FORMS - Generic/Trade: suspension 1% (5, 10,15 mL), solution 0.125% (5 mL), 1% (5,10, 15 mL). Trade only: suspension 0.12% (5,10 mL), solution 0.125% (5,10 mL)

NOTES - Prednisolone acetate (Pred Mild, Pred Forte) is more potent than prednisolone sodium phosphate (AK-Pred, Inflamase Forte).

rimexolone (Vexol) ▶L ♀C ▶? $$

ADULT - Post-operative inflammation: 1-2 gtts qid x 2 weeks. Uveitis: 1-2 gtts q1h while awake x 1 week, then 1 gtt q2h while awake x 1 week, then taper.

PEDS - Not approved in children.

FORMS - Trade only: suspension 1% (5,10 mL).

NOTES - Prolonged use associated with corneal/scleral perforation and cataracts.

OPHTHALMOLOGY: Glaucoma Agents – Beta Blockers

NOTE: May be absorbed and cause side effects and drug interactions associated with systemic beta-blocker therapy. Use caution in cardiac conditions and asthma.

betaxolol (Betoptic, Betoptic S) ▶LK♀C▶?$$

ADULT, PEDS - Chronic open angle glaucoma or ocular hypertension: 1-2 gtts bid.

FORMS - Trade only: suspension 0.25% (5,10 mL). Generic only: solution 0.5% (5,10,15 mL).

NOTES - Selective beta1-blocking agent. Shake suspension before use.

carteolol (Ocupress) ▶KL ♀C ▶? $

ADULT - Chronic open angle glaucoma or ocular hypertension: 1 gtt bid.

PEDS - Not approved in children.

FORMS - Generic/Trade: soln 1% (5,10,15 mL).

NOTES - Nonselective beta-blocker but has intrinsic sympathomimetic activity.

levobunolol (Betagan) ▶? ♀C ▶- $

ADULT - Chronic open angle glaucoma or ocular hypertension: 1-2 gtts (0.5%) daily-bid or 1-2 gtts (0.25%) bid.

PEDS - Not approved in children.
FORMS - Generic/Trade: solution 0.25% (5,10 mL) 0.5% (5,10,15 mL - Trade only 2 mL).
NOTES - Nonselective beta blocker.

metipranolol (*Optipranolol*) ▶? ♀C ▶? $
ADULT - Chronic open angle glaucoma or ocular hypertension: 1 gtt bid.
PEDS - Not approved in children.
FORMS - Generic/Trade: soln 0.3% (5,10 mL).
NOTES - Nonselective beta blocker.

timolol (*Betimol, Timoptic, Timoptic XE, Istalol, Timoptic Ocudose*) ▶LK ♀C ▶+ $
ADULT - Chronic open angle glaucoma or ocular HTN: 1 gtt (0.25 or 0.5%) bid or 1 gtt of gel-forming solution (0.25 or 0.5% Timoptic XE) daily or 1 gtt (0.5% Istalol solution) daily.
PEDS - Chronic open angle glaucoma or ocular HTN: 1 gtt (0.25 or 0.5%) of gel-forming solution daily.
FORMS - Generic/Trade: solution 0.25, 0.5% (5,10,15 mL), preservative free 0.2 mL. Generic/Trade: gel forming solution 0.25, 0.5% (2.5*, 5 mL). Trade (Istalol): solution 0.5% 2.5, 5 mL. Note: *0.25% Timoptic XE.
NOTES - Administer other eye meds ≥10 minutes before Timoptic XE, which has greatest effect if administered in the morning. Nonselective beta blocker.

OPHTHALMOLOGY: Glaucoma Agents – Carbonic Anhydrase Inhibitors

NOTE: Sulfonamide derivatives; verify absence of sulfa allergy before prescribing.

brinzolamide (*Azopt*) ▶LK ♀C ▶? $$
ADULT - Chronic open angle glaucoma or ocular hypertension: 1 gtt tid.
PEDS - Not approved in children.
FORMS - Trade: suspension 1% (5,10,15 mL).
NOTES - Do not administer while wearing soft contact lenses. Wait 10 minutes after use before inserting contact lenses.

dorzolamide (*Trusopt*) ▶KL ♀C ▶- $$
ADULT, PEDS - Chronic open angle glaucoma or ocular hypertension: 1 gtt tid.
FORMS - Trade only: solution 2% (5,10 mL).
NOTES - Do not administer while wearing soft contact lenses. Keep bottle tightly capped to avoid crystal formation. Wait 10 minutes after use before inserting contact lenses.

methazolamide (*Neptazane*) ▶LK ♀C ▶? $
ADULT - Glaucoma: 100-200 mg PO initially, then 100 mg PO q 12h until desired response. Maintenance dose: 25-50 mg PO daily-tid.
PEDS - Not approved in children.
FORMS - Generic only: Tabs 25, 50 mg.
NOTES - Mostly metabolized by liver thus less risk of renal calculi than with acetazolamide.

OPHTHALMOLOGY: Glaucoma Agents – Miotics

NOTE: Observe for cholinergic systemic effects (eg, salivation, lacrimation, urination, diarrhea, gastrointestinal upset, excessive sweating).

acetylcholine (*Miochol-E*) ▶Acetylcholinesterases ♀? ▶? $$
ADULT - Intraoperative miosis or pressure lowering: 0.5 mL to 3 mL injected intraocularly.
PEDS - Not approved in children.

carbachol (*Isopto Carbachol, Miostat*) ▶? ♀C ▶? $$
ADULT - Glaucoma: 1 gtt tid. Intraoperative miosis or pressure lowering: 0.5 mL injected intraocularly.
PEDS - Not approved in children.
FORMS - Solution (Isopto Carbachol) 0.75%, 3%. Intraocular solution (Miostat) 0.01%.

echothiophate iodide (*Phospholine Iodide*) ▶? ♀C ▶? $$$
ADULT - Glaucoma: 1 gtt bid.
PEDS - Accommodative estropia: 1 gtt daily (0.06%) or 1 gtt qod (0.125%).
FORMS - Solution 0.03%, 0.06%, 0.125%, 0.25%, 5 mL.
NOTES - Use lowest effective strength. Caution if asthma, spastic GI diseases, GI ulcers, bradycardia, hypotension, recent MI, epilepsy, Parkinson's Disease, history of retinal detachment. Stop 3 weeks before general anesthesia as may cause prolonged succinylcholine paralysis. Discontinue if cardiac effects noted.

pilocarpine (*Pilocar, Pilopine HS, Isopto Carpine, Ocusert, Ocu Carpine, ✦Diocarpine, Akarpine*) ▶Plasma ♀C ▶? $
ADULT - Glaucoma: 1-2 gtts up to tid-qid up to 6 times/day or ½ inch ribbon (4% gel) qhs.
PEDS - Glaucoma: 1-2 gtts up to tid-qid up to 6 times/day.
FORMS - Generic/Trade: solution 0.5, 1, 2, 3, 4,

6% (15mL). Trade only: 5%, 8% (15 mL), gel 4% (4 g tube).
NOTES - Do not administer while wearing soft

contact lenses; wait ≥15 minutes after use before inserting. Causes miosis. May cause blurred vision and difficulty with night vision.

OPHTHALMOLOGY: Glaucoma Agents – Prostaglandin Analogs

NOTE: Do not administer while wearing soft contact lenses. Wait 10 minutes after use before inserting contact lenses. May aggravate intraocular inflammation. None approved in children.

bimatoprost (*Lumigan*) ▶LK ♀C ▶? $$$
ADULT - Chronic open angle glaucoma or ocular hypertension: 1 gtt qhs.
FORMS - Trade: solution 0.03% (2.5,5,7.5 mL).

latanoprost (*Xalatan*) ▶LK ♀C ▶? $$$
ADULT - Chronic open angle glaucoma or ocular hypertension: 1 gtt qhs.

FORMS - Trade only: solution 0.005% (2.5 mL).
travoprost (*Travatan, Travatan Z*) ▶L ♀C ▶? $$
ADULT - Chronic open angle glaucoma or ocular hypertension: 1 gtt qhs.
FORMS - Trade only: solution (Travatan) & benzalkonium chloride-free (Travatan Z) 0.004% (2.5, 5 mL).
NOTES - Wait 10 minutes after use before inserting contact lenses. Avoid if prior or current intraocular inflammation.

OPHTHALMOLOGY: Glaucoma Agents – Sympathomimetics

NOTE: Do not administer while wearing soft contact lenses. Wait 10 minutes after use before inserting contact lenses.

apraclonidine (*Iopidine*) ▶KL ♀C ▶? $$$
ADULT - Perioperative IOP elevation: 1 gtt (1%) 1h prior to surgery then 1 gtt immediately after.
PEDS - Not approved in children.
FORMS - Trade only: solution 0.5% (5,10 mL), 1% (0.1 mL).
NOTES - Rapid tachyphylaxis may occur. Do not use long-term.

brimonidine (*Alphagan P, ✦Alphagan*) ▶L ♀B ▶? $$
ADULT - Chronic open angle glaucoma or ocular hypertension: 1 gtt tid.
PEDS - Glaucoma >2 yo: 1 gtt tid.

FORMS - Trade only: solution 0.1% (5,10,15 mL). Generic/Trade: solution 0.15% (5,10,15 mL). Generic only: 0.2% solution (5,10,15 mL).
NOTES - Contraindicated with MAO inhibitors. BID dosing may have similar efficacy.

dipivefrin (*Propine*) ▶Eye/plasma/L ♀B ▶? $
ADULT - Chronic open angle glaucoma or ocular hypertension: 1 gtt bid.
PEDS - Glaucoma: 1 gtt bid.
FORMS - Generic/Trade: solution 0.1% (5,10,15 mL).

epinephrine (*Epifrin, Glaucon, Epinal, Eppy/N, Epitrate*) ▶Eye/plasma/L ♀C ▶? $$
ADULT - Chronic open angle glaucoma or ocular hypertension: 1 gtt bid.
FORMS - Generic/Trade: sol 0.1%(5,10,15 mL).

OPHTHALMOLOGY: Glaucoma Agents – Other

Cosopt (dorzolamide + timolol) ▶LK ♀D ▶- $$$$
ADULT - Chronic open angle glaucoma or ocular hypertension: 1 gtt bid.
PEDS - Not approved in children.
FORMS - Trade only: solution dorzolamide 2%

+ timolol 0.5% (5, 7.5, 10, 18 mL).
NOTES - Do not administer while wearing soft contact lenses; wait 10 minutes after use before inserting. Not recommended if severe renal or hepatic dysfunction. Caution in sulfa allergy. See beta-blocker warnings.

OPHTHALMOLOGY: Macular Degeneration

NOTE: None approved in children.
pegaptanib (*Macugen*) ▶Minimal absorption ♀B ▶? $$$$$

ADULT - "Wet" macular degeneration: 0.3 mg intravitreal injection q 6 weeks.
ranibizumab (*Lucentis*) ▶Intravitreal ♀C ▶?

$$$$$
ADULT - Treatment of neovascular (wet) macular degeneration: 0.5 mg intravitreal injection once a month. If monthly injections not feasible, can administer every 3 months, but this regimen is less effective.
NOTES - Increased stroke risk noted with higher doses (0.5 mg) and with prior stroke.

verteporfin (*Visudyne*) ▶L/plasma ♀C ▶?
$$$$$
ADULT - Treatment of exudative age-related macular degeneration: 6 mg/m^2 IV over 10 minutes; laser light therapy 15 minutes after start of infusion.
NOTES - Severe risk of photosensitivity x 5 days; must avoid exposure to sunlight.

OPHTHALMOLOGY: Mydriatics & Cycloplegics

NOTE: Use caution in infants.

atropine (*Isopto Atropine*) ▶L ♀C ▶+ $
ADULT - Uveitis: 1-2 gtts (0.5 or 1% solution) up to qid or ¼ inch ribbon (1% ointment) up to tid. Refraction: 1-2 gtts (1% solution) 1 h before procedure or 1/8-1/4 inch ribbon daily-tid.
PEDS - Uveitis: 1-2 gtts (0.5%) up to tid or 1/8-1/4 inch ribbon up to tid. Refraction: 1-2 gtts (0.5%) bid x 1-3 days before procedure or 1/8 inch ribbon (1% ointment) x 1-3 days before procedure.
UNAPPROVED PEDS - Amblyopia: 1 gtt in good eye daily.
FORMS - Generic/Trade: solution 1% (5,15 mL) Generic only: ointment 1% (3.5 g tube).
NOTES - Cycloplegia may last up to 5-10d and mydriasis may last up to 7-14d. Each drop of a 1% solution contains 0.5 mg atropine. Treat atropine overdose with physostigmine 0.25 mg every 15 minutes until symptoms resolve.

cyclopentolate (*AK-Pentolate, Cyclogyl, Pentolair*) ▶? ♀C ▶? $
ADULT - Refraction: 1-2 gtts (1-2%), repeat in 5-10 minutes prn. Give 45 min before procedure.
PEDS - May cause CNS disturbances. Refraction: 1-2 gtts (0.5,1, or 2%), repeat in 5-10 minutes prn. Give 45 mins before procedure.
FORMS - Generic/Trade: solution 1% (2,15 mL). Trade only: 0.5% (15 mL) and 2% (2,5,15 mL)
NOTES - Cycloplegia may last 6-24h; mydriasis may last 1 day.

homatropine (*Isopto Homatropine*) ▶? ♀C ▶? $
ADULT - Refraction: 1-2 gtts (2%) or 1 gtt (5%)

in eye(s) immediately before procedure, repeat q5-10 minutes prn. Max 3 doses. Uveitis: 1-2 gtts (2-5%) bid-tid or as often as q3-4h.
PEDS - Refraction: 1 gtt (2%) in eye(s) immediately before procedure, repeat q10 minutes prn. Uveitis: 1 gtt (2%) bid-tid.
FORMS - Trade only: solution 2% (5 mL), 5% (15 mL). Generic/Trade: solution 5% (5 mL)
NOTES - Cycloplegia & mydriasis last 1-3 days.

phenylephrine (*Neo-Synephrine, Mydfrin, Relief*) ▶Plasma, L ♀C ▶? $
ADULT - Ophthalmologic exams: 1-2 gtts (2.5, 10%) before procedure. Ocular surgery: 1-2 gtts (2.5, 10%) before surgery.
PEDS - Not routinely used in children.
UNAPPROVED PEDS - Ophthalmologic exams: 1 gtt (2.5%) before procedure. Ocular surgery: 1 gtt (2.5%) before surgery.
FORMS - Generic/Trade: solution 2.5,10% (3*, 5, 15 mL) Note: * 2.5% Mydfrin.
NOTES - Overuse can cause rebound dilation of blood vessels. No cycloplegia; mydriasis may last up to 5 hours. Systemic absorption, especially with 10% solution, may be associated with sympathetic stimulation (eg, increased blood pressure).

tropicamide (*Mydriacyl*) ▶? ♀? ▶? $
ADULT - Dilated eye exam: 1-2 gtts (0.5%) in eye(s) 15- 20 minutes before exam, repeat q30 minutes prn.
PEDS - Not approved in children.
FORMS - Generic/Trade: solution 0.5% (15 mL), 1% (2, 3, 15 mL)
NOTES - Mydriasis may last 6 hours and has weak cycloplegic effects.

OPHTHALMOLOGY: Nonsteroidal Anti-Inflammatories

bromfenac (*Xibrom*) ▶Minimal absorption ♀C, D (3rd trimester) ▶? $$$$
ADULT - Post-op inflammation and pain follow-

ing cataract surgery: 1 gtt bid beginning 24 hours after cataract surgery x 2 weeks.
PEDS - Not approved in children.

FORMS - Trade: solution 0.09% (2.5, 5 mL).

NOTES - Not for use with contact lenses. Contains sodium sulfite and may cause allergy.

diclofenac (*Voltaren*, ✿*Voltaren Ophtha*) ▶L ♀B, D (3rd trimester) ▶? $$$

ADULT - Post-op inflammation following cataract surgery: 1 gtt qid x 1-2 weeks. Ocular photophobia and pain associated with corneal refractive surgery: 1-2 gtt to operative eye(s) 1 h prior to surgery and 1-2 gtt within 15 minutes after surgery, then 1 gtt qid prn for ≤3 days.

PEDS - Not approved in children.

FORMS - Trade only: solution 0.1% (2.5,5 mL).

NOTES - Contraindicated with soft contacts.

flurbiprofen (*Ocufen*) ▶L ♀C ▶? $

ADULT - Inhibition of intraoperative miosis: 1 gtt q30 min beginning 2h prior to surgery (total of 4 gtts).

PEDS - Not approved in children.

UNAPPROVED ADULT - Treatment of cystoid macular edema, inflammation after glaucoma or cataract laser surgery, uveitis syndromes.

FORMS - Generic/Trade: soln 0.03% (2.5 mL).

ketorolac (*Acular, Acular LS*) ▶L ♀C ▶? $$$

ADULT - Allergic conjunctivitis: 1 gtt (0.5%) qid. Post-op inflammation following cataract surgery: 1 gtt (0.5%) qid beginning 24 h after surgery x 1-2 weeks. Post-op corneal refractive surgery: 1 gtt (0.4%) prn for up to 4 days.

PEDS - ≥3 yo: Adult dose. <3 yo: Not approved.

FORMS - Trade only: solution Acular LS 0.4% (5 mL), Acular 0.5% (3, 5, 10 mL), preservative free Acular 0.5% unit dose (0.4 mL).

NOTES - Do not administer with soft contact lenses; wait 10 minutes after use before inserting. Avoid use in late pregnancy.

nepafenac (*Nevanac*) ▶Minimal absorption ♀C ▶? $$$

ADULT - Post-op inflammation following cataract surgery: 1 gtt tid beginning 24 hours before cataract surgery and continued for 2 weeks after surgery.

PEDS - Not approved in children.

FORMS - Trade only: suspension 0.1% (3 mL).

NOTES - Not for use with contact lenses. Caution if previous allergy to ASA or other NSAIDs.

OPHTHALMOLOGY: Other

artificial tears (*Tears Naturale, Hypotears, Refresh Tears, GenTeal, Systane*) ▶Minimal absorption ♀A ▶+ $

ADULT, PEDS - Ophthalmic lubricant: 1-2 gtts tid-qid prn.

FORMS - OTC soln (15, 30 mL among others).

cyclosporine (*Restasis*) ▶Minimal absorption ♀C ▶? $$$$

ADULT - Keratoconjunctivitis sicca (chronic dry eye disease): 1 gtt in each eye q12h.

PEDS - Not approved in children.

FORMS - Trade only: emulsion 0.05% (0.4 mL single-use vials).

NOTES - Wait 10 min after use before inserting contact lenses.

dapiprazole (*Rev-Eyes*) ▶Minimal absorption ♀B ▶? $

ADULT - Reversal of diagnostic phenylephrine mydriasis: 2 gtts in each eye, repeat in 5 mins.

PEDS - ≥4 yo: Adult dose. <4 yo: Not approved.

FORMS - Trade: powder for soln 0.5% (5 mL).

NOTES - Wait 10 minutes after use before inserting contact lenses.

hydroxypropyl cellulose (*Lacrisert*) ▶Minimal absorption ♀+ ▶+ $$$

ADULT - Moderate-severe dry eyes: One insert in each eye daily. Some patients may require bid use.

PEDS - Not approved in children.

FORMS - Trade only: ocular insert 5 mg.

NOTES - Do not use with soft contact lenses.

petrolatum (*Lacrilube, Dry Eyes, Refresh PM, ✿Duolube*) ▶Minimal absorption ♀A ▶+ $

ADULT, PEDS - Ophthalmic lubricant: Apply ¼-½ inch ointment to inside of lower lid prn.

FORMS - OTC ointment 3.5g tube.

proparacaine (*Ophthaine, Ophthetic, ✿Alcaine*) ▶L ♀C ▶? $

ADULT - Do not prescribe for unsupervised use. Corneal toxicity may occur with repeated use. Local anesthetic: 1-2 gtts before procedure. Repeat q5-10 minutes x 1-3 doses (suture or foreign body removal) or x 5-7 doses (ocular surgery).

PEDS - Not approved in children.

FORMS - Generic/Trade: solution 0.5% (15 mL).

tetracaine (*Pontocaine*) ▶Plasma ♀C ▶? $

ADULT - Do not prescribe for unsupervised use. Corneal toxicity may occur with repeated use. Local anesthetic: 1-2 gtts or ½-1 inch ribbon of ointment before procedure.

PEDS - Not approved in children.

FORMS - Generic/Trade: solution 0.5% (15 mL).

trypan blue (*Vision Blue*) ▶Not absorbed ♀C

▶? $$
ADULT - Aid during ophthalmic surgery by staining anterior capsule: inject into anterior chamber of eye.
PEDS - Not approved in children.
FORMS - Trade: 0.06% ophthalmic solution.

PSYCHIATRY: Antidepressants – Heterocyclic Compounds

NOTE: Gradually taper when discontinuing to avoid withdrawal symptoms. Seizures, orthostatic hypotension, arrhythmias, and anticholinergic side effects may occur. Don't use with MAOIs. Antidepressants increase the risk of suicidal thinking and behavior in children, adolescents, and young adults; carefully weigh the risks and benefits before starting and monitor closely.

amitriptyline (*Elavil*) ▶L ♀D ▶- $$
ADULT - Depression: Start 25-100 mg PO qhs; gradually increase to usual effective dose of 50-300 mg/day.
PEDS - Depression, adolescents: Use adult dosing. Not approved in children <12 yo.
UNAPPROVED ADULT - Migraine prophylaxis and/or chronic pain: 10-100 mg/day. Fibromyalgia: 25-50 mg/day.
UNAPPROVED PEDS - Depression, <12 yo: Start 1 mg/kg/day PO divided tid x 3 days, then increase to 1.5 mg/kg/day. Max 5 mg/kg/day.
FORMS - Generic: Tabs 10, 25, 50, 75, 100,150 mg. Elavil brand name no longer available; retained here for name recognition only.
NOTES - Tricyclic, tertiary amine - primarily inhibits serotonin reuptake. Demethylated to nortriptyline, which primarily inhibits norepinephrine reuptake. Usual therapeutic range is 150-300 ng/ml (amitriptyline + nortriptyline).

amoxapine ▶L ♀C ▶- $$$
ADULT - Rarely used; other drugs preferred. Depression: Start 25-50 mg PO bid-tid; increase by 50-100 mg bid-tid after 1 week. Usual effective dose is 150-400 mg/day. Max 600 mg/day.
PEDS - Not approved in children <16 yo.
FORMS - Generic: Tabs 25, 50, 100, 150 mg.
NOTES - Tetracyclic - primarily inhibits norepinephrine reuptake. Dose ≤300 mg/day may be given once daily at bedtime.

clomipramine (*Anafranil*) ▶L ♀C ▶+ $$$
ADULT - OCD: Start 25 mg PO qhs; gradually increase over 2 weeks to usual effective dose of 150-250 mg/day. Max 250 mg/day.
PEDS - OCD, ≥10 yo: Start 25 mg PO qhs, then increase gradually over 2 weeks to 3 mg/kg/day or 100 mg/day, max 200 mg/day.
UNAPPROVED ADULT - Depression: 100- 250 mg/day. Panic disorder: 12.5- 150 mg/day.

Chronic pain: 100- 250 mg/day.
FORMS - Generic/Trade: Caps 25, 50, 75 mg.
NOTES - Tricyclic, tertiary amine - primarily inhibits serotonin reuptake.

desipramine (*Norpramin*) ▶L ♀C ▶+ $$
ADULT - Depression: Start 25-100 mg PO given once daily or in divided doses. Gradually increase to usual effective dose of 100-200 mg/day, max 300 mg/day.
PEDS - Adolescents: 25-100 mg/day. Not approved in children.
FORMS - Generic/Trade: Tabs 10, 25, 50, 75, 100, 150 mg.
NOTES - Tricyclic, secondary amine - primarily inhibits norepinephrine reuptake. Usual therapeutic range is 125-300 ng/ml. May cause fewer anticholinergic side effects than tertiary amines. Lower doses in adolescents or elderly.

doxepin (*Sinequan*) ▶L ♀C ▶- $$
ADULT - Depression and/or anxiety: Start 75 mg PO qhs. Gradually increase to usual effective dose of 75-150 mg/day, max 300 mg/day.
PEDS - Adolescents: Use adult dosing. Not approved in children <12 yo.
UNAPPROVED ADULT - Chronic pain: 50-300 mg/day. Pruritus: Start 10-25 mg at bedtime. Usual effective dose is 10-100 mg/day.
FORMS - Generic/Trade: Caps 10, 25, 50, 75, 100, 150 mg. Oral concentrate 10 mg/mL.
NOTES - Tricyclic, tertiary amine - primarily inhibits norepinephrine reuptake. Do not mix oral concentrate with carbonated beverages. Some patients with mild symptoms may respond to 25-50 mg/day.

imipramine (*Tofranil, Tofranil PM*) ▶L ♀D ▶- $$$
ADULT - Depression: Start 75-100 mg PO qhs or in divided doses; gradually increase to max 300 mg/day.
PEDS - Not approved for depression if <12 yo. Enuresis ≥6 yo: 10- 25 mg/day PO given 1h before bedtime, then increase in increments of 10-25 mg at 1-2 week intervals not to exceed 50 mg/day in 6-12 yo children or 75 mg/day if >12 yo. Do not exceed 2.5 mg/kg/day.
UNAPPROVED ADULT - Panic disorder: Start 10 mg PO qhs, titrate to usual effective dose of

50-300 mg/day. Enuresis: 25-75 mg PO qhs.
UNAPPROVED PEDS - Depression, children: Start 1.5 mg/kg/day PO divided tid; increase by 1-1.5 mg/kg/day q3-4 days to max 5 mg/kg/d.
FORMS - Generic/Trade: Tabs 10, 25, 50 mg. Trade only: Caps 75, 100, 125, 150 mg (as pamoate salt).
NOTES - Tricyclic, tertiary amine - inhibits serotonin and norepinephrine reuptake. Demethylated to desipramine, which primarily inhibits norepinephrine reuptake.

nortriptyline (*Aventyl, Pamelor*) ▶L ♀D ▶+ $$$
ADULT - Depression: Start 25 mg PO given once daily or divided bid-qid. Gradually increase to usual effective dose of 75-100 mg/day, max 150 mg/day.
PEDS - Not approved in children.
UNAPPROVED ADULT - Panic disorder: Start 25 mg PO qhs, titrate to usual effective dose of 50-150 mg/day. Smoking cessation: Start 25 mg PO daily 14 days prior to quit date. Titrate

to 75 mg/day as tolerated. Continue for ≥6 weeks after quit date.
UNAPPROVED PEDS - Depression 6-12 yo: 1-3 mg/kg/day PO divided tid-qid or 10-20 mg/day PO divided tid-qid.
FORMS - Generic/Trade: Caps 10, 25, 50, 75 mg. Oral Solution 10 mg/5 mL.
NOTES - Tricyclic, secondary amine - primarily inhibits norepinephrine reuptake. Usual therapeutic range is 50-150 ng/ml. May cause fewer anticholinergic side effects than tertiary amines. May be used in combination with nicotine replacement for smoking cessation.

protriptyline (*Vivactil*) ▶L ♀C ▶+ $$$$
ADULT - Depression: 15-40 mg/day PO divided tid-qid. Maximum dose is 60 mg/day.
PEDS - Not approved in children.
FORMS - Trade only: Tabs 5, 10 mg.
NOTES - Tricyclic, secondary amine - primarily inhibits norepinephrine reuptake. May cause fewer anticholinergic side effects than tertiary amines. Dose increases should be in morning.

PSYCHIATRY: Antidepressants – Monoamine Oxidase Inhibitors (MAOIs)

NOTE: May interfere with sleep; avoid qhs dosing. Must be on tyramine-free diet throughout treatment, and for 2 weeks after discontinuation. Numerous drug interactions; risk of hypertensive crisis and serotonin syndrome with many medications, including OTC. Allow ≥2 weeks wash-out when converting from an MAOI to an SSRI (6 weeks after fluoxetine), TCA, or other antidepressant. Contraindicated with carbamazepine or oxcarbazepine. Antidepressants increase the risk of suicidal thinking and behavior in children, adolescents, and young adults; carefully weigh the risks & benefits before starting & monitor closely.

isocarboxazid (*Marplan*) ▶L ♀C ▶? $$$
ADULT - Depression: Start 10 mg PO bid; increase by 10 mg q2-4 days. Usual effective dose is 20- 40 mg/day. Max 60 mg/day divided bid-qid.
PEDS - Not approved in children <16 yo.
FORMS - Trade only: Tabs 10 mg.
NOTES - Requires MAOI diet.

moclobemide (✣*Manerix*) ▶L ♀C ▶- $$
ADULT - Canada only. Depression: Start 300 mg/day PO divided bid after meals. May increase after 1 week to max 600 mg/day.
PEDS - Not approved in children.
FORMS - Generic/Trade: Tabs 150, 300 mg. Generic only: Tabs 100 mg.

NOTES - No dietary restrictions. Don't use with tricyclic antidepressants; use caution with conventional MAOIs, other antidepressants, epinephrine, thioridazine, sympathomimetics, dextromethorphan, meperidine, and other opiates. Reduce dose in severe hepatic dysfunction.

phenelzine (*Nardil*) ▶L ♀C ▶? $$$
ADULT - Depression: Start 15 mg PO tid. Usual effective dose 60-90 mg/day in divided doses.
PEDS - Not approved in children <16 yo.
FORMS - Trade only: Tabs 15 mg.
NOTES - Requires MAOI diet. May increase insulin sensitivity. Don't use with meperidine.

selegiline (*Emsam*) ▶L ♀C ▶? $$$$$
ADULT - Depression: start 6 mg/24hr patch q 24 hr. Adjust in ≥2 wk intervals to max 12 mg/day.
PEDS - Not approved in children.
FORMS - Trade only: Transdermal patch 6 mg/24hr, 9 mg/24hr, 12 mg/24hr.
NOTES - MAOI diet if ≥9 mg/24 hours.

tranylcypromine (*Parnate*) ▶L ♀C ▶- $$
ADULT - Depression: Start 10 mg PO qam; increase by 10 mg/day at 1-3 week intervals to usual effective dose of 10-40 mg/day divided bid. Max 60 mg/day.
PEDS - Not approved in children <16 yo.
FORMS - Generic/Trade: Tabs 10 mg.
NOTES - Requires MAOI diet.

PSYCHIATRY: Antidepressants – Selective Serotonin Reuptake Inhibitors (SSRIs)

NOTE: Gradually taper when discontinuing to avoid withdrawal symptoms. Observe for worsening depression or the emergence of suicidality, anxiety, agitation, panic attacks, insomnia, irritability, hostility, impulsivity, akathisia, mania, or hypomania, particularly early in therapy or after increases in dose. Antidepressants increase the risk of suicidal thinking and behavior in children, adolescents, and young adults; carefully weigh the risks and benefits before starting treatment and then monitor closely. Use during the third trimester of pregnancy has been associated with neonatal complications including respiratory (including persistent pulmonary hypertension), gastrointestinal, & feeding problems, as well as seizures and withdrawal symptoms. Balance these risks against those of withdrawal and depression for the mother. Paroxetine should be avoided throughout pregnancy. Don't use sibutramine with SSRIs. Increased risk of gastrointestinal bleeding; caution when combined with NSAIDs or aspirin. Use cautiously and observe closely for serotonin syndrome if SSRI is used with a triptan.

citalopram (Celexa) ▶LK ♀C but - in 3rd trimester ▶- $$$

ADULT - Depression: Start 20 mg PO daily; increase by 20 mg/day at >1 week intervals. Usual effective dose is 20-40 mg/day, max 60 mg/day.

PEDS - Not approved in children.

FORMS - Generic/Trade: Tabs 10, 20, 40 mg. Oral solution 10 mg/5 mL. Generic only: Oral disintegrating tab 10, 20, 40 mg.

NOTES - Don't use with MAOIs or tryptophan.

escitalopram (Lexapro, ♥Cipralex) ▶LK ♀C but - in 3rd trimester ▶- $$$

ADULT - Depression, generalized anxiety disorder: Start 10 mg PO daily; may increase to max 20 mg PO daily after >1 week.

PEDS - Not approved in children.

UNAPPROVED ADULT - Social anxiety disorder: 5-20 mg PO daily.

FORMS - Trade only: Tabs 5, 10, 20 mg (10 & 20 mg scored), Oral solution 1 mg/mL.

NOTES - Don't use with MAOIs. Doses >20 mg daily are not superior to 10 mg daily. Escitalopram is the active isomer of citalopram.

fluoxetine (Prozac, Prozac Weekly, Sarafem) ▶L ♀C but - in 3rd trimester ▶- $$$

ADULT - Depression, OCD: Start 20 mg PO q am; may increase after several weeks to usual effective dose of 20-40 mg/day, max 80 mg/day. Depression, maintenance therapy: 20-40 mg/day (standard-release) or 90 mg PO once weekly (Prozac Weekly) starting 7 days after last standard-release dose. Bulimia: 60 mg PO qam; may need to titrate up to this dose slowly over several days. Panic disorder: Start 10 mg PO q am; titrate to 20 mg/day after one week, max 60 mg/day. Premenstrual Dysphoric Disorder (Sarafem): 20 mg PO daily given continuously throughout the menstrual cycle (continuous dosing) or 20 mg PO daily for 14 days prior to menses (intermittent dosing); max 80 mg daily. Doses >20 mg/day can be divided bid (q am and q noon).

PEDS - Depression 7-17 yo: 10-20 mg PO q am (10 mg for smaller children), max 20 mg/day. OCD: Start 10 mg PO q am; max 60 mg/day (30 mg/day for smaller children).

UNAPPROVED ADULT - Hot flashes: 20 mg PO daily. Post-traumatic stress disorder: 20-80 mg PO daily. Social anxiety disorder: 10-60 mg PO daily.

FORMS - Generic/Trade: Tabs 10 mg. Caps 10, 20, 40 mg. Oral solution 20 mg/5 mL. Trade only: Caps (Sarafem) 10, 15, 20 mg. Caps, delayed-release (Prozac Weekly) 90 mg. Generic only: Tabs 20, 40 mg.

NOTES - Half-life of parent is 1-3 days and for active metabolite norfluoxetine is 6-14 days. Don't use with thioridazine, MAOIs, cisapride, or tryptophan; use caution with lithium, phenytoin, TCAs, and warfarin. Pregnancy exposure has been associated with premature delivery, low birth weight, and lower Apgar scores. Decrease dose with liver disease. Increases risk of mania with bipolar disorder.

fluvoxamine (♥Luvox) ▶L ♀C but - in 3rd trimester ▶- $$$$

ADULT - OCD: Start 50 mg PO qhs, then increase by 50 mg/day q4-7 days to usual effective dose of 100-300 mg/day divided bid. Max 300 mg/day.

PEDS - OCD (≥8 yo): Start 25 mg PO qhs; increase by 25 mg/day q4-7 days to usual effective dose of 50-200 mg/day divided bid. Max 200 mg/day (8-11 yo) or 300 mg/day (>11 yo). Therapeutic effect may be seen with lower doses in girls.

FORMS - Generic only: Tabs 25, 50, 100 mg.
NOTES - Don't use with thioridazine, pimozide, alosetron, cisapride, tizanidine, tryptophan, or MAOIs; use caution with benzodiazepines, theophylline, TCAs, and warfarin. Luvox brand not currently on US market.

paroxetine (*Paxil, Paxil CR, Pexeva*) ▶LK ♀D ▶? $$$

ADULT - Depression: Start 20 mg PO qam; increase by 10 mg/day at intervals ≥1 week to usual effective dose of 20-50 mg/day, max 50 mg/day. Depression, controlled-release tabs: Start 25 mg PO qam; may increase by 12.5 mg/day at intervals ≥1 week to usual effective dose of 25-62.5 mg/day; max 62.5 mg/day. OCD: Start 20 mg PO qam; increase by 10 mg/day at intervals ≥1 week to usual recommended dose of 40 mg/day; max 60 mg/day. Panic disorder: Start 10 mg PO qam; increase by 10 mg/day at intervals ≥1 week to target dose of 40 mg/day; max 60 mg/day. Panic disorder, controlled-release tabs: start 12.5 mg/day; increase by 12.5 mg/day at intervals ≥1 week to usual effective dose of 12.5-75 mg/day; max 75 mg/day. Social anxiety disorder: Start 20 mg PO qam (which is the usual effective dose); max 60 mg/day. Social anxiety disorder, controlled-release tabs: Start 12.5 mg PO qam; may increase at intervals ≥1 week to max 37.5 mg/day. Generalized anxiety disorder: Start 20 mg PO qam (which is the usual effective dose); max 50 mg/day. Post-traumatic stress disorder: Start 20 mg PO qam; usual effective dose is 20-40 mg/day; max 50 mg/day. Premenstrual dysphoric disorder (PMDD), continuous dosing: Start 12.5 mg PO qam (controlled-release tabs); may increase dose after 1 wk to max 25 mg qam. PMDD, intermittent dosing (given for 2 weeks prior to menses): Start 12.5 mg PO qam (controlled-release tabs), max 25 mg/day.
PEDS - Not recommended for use in children or adolescents due to increased risk of suicidality.
UNAPPROVED ADULT - Hot flashes related to menopause or breast cancer: 20 mg PO daily (tabs), or 12.5-25 mg PO daily (controlled-release tabs).

FORMS - Generic/Trade: Tabs 10, 20, 30, 40 mg. Oral susp 10 mg/5 mL. Controlled-release tabs 12.5, 25 mg. Trade: (Paxil CR) 37.5 mg.
NOTES - Start at 10 mg/day and do not exceed 40 mg/day in elderly or debilitated or those with renal or hepatic impairment. Paroxetine is an inhibitor of CYP2D6, and is contraindicated with thioridazine, pimozide, MAOIs, and tryptophan; use caution with barbiturates, cimetidine, phenytoin, theophylline, TCAs, risperidone, atomoxetine, and warfarin. Taper gradually after long-term use; reduce by 10 mg/day q week to 20 mg/day; continue for 1 week at this dose, and then stop. If withdrawal symptoms develop, then restart at prior dose and taper more slowly. Pexeva is paroxetine mesylate and is a generic equivalent for paroxetine HCl.

sertraline (*Zoloft*) ▶LK ♀C but - in 3rd trimester ▶+ $$$

ADULT - Depression, OCD: Start 50 mg PO daily; may increase after 1 week. Usual effective dose is 50-200 mg/day, max 200 mg/day. Panic disorder, post-traumatic stress disorder, social anxiety disorder: Start 25 mg PO daily; may increase after 1 week to 50 mg PO daily. Usual effective dose is 50-200 mg/day; max 200 mg/day. Premenstrual dysphoric disorder (PMDD), continuous dosing: Start 50 mg PO daily; max 150 mg/day. PMDD, intermittent dosing (given for 14 days prior to menses): Start 50 mg PO daily x 3 days, then increase to max 100 mg/day.
PEDS - OCD, 6-12 yo: Start 25 mg PO daily, max 200 mg/day. OCD, ≥13 yo: Adult dosing.
UNAPPROVED PEDS - Major depressive disorder: Start 25 mg PO daily; usual effective dose is 50-200 mg/day.
FORMS - Generic/Trade: Tabs 25, 50, 100 mg. Oral concentrate 20 mg/mL.
NOTES - Don't use with cisapride, tryptophan, or MAOIs; use caution with cimetidine, warfarin, pimozide, or TCAs. Must dilute oral concentrate before administration. Administration during pregnancy has been associated with premature delivery, low birth weight, and lower Apgar scores.

PSYCHIATRY: Antidepressants – Serotonin-Norepinephrine Reuptake Inhibitors (SNRIs)

NOTE: Monitor for the emergence of anxiety, agitation, panic attacks, insomnia, irritability, hostility, impulsivity, akathisia, mania, or hypomania, and for worsening depression or the emergence of suicidality, particularly early in therapy or after increases in dose. Antidepressants increase the risk of suicidal thinking and behavior in children, adolescents, and young adults; carefully weigh the risks and benefits before starting treatment, and then monitor closely.

duloxetine (Cymbalta) ▶L ♀C ▶? $$$$
ADULT - Depression: 20 mg PO bid; max 60 mg/day given once daily or divided bid. Generalized anxiety disorder: Start 30-60 mg PO daily, max 120 mg/d. Diabetic peripheral neuropathic pain: 60 mg PO daily, max 60 mg/day.
PEDS - Not approved in children.
FORMS - Trade only: Caps 20, 30, 60 mg.
NOTES - Avoid in renal insufficiency (CrCl <30 ml/min), hepatic insufficiency, or substantial alcohol use. Don't use with thioridazine, MAOIs, or potent inhibitors of CYP1A2; use caution with inhibitors of CYP2D6. Small BP increases (2 mmHg systolic, 0.5 mmHg diastolic) have been observed. Exposure during the third trimester of pregnancy has been associated with neonatal complications including respiratory, gastrointestinal, and feeding problems, as well as seizures, and withdrawal symptoms; balance these risks against those of withdrawal and depression for the mother.

venlafaxine (Effexor, Effexor XR) ▶LK ♀C but - in 3rd trimester ▶? $$$$
ADULT - Depression: Start 37.5-75 mg PO daily (Effexor XR) or 75 mg/day divided bid-tid (Effexor). Increase in 75 mg increments q4 days to usual effective dose of 150-225 mg/day, max 225 mg/day (Effexor XR) or 375 mg/day (Effexor). Generalized anxiety disorder or social anxiety disorder: Start 37.5-75 mg PO daily (Effexor XR); increase in 75 mg increments q4 days to max 225 mg/day. Panic disorder: Start 37.5 mg daily (Effexor XR), may titrate by 75 mg/day at weekly intervals to max 225 mg/day.
PEDS - Not approved in children. May increase the risk of suicidality in children and teenagers.
UNAPPROVED ADULT - Hot flashes (primarily in cancer patients): 37.5-75 mg/day of the extended-release form.
FORMS - Trade only: Caps, extended release 37.5, 75, 150 mg. Generic/Trade: Tabs 25, 37.5, 50, 75, 100 mg.
NOTES - Non-cyclic, serotonin-norepinephrine reuptake inhibitor. Decrease dose in renal or hepatic impairment. Monitor for increases in BP. Don't give with MAOIs; caution with cimetidine, haloperidol. Use caution and monitor for serotonin syndrome if used with triptans. Gradually taper when discontinuing to avoid withdrawal symptoms after prolonged use. Hostility, suicidal ideation, and self-harm have been reported when used in children. Exposure during the third trimester of pregnancy has been associated with neonatal complications including respiratory, gastrointestinal, and feeding problems, as well as seizures and withdrawal symptoms. Balance these risks against those of withdrawal and depression for the mother. Mydriasis and increased intraocular pressure can occur; use caution in glaucoma.

PSYCHIATRY: Antidepressants – Other

NOTE: Monitor for the emergence of anxiety, agitation, panic attacks, insomnia, irritability, hostility, impulsivity, akathisia, mania, or hypomania, and for worsening depression or the emergence of suicidality, particularly early in therapy or after increases in dose. Antidepressants increase the risk of suicidal thinking and behavior in children, adolescents, and young adults; carefully weigh the risks and benefits before starting treatment, and then monitor closely.

bupropion (Wellbutrin, Wellbutrin SR, Wellbutrin XL, Zyban, Buproban) ▶LK ♀C ▶- $$$$
ADULT - Depression: Start 100 mg PO bid (immediate-release tabs); can increase to 100 mg tid after 4-7 days. Usual effective dose is 300-450 mg/day, max 150 mg/dose and 450 mg/day. Depression, sustained-release tabs (Wellbutrin SR): Start 150 mg PO q am; may increase to 150 mg bid after 4-7 days, max 400 mg/day. Give the last dose no later than 5 pm. Depression, extended-release tabs (Wellbutrin XL): Start 150 mg PO q am; may increase to 300 mg q am after 4 days, max 450 mg q am. Seasonal affective disorder, extended-release tabs (Wellbutrin XL): Start 150 mg PO q am in autumn; may increase after 1 week to target dose of 300 mg q am, max 300 mg/day. In the spring, decrease to 150 mg/day for 2 weeks and then discontinue. Smoking cessation (Zyban, Buproban): Start 150 mg PO qam x 3 days, then increase to 150 mg PO bid x 7-12 wks. Allow 8 h between doses, with the last dose given no later than 5 pm. Max 150 mg PO bid. Target quit date should be after >1 week of therapy. Stop if there is no progress towards

abstinence by the 7th week. Write "dispense behavioral modification kit" on first script.

PEDS - Not approved in children.

UNAPPROVED ADULT - ADHD: 150-450 mg/day PO.

UNAPPROVED PEDS - ADHD: 1.4-5.7 mg/kg/day PO.

FORMS - Generic/Trade (for depression): Tabs 75,100 mg. Sustained release tabs 100, 150, 200 mg. Extended-release tabs 150, 300 mg (Wellbutrin XL). Generic/Trade (smoking cessation): Sustained-release tabs 150 mg (Zyban, Buproban).

NOTES - Weak inhibitor of dopamine reuptake. Don't use with MAOIs. Seizures occur in 0.4% taking 300-450 mg per day. Contraindicated in seizure or eating disorders, or with abrupt alcohol/sedative withdrawal. Wellbutrin SR, Zyban, and Buproban are all the same formulation.

mirtazapine (*Remeron, Remeron SolTab*) ►LK ♀C ▶? $$

ADULT - Depression: Start 15 mg PO qhs, increase after 1-2 weeks to usual effective dose of 15-45 mg/day.

PEDS - Not approved in children.

FORMS - Generic/Trade: Tabs 15, 30, 45 mg. Tabs, orally disintegrating (SolTab) 15, 30, 45 mg. Generic: Tabs 7.5 mg.

NOTES - 0.1% risk of agranulocytosis. May cause drowsiness, increased appetite, and weight gain. Don't use with MAOIs.

nefazodone ►L ♀C ▶? $$$

WARNING - Rare reports of life-threatening liver failure. Discontinue if evidence of liver dysfunction. Brand name product withdrawn from the market in USA and Canada.

ADULT - Depression: Start 100 mg PO bid. Increase by 100-200 mg/day at ≥1 week intervals to usual effective dose of 150-300 mg PO bid, max 600 mg/day. Start 50 mg PO bid in elderly or debilitated patients.

PEDS - Not approved in children.

FORMS - Generic only: Tabs 50, 100, 150, 200, 250 mg.

NOTES - Don't use with cisapride, MAOIs, pimozide, or triazolam; use caution with alprazolam. Many other drug interactions.

trazodone ►L ♀C ▶- $$$$

ADULT - Depression: Start 50-150 mg/day PO in divided doses, increase by 50 mg/day q3-4 days. Usual effective dose is 400-600 mg/day.

PEDS - Not approved in children.

UNAPPROVED ADULT - Insomnia: 50-100 mg PO qhs, max 150 mg/day.

UNAPPROVED PEDS - Depression, 6-18 yo: Start 1.5-2 mg/kg/day PO divided bid-tid; may increase q3-4 days to max 6 mg/kg/day.

FORMS - Generic: Tabs 50, 100, 150, 300 mg.

NOTES - May cause priapism. Rarely used as monotherapy for depression; most often used as a sleep aid and adjunct to another antidepressant. Use caution with CYP3A4 inhibitors or inducers.

tryptophan (♥*Tryptan*) ►K ♀? ▶? $$

ADULT - Canada only. Adjunct to antidepressant treatment for affective disorders: 8-12 g/day in 3-4 divided doses.

PEDS - Not indicated.

FORMS - Trade only: L-tryptophan tabs 250, 500, 750, 1000 mg.

NOTES - Caution in diabetics; may worsen glycemic control.

PSYCHIATRY: Antimanic (Bipolar) Agents

lamotrigine (*Lamictal, Lamictal CD*) ►LK ♀C (see notes) ▶- $$$$

WARNING - Potentially life-threatening rashes (eg, Stevens-Johnson Syndrome, toxic epidermal necrolysis) have been reported in 0.3% of adults and 0.8% of children, usually within 2-8 weeks of initiation; discontinue at first sign of rash. Drug interaction with valproate – see adjusted dosing guidelines.

ADULT - Bipolar disorder (maintenance): Start 25 mg PO daily, 50 mg PO daily if on carbamazepine or other enzyme-inducing drugs, or 25 mg PO qod if on valproate. Increase for weeks 3-4 to 50 mg/day, 50 mg bid if on en-zyme-inducing drugs, or 25 mg/day if on valproate, then adjust over weeks 5-7 to target doses of 200 mg/day, 400 mg/day divided bid if on enzyme-inducing drugs, or 100 mg/day if on valproate. See neurology section for epilepsy dosing.

PEDS - Not approved in children.

FORMS - Generic/Trade: Chewable dispersible tabs 5, 25 mg. Trade only: Tabs 25, 100, 150, 200 mg.

NOTES - Drug interactions with valproate and enzyme-inducing antiepileptic drugs (ie, carbamazepine, phenobarbital, phenytoin, primidone); may need to adjust dose. May increase carbamazepine toxicity. Preliminary evidence suggests that exposure during the first trimester of pregnancy is associated with a risk for cleft palate and/or cleft lip. Please report all fetal exposure to the Lamotrigine Pregnancy Registry (800-336-2176) and the North American Antiepileptic Drug Pregnancy Registry (888-233-2334).

lithium (*Eskalith, Eskalith CR, Lithobid,* ♥*Lithane*) ▶K ♀D ▶- $

WARNING - Lithium toxicity can occur at therapeutic levels.

ADULT - Acute mania: Start 300-600 mg PO bid-tid; usual effective dose is 900-1,800 mg/day. Bipolar maintenance usually 900-1,200 mg/day titrated to therapeutic trough level of 0.6-1.2 mEq/L.

PEDS - Adolescents ≥12 yo: Use adult dosing.

UNAPPROVED PEDS - Mania (<12 yo): Start 15-60 mg/kg/day PO divided tid-qid. Adjust weekly to achieve therapeutic levels.

FORMS - Generic/Trade: Caps 300, Extended release tabs 300, 450 mg. Generic only: Caps 150, 600 mg, Tabs 300 mg, Syrup 300/5 mL.

NOTES - Steady state levels occur in 5 days (later in elderly or renally-impaired patients). Usual therapeutic trough levels are 1.0-1.5 mEq/L (acute mania) or 0.6-1.2 mEq/L (maintenance). 300 mg = 8 mEq or mmol. A dose increase of 300 mg/day will increase the level by approx 0.2 mEq/L. Monitor renal and thyroid function, avoid dehydration or salt restriction, and watch closely for polydipsia or polyuria. Diuretics, ACE inhibitors, angiotensin receptor blockers, and NSAIDs may increase lithium levels (ASA & sulindac OK). Dose-related side effects (e.g. tremor, GI upset) may improve by dividing doses tid-qid or using extended-release tabs. Monitor renal function and electrolytes.

topiramate (*Topamax*) ▶K ♀C ▶? $$$$$

ADULT - See neurology section

PEDS - Not approved for psychiatric use in children; see Neurology section.

UNAPPROVED ADULT - Bipolar disorder: Start 25-50 mg/day PO; titrate prn to max 400 mg/day divided bid. Alcohol dependence: Start 25 mg/day PO; titrate weekly to max 150 mg bid.

FORMS - Trade only: Tabs 25, 50, 100, 200 mg. Sprinkle caps 15, 25 mg.

NOTES - Give ½ usual adult dose to patients with renal impairment (CrCl <70 ml/ min). Cognitive symptoms, confusion, renal stones, glaucoma, and weight loss may occur. Risk of oligohidrosis and hyperthermia, particularly in children; use caution in warm ambient temperatures and/or with vigorous physical activity. Hyperchloremic, non-anion gap metabolic acidosis may occur; monitor serum bicarbonate and reduce dose or taper off if this occurs.

valproic acid (*Depakote, Depakote ER, divalproex,* ♥*Epiject, Epival, Deproic*) ▶L ♀D ▶+ $$$$

WARNING - Fatal hepatic failure has occurred, especially in children <2 yo with multiple anticonvulsants and co-morbidities. Monitor LFTs frequently during first 6 months. Life-threatening pancreatitis has been reported after initial or prolonged use. Evaluate for abdominal pain, N/V, and/or anorexia and discontinue if pancreatitis occurs. May be more teratogenic than other anticonvulsants (eg, carbamazepine, lamotrigine, and phenytoin). Hepatic failure and clotting disorders have also occurred when used during pregnancy.

ADULT - Mania: Start 250 mg PO tid (Depakote) or 25 mg/kg once daily (Depakote ER); titrate to therapeutic level. Max 60 mg/kg/day.

PEDS - Not approved for mania in children.

UNAPPROVED PEDS - Bipolar disorder, manic or mixed phase (>2 yo): Start 125-250 mg PO bid or 15 mg/kg/day in divided doses. Titrate to therapeutic trough level of 45-125 mcg/ml, max 60 mg/kg/day.

FORMS - Generic/Trade: Caps 250mg (Depakene), syrup (Depakene, valproic acid) 250 mg/5 mL. Trade only (Depakote): Caps, sprinkle 125 mg, delayed release tabs 125, 250, 500 mg; extended release tabs (Depakote ER) 250, 500mg.

NOTES - Contraindicated in urea cycle disorders or hepatic dysfunction. Reduce dose in the elderly. Recommended therapeutic trough level is 50-125 mcg/ml for Depakote and 85-125 mcg/ml for Depakote ER, though higher levels have been used. Many drug interactions. Hyperammonemia, GI irritation, or thrombocytopenia may occur. Depakote ER is about 10% less bioavailable than Depakote. Depakote releases divalproex sodium over 8-12h (daily-qid dosing) and Depakote ER releases divalproex sodium over 18-24h (daily dosing).

PSYCHIATRY: Antipsychotics – First Generation (Typical)

NOTE: Antipsychotic potency is determined by D2 receptor affinity. Extrapyramidal side effects (EPS) including tardive dyskinesia may occur. High potency agents are more likely to cause EPS and hyperprolactinemia. Can be given in qhs doses, but may be divided initially to decrease side effects and increase daytime sedation. Antipsychotics have been associated with an increased risk of venous thromboembolism, especially early in therapy. Assess for other risk factors and monitor carefully.

chlorpromazine (*Thorazine*) ▶LK ♀C ▶- $$$
ADULT - Psychotic disorders: 10-50 mg PO bid-qid or 25-50 mg IM, can repeat in 1 hour. Severe cases may require 400 mg IM q4-6h up to max of 2,000 mg/day IM. Hiccups: 25-50 mg PO/IM tid-qid. Persistent hiccups may require 25-50 mg in 0.5-1 L NS by slow IV infusion.
PEDS - Severe behavioral problems/ psychotic disorders age 6 months-12 yo: 0.5 mg/kg PO q4-6h prn or 1 mg/kg PR q6-8h prn or 0.5 mg/kg IM q6-8h prn.
FORMS - Generic only: Tabs 10, 25, 50, 100, 200 mg. Generic/Trade: Oral concentrate 30 mg/mL, 100 mg/mL. Trade only: Syrup 10 mg/5 mL. Suppositories 25, 100 mg.
NOTES - Monitor for hypotension if IM/IV use.

flupenthixol (✤*Fluanxol, Fluanxol Depot*) ▶? ♀? ▶- $$
ADULT - Canada only. Schizophrenia/psychosis: Tablets: Start 3 mg PO daily in divided doses, maintenance 3-12 mg daily in divided doses. IM initial dose 5-20 mg IM q2-4 weeks, maintenance 20-40 mg q 2-4 weeks. Higher doses may be necessary in some patients.
PEDS - Not approved in children.
FORMS - Trade only: tabs 0.5, 3 mg.
NOTES - Relatively non-sedating antipsychotic.

fluphenazine (*Prolixin*, ✤*Modecate, Modeten*) ▶LK ♀C ▶ $$$
ADULT - Psychotic disorders: Start 0.5-10 mg/day PO divided q6-8h. Usual effective dose 1-20 mg/day. Maximum dose is 40 mg/day PO or 1.25-10 mg/day IM divided q6-8h. Maximum dose is 10 mg/day IM. May use long-acting formulations (enanthate/ decanoate) when patients are stabilized on a fixed daily dose. Approximate conversion ratio: 12.5- 25 mg IM/ SC (depot) q3 weeks = 10- 20 mg/day PO.
PEDS - Not approved in children.
FORMS - Generic/Trade: Tabs 1, 2.5, 5, 10 mg.

Elixir 2.5 mg/5 mL. Oral concentrate 5 mg/mL.
NOTES - Do not mix oral concentrate with coffee, tea, cola, or apple juice.

haloperidol (*Haldol*) ▶LK ♀C ▶- $$
ADULT - Psychotic disorders/ Tourette's: 0.5- 5 mg PO bid-tid. Usual effective dose is 6-20 mg/day, maximum dose = 100 mg/day or 2-5 mg IM q1-8h prn. May use long-acting (depot) formulation when stabilized on a fixed daily dose. Approximate conversion ratio: 100- 200 mg IM (depot) q4 weeks = 10 mg/day PO haloperidol.
PEDS - Psychotic disorders, 3-12 yo: 0.05- 0.15 mg/kg/day PO divided bid-tid. Tourette's or non-psychotic behavior disorders, 3-12 yo: 0.05-0.075 mg/kg/day PO divided bid-tid. Increase by 0.5 mg q week to maximum dose of 6 mg/day. Not approved for IM route in children.
UNAPPROVED ADULT - Acute psychoses and combative behavior: 5-10 mg IV/IM, repeat prn in 10-30 min.
UNAPPROVED PEDS - Psychosis 6-12 yo: 1-3 mg/dose IM q4-8h, max 0.15 mg/kg/day.
FORMS - Generic only: Tabs 0.5, 1, 2, 5, 10, 20 mg. Oral concentrate 2 mg/mL.
NOTES - Therapeutic range is 2- 15 ng/mL.

loxapine (*Loxitane*, ✤*Loxapac*) ▶LK ♀C ▶- $$$$
ADULT - Psychotic disorders: Start 10 mg PO bid, usual effective dose is 60-100 mg/day divided bid- qid. Maximum dose is 250 mg/day.
PEDS - Not approved in children.
FORMS - Generic/Trade: Caps 5,10, 25, 50 mg.

methotrimeprazine (✤*Nozinan*) ▶L ♀? ▶? $
ADULT - Canada only. Anxiety/analgesia: 6-25 mg PO per day given tid. Sedation: 10-25 mg hs. Psychoses/intense pain: Start 50-75 mg PO per day given in 2-3 doses, max 1000 mg/day. Postoperative pain: 20-40 mg PO or 10-25 mg IM q 8h. Anesthesia premedication: 10-25 mg IM or 20-40 mg PO q 8h with last dose of 25-50 mg IM 1h before surgery. Limit therapy to ≤30 days.
PEDS - Canada only. 0.25 mg/kg/day given in 2-3 doses, max 40 mg/day for child <12 yo.
FORMS - Canada only - Generic/Trade: Tabs 2, 5, 25, 50 mg.

molindone (*Moban*) ▶LK ♀C ▶? $$$$$
ADULT - Psychotic disorders: Start 50-75 mg/day PO divided tid- qid, usual effective dose is 50-100 mg/day. Maximum dose is 225 mg/day.
PEDS - >12 yo: Adult dosing.

FORMS - Trade only: Tabs 5,10,25,50 mg.

perphenazine ▸LK ♀C ▸? $$$
ADULT - Psychotic disorders: Start 4-8 mg PO tid or 8-16 mg PO bid-qid (hospitalized patients), maximum PO dose is 64 mg/day. Can give 5-10 mg IM q6h, max IM dose 30 mg/day.
PEDS - Not approved for children <12 yo.
FORMS - Generic only: Tabs 2, 4, 8, 16 mg. Oral concentrate 16 mg/5 mL.
NOTES - Do not mix oral concentrate with coffee, tea, cola, or apple juice.

pimozide (*Orap*) ▸L ♀C ▸- $$$
ADULT - Tourette's: Start 1-2 mg/day PO in divided doses, increase q2 days to usual effective dose of 1-10 mg/day. Maximum dose is 0.2 mg/kg/day up to 10 mg/day.
PEDS - Tourette's age >12 yo: 0.05 mg/kg PO qhs, increase q3 days to maximum of 0.2 mg/kg/day up to 10 mg/day.
FORMS - Trade only: Tabs 1, 2 mg.
NOTES - QT prolongation may occur. Monitor ECG at baseline and periodically throughout therapy. Contraindicated with macrolide antibiotics, nefazodone, and sertraline. Use caution with inhibitors of CYP3A4.

thioridazine (*Mellaril*, ✤*Rideril*) ▸LK ♀C ▸? $$
WARNING - Can cause QTc prolongation, torsade de pointes, and sudden death.
ADULT - Psychotic disorders: Start 50-100 mg PO tid, usual effective dose is 200-800 mg/day divided bid-qid. Maximum dose is 800 mg/day.
PEDS - Behavioral disorders 2- 12 yo: 10- 25 mg PO bid-tid, maximum dose is 3 mg/kg/day.
FORMS - Generic: Tabs 10, 15, 25, 50, 100, 150, 200 mg. Oral concentrate 30, 100 mg/mL.
NOTES - Not recommended as first-line therapy. Contraindicated with a history of cardiac arrhythmias, long QT syndrome, or when taking fluvoxamine, propranolol, pindolol, drugs that inhibit CYP 2D6 (e.g. fluoxetine, paroxetine), and other drugs that prolong the QTc interval. Only use for patients with schizophrenia who do not respond to other antipsychotics. Monitor baseline ECG and potassium. Pigmentary retinopathy with doses >800 mg/day.

thiothixene (*Navane*) ▸LK ♀C ▸? $$$
ADULT - Psychotic disorders: Start 2 mg PO tid. Usual effective dose is 20-30 mg/day, maximum dose is 60 mg/day PO.
PEDS - >12 yo: Adult dosing.
FORMS - Generic/Trade: Caps 1, 2, 5, 10. Oral concentrate 5 mg/mL. Trade only: Caps 20 mg.

trifluoperazine (*Stelazine*) ▸LK ♀C ▸- $$$
ADULT - Psychotic disorders: Start 2-5 mg PO bid. Usual effective dose is 15-20 mg/day, some may require ≥40 mg/day. Anxiety: 1-2 mg PO bid for up to 12 weeks. Maximum dose is 6 mg/day.
PEDS - Psychotic disorders 6-12 yo: 1 mg PO daily-bid, gradually increase to maximum dose of 15 mg/day.
FORMS - Generic/Trade: Tabs 1, 2, 5, 10 mg. Trade only: Oral concentrate 10 mg/mL.
NOTES - Dilute oral concentrate before giving.

zuclopenthixol (✤*Clopixol, Clopixol Accuphase, Clopixol Depot*) ▸L ♀? ▸? $$$$
ADULT - Canada only. Tabs: Start 10-50 mg PO daily, maintenance 20-60 mg daily. Injectable: Accuphase (acetate) 50-150 mg IM q2-3 days, Depot (decanoate) 150-300 mg IM q2-4 weeks.
PEDS - Not approved in children.
FORMS - Trade, Canada-only: Tab 10, 20 mg (Clopixol).

PSYCHIATRY: Antipsychotics – Second Generation (Atypical)

NOTE: Tardive dyskinesia, neuroleptic malignant syndrome, drug-induced parkinsonism, and other extrapyramidal side effects may occur. Atypical antipsychotics have been associated with weight gain, dyslipidemia, hyperglycemia, diabetes mellitus; monitor closely. Off-label use for dementia-related psychosis in the elderly has been associated with increased mortality. Antipsychotics have been associated with an increased risk of venous thromboembolism, particularly early in therapy; assess for other risk factors & monitor.

aripiprazole (*Abilify, Abilify Discmelt*) ▸L ♀C ▸? $$$$$
ADULT - Schizophrenia: Start 10-15 mg PO daily. Max 30 mg daily. Bipolar disorder (acute and maintenance for manic or mixed episodes): Start 30 mg PO daily; reduce dose to 15 mg/day if higher dose poorly tolerated. Agitation associated with schizophrenia or bipolar disorder: 9.75 mg IM recommended. May consider 5.25 to 15 mg if indicated. May repeat in >2 hrs up to max 30 mg/day.
PEDS - Not approved in children.
FORMS - Trade only: Tabs 2,5,10,15,20,30 mg. Oral solution 1 mg/mL (150 mL). Orally disintegrating tabs (Discmelt) 10, 15, 20, 30 mg.

ANTIPSYCHOTIC RELATIVE ADVERSE EFFECTS[a]

Antipsychotic	Anti-cholinergic	Sedation	Hypoten-sion	EPS[b]	Weight gain	DM / ↑ glucose	Dyslipi-demia
First Generation							
chlorpromazine	+++	+++	++	++	++	?	?
fluphenazine	++	+	+	++++	++	?	?
haloperidol	+	+	+	++++	++	0	?
loxapine	++	+	+	++	+	?	?
molindone	++	++	+	++	+	?	?
perphenazine	++	++	+	++	+	+/?	?
pimozide	+	+	+	+++	?	?	?
thioridazine	++++	+++	+++	+	+++	+/?	?
thiothixene	+	++	++	+++	++	?	?
trifluoperazine	++	+	+	+++	++	?	?
Second Generation							
aripiprazole[c]	++	+	0	0	0/+	0	0
clozapine	++++	+++	+++	0	+++	+	+
olanzapine	+++	++	+	0[b]	+++	+	+
risperidone	+	++	+	+[b]	++	?	?
quetiapine	+	+++	++	0	++	?	?
ziprasidone	+	+	0	0	0/+	0	0

a. Risk: 0 (absent) to ++++ (high). ? = Limited or inconsistent comparative data. DM = diabetes. References: Goodman & Gilman 11e p461-500, Applied Therapeutics 8e p78, APA schizophrenia practice guideline, Psychiatry Q 2002; 73:297, Diabetes Care 2004; 27:596. **b.** EPS (extrapyramidal symptoms) are dose-related and are more likely for risperidone >6-8 mg/day / olanzapine >20 mg/day. Akathisia risk remains unclear and may not be reflected in these ratings. **c.** Limited comparative data to other second generation antipsychotics.

NOTES - Low EPS and tardive dyskinesia risk. Increase dose when used with CYP3A4 inducers such as carbamazepine. Decrease usual dose by at least half when used with CYP3A4 or CYP2D6 inhibitors such as ketoconazole, fluoxetine or paroxetine. Increase dose by one-half to 20-30 mg/day when used with CYP3A4 inducers such as carbamazepine. Reduce when inducer is stopped.

clozapine (*Clozaril, FazaClo ODT*) ▶L ♀B ▶- $$$$$
WARNING - Agranulocytosis risk 1-2%, monitor WBC and ANC q week x 6 months, then q2 weeks thereafter, and weekly for 4 weeks after discontinuation. Contraindicated if WBC <3,500 or ANC <2,000/mm3. Discontinue if WBC <3,000/mm3. May decrease monitoring to q4 weeks after 12 months if WBC >3,500/mm3 and ANC >2,000/mm3. See package insert for more details. Risk of myocarditis (particularly during the first month), seizures, orthostatic hypotension, and cardiopulmonary arrest.
ADULT - Severe, medically-refractory schizophrenia or schizophrenia/schizoaffective disorder with suicidal behavior: Start 12.5 mg PO daily or bid; increase by 25-50 mg/day to usual effective dose of 300-450 mg/day, max 900 mg /day. Retitrate if stopped for >3-4 days.
PEDS - Not approved in children.
FORMS - Generic/Trade: Tabs 25, 100 mg. Generic only: Tabs 12.5, 50, 200 mg. Trade only: Orally disintegrating tab (Fazaclo ODT) 12.5, 25, 100 mg (scored).
NOTES - Patients rechallenged after an episode of leukopenia are at increased risk of agranulocytosis, and must undergo weekly monitoring x 12 months. Register all occurrences of leukopenia, discontinuation, and/or rechallenge to the Clozaril National Registry at 1-800-448-5938. Much lower risk of EPS and tardive dyskinesia than other neuroleptics. May be effective for treatment-resistant patients who have not responded to conventional agents. May cause significant weight gain, dyslipidemia, hyperglycemia, or new onset diabetes - monitor weight, fasting blood glucose, and triglycerides before initiation and at regular intervals during treatment. Excessive sedation or respiratory depression may occur when used with CNS depressants, particularly benzodiazepines. If

an orally-disintegrating tab is split, then discard the remaining portion.

olanzapine (*Zyprexa, Zyprexa Zydis*) ▶L ♀C ▶- $$$$$

ADULT - Agitation in acute bipolar mania or schizophrenia: Start 10 mg IM (2.5-5 mg in elderly or debilitated); may repeat in ≥2h to max 30 mg/day. Psychotic disorders, oral therapy: Start 5-10 mg PO daily. Increase weekly to usual effective dose of 10-15 mg/day, max 20 mg/day. Bipolar disorder, maintenance treatment or monotherapy for acute manic or mixed episodes: Start 10-15 mg PO daily. Increase by 5 mg/day at intervals ≥24 h. Clinical efficacy seen at doses of 5-20 mg/day, max 20 mg/day. Bipolar disorder, adjunctive therapy for acute mixed/manic episodes: Start 10 mg daily; usual effective dose is 5-20 mg/day, max 20 mg/day.

PEDS - Not approved in children.

UNAPPROVED ADULT - Augmentation of SSRI therapy for OCD: Start 2.5-5.0 mg PO daily, max 20 mg/day. Post-traumatic stress disorder, adjunctive therapy: Start 5 mg PO daily, max 20 mg/day.

UNAPPROVED PEDS - Bipolar disorder, manic /mixed phase: Start 2.5 mg PO daily; increase by 2.5 mg/day every 3 days to max 20 mg/day.

FORMS - Trade only: Tabs 2.5, 5, 7.5, 10, 15, 20 mg. Tabs, orally-disintegrating (Zyprexa Zydis) 5,10,15,20 mg.

NOTES - Use for short-term (3-4 weeks) acute manic episodes associated with bipolar disorder. May cause significant weight gain, dyslipidemia, hyperglycemia, or new onset diabetes; monitor weight, blood glucose, and triglycerides before initiation and at regular intervals. Monitor for orthostatic hypotension, particularly when given IM. IM injection can also be associated with bradycardia & hypoventilation especially if used with other drugs with these effects. Use caution with benzodiazepines.

paliperidone (*Invega*, 9-hydroxyrisperidone) ▶KL ♀C ▶- $$$$$

ADULT - Schizophrenia: Start 6 mg PO qam. 3 mg/day may be sufficient. Max 12 mg/day.

PEDS - Not approved in children.

FORMS - Trade only: Extended-release tabs 3, 6, 9, 12 mg.

NOTES - Active metabolite of risperidone. Maximum 3 mg/d if CrCl is 10-49 mL/min.

quetiapine (*Seroquel, Seroquel XR*) ▶LK ♀C ▶- $$$$$

WARNING - Antidepressants including quetiapine when used for bipolar depression increase

the risk of suicidal thinking and behavior in children, adolescents, and young adults; carefully weigh the risks and benefits before starting treatment, and then monitor closely.

ADULT - Schizophrenia: Start 25 mg PO bid (regular tabs); increase by 25-50 mg bid-tid on days 2 and 3, and then to target dose of 300-400 mg/day divided bid-tid on day 4. Usual effective dose is 150-750 mg/day, max 800 mg/day. Schizophrenia, extended release tabs: Start 300 mg PO daily in evening, increase by up to 300 mg/day at intervals of >1 day to usual effective range of 400-800 mg/day. Acute bipolar mania, monotherapy or adjunct: Start 50 mg PO bid on day 1, then increase to no higher than 100 mg bid on day 2, 150 mg bid on day 3, and 200 mg bid on day 4. May increase prn to 300 mg bid on day 5 and 400 mg bid thereafter. Usual effective dose is 400-800 mg/day. Bipolar depression: 50 mg PO hs on day 1, 100 mg hs day 2, 200 mg hs day 3, and 300 mg hs day 4. May increase prn to 400 mg hs on day 5 and 600 mg hs on day 8.

PEDS - Not approved in children.

UNAPPROVED ADULT - Augmentation of SSRI therapy for OCD: Start 25 mg PO bid, max 300 mg/day. Adjunctive for post-traumatic stress disorder: Start 25 mg daily, max 300 mg/day.

UNAPPROVED PEDS - Bipolar disorder (manic or mixed phase): Start 12.5 mg PO bid (children) or 25 mg PO bid (adolescents); max 150 mg PO tid.

FORMS - Trade: Tabs 25,50,100,200,300,400 mg. Extended-release tabs 200, 300, 400 mg.

NOTES - Eye exam for cataracts recommended q 6 months. Low risk of EPS & tardive dyskinesia. May cause significant weight gain, dyslipidemia, hyperglycemia, or new onset diabetes; monitor weight, fasting blood glucose, and triglycerides before initiation and at regular intervals during treatment. Use lower doses and slower titration in elderly patients or hepatic dysfunction. Extended-release tabs should be taken without food or after light meal.

risperidone (*Risperdal, Risperdal Consta*) ▶LK ♀C ▶- $$$$$

ADULT - Psychotic disorders: Start 1 mg PO bid; increase by 1 mg bid on the 2nd and 3rd day, and then at intervals ≥1 week. Start 0.5 mg/dose and titrate by ≤0.5 mg bid in elderly, debilitated, hypotensive, or renally or hepatically impaired. Usual effective dose is 4-8 mg/day given once daily or divided bid; max 16 mg/day. Long-acting injection (Consta) for schizophrenia: Start 25 mg IM q 2 weeks while continuing oral dose x 3 weeks. May increase q 4 weeks to max 50 mg q 2 weeks. Bipolar mania: Start 2-3 mg PO daily; may adjust by 1 mg/day at 24 hour intervals to max 6 mg/day.

PEDS - Autistic disorder irritability (≥5 yo): Start 0.25 mg (<20 kg) or 0.5 mg (≥20 kg) PO daily. May increase after ≥4 days to 0.5 mg/d (<20 kg) or 1.0 mg/d (≥20 kg). Maintain ≥14 days. May then increase at ≥14 day intervals by increments of 0.25 mg/d (<20 kg) or 0.5 mg/d (≥20 kg) to max 1.0 mg/d (<20 kg), 2.5 mg/d (20-44 kg) or 3.0 mg/d (>45 kg).

UNAPPROVED ADULT - Augmentation of SSRI therapy for OCD: Start 1 mg/day PO, max 6 mg/day. Adjunctive therapy for post-traumatic stress disorder: Start 0.5 mg PO qhs, max 3 mg/day.

UNAPPROVED PEDS - Psychotic disorders, mania, aggression: 0.5-1.5 mg/day PO.

FORMS - Trade only: Tabs 0.25, 0.5, 1, 2, 3, 4 mg. Orally disintegrating tablets (M-TAB) 0.5, 1, 2 mg. Oral solution 1 mg/mL.

NOTES - Has a greater tendency to produce extrapyramidal side effects (EPS) than other atypical neuroleptics. EPS reported in neonates following use in third trimester of pregnancy. May cause weight gain, hyperglycemia,

or new onset diabetes - monitor closely. Patients with Parkinson's disease and dementia have increased sensitivity to side effects such as EPS, confusion, falls, and neuroleptic malignant syndrome. Solution is compatible with water, coffee, orange juice, and low-fat milk; is NOT compatible with cola or tea. Place orally disintegrating tablets on tongue and do not chew. Establish tolerability with oral form before starting long-acting injection. Alternate injections between buttocks.

ziprasidone (Geodon) ▶L ♀C ▶- $$$$$
WARNING - May prolong QTc. Avoid with drugs that prolong QTc or in those with long QT syndrome or cardiac arrhythmias.

ADULT - Schizophrenia: Start 20 mg PO bid with food; may increase at >2 day intervals to max 80 mg PO bid. Acute agitation in schizophrenia: 10-20 mg IM. May repeat 10 mg dose q 2 hours or 20 mg dose q 4 hours, to max 40 mg/day. Bipolar mania: Start 40 mg PO bid with food; may increase to 60-80 mg bid on day 2. Usual effective dose is 40-80 mg bid.

PEDS - Not approved in children.

FORMS - Trade only: Caps 20, 40, 60, 80 mg, Susp 10 mg/mL.

NOTES - Drug interactions with carbamazepine and ketoconazole.

PSYCHIATRY: Anxiolytics / Hypnotics – Benzodiazepines – Long Half-Life (25-100 hours)

NOTE: To avoid withdrawal, gradually taper when discontinuing after prolonged use. Use cautiously in the elderly; may accumulate and lead to side effects, psychomotor impairment. Sedative-hypnotics have been associated with severe allergic reactions and complex sleep behaviors including sleep driving. Use caution and discuss with patients.

bromazepam (♣Lectopam) ▶L ♀D ▶- $
ADULT - Canada only. 6-18 mg PO in equally divided doses.

PEDS - Not approved in children.

FORMS - Generic/Trade: Tabs 1.5, 3, 6 mg.

NOTES - Do not exceed 3 mg/day initially in the elderly or debilitated. Gradually taper when discontinuing after prolonged use. Half life ~20 hours in adults but increased in elderly. Cimetidine may prolong elimination.

chlordiazepoxide (Librium) ▶LK♀D▶- ©IV $$
ADULT - Anxiety: 5-25 mg PO tid- qid or 25-50 mg IM/IV tid-qid (acute/severe anxiety). Acute

alcohol withdrawal: 50-100 mg PO/IM/IV, repeat q3-4h prn up to 300 mg/day.

PEDS - Anxiety and >6 yo: 5-10 mg PO bid-qid.

FORMS - Generic/Trade: Caps 5, 10, 25 mg.

NOTES - Half-life 5-30 h.

clonazepam (Klonopin, Klonopin Wafer, ♣Rivotril, Clonapam) ▶LK ♀D ▶- ©IV $
ADULT - Panic disorder: 0.25 mg PO bid, increase by 0.125- 0.25 mg q3 days to maximum dose of 4 mg/day. Akinetic or myoclonic seizures: Start 0.5 mg PO tid. Increase by 0.5-1 mg q3 days prn. Max 20 mg/day.

PEDS - Akinetic or myoclonic seizures, Lennox-Gastaut syndrome (petit mal variant), or absence seizures (≤10 yo or ≤30 kg): 0.01- 0.03 mg/kg/day PO divided bid-tid. Increase by 0.25-0.5 mg q3 days prn. Max 0.1-0.2 mg/kg/ day divided tid.

UNAPPROVED ADULT - Neuralgias: 2-4 mg PO daily. Restless legs syndrome: Start 0.25 mg PO qhs. Max 2 mg qhs. REM sleep behav-

ior disorder: 1-2 mg PO qhs.
FORMS - Generic/Trade: Tabs 0.5, 1, 2 mg. Orally disintegrating tabs (approved for panic disorder only) 0.125, 0.25, 0.5, 1, 2 mg.
NOTES - Usual therapeutic range = 20-80 ng/mL. Contraindicated in hepatic failure or acute narrow angle glaucoma.

clorazepate (*Tranxene, Tranxene SD*) ▶LK ♀D ▶- ©IV $$
ADULT - Anxiety: Start 7.5-15 mg PO qhs or bid-tid, usual effective dose 15-60 mg/day. Acute alcohol withdrawal: 60-90 mg/day on first day divided bid-tid, gradually reduce dose to 7.5-15 mg/day over 5 days. Maximum dose is 90 mg/day. May transfer patients to single-dose Tabs (Tranxene-SD) when dose stabilized.
PEDS - Not approved in children <9 yo.
FORMS - Generic/Trade: Tabs 3.75, 7.5, 15 mg. Trade only (Tranxene SD): Extended release Tabs 11.25, 22.5 mg.
NOTES - Half-life 40-50 h.

diazepam (*Valium, Diastat, Diastat Acu-Dial, ♥Vivol, E Pam, Diazemuls*) ▶LK ♀D ▶- ©IV $
ADULT - Status epilepticus: 5-10 mg IV. Repeat q10-15 minutes prn to max 30 mg. Epilepsy, adjunctive therapy: 2-10 mg PO bid-qid. Increased seizure activity: 0.2-0.5 mg/kg PR (rectal gel) to max 20 mg/day. Skeletal muscle spasm, spasticity related to cerebral palsy, paraplegia, athetosis, stiff man syndrome: 2-10 mg PO/PR tid-qid. 5-10 mg IM/IV initially, then 5-10 mg q 3-4h prn. Decrease dose in elderly. Anxiety: 2-10 mg PO bid-qid or 2-20 mg IM/IV, repeat dose in 3-4h prn. Alcohol withdrawal: 10 mg PO tid-qid x 24 hr then 5 mg PO tid-qid prn.
PEDS - Skeletal muscle spasm: 0.1-0.8 mg/kg/day PO/PR divided tid-qid. 0.04-0.2 mg/kg/dose IV/IM q2-4h. Max dose 0.6 mg/kg within 8 hours. Status epilepticus, age 1 m to 5 yo: 0.2-

0.5 mg IV slowly q2-5 minutes to max 5 mg. Status epilepticus, >5 yo: 1 mg IV slowly q2-5 minutes to max 10 mg. Repeat q2-4 hours prn. Epilepsy, adjunctive therapy, age >6 months: 1-2.5 mg PO tid-qid; gradually increase to max 30 mg/day. Increased seizure activity (rectal gel, age >2 yo): 0.5 mg/kg PR (2-5 yo), 0.3 mg/kg PR (6-11 yo), or 0.2 mg/kg PR (>12 yo). Max 20 mg. May repeat in 4-12 hours prn.
UNAPPROVED ADULT - Loading dose strategy for alcohol withdrawal: 10-20 mg PO or 10 mg slow IV in closely monitored setting, then repeat similar or lower doses q1-2 hr prn until sedated. Further doses should be unnecessary due to long half-life. Restless legs syndrome: 0.5-4.0 mg PO qhs.
FORMS - Generic/Trade: Tabs 2, 5, 10 mg. Generic only: Oral solution 5 mg/5 mL. Oral concentrate (Intensol) 5 mg/mL. Trade only: Rectal gel (Diastat) 2.5, 5, 10, 15, 20 mg. Rectal gel (Diastat AcuDial) 10, 20 mg.
NOTES - Half-life 20-80h. Respiratory and CNS depression may occur. Caution in liver disease. Abuse potential. Long half-life may increase the risk of adverse effects in the elderly. Cimetidine, oral contraceptives, disulfiram, fluoxetine, isoniazid, ketoconazole, metoprolol, propoxyphene, propranolol, & valproic acid may increase diazepam concentrations. Diazepam may increase digoxin & phenytoin concentrations. Rifampin may increase diazepam metabolism. Avoid with protease inhibitors. Diastat AcuDial is for home use and allows dosing from 5-20 mg in 2.5 mg increments.

flurazepam (*Dalmane*) ▶LK ♀X ▶- ©IV $
ADULT - Insomnia: 15-30 mg PO qhs.
PEDS - Not approved in children <15 yo.
FORMS - Generic/Trade: Caps 15, 30 mg.
NOTES - Half-life 70-90h. For short term treatment of insomnia.

PSYCHIATRY: Anxiolytics / Hypnotics – Benzodiazepines – Medium Half-Life (10-15 hours)

NOTE: To avoid withdrawal, gradually taper when discontinuing after prolonged use. Sedative-hypnotics have been associated with severe allergic reactions and complex sleep behaviors including sleep driving. Use caution and discuss with patients.

estazolam (*ProSom*) ▶LK ♀X - ©IV $$
ADULT - Insomnia: 1-2 mg PO qhs for up to 12 weeks. Reduce dose to 0.5 mg in elderly,

small, or debilitated patients.
PEDS - Not approved in children.
FORMS - Generic/Trade: Tabs 1, 2 mg.
NOTES - For short term treatment of insomnia. Avoid with ketoconazole or itraconazole; caution with less potent inhibitors of CYP3A4.

lorazepam (*Ativan*) ▶LK ♀D ▶- ©IV $
ADULT - Anxiety: Start 0.5-1 mg PO bid-tid, usual effective dose is 2-6 mg/day. Max dose

10 mg/day PO. Anxiolytic/sedation: 0.04-0.05 mg/kg IV/IM; usual dose 2 mg, max 4 mg. Insomnia: 2-4 mg PO qhs. Status epilepticus: 4 mg IV over 2 mins. May repeat in 10-15 mins.
PEDS - Not approved in children.
UNAPPROVED ADULT - Alcohol withdrawal: 1-2 mg PO/IM/IV q 2-4 hr prn or 2 mg PO/IM/IV q6h x 24 hr then 1 mg q6h x 8 doses. Chemotherapy-induced N/V: 1-2 mg PO/SL/IV/IM q6h.
UNAPPROVED PEDS - Status epilepticus: 0.05 -0.1 mg/kg IV over 2-5 minutes. May repeat 0.05 mg/kg x 1 in 10-15 minutes. Do not exceed 4 mg as single dose. Anxiolytic/Sedation: 0.05 mg/kg/dose q4-8h PO/IV, max 2 mg/dose. Chemotherapy-induced N/V: 0.05 mg/kg PO/IV q8-12h prn, max 3 mg/dose; or 0.02-0.05 mg/kg IV q6h prn, max 2 mg/dose.

FORMS - Generic/Trade: Tabs 0.5, 1, 2 mg. Generic only: Oral concentrate 2 mg/mL.
NOTES - Half-life 10-20h. No active metabolites. For short term treatment of insomnia.

nitrazepam (✤*Mogadon*) ▶L ♀C ▶- $
ADULT - Canada. Insomnia: 5-10 mg PO qhs.
PEDS - Canada only. Myoclonic seizures: 0.3-1 mg/kg/day in 3 divided doses.
FORMS - Generic/Trade: Tabs 5, 10 mg.
NOTES - Use lower doses in elderly/debilitated.

temazepam (*Restoril*) ▶LK ♀X ▶- ©IV $
ADULT - Insomnia: 7.5- 30 mg PO qhs x 7-10 d.
PEDS - Not approved in children.
FORMS - Generic/Trade: Caps 15, 30 mg. Trade only: Caps 7.5, 22.5 mg.
NOTES - Half-life 8-25h. For short term treatment of insomnia.

PSYCHIATRY: Anxiolytics / Hypnotics – Benzodiazepines – Short Half-Life (<12 hours)

NOTE: To avoid withdrawal, gradually taper when discontinuing after prolonged use. Sedative-hypnotics have been associated with severe allergic reactions and complex sleep behaviors including sleep driving. Use caution and discuss with patients.

alprazolam (*Xanax, Xanax XR, Niravam*) ▶LK ♀D ▶- ©IV $
ADULT - Anxiety: Start 0.25-0.5 mg PO tid, may increase q3-4 days to a maximum dose of 4 mg/day. Use 0.25 mg PO bid in elderly or debilitated patients. Panic disorder: Start 0.5 mg PO tid (or 0.5-1.0 mg PO daily of Xanax XR), may increase by up to 1 mg/day q3-4 days to usual effective dose of 5-6 mg/day (3-6 mg/day for Xanax XR), maximum dose is 10 mg/day.
PEDS - Not approved in children.
FORMS - Trade only: Orally disintegrating tab (Niravam) 0.25, 0.5, 1, 2 mg. Generic/Trade: Tabs 0.25, 0.5, 1, 2 mg. Extended release tabs: 0.5, 1, 2, 3 mg. Generic only: Oral concentrate (Intensol) 1 mg/mL.
NOTES - Half-life 12h, but need to give tid. Divide administration time evenly during waking hours to avoid interdose symptoms. Don't give with antifungals (i.e. ketoconazole, itracona-

zole); use caution with macrolides, propoxyphene, oral contraceptives, TCAs, cimetidine, antidepressants, anticonvulsants, paroxetine, sertraline, and others that inhibit CYP 3A4.

oxazepam (*Serax*) ▶LK ♀D ▶- ©IV $$$
ADULT - Anxiety: 10-30 mg PO tid-qid. Acute alcohol withdrawal: 15-30 mg PO tid-qid.
PEDS - Not approved in children <6 yo.
UNAPPROVED ADULT - Restless legs syndrome: start 10 mg PO qhs. Max 40 mg qhs.
FORMS - Generic/Trade: Caps 10, 15, 30 mg. Trade only: Tabs 15 mg.
NOTES - Half-life 8 hours.

triazolam (*Halcion*) ▶LK ♀X ▶- ©IV $
ADULT - Hypnotic: 0.125- 0.25 mg PO qhs x 7-10 days, maximum dose is 0.5 mg/day. Start 0.125 mg/day in elderly or debilitated patients.
PEDS - Not approved in children.
UNAPPROVED ADULT - Start 0.125mg PO qhs for restless legs syndrome; max 0.5 mg qhs.
FORMS - Generic/Trade: Tabs 0.125, 0.25 mg.
NOTES - Half-life 2-3 hours. Anterograde amnesia may occur. Don't use with protease inhibitors, ketoconazole, itraconazole, or nefazodone; use caution with macrolides, cimetidine, and other CYP 3A4 inhibitors.

PSYCHIATRY: Anxiolytics / Hypnotics – Other

NOTE: Sedative-hypnotics have been associated with severe allergic reactions and complex sleep behaviors including sleep driving. Use caution and discuss with patients.

buspirone (*BuSpar, Vanspar*) ▶K ♀B ▶- $$$
ADULT - Anxiety: Start 15 mg "dividose" daily (7.5 mg PO bid), increase by 5 mg/day q2-3 days to usual effective dose of 30 mg/day, maximum dose is 60 mg/day.
PEDS - Not approved in children.
FORMS - Generic/Trade: Tabs 5, 10, 15 mg. Trade only: Dividose tab 15, 30 mg (scored to be easily bisected or trisected). Generic only: Tabs 7.5 mg.
NOTES - Slower onset than benzodiazepines; optimum effect requires 3-4 wks of therapy. Don't use with MAOIs; caution with itraconazole, cimetidine, nefazodone, erythromycin, and other CYP 3A4 inhibitors.

chloral hydrate (*Aquachloral Supprettes, Somnote*) ▶LK ♀C ▶+ ©IV $
ADULT - Sedative: 250 mg PO/PR tid after meals. Hypnotic: 500-1,000 mg PO/PR qhs. Acute alcohol withdrawal: 500-1,000 mg PO/PR q6h prn.
PEDS - Sedative: 25 mg/kg/day PO/PR divided tid-qid, up to 500 mg tid. Hypnotic: 50 mg/kg PO/PR qhs, up to max of 1 g. Pre-anesthetic: 25- 50 mg/kg PO/PR before procedure.
UNAPPROVED PEDS - Sedative: higher than approved doses 75-100 mg/kg PO/PR.
FORMS - Generic only: Syrup 500 mg/5 mL, rectal suppositories 500 mg. Trade only: Caps 500 mg. Rectal suppositories: 325, 650 mg.
NOTES - Give syrup in ½ glass fruit juice, water.

eszopiclone (*Lunesta*) ▶L ♀C ▶? ©IV $$$$
ADULT - Insomnia: 2 mg PO qhs prn, max 3 mg. Elderly: 1 mg PO qhs prn, max 2 mg.
PEDS - Not approved for children.
FORMS - Trade only: Tabs 1, 2, 3 mg.
NOTES - Half-life = 6 hours. Take immediately before bedtime.

ramelteon (*Rozerem*) ▶L ♀C ▶? $$$
ADULT - Insomnia: 8 mg PO qhs.
PEDS - Not approved for children.
FORMS - Trade only: Tabs 8 mg.
NOTES - Do not take with/after high-fat meal. No evidence of dependence or abuse liability. Inhibitors or CYP 1A2, 3A4, and 2C9 may increase serum level and effect. Avoid with severe liver disease. May decrease testosterone and increase prolactin.

zaleplon (*Sonata, ✦Starnoc*) ▶L ♀C ▶- ©IV $$$
ADULT - Insomnia: 5-10 mg PO qhs prn, maximum 20 mg.
PEDS - Not approved in children.
FORMS - Trade only: Caps 5, 10 mg.
NOTES - Half-life = 1 hour. Useful if problems with sleep initiation or morning grogginess. For short term treatment of insomnia. Take immediately before bedtime or after going to bed and experiencing difficulty falling asleep. Use 5 mg dose in patients with mild to moderate hepatic impairment, elderly patients, and in patients taking cimetidine. Possible drug interactions with rifampin, phenytoin, carbamazepine, and phenobarbital. Do not use for benzodiazepine or alcohol withdrawal.

zolpidem (*Ambien, Ambien CR*) ▶L ♀B ▶+ ©IV $$$$
ADULT - Hypnotic: 5-10 mg PO qhs (standard tabs) or 6.25-12.5 mg PO qhs (controlled release tabs). Maximum dose is 10 mg (regular release) or 12.5 mg (controlled release). Start with 5 mg (regular release) in elderly or debilitated.
PEDS - Not approved in children.
FORMS - Generic/Trade: Tabs 5, 10 mg. Trade only: Controlled release tabs 6.25, 12.5 mg.
NOTES - Half-life = 2.5 hours. CR useful if problems with early morning awakening. Ambien regular release is for short term treatment of insomnia characterized by problems with sleep initiation. Do not use for benzodiazepine or alcohol withdrawal.

zopiclone (*✦Imovane*) ▶L ♀D ▶- $
ADULT - Canada only. Short-term treatment of insomnia: 5-7.5 mg PO qhs. In elderly or debilitated, use 3.75 mg qhs initially, and increase prn to 5-7.5 mg qhs. Maximum 7.5 mg qhs.
PEDS - Not approved in children.
FORMS - Generic/Trade: Tabs 5, 7.5 mg. Generic only: Tabs 3.75 mg.
NOTES - Treatment should usually not exceed 7-10 days without re-evaluation.

PSYCHIATRY: Combination Drugs

Limbitrol (chlordiazepoxide + amitriptyline, *Limbitrol DS*) ▶LK ♀D ▶- ©IV $$$
ADULT - Rarely used; other drugs preferred. Depression/ Anxiety: 1 tab PO tid-qid, may increase up to 6 tabs/day.
PEDS - Not approved in children <12 yo.
FORMS - Generic/Trade: Tabs 5/12.5, 10/25 mg chlordiazepoxide/amitriptyline.

***Symbyax* (olanzapine + fluoxetine)** ▶LK ♀C ▶- $$$$$
WARNING - Observe SSRI patients for worsening depression/emergence of suicidal thoughts or behaviors especially early in therapy or after increases in dose. Monitor for anxiety, agitation, panic attacks, insomnia, irritability, hostility, impulsivity, akathisia, mania and hypomania. Antidepressants increase the risk of suicidal thinking and behavior in children, adolescents, and young adults; carefully weigh risks and benefits before starting and then monitor closely. The use of atypical antipsychotics to treat behavioral problems in dementia has been associated with higher mortality rates.
ADULT - Bipolar depression: Start 6/25 mg PO qhs. Max 18/75 mg/day.
PEDS - Not approved in children <12 yo.
FORMS - Trade only: Caps (olanzapine/fluoxetine) 6/25, 6/50, 12/25, 12/50 mg.
NOTES - Efficacy beyond 8 weeks not established. Monitor weight, glucose, triglycerides before initiation and periodically during treatment. Contraindicated with thioridazine; don't use with cisapride, thioridazine, tryptophan, or MAOIs; caution with lithium, phenytoin, TCAs, ASA, NSAIDs and warfarin. Pregnancy exposure to fluoxetine associated with premature delivery, low birth weight, and lower Apgar scores. Decrease dose with liver disease.

***Triavil* (perphenazine + amitriptyline)** ▶LK ♀D ▶? $$
ADULT - Rarely used; other drugs preferred. Depression/ Anxiety: 1 tab (2-25 or 4-25) PO tid-qid. Max 8 tabs/day (2-25 or 4-25).
PEDS - Not approved in children.
FORMS - Generic only: Tabs (perphenazine/amitriptyline) 2/10, 2/25, 4/10, 4/25, 4/50 mg.

PSYCHIATRY: Drug Dependence Therapy

acamprosate (*Campral*) ▶K ♀C ▶? $$$$
ADULT - Maintenance of abstinence from alcohol: 666 mg (2 tabs) PO tid. Start after alcohol withdrawal and when patient is abstinent.
PEDS - Not approved in children.
FORMS - Trade: delayed-release tabs 333 mg.
NOTES - Reduce dose to 333 mg if CrCl 30-50 mL/min. Contraindicated if CrCl <30 mL/min.

disulfiram (*Antabuse*) ▶L ♀C ▶? $$$
WARNING - Never give to the intoxicated.
ADULT - Sobriety: 125-500 mg PO daily.
PEDS - Not approved in children.
FORMS - Trade only: Tabs 250, 500 mg.
NOTES - Must abstain from any alcohol for ≥12 h before using. Disulfiram reaction may occur for up to 2 weeks after discontinuing. Metronidazole and alcohol in any form (eg, cough syrups, tonics) contraindicated. Hepatotoxicity.

naltrexone (*ReVia, Depade, Vivitrol*) ▶LK ♀C ▶? $$$$
WARNING - Hepatotoxicity with higher than approved doses.
ADULT - Alcohol dependence: 50 mg PO daily. Extended-release injectable suspension: 380 mg IM q 4 wks or monthly. Opioid dependence: Start 25 mg PO daily, increase to 50 mg PO daily if no signs of withdrawal.
PEDS - Not approved in children.
FORMS - Generic/Trade: Tabs 50 mg. Trade only (Vivitrol): extended-release injectable suspension kits 380 mg.
NOTES - Avoid if recent (past 7-10 days) ingestion of opioids. Conflicting evidence of efficacy for chronic, severe alcoholism.

nicotine gum (*Nicorette, Nicorette DS*) ▶LK ♀X ▶- $$$$$
ADULT - Smoking cessation: Gradually taper 1 piece (2 mg) q1-2h x 6 weeks, 1 piece (2 mg) q2-4h x 3 weeks, then 1 piece (2 mg) q4-8h x 3 weeks. Max 30 pieces/day of 2 mg gum or 24 pieces/day of 4 mg gum. Use 4 mg pieces (Nicorette DS) for high cigarette use (>24 cigarettes/day).
PEDS - Not approved in children.
FORMS - OTC/Generic/Trade: gum 2, 4 mg.
NOTES - Chew slowly and park between cheek and gum periodically. May cause N/V, hiccups. Coffee, juices, wine, and soft drinks may reduce absorption. Avoid eating/drinking x 15 minutes before/during gum use. Available in original, orange, or mint flavor. Do not use beyond 6 months.

nicotine inhalation system (*Nicotrol Inhaler,* ✦*Nicorette inhaler*) ▶LK ♀D ▶- $$$$$
ADULT - Smoking cessation: 6-16 cartridges/day x 12 weeks.
PEDS - Not approved in children.
FORMS - Trade: Oral inhaler 10 mg/cartridge (4 mg nicotine delivered), 42 cartridges/box.

nicotine lozenge (*Commit*) ▶LK ♀D ▶- $$$$$
ADULT - Smoking cessation: In those who smoke <30 min after waking use 4 mg lozenge;

others use 2 mg. Take 1-2 lozenges q1-2 h x 6 weeks, then q2-4h in weeks 7-9, then q4-8h in weeks 10-12. Length of therapy 12 weeks.

PEDS - Not approved in children.

FORMS - OTC Generic/Trade: lozenge 2,4 mg in 72,168-count packages

NOTES - Allow lozenge to dissolve and do not chew. Do not eat or drink within 15 minutes before use. Avoid other sources of nicotine.

nicotine nasal spray (Nicotrol NS) ▶LK ♀D ▶- $$$$$

ADULT - Smoking cessation: 1-2 doses q hour, with each dose = 2 sprays, one in each nostril (1 spray = 0.5 mg nicotine). Minimum recommended: 8 doses/day, max 40 doses/day.

PEDS - Not approved in children.

FORMS - Trade only: nasal solution 10 mg/mL (0.5 mg/inhalation); 10 mL bottles.

nicotine patches (Habitrol, NicoDerm CQ, Nicotrol, ✚Prostep) ▶LK ♀D ▶- $$$$

ADULT - Smoking cessation: Start one patch (14- 22 mg) daily and taper after 6 weeks. Total duration of therapy is 12 weeks.

PEDS - Not approved in children.

FORMS - OTC/Rx/Generic/Trade: patches 11, 22 mg/ 24 hours. 7, 14, 21 mg/ 24 h (Habitrol & NicoDerm). OTC/Trade: 15 mg/ 16 h (Nicotrol).

NOTES - Ensure patient has stopped smoking.

Dispose of safely; can be toxic to kids, pets. Remove opaque NicoDerm CQ patch prior to MRI procedures to avoid possible burns.

Suboxone (buprenorphine + naloxone) ▶L ♀C ▶- ©III $$$$$

ADULT - Treatment of opioid dependence: Maintenance: 16 mg SL daily. Can individualize to range of 4-24 mg SL daily.

PEDS - Not approved in children.

FORMS - Trade only: SL tabs 2/0.5 and 8/2 mg buprenorphine / naloxone

NOTES - Suboxone preferred over Subutex for unsupervised administration. Titrate in 2-4 mg increments / decrements to maintain therapy compliance and prevent withdrawal. Prescribers must complete training and apply for special DEA number. See www.suboxone.com.

varenicline (Chantix) ▶K ♀C ▶? $$$$

ADULT - Smoking cessation: Start 0.5 mg PO daily for days 1-3, then 0.5 mg bid days 4-7, then 1 mg bid thereafter. Take after meals with full glass of water. Start 1 wk prior to cessation and continue x 12 wks.

PEDS - Not approved in children.

FORMS - Trade only: Tabs 0.5, 1 mg.

NOTES - In severe renal dysfunction reduce max dose to 0.5 mg bid. For hemodialysis may use 0.5 mg once daily if tolerated.

PSYCHIATRY: Stimulants / ADHD / Anorexiants

NOTE: Sudden cardiac death has been reported with stimulants at usual ADHD doses; carefully assess prior to treatment and avoid if cardiac conditions or structural abnormalities. Amphetamines are associated with high abuse potential and dependence with prolonged administration. Stimulants may also cause or worsen underlying psychosis or induce a manic or mixed episode in bipolar disorder. Problems with visual accommodation have also been reported with stimulants.

Adderall (dextroamphetamine + amphetamine, Adderall XR) ▶L ♀C ▶- ©II $$$$

ADULT - Narcolepsy, standard-release: Start 10 mg PO q am, increase by 10 mg q week, maximum dose is 60 mg/day divided bid-tid at 4-6h intervals. ADHD, extended-release caps (Adderall XR): 20 mg PO daily.

PEDS - ADHD, standard-release tabs: Start 2.5 mg (3-5 yo) or 5 mg (≥6 yo) PO daily-bid, increase by 2.5-5 mg every week, max 40 mg/day. ADHD, extended-release caps (Adderall XR): If 6-12 yo, then start 5-10 mg PO daily to

a max of 30 mg/day. If 13-17 yo, then start 10 mg PO daily to a max of 20 mg/d. Not recommended if <3 yo. Narcolepsy, standard-release: 6-12 yo: Start 5 mg PO daily, increase by 5 mg q week. Age >12 yo: Start 10 mg PO q am, increase by 10 mg q week, maximum dose is 60 mg/day divided bid-tid at 4-6h intervals.

FORMS - Generic/Trade: Tabs 5, 7.5, 10, 12.5, 15, 20, 30 mg. Trade only: Capsules, extended release (Adderall XR) 5, 10, 15, 20, 25, 30 mg.

NOTES - Capsules may be opened and the beads sprinkled on applesauce; do not chew beads. Adderall XR should be given upon awakening. Avoid evening doses. Monitor growth and use drug holidays when appropriate. May increase pulse and BP. May exacerbate bipolar or psychotic conditions.

armodafinil (Nuvigil) ▶L ♀C ▶? ©IV ?

ADULT - Obstructive sleep apnea/hypopnea syndrome and narcolepsy: 150-250 mg PO q am. Inconsistent evidence for improved efficacy of 250 mg/day dose. Shift work sleep disor-

der: 150 mg PO 1 hr prior to start of shift.
PEDS - Not approved in children.
FORMS - Trade only: tabs 50, 150, 250 mg.
NOTES - Weak inducer for substrates of CYP 3A4/5 (e.g. carbamazepine, cyclosporine) which may require dose adjustments. May inhibit metabolism of substrates of CYP2C19 (e.g. omeprazole, diazepam, phenytoin). May reduce efficacy of oral contraceptives; consider alternatives during treatment. Reduce dose with severe liver impairment.

atomoxetine (*Strattera*) ▶K ♀C ▶? $$$$$
WARNING - Severe liver injury and failure have been reported; discontinue if jaundice or elevated LFTs. Increases risk of suicidal thinking or behavior in children and adolescents; carefully weigh risks/benefits before starting and then monitor closely for worsening depression or emergence of suicidal thoughts or behaviors especially early in therapy or after dose increases. Monitor for anxiety, agitation, panic attacks, insomnia, irritability, hostility, impulsivity, akathisia, mania and psychosis.
ADULT - ADHD: Start 40 mg PO daily, then increase after >3 days to target of 80 mg/day divided daily-bid. Max dose 100 mg/day.
PEDS - ADHD: Children/adolescents ≤70 kg: Start 0.5 mg/kg daily, then increase after >3 days to target dose of 1.2 mg/kg/day divided daily-bid. Max dose 1.4 mg/kg or 100 mg per day. If >70 kg use adult dose.
FORMS - Trade only: caps 10, 18, 25, 40, 60, 80, 100 mg.
NOTES - If taking strong CYP2D6 inhibitors, use same starting dose but only increase if well-tolerated at 4 weeks and symptoms unimproved. Caution when co-administered with oral or parenteral albuterol or other beta-2 agonists, as increases in heart rate and blood pressure may occur. May be stopped without tapering. Monitor growth. Give "Patient Medication Guide" when dispensed.

benzphetamine (*Didrex*) ▶K ♀X ▶? ©III $$$
WARNING - Chronic overuse/abuse can lead to marked tolerance and psychic dependence; caution with prolonged use.
ADULT - Short-term treatment of obesity: Start with 25-50 mg once daily in the morning and increase if needed to 1-3 times daily.
PEDS - Not approved for children <12 yo.
FORMS - Generic/Trade: Tabs 50 mg.
NOTES - Tolerance to anorectic effect develops within weeks and cross-tolerance to other drugs in class common.

caffeine (*NoDoz, Vivarin, Caffedrine, Stay Awake, Quick-Pep, Cafcit*) ▶L ♀B/C ▶? $
ADULT - Fatigue: 100- 200 mg PO q3-4h prn.
PEDS - Not approved in children <12 yo, except apnea of prematurity in infants between 28 & <33 weeks gestational age (Cafcit): Load 20 mg/kg IV over 30 min. Maintenance 5 mg/kg PO q 24h. Monitor for necrotizing enterocolitis.
FORMS - OTC/Generic/Trade: Tabs/Caps 200 mg. OTC/Trade: Extended-release tabs 200 mg. Lozenges 75 mg. Oral solution caffeine citrate (Cafcit): 20 mg/mL in 3 mL vials.
NOTES - 2 mg caffeine citrate = 1 mg caffeine base.

dexmethylphenidate (*Focalin, Focalin XR*) ▶LK ♀C ▶? ©II $$$
ADULT - ADHD, not already on stimulants: Start 10 mg PO q am (extended release) or 2.5 mg PO bid (immediate release). Max 20 mg/day for both. If taking racemic methylphenidate use conversion of 2.5 mg for each 5 mg of methylphenidate, max 20 mg/day. Doses should be ≥4h apart for immediate release.
PEDS - ADHD and ≥6 yo and not already on stimulants: Start 5 mg PO q am (extended release) or 2.5 mg PO bid (immediate release), max 20 mg/24 hr. If already on racemic methylphenidate, use conversion of 2.5 mg for each 5 mg of methylphenidate given bid, max 20 mg/day. Doses should be ≥4h apart.
FORMS - Generic/Trade: Immediate release tabs 2.5, 5, 10 mg. Trade only: Extended release caps (Focalin XR) 5, 10, 15, 20 mg.
NOTES - Avoid evening doses. Monitor growth and use drug holidays when appropriate. May increase pulse and BP. 2.5 mg is equivalent to 5 mg racemic methylphenidate. Focalin XR capsules may be opened and sprinkled on applesauce, but beads must not be chewed. May exacerbate bipolar or psychotic conditions.

dextroamphetamine (*Dexedrine, Dextrostat*) ▶L ♀C ▶- ©II $$$
ADULT - Narcolepsy: Start 10 mg PO qam, increase by 10 mg q week, max 60 mg/day divided daily (sustained release) or bid-tid at 4-6h intervals.
PEDS - Narcolepsy: 6-12 yo: Start 5 mg PO q am, increase by 5 mg q week. >12 yo: Start 10 mg PO q am, increase by 10 mg q week, max 60 mg/day divided daily (sustained release) or bid-tid at 4-6h intervals. ADHD, 3-5 yo: Start 2.5 mg PO daily, increase by 2.5 mg q week. ≥6 yo: Start 5 mg PO daily-bid, increase by 5 mg q week, max 40 mg/day divided daily-tid at

4-6h intervals. Not recommended if <3 yo.
FORMS - Generic/Trade: Tabs 5, 10 mg. Extended Release caps 5, 10, 15 mg.
NOTES - Avoid evening doses. Monitor growth and use drug holidays when appropriate. May exacerbate bipolar or psychotic conditions.

diethylpropion (*Tenuate, Tenuate Dospan*) ▶K ♀B ▶? ©IV $
WARNING - Chronic overuse/abuse can lead to marked tolerance and psychic dependence; caution with prolonged use.
ADULT - Short-term treatment of obesity: 25 mg PO tid 1 hour before meals and mid evening if needed or 75 mg sustained-release daily at midmorning.
PEDS - Not approved for <12 yo.
FORMS - Generic/Trade: Tabs 25 mg, sustained-release tabs 75 mg.
NOTES - Tolerance to anorectic effect develops within weeks and cross-tolerance to other drugs in class common.

lisdexamfetamine (*Vyvanse*) ▶L ♀C ▶- ©II $$$$
ADULT - Not approved for use in adults.
PEDS - ADHD ages 6-12 yo: Start 30 mg PO q am. May increase weekly by 20 mg/day to max 70 mg/day.
FORMS - Trade: Caps 30, 50, 70 mg.
NOTES - May open capsule and place contents in water for administration. Avoid evening doses. Monitor growth and use drug holidays when appropriate.

methylphenidate (*Ritalin, Ritalin LA, Ritalin SR, Methylin, Methylin ER, Metadate ER, Metadate CD, Concerta, Daytrana, ♣Biphentin*) ▶LK ♀C ▶? ©II $$
ADULT - Narcolepsy: 10 mg PO bid-tid before meals. Usual effective dose is 20-30 mg/day, max 60 mg/day. Use sustained release Tabs when the 8-hour dosage corresponds to the titrated 8-hour dosage of the conventional tabs.
PEDS - ADHD ≥6 yo: Start 5 mg PO bid before breakfast and lunch, increase gradually by 5-10 mg/day at weekly interval to max 60 mg/day. Sustained and extended release: start 20 mg PO daily, max 60 mg daily. Concerta (extended release) start 18 mg PO qam; titrate in 9-18 mg increments at weekly intervals to max 72 mg/day. Consult product labeling for dose conversion from other methylphenidate regimens. Discontinue after 1 month if no improvement. Transdermal patch 6-12 yo: Start 10 mg/9 hrs, may increase at weekly intervals to max 30 mg/9 hrs. Apply 2h prior to desired onset

and remove 9h later. Effect may last up to 12 hrs after application. Must alternate sites daily.
FORMS - Trade only: tabs 5, 10, 20 mg (Ritalin, Methylin, Metadate). Extended release tabs 10, 20 mg (Methylin ER, Metadate ER). Extended release tabs 18, 27, 36, 54 mg (Concerta). Extended release caps 10, 20, 30, 40, 50, 60 mg (Metadate CD) May be sprinkled on food. Sustained-release tabs 20 mg (Ritalin SR). Extended release caps 10, 20, 30, 40 mg (Ritalin LA). Chewable tabs 2.5, 5, 10 mg (Methylin). Oral soln 5 mg/5ml, 10 mg/5 ml (Methylin). Transdermal patch (Daytrana) 10 mg/9 hrs, 15 mg/9 hrs, 20 mg/9 hrs, 30 mg/9 hrs. Generic only: tabs 5, 10, 20 mg, extended release tabs 10, 20 mg, sustained-release tabs 20 mg.
NOTES - Avoid evening doses. Monitor growth and use drug holidays when appropriate. May increase pulse and BP. Ritalin LA may be opened and sprinkled on applesauce. Apply transdermal patch to hip below beltline to avoid rubbing it off. My exacerbate bipolar or psychotic conditions.

modafinil (*Provigil, ♣Alertec*) ▶L ♀C ▶? ©IV $$$$$
ADULT - Narcolepsy and sleep apnea/hypopnea: 200 mg PO qam. Shift work sleep disorder: 200 mg PO one hour before shift.
PEDS - Not approved in children <16 yo.
FORMS - Trade only: Tabs 100, 200 mg.
NOTES - May increase levels of diazepam, phenytoin, TCAs, warfarin, or propranolol; may decrease levels of cyclosporine, oral contraceptives, or theophylline. Reduce dose in severe liver impairment.

phendimatrizine (*Bontril SR, Melfiat, Prelu-2*) ▶K ♀C ▶? ©III $$
WARNING - Chronic overuse/abuse can lead to marked tolerance and psychic dependence; caution with prolonged use.
ADULT - Short-term treatment of obesity: Start 35 mg 2 or 3 times daily 1 hr before meals. Sustained-release 105 mg once in the morning before breakfast.
PEDS - Not approved in children <12 yo.
FORMS - Generic/Trade: tabs/caps 35 mg, sustained-release caps 105 mg.
NOTES - Tolerance to anorectic effect develops within weeks and cross-tolerance to other drugs in class common.

phentermine (*Adipex-P, Ionamin, ProFast*) ▶KL ♀C ▶- ©IV $$
WARNING - Chronic overuse/abuse can lead to marked tolerance and psychic dependence;

caution with prolonged use.

ADULT - Obesity: 8 mg PO tid before meals or 1-2 h after meals. May give 15-37.5 mg PO q am or 10-14 h before bedtime.

PEDS - Not approved in children <16 yo.

FORMS - Generic/Trade: Caps 15, 18.75, 30, 37.5 mg. Tabs 8, 30, 37.5 mg. Trade only: extended release Caps 15, 30 mg (Ionamin).

NOTES - Indicated for short term (8-12 weeks) use only. Contraindicated for use during or within 14 days of MAOIs (hypertensive crisis).

sibutramine (*Meridia*) ▶KL ♀C ▶- ©IV $$$$

WARNING - Chronic overuse/abuse can lead to marked tolerance and psychic dependence; caution with prolonged use.

ADULT - Obesity: Start 10 mg PO q am, may titrate to 15 mg/day after one month. Maximum dose is 15 mg/day.

PEDS - Not approved in children <16 yo.

FORMS - Trade only: Caps 5, 10, 15 mg.

NOTES - Indicated for BMI >30 kg/m² or >27 kg/m² with risk factors for cardiovascular disease or diabetes. Monitor pulse and BP. Don't use if uncontrolled HTN, heart disease, or severe renal impairment or end-stage renal disease. Caution using with SSRIs or other antidepressants, sumatriptan, ergotamine and other serotonin agents to avoid development of serotonin syndrome. Contraindicated for use during or within 14 days of MAOIs (hypertensive crisis).

BODY MASS INDEX*		Heights are in feet and inches; weights are in pounds				
BMI	*Classification*	*4'10"*	*5'0"*	*5'4"*	*5'8"*	*6'0"*	*6'4"*
<19	Underweight	<91	<97	<110	<125	<140	<156
19-24	Healthy Weight	91-119	97-127	110-144	125-163	140-183	156-204
25-29	Overweight	120-143	128-152	145-173	164-196	184-220	205-245
30-40	Obese	144-191	153-204	174-233	197-262	221-293	246-328
>40	Very Obese	>191	>204	>233	>262	>293	>328

*BMI = kg/m² = (weight in pounds)(703)/(height in inches)². Anorectants appropriate if BMI ≥30 (with comorbidities ≥27); surgery an option if BMI >40 (with comorbidities 35-40). www.nhlbi.nih.gov

PULMONARY: Beta Agonists

NOTE: Palpitations, tachycardia, tremor, lightheadedness, nervousness, headache, & nausea may occur; these effects may be more pronounced with systemic administration. Decreases in serum potassium can occur, rarely leading to adverse cardiovascular effects; monitor accordingly. Potential for tolerance with continued use of short-acting beta agonists.

albuterol (*Ventolin, Ventolin HFA, Proventil, Proventil HFA, ProAir HFA, Volmax, VoSpire ER, Ventodisk, ✦Airomir, Asmavent, salbutamol*) ▶L ♀C ▶? $

ADULT - Acute asthma: MDI: 2 puffs q4-6h prn. Soln for inhalation: 2.5 mg nebulized tid-qid. Dilute 0.5 mL 0.5% soln with 2.5 mL NS. Deliver over ~ 5-15 min. One 3 mL unit dose (0.083%) nebulized tid-qid. Caps for inhalation: 200-400 mcg inh q4-6h via a Rotahaler device. Asthma: 2-4 mg PO tid-qid or extended release 4-8 mg PO q12h up to 16 mg PO q12h.

PEDS - Acute asthma: MDI: ≥4 yo: 1-2 puffs q4-6 h prn. Soln for inhalation (0.5%): 2-12 yo: 0.1-0.15 mg/kg/dose not to exceed 2.5 mg tid-qid, diluted with NS to 3 mL. Caps for inhalation: ≥4 yo 200-400 mcg inhaled q4-6h via a

Rotahaler device. Asthma: Tabs, syrup 6-12 yo: 2-4 mg PO tid-qid, max dose 24 mg/d in divided doses or extended release 4 mg PO q12h. Syrup 2-5 yo: 0.1-0.2 mg/kg/dose PO tid up to 4 mg tid. Prevention of exercise-induced bronchospasm ≥4 yo (Proventil HFA, Ventolin HFA): 2 puffs 15-30 minutes before exercise.

UNAPPROVED ADULT - COPD: MDI, soln for inhalation: use asthma dose. Acute asthma: MDI, soln for inhalation: dose as above q20 min X 3 or until improvement. Continuous nebulization: 10-15 mg/h until improvement.

UNAPPROVED PEDS - Acute asthma: Soln for inhalation: 0.15 mg/kg (minimum dose = 2.5 mg) q 20 minutes x 3 doses then 0.15-0.3 mg/kg up to 10 mg q1-4 hrs as needed, or 0.5 mg/kg/hour continuous nebulization. MDI: 4-8 puffs q 20 minutes for 3 doses then q1-4 hours prn. Soln for inhalation (0.5%): <2 yo: 0.05-0.15 mg/kg/dose q4-6h. Syrup <2 yo: 0.3 mg/ kg/24h PO divided tid, max dose 12 mg/24h. Prevention of exercise-induced bronchospasm: MDI: ≥4 yo 2 puffs 15-30 minutes before exercise.

FORMS - Generic/Trade: MDI 90 mcg/actuation, 17g-200/canister. "HFA" inhalers use hydrofluoroalkane propellant instead of CFCs but are otherwise equivalent. Soln for inhalation 0.042% and 0.083% in 3 mL vial, 0.5% (5 mg/mL) in 20 mL with dropper. Tabs 2, 4 mg, Extended release tabs 4, 8 mg. Generic only: Syrup 2 mg/5 mL. Trade only: (AccuNeb) Soln for inhalation 0.021% in 3 mL vial.

NOTES - Do not crush or chew extended release tablets. Volmax must be stored in the refrigerator. Use with caution in patients on MAO inhibitors or cyclic antidepressants -- may increase cardiovascular side effects.

arformoterol (*Brovana*) ▶L ♀C ▶? ?

WARNING - Long-acting beta agonists may increase the risk of asthma-related death; it is unclear if this also applies to COPD. Do not use for rescue therapy.

ADULT - COPD: 15 mcg nebulized bid.

PEDS - Not approved in children.

FORMS - Trade only: Solution for inhalation 15 mcg in 2mL vial.

NOTES - Not for acute COPD exacerbations.

fenoterol (*♥Berotec*) ▶L ♀C ▶? $

ADULT - Canada only. Acute asthma: MDI 1-2 puffs tid-qid; maximum 8 puffs/day. Soln for nebulization: up to 2.5 mg q6 hours.

PEDS - Not approved in children.

FORMS - Trade: MDI 100 mcg/actuation. Soln for inhalation: 20 mL bottles of 1 mg/mL (with preservatives that may cause bronchoconstriction in those with hyperreactive airways).

formoterol (*Foradil, Perforomist, ♥Oxeze Turbuhaler*) ▶L ♀C ▶? $$$

WARNING - May increase the risk of asthma-related death. Use only as a 2nd agent if inadequate control with an optimal dose of inhaled corticosteroids. Avoid in significantly worsening or acute asthma. Not for rescue therapy.

ADULT - Chronic asthma, COPD: 1 puff bid. Prevention of exercise-induced bronchospasm: 1 puff 15 min prior to exercise. COPD: 20 mcg nebulized q12h.

PEDS - Chronic asthma ≥5 yo: 1 puff bid. Prevention of exercise-induced bronchospasm ≥12 yo: Use adult dose.

FORMS - Trade only: DPI 12 mcg, 12 & 60 blisters/pack. Soln for inhalation: 20 mcg in 2 mL vial. Canada only (Oxeze): DPI 6 & 12 mcg 60 blisters/pack.

NOTES - Do not use additional doses for exercise if on maintenance.

levalbuterol (*Xopenex, Xopenex HFA*) ▶L ♀C ▶? $$$

ADULT - Acute asthma: MDI 2 puffs q4-6h prn.

Inhalation soln: 0.63-1.25 mg nebulized q6-8h.

PEDS - Acute asthma: MDI ≥4 yo: 2 puffs q4-6h prn. Soln for inhalation ≥12 yo: Use adult dose. 6-11 yo: 0.31 mg nebulized tid.

FORMS - Trade only: MDI 45 mcg/actuation, 15g 200/canister. "HFA" inhalers use hydrofluoroalkane propellant. Soln for inhalation 0.31, 0.63, 1.25 mg in 3 mL and 1.25mg in 0.5 mL unit-dose vials.

NOTES - R-isomer of albuterol. Dyspepsia may occur. Caution with MAO inhibitors or cyclic antidepressants.

metaproterenol (*Alupent, ♥orciprenaline*) ▶L ♀C ▶? $$

ADULT - Acute asthma: MDI: 2-3 puffs q3-4h; max dose 12 puffs/day. Soln for inhalation: 0.2-0.3 mL of the 5% soln in 2.5 mL NS. 20 mg PO tid-qid.

PEDS - Acute asthma: soln for inhalation: >6 yo 0.1-0.3 mL of the 5% soln in 2.5 mL NS. Tabs or syrup: >9 yo or >60 lbs: 20 mg PO tid-qid. 6-9 yo or <60 lbs: 10 mg PO tid-qid. 2-5 yo: 1.3-2.6 mg/kg/day PO in divided doses tid-qid.

UNAPPROVED PEDS - Acute asthma: MDI: >6 yo 2-3 puffs q3-4h; max dose 12 puffs/day. Soln for inhalation: 0.1-0.3 mL of the 5% soln in 2.5 mL NS q4-6h prn or q20 min until improvement. Tabs or syrup: <2 yo: 0.4 mg/kg/dose PO tid-qid.

FORMS - Trade only: MDI 0.65 mg/actuation, 14g-200/canister. Generic/Trade: Soln for inhalation 0.4% & 0.6% in 2.5 mL unit-dose vials. Generic: Syrup 10 mg/5 mL, Tabs 10 & 20 mg.

pirbuterol (*Maxair, Maxair Autohaler*) ▶L ♀C ▶? $$$$

ADULT - Acute asthma: MDI: 1-2 puffs q4-6h. Max dose 12 puffs/day.

PEDS - Not approved in children.

UNAPPROVED PEDS - ≥12 yo: Adult dose.

FORMS - Trade only: MDI 0.2 mg/actuation, 14g 400/canister.

NOTES - Breath-actuated autohaler.

salmeterol (*Serevent Diskus*) ▶L ♀C ▶? $$$$

WARNING - May increase the risk of asthma-related death. Use only as a 2nd agent if inadequate control with an optimal dose of inhaled corticosteroids. Avoid in significantly worsening or acute asthma. Not for rescue therapy.

ADULT - Chronic asthma/ COPD: 1 puff bid. Prevention of exercise-induced bronchospasm: 1 puff 30 minutes before exercise.

PEDS - Chronic asthma ≥4 yo: 1 puff bid. Prevention of exercise-induced bronchospasm: 1 puff 30 minutes before exercise.

FORMS - Trade only: DPI (Diskus): 50 mcg, 60 blisters.

NOTES - Do not use additional doses for exercise if on maintenance

terbutaline (*Brethine*, ✚*Bricanyl Turbuhaler*) ▶L ♀B ▶- $$

ADULT - Asthma: 2.5-5 mg PO q6h while awake. Max dose 15 mg/24h. Acute asthma: 0.25 mg SC into lateral deltoid area; may repeat x1 within 15-30 min. Max dose 0.5 mg/4h.

PEDS - Not approved in children.

UNAPPROVED ADULT - Preterm labor: 0.25 mg SC q30 min up to 1 mg in four hours. Infusion: 2.5-10 mcg/min IV, gradually increased to effective max doses of 17.5-30 mcg/min.

UNAPPROVED PEDS - Asthma, >12 yo: Use adult dose, max 7.5 mg/24h. If ≤12 yo: 0.05 mg/kg/dose PO tid, increase to max of 0.15 mg/kg/dose tid, max 5 mg/day. Acute asthma: 0.01 mg/kg SC q 20 minutes x 3 doses then q 2-6 hrs as needed.

FORMS - Generic/Trade: Tabs 2.5 & 5 mg (Brethine scored). Canada only (Bricanyl): DPI 0.5 mg/actuation, 200 per DPI.

NOTES - Give 50% normal dose in renal insufficiency; avoid in renal failure. Concomitant use with magnesium sulfate may lead to fatal pulmonary edema.

PREDICTED PEAK EXPIRATORY FLOW (liters/min)   *Am Rev Resp Dis* 1963; 88:644

Age (yrs)	Women (height in inches)					Men (height in inches)					Child (height in inches)	
	55"	60"	65"	70"	75"	60"	65"	70"	75"	80"		
20	390	423	460	496	529	554	602	649	693	740	44"	160
30	380	413	448	483	516	532	577	622	664	710	46"	187
40	370	402	436	470	502	509	552	596	636	680	48"	214
50	360	391	424	457	488	486	527	569	607	649	50"	240
60	350	380	412	445	475	463	502	542	578	618	52"	267
70	340	369	400	432	461	440	477	515	550	587	54"	293

PULMONARY: Combinations

Advair (fluticasone + salmeterol, *Advair HFA*) ▶L ♀C ▶? $$$$

WARNING - Long-acting beta agonists may increase the risk of asthma-related death; use as an adjunct only if inadequate control with an optimal dose of inhaled corticosteroids. Avoid in significantly worsening or acute asthma. Not for rescue therapy. Do not stop abruptly.

ADULT - Chronic asthma: DPI: 1 puff bid (all strengths). MDI: 2 puffs bid (all strengths). COPD with chronic bronchitis: DPI: 1 puff bid (250/50 only).

PEDS - Chronic asthma ≥12 yo: DPI: Use adult dose. 4-11 yo: 1 puff bid (100/50 only).

FORMS - Trade only: DPI: 100/50, 250/50, 500/50 mcg fluticasone/salmeterol per actuation; 60 doses per DPI. MDI: 45/21, 115/21, 230/21 mcg fluticasone/salmeterol per actuation; 120 doses/canister.

NOTES - See individual components for additional information. Ritonavir & other CYP3A4 inhibitors such as ketoconazole significantly increase fluticasone concentrations, resulting in systemic effects, including adrenal suppression. Very rare anaphylactic reaction in patients with severe milk protein allergy.

Combivent (albuterol + ipratropium) ▶L ♀C ▶? $$$$

ADULT - COPD: MDI: 2 puffs qid. Max dose 12 puffs/24 hours.

PEDS - Not approved in children.

FORMS - Trade only: MDI: 90 mcg albuterol/18 mcg ipratropium per actuation, 200/canister.

NOTES - Contraindicated with soy or peanut allergy. Refer to components.

DuoNeb (albuterol + ipratropium, ✚*Combivent inhalation soln*) ▶L ♀C ▶? $$$$$

ADULT - COPD: One unit dose nebulized qid; may add 2 doses/day prn to max 6 doses/day.

PEDS - Not approved in children.

FORMS - Generic/Trade: Unit dose: 2.5 mg albuterol/0.5 mg ipratropium per 3 mL vial, premixed; 30 & 60 vials/carton.

NOTES - Refer to components

Duovent UDV (ipratropium + fenoterol) ▶L ♀? ▶? $$

ADULT - Canada only. Bronchospasm with asthma/COPD: 1 vial (via nebulizer) q6h prn.

PEDS - Canada only. ≥12 yo: Adult dose.

FORMS - Trade: unit dose vial (for neb) 0.5 mg ipratropium & 1.25 mg fenoterol in 4 ml NS.

Symbicort (budesonide + formoterol) ▶L

♀C ▶? $$$$

WARNING - Long-acting beta agonists may increase the risk of asthma-related death; use as an adjunct only if inadequate control with an optimal dose of inhaled corticosteroids. Avoid in significantly worsening or acute asthma. Not for rescue therapy. Do not stop abruptly.

ADULT - Chronic asthma: 2 puffs bid (both strengths).

PEDS - Chronic asthma ≥12 yo: Adult dose.

FORMS – Trade only: MDI: 80/4.5, 160/4.5 mcg budesonide/formoterol per actuation; 120 doses/canister.

NOTES - See individual components for additional information. Ritonavir & other CYP3A4 inhibitors such as ketonazole significantly increase concentrations, resulting in systemic effects, including adrenal suppression.

WHAT COLOR IS WHAT INHALER? (Body then cap - Generics may differ)

Advair	purple	Combivent	clear/orange	Pulmicort	white/brown
Advair HFA	purple/light purple	Flovent HFA	orange/peach	QVAR 40 mcg	beige/grey
		Foradil	grey/beige	QVAR 80 mcg	mauve/grey
Aerobid	grey/purple	Intal	white/blue	Serevent Diskus	green
Aerobid-M	grey/green	Maxair	white/white	Spiriva	grey
Alupent	clear/blue	Maxair Autohaler	white/white	Symbicort	red/grey
Asmanex	pink/white			Tilade	white/white
Atrovent HFA	clear/green	ProAir HFA	red/white	Ventolin HFA	light blue/navy
Azmacort	white/white	Proventil HFA	yellow/orange	Xopenex HFA	blue/red

PULMONARY: Inhaled Steroids

NOTE: See Endocrine-Corticosteroids for oral steroids. Beware of adrenal suppression when changing from systemic to inhaled. Inhaled steroids are not for treatment of acute asthma; higher doses may be needed for severe asthma and exacerbations. Adjust to lowest effective dose for maintenance. Use of a DPI, a spacing device, & rinsing the mouth with water after each use may decrease the incidence of thrush & dysphonia. Pharyngitis & cough may occur with all products. Use with caution in patients with active or quiescent TB, untreated systemic fungal, bacterial, viral or parasitic infections or in patients with ocular HSV. Inhaled steroids produce small, transient reductions in growth velocity in children.

beclomethasone (*QVAR*) ▶L ♀C ▶? $$$

ADULT - Chronic asthma: 40 mcg: 1-4 puffs bid. 80 mcg: 1-2 puffs bid.

PEDS - 5-11 yo: 40 mcg 1-2 puffs bid.

UNAPPROVED ADULT - Chronic asthma: NHLBI dosing schedule (puffs/day divided bid): Low dose 2-6 puffs of 40 mcg or 1-3 puffs of 80 mcg. Medium dose: 6-12 puffs of 40 mcg or 3-6 puffs of 80 mcg. High dose: >12 puffs of 40 mcg or >6 puffs 80 mcg.

UNAPPROVED PEDS - Chronic asthma: NHLBI dosing schedule (puffs/day divided bid): 2-4 puffs of 40 mcg or 1-2 puffs of 80 mcg. Medium dose: 4-8 puffs of 40 mcg or 2-4 puffs of 80 mcg. High dose: >8 puffs of 40 mcg or >4 puffs

of 80 mcg.

FORMS - Trade: MDI (non-CFC): 40 mcg & 80 mcg/actuation, 7.3g-100 actuations/canister.

budesonide (*Pulmicort Respules, Pulmicort Flexhaler*) ▶L ♀B ▶? $$$$

ADULT - Chronic asthma: DPI: 1-2 puffs daily-bid up to 4 puffs bid.

PEDS - Chronic asthma 6-12 yo: DPI: 1-2 puffs daily-bid. 12 mo - 8 yo: Suspension for inhalation (Respules): 0.5-1 mg daily or divided bid.

UNAPPROVED ADULT - Chronic asthma: NHLBI dosing schedule (puffs/day daily or divided bid): DPI: Low dose: 1-3 puffs. Medium dose: 3-6 puffs. High dose: >6 puffs.

UNAPPROVED PEDS - Chronic asthma: NHLBI dosing schedule (puffs/day daily or divided bid) DPI: Low dose: 1-2 puffs. Medium dose: 2-4 puffs. High dose: >4 puffs. Suspension for inhalation (daily or divided bid): Low dose: 0.5 mg. Medium dose: 1 mg. High dose: 2 mg.

FORMS - Trade: DPI: (Flexhaler) 90 & 180mcg powder/actuation 60 & 120/canister. Respules: 0.25 mg/2 mL & 0.5 mg/2 mL unit dose.

NOTES - Respules should be delivered via a jet nebulizer with a mouthpiece or face mask. CYP3A4 inhibitors such as ketoconazole, erythromycin, ritonavir, etc may significantly increase systemic concentrations, possibly causing adrenal suppression.

flunisolide (*Aerobid, Aerobid-M, Aero-

span) ▶L ♀C ▶? $$$

ADULT - Chronic asthma: MDI: 2 puffs bid up to 4 puffs bid.

PEDS - 6-15 yo: MDI: 2 puffs bid.

UNAPPROVED ADULT - Chronic asthma: NHLBI dosing schedule (puffs/day divided bid): Low dose: 2-4 puffs. Medium dose: 4-8 puffs. High dose: >8 puffs.

UNAPPROVED PEDS - Chronic asthma: NHLBI dosing schedule (puffs/day divided bid): Low dose: 2-3 puffs. Medium dose: 4-5 puffs. High dose: >5 puffs.

FORMS - Trade only: MDI: 250 mcg/actuation, 100/canister. AeroBid-M: menthol flavor. Aerospan (HFA) MDI: 80 mcg/actuation, 60 & 120/canister.

fluticasone (*Flovent, Flovent HFA, Flovent Rotadisk***)** ▶L ♀C ▶? $$$$

ADULT - Chronic asthma: MDI: 2 puffs bid up to 4 puffs bid. Max dose 880 mcg bid.

PEDS - Chronic asthma: >12 yo: Use adult dose. 4-11 yo: 2 puffs bid of 44 mcg/puff.

UNAPPROVED ADULT - Chronic asthma: NHLBI dosing schedule (puffs/day divided bid): Low dose: 2-6 puffs of 44 mcg MDI. Medium dose: 6-15 puffs of 44 mcg MDI. 3-6 puffs of 110 mcg MDI. 2-3 puffs of 220 mcg MDI. High dose: >6 puffs 110 mcg MDI.

UNAPPROVED PEDS - Chronic asthma: NHLBI dosing schedule (puffs/day divided bid): Low dose: 2-4 puffs of 44 mcg MDI. Medium dose: 4-10 puffs of 44 mcg MDI. 1-4 puffs of 110 mcg MDI. 1-2 puffs of 220 mcg MDI. High dose: >10 puffs 44 mcg MDI. >4 puffs 110 mcg MDI.

FORMS - Trade only: MDI: 44, 110, 220 mcg/ actuation in 60 & 120/canister. HFA MDI: 44, 110, 220 mcg/actuation in 120/canister. DPI: 50, 100, 250 mcg/actuation delivering 44, 88, 220 mcg respectively.

NOTES - Ritonavir & other CYP3A4 inhibitors such as ketoconazole significantly increase fluticasone concentrations, resulting in systemic effects, including adrenal suppression.

mometasone (*Asmanex Twisthaler***)** ▶L ♀C ▶? $$$$

ADULT - Chronic asthma: 1-2 puffs q pm or 1 puff bid. If prior oral corticosteroids: 2 puffs bid.

PEDS - Chronic asthma: ≥ 12 yo: Adult dose.

FORMS - Trade only: DPI: 220 mcg/actuation, 30, 60 & 120/canister.

NOTES - CYP3A4 inhibitors such as ketoconazole may significantly increase concentrations.

triamcinolone (*Azmacort***)** ▶L ♀D ▶? $$$$

ADULT - Chronic asthma: MDI: 2 puffs tid-qid or 4 puffs bid. Max dose 16 puffs/day. Severe asthma: 12-16 puffs/day and adjust downward.

PEDS - >12 yo: Adult dose. 6-12 yo: 1-2 puffs tid-qid or 2-4 puffs bid. Max dose 12 puffs/day.

UNAPPROVED ADULT - Chronic asthma: NHLBI dosing schedule (puffs/day divided bid): Low dose: 4-10 puffs. Medium dose: 10-20 puffs. High dose: >20 puffs.

UNAPPROVED PEDS - Chronic asthma: NHLBI dosing schedule (puffs/day divided bid): Low dose: 4-8 puffs. Medium dose: 8-12 puffs. High dose: >12 puffs.

FORMS - Trade only: MDI: 100 mcg/actuation, 240/canister. Built-in spacer.

INHALED STEROIDS: ESTIMATED COMPARATIVE DAILY DOSES*

Drug	Form	ADULT			CHILD (≤12 yo)		
		Low	Medium	High	Low	Medium	High
beclomethasone MDI	40 mcg/puff	2-6	6-12	>12	2-4	4-8	>8
	80 mcg/puff	1-3	3-6	>6	1-2	2-4	>4
budesonide DPI	200 mcg/dose	1-3	3-6	>6	1-2	2-4	>4
	Soln for nebs	-	-	-	0.5 mg	1 mg	2 mg
flunisolide MDI	250 mcg/puff	2-4	4-8	>8	2-3	4-5	>5
fluticasone MDI	44 mcg/puff	2-6	6-15	>15	2-4	4-10	>10
	110 mcg/puff	1-2	3-6	>6	1	1-4	>4
	220 mcg/puff	1	2-3	>3	n/a	1-2	>2
fluticasone DPI	50 mcg/dose	2-6	6-12	>12	2-4	4-8	>8
	100 mcg/dose	1-3	3-6	>6	1-2	2-4	>4
	250 mcg/dose	1	2	>2	n/a	1	>1
mometasone DPI	220 mcg/dose	1-2	3-4	>4	1	2	>2
triamcinolone MDI	100 mcg/puff	4-10	10-20	>20	4-8	8-12	>12

*MDI=metered dose inhaler. DPI=dry powder inhaler. All doses in puffs (MDI) or inhalations (DPI).
Reference: http://www.nhlbi.nih.gov/guidelines/asthma/execsumm.pdf

PULMONARY: Leukotriene Inhibitors

NOTE: Not for treatment of acute asthma. Abrupt substitution for corticosteroids may precipitate Churg-Strauss syndrome.

montelukast (*Singulair*) ▶L ♀B ▶? $$$$
ADULT - Chronic asthma, allergic rhinitis: 10 mg PO daily. Prevention of exercise-induced bronchoconstriction: 10 mg PO 2 h before exercise.
PEDS - Chronic asthma, allergic rhinitis: 6-14 yo: 5 mg PO daily. 2-5 yo: 4 mg (chew tab or oral granules) PO daily. Asthma 12-23 months: 4 mg (oral granules) PO daily. Allergic rhinitis 6-23 months: 4 mg (oral granules) PO daily. Prevention of exercise-induced bronchoconstriction: ≥ 15 yo: Use adult dose.
FORMS - Trade only: Tabs 10 mg. Oral granules 4 mg packet, 30/box. Chewable tabs (cherry flavored) 4 & 5 mg.
NOTES - Chew tabs contain phenylalanine. Oral granules may be taken directly or mixed with a spoonful of breast milk, baby formula, applesauce, carrots, rice or ice cream. If mixed with food, eat in <15 minutes. Do not mix with liquids. Levels decreased by phenobarbital & rifampin. Dyspepsia may occur. Do not take an additional dose for exercise-induced bronchospasm if already taking chronically.

zafirlukast (*Accolate*) ▶L ♀B ▶- $$$
WARNING - Hepatic failure has been reported.
ADULT - Chronic asthma: 20 mg PO bid, 1h ac or 2h pc.
PEDS - Chronic asthma ≥12 yo: use adult dose. 5-11 yo: 10 mg PO bid, 1h ac or 2h pc.
UNAPPROVED ADULT - Allergic rhinitis: 20 mg PO bid, 1h ac or 2h pc.
FORMS - Trade only: Tabs 10, 20 mg.
NOTES - Potentiates warfarin & theophylline. Levels decreased by erythromycin & increased by high-dose aspirin. Nausea may occur. If liver dysfunction is suspected, then discontinue drug. Consider monitoring LFTs.

zileuton (*Zyflo CR*) ▶L ♀C ▶? $$$$$
WARNING - Contraindicated in active liver dz.
ADULT - Chronic asthma: 1200 mg PO bid.
PEDS - Chronic asthma ≥12 yo: use adult dose.
FORMS - Trade: Tabs, ext'd release 600 mg.
NOTES - Monitor LFTs for elevation. Potentiates warfarin, theophylline, & propranolol. Dyspepsia & nausea may occur.

PULMONARY: Other

acetylcysteine (*Mucomyst*) ▶L ♀B ▶? $
ADULT - Mucolytic nebulization: 3-5 mL of the 20% soln or 6-10 mL of the 10% soln tid-qid. Instillation, direct or via tracheostomy: 1-2 mL of a 10% to 20% soln q1-4h; via percutaneous intratracheal catheter: 1-2 mL of the 20% soln or 2-4 mL of the 10% soln q1-4h.
PEDS - Mucolytic nebulization: Adult dosing.
FORMS - Generic/Trade: Soln for inhalation 10 & 20% in 4,10 & 30 mL vials.
NOTES - Increased volume of liquefied bronchial secretions may occur; maintain an open airway. Watch for bronchospasm in asthmatics. Stomatitis, N/V, fever, & rhinorrhea may occur. A slight disagreeable odor may occur & should soon disappear. Mask may cause facial stickiness after nebulization; wash with water. Dilute 20% soln with NaCl or sterile water.

alpha-1 proteinase inhibitor (alpha-1 antitrypsin, *Aralast, Prolastin, Zemaira*) ▶Plasma ♀C ▶? $
WARNING - Possible transmission of viruses, et, Creutzfeldt-Jakob disease.
ADULT - Congenital alpha-1 proteinase inhibitor deficiency with emphysema: 60 mg/kg IV q wk.
PEDS - Not approved in children.
NOTES - Contraindicated in selected IgA deficiencies with known antibody to IgA. Hepatitis B vaccine recommended before Prolastin use.

aminophylline (✿*Phyllocontin*) ▶L ♀C ▶? $
ADULT - Acute asthma: loading dose if currently not receiving theophylline: 6 mg/kg IV over 20-30 min. Maintenance IV infusion 1g in 250 mL D5W (4 mg/mL) at 0.5-0.7 mg/kg/h (70 kg: 0.7 mg/kg/h = 11 mL/h). In cor pulmonale, heart failure, liver failure, use 0.25 mg/kg/h. If currently on theophylline, each 0.6 mg/kg aminophylline will increase the serum theophylline concentration by approximately 1 mcg/mL. Maintenance: 200 mg PO bid-qid.
PEDS - Acute asthma: loading dose if currently not receiving theophylline: 6 mg/kg IV over 20-30 min. Maintenance >6 mo: 0.8-1 mg/kg/hr IV infusion. >1 yo: 3-4 mg/kg/dose PO q6h.
UNAPPROVED PEDS - Neonatal apnea of prematurity: loading dose 5-6 mg/kg IV/PO. Main-

tenance: 1-2 mg/kg/dose q6-8 h IV/PO.
FORMS - Generic: Tabs 100 & 200 mg. Oral liquid 105 mg/5 mL. Canada Trade only: Tabs controlled release (12 hr) 225, 350 mg, scored.
NOTES - Aminophylline is 79% theophylline. Administer IV infusion ≤25 mg/min. Multiple drug interactions (especially ketoconazole, rifampin, carbamazepine, isoniazid, phenytoin, macrolides, zafirlukast & cimetidine). Review meds before initiating treatment. Irritability, nausea, palpitations & tachycardia may occur. Overdose may be life-threatening.

beractant (*Survanta*) ▶Lung ♀? ▶? $$$$$
PEDS - RDS (hyaline membrane disease) in premature infants: Specialized dosing.

calfactant (*Infasurf*) ▶Lung ♀? ▶? $$$$$
PEDS - RDS (hyaline membrane disease) in premature infants: Specialized dosing.
FORMS - Trade only: Oral suspension: 35 mg/mL in 3 & 6 mL vials. Preservative-free.

cromolyn (*Intal, Gastrocrom, ✦Nalcrom*) ▶LK ♀B ▶? $$$
ADULT - Chronic asthma: MDI: 2-4 puffs qid. Soln for inhalation: 20 mg inh qid. Prevention of exercise-induced bronchospasm: MDI: 2 puffs 10-15 min prior to exercise. Soln for nebulization: 20 mg 10-15 min prior. Mastocytosis: 200 mg PO qid, 30 min ac & qhs.
PEDS - Chronic asthma >5 yo: MDI: 2 puffs qid. >2 yo: soln for nebulization: 20 mg inh qid. Prevention of exercise-induced bronchospasm >5 yo: MDI: 2 puffs 10-15 min prior to exercise. >2 yo soln for nebulization: 20 mg 10-15 min prior. Mastocytosis: 2-12 yo: 100 mg PO qid 30 min ac & qhs.
FORMS - Trade only: MDI 800 mcg/actuation, 112 & 200/canister. Oral concentrate 100 mg/5 mL in 8 amps/foil pouch (Gastrocrom). Generic/Trade: Soln for nebs: 20 mg/2 mL.
NOTES - Not for treatment of acute asthma. Pharyngitis may occur. Directions for oral concentrate: 1) Break open and squeeze liquid contents of ampule(s) into a glass of water. 2) Stir soln. 3) Drink all of the liquid.

dornase alfa (*Pulmozyme*) ▶L ♀B ▶? $$$$$
ADULT - Cystic fibrosis: 2.5 mg neb daily-bid.
PEDS - Cystic fibrosis ≥6 yo: 2.5 mg nebulized daily-bid.
UNAPPROVED PEDS - Has been used in a small number of children as young as 3 mo with similar efficacy & side effects.
FORMS - Trade only: soln for inhalation: 1 mg/ mL in 2.5 mL vials.
NOTES - Voice alteration, pharyngitis, laryngitis,

& rash may occur. Do not mix with other drugs.
doxapram (*Dopram*) ▶L ♀B ▶? $$$
ADULT - Acute hypercapnia due to COPD: 1-2 mg/min IV, max 3 mg/min. Maximum infusion time: 2 hours.
PEDS - Not approved in children.
UNAPPROVED PEDS - Apnea of prematurity unresponsive to methylxanthines: Load 2.5-3 mg/kg over 15 min, then 1 mg/kg/h titrated to lowest effective dose. Max: 2.5 mg/kg/h. Contains benzyl alcohol; caution in neonates.
NOTES - Monitor arterial blood gases at baseline and q30 min during infusion. Do not use with mechanical ventilation. Contraindicated with seizure disorder, severe HTN, CVA, head injury, CAD and severe heart failure.

epinephrine racemic (*S-2, ✦Vaponefrin*) ▶Plasma ♀C ▶- $
ADULT - See cardiovascular section
PEDS - Severe croup: soln for inhalation: 0.05 mL/kg/dose diluted to 3 mL w/NS over 15 min prn not to exceed q1-2h dosing. Max 0.5 mL.
FORMS - Trade only: soln for inhalation: 2.25% epinephrine in 15 & 30 mL.
NOTES - Cardiac arrhythmias, HTN may occur.

ipratropium (*Atrovent, Atrovent HFA*) ▶Lung ♀B ▶? $$$
ADULT - COPD: MDI (Atrovent, Atrovent HFA): 2 puffs qid; may use additional inhalations not to exceed 12 puffs/day. Soln for inhalation: 500 mcg nebulized tid-qid.
PEDS - Not approved in children <12 yo.
UNAPPROVED PEDS - Acute asthma: MDI (Atrovent, Atrovent HFA): >12 yo: Adult dose. ≤12 yo: 1-2 puffs tid-qid. Soln for inhalation: >12 yo: 250-500 mcg/dose tid-qid; ≤12 yo: 250 mcg/ dose tid-qid. Acute asthma: 2-18yo: 500 mcg nebulized with 2nd & 3rd doses of albuterol.
FORMS - Trade: Atrovent HFA MDI: 17 mcg/actuation, 200/canister. Generic/Trade: Soln for neb: 0.02% (500 mcg/vial) in unit dose vials.
NOTES - Atrovent MDI is contraindicated with soy or peanut allergy; HFA not contraindicated. Caution with glaucoma, myasthenia gravis, BPH, or bladder neck obstruction. Cough, dry mouth & blurred vision may occur.

ketotifen (*✦Zaditen*) ▶L ♀C ▶- $$
ADULT - Not approved.
PEDS - Canada. Chronic asthma: 6 mo to 3 yo: 0.05 mg/kg PO bid. >3 yo: 1 mg PO bid.
FORMS - Generic/Trade: Tabs 1 mg. Syrup 1 mg/5 mL.
NOTES - Several weeks may be necessary before therapeutic effect. Full clinical effective-

ness is generally reached after 10 weeks.

methacholine (*Provocholine*) ▶Plasma ♀C ▶? $$

WARNING - Life-threatening bronchoconstriction can result; have resuscitation capability available.

ADULT - Diagnosis of bronchial airway hyperreactivity in non-wheezing patients with suspected asthma: 5 breaths each of ascending serial concentrations, 0.025 mg/mL to 25 mg/mL, via nebulization. The procedure ends when there is a ≥20% reduction in the FEV1 compared with baseline.

PEDS - Diagnosis of bronchial airway hyperreactivity: use adult dose.

NOTES - Avoid with epilepsy, bradycardia, peptic ulcer disease, thyroid disease, urinary tract obstruction or other conditions that could be adversely affected by a cholinergic agent. Hold beta-blockers. Do not inhale powder.

nedocromil (*Tilade*) ▶L ♀B ▶? $$$

ADULT - Chronic asthma: MDI: 2 puffs qid. Reduce dose to bid-tid as tolerated.

PEDS - Chronic asthma >6yo: MDI: 2 puffs qid.

FORMS - Trade only: MDI: 1.75 mg/actuation, 112/canister.

NOTES - Not for treatment of acute asthma. Unpleasant taste & dysphonia may occur.

nitric oxide (*INOmax*) ▶Lung, K ♀C ▶? $$$$

PEDS - Respiratory failure with pulmonary HTN in infants >34 weeks old: Specialized dosing.

NOTES - Risk of methemoglobinemia increases with concomitant nitroprusside or nitroglycerin.

omalizumab (*Xolair*) ▶Plasma, L ♀B ▶? $$$$$

WARNING - Anaphylaxis may occur within 2 hours of administration; monitor closely and be prepared to treat.

ADULT - Moderate to severe asthma with perennial allergy: 150-375 mg SC q 2-4 weeks, based on pretreatment serum total IgE level & body weight.

PEDS - ≥12 yo: Use adult dose.

NOTES - Not for treatment of acute asthma. Divide doses >150 mg over more than 1 injection site. Monitor for signs of anaphylaxis.

poractant (*Curosurf*) ▶Lung ♀? ▶? $$$$$

PEDS - RDS (hyaline membrane disease) in premature infants: Specialized dosing.

theophylline (*Elixophyllin, Uniphyl, Theo-24, T-Phyl, ♣Theo-Dur, Theolair*) ▶L ♀C ▶+ $

ADULT - Chronic asthma: 5-13 mg/kg/day PO in divided doses. Max dose 900 mg/day.

PEDS - Initial: >1 yo & <45 kg: 12-14 mg/kg/day PO divided q4-6h to max of 300 mg/24h. Maintenance: 16-20 mg/kg/day PO divided q4-6h to max of 600 mg/24h. >1 yo & ≥45 kg: Initial: 300 mg/24h PO divided q6-8h. Maintenance: 400-600 mg/24h PO divided q6-8h. Infants 6-52 weeks: [(0.2 x age in weeks) + 5] x kg = 24hr dose in mg PO divided q6-8h.

UNAPPROVED ADULT - COPD: 10 mg/kg/day PO in divided doses.

UNAPPROVED PEDS - Apnea & bradycardia of prematurity: 3-6 mg/kg/day PO divided q6-8h. Maintain serum concentrations 3-5 mcg/mL.

FORMS - Generic/Trade: Elixir 80 mg/15 mL. Trade: Caps - Theo-24: 100, 200, 300, 400 mg. T-Phyl - 12 Hr SR tabs 200 mg. Theolair - tabs 125, 250 mg. Generic: 12 Hr tabs 100, 200, 300, 450 mg, 12 Hr caps 125, 200, 300 mg.

NOTES - Multiple drug interactions (especially ketoconazole, rifampin, carbamazepine, isoniazid, phenytoin, macrolides, zafirlukast & cimetidine). Review meds before initiating treatment. Overdose may be life-threatening.

tiotropium (*Spiriva*) ▶K ♀C ▶- $$$$

ADULT - COPD: Handihaler: 18 mcg inhaled daily.

PEDS - Not approved in children.

FORMS - Trade only: Capsule for oral inhalation 18 mcg. To be used with "Handihaler" device only. Packages of 6 or 30 capsules with Handihaler device.

NOTES - Not for acute bronchospasm. Administer at the same time each day. Caution in narrow-angle glaucoma, myasthenia gravis, BPH, bladder-neck obstruction. Avoid touching opened capsule. Glaucoma, eye pain, or blurred vision may occur if powder enters eyes. May increase dosing interval in patients with CrCl <50 mL/min. Avoid if severe lactose allergy.

TOXICOLOGY

acetylcysteine (*Mucomyst, Acetadote, ♣Parvolex*) ▶L ♀B ▶? $$$$

ADULT - Acetaminophen toxicity: Mucomyst – loading dose 140 mg/kg PO or NG, then 70

mg/kg q4h x 17 doses. May be mixed in water or soft drink diluted to a 5% solution. Acetadote (IV) – loading dose 150 mg/kg in 200 mL of D5W infused over 60 min; maintenance dose

50 mg/kg in 500 mL of D5W infused over 4 hours followed by 100 mg/kg in 1000 mL of D5W infused over 16 hours.

PEDS - Acetaminophen toxicity: Adult dosing.

UNAPPROVED ADULT - Prevention of contrast-induced nephropathy: 600-1200 mg PO bid for 2 doses before procedure and 2 doses after procedure.

FORMS - Generic/Trade: solution 10%, 20%. Trade only: IV (Acetadote)

NOTES - May be diluted with water or soft drink to a 5% solution; use within 1 hour. Repeat loading dose if vomited within 1 hour. Critical ingestion-treatment interval for maximal protection against severe hepatic injury is between 0-8 hours. Efficacy diminishes after 8 hours & treatment initiation between 15 & 24 hours post ingestion yields limited efficacy. However, treatment should not be withheld, since the reported time of ingestion may not be correct. Anaphylactoid reactions usually occurs 30-60 mins after initiating infusion. Stop infusion, administer antihistamine or epinephrine, restart infusion slowly. If anaphylactoid reactions return or severity increases, then stop treatment.

charcoal (activated charcoal, *Actidose-Aqua, CharcoAid, EZ-Char, ✚Charcodate*) ▶Not absorbed ♀+ ▶+ $

ADULT - Gut decontamination: 25-100 g (1-2 g/kg or 10 times the amount of poison ingested) PO or NG as soon as possible. May repeat q1-4h prn at doses equivalent to 12.5g/hr. When sorbitol is coadministered, use only with the first dose if repeated doses are to be given.

PEDS - Gut decontamination: <1 yo - 1 g/kg; 15-30 g or 1-2 g/kg if 1-12 yo PO or NG as soon as possible. Repeat doses in children have not been established, but half the initial dose is recommended. Repeat q 2-6h prn. When sorbitol is coadministered, use only with the first dose if repeated doses are to be given.

FORMS - OTC/Generic/Trade: Powder 15,30, 40,120,240 g. Solution 12.5 g/60 mL, 15 g/75 mL, 15g/120 mL, 25 g/120 mL, 30 g/120 mL, 50 g/240 mL. Suspension 15g/120 mL, 25g/120 ml, 30g/150 mL, 50g/240 mL. Granules 15g/120 mL.

NOTES - Some products contain sorbitol to improve taste and reduce GI transit time. Chocolate milk/powder may enhance palatability for children. Not usually effective for toxic alcohols (methanol, ethylene glycol, isopropanol), heavy metals (lead, iron, bromide), arsenic, lithium, potassium, hydrocarbons, and caustics (acids, alkalis). Mix powder with 8 oz water. Greatest effect when administered <1 hour of ingestion.

Cyanide Antidote Kit (amyl nitrite + sodium nitrite + sodium thiosulfate) ▶? ♀-▶? $$$$$

ADULT - Cyanide toxicity: Induce methemoglobinemia with inhaled amyl nitrite 0.3 mL followed by sodium nitrite 300 mg IV over 2-4 minutes. Then administer sodium thiosulfate 12.5 g IV.

PEDS - Induce methemoglobinemia with inhaled amyl nitrite followed by sodium nitrite 240 mg/m^2 (max 300 mg) IV over 2-4 minutes. Then administer sodium thiosulfate 7 g/m^2 (max 12.5 g) IV.

FORMS - Package contains amyl nitrite inhalant (0.3mL), sodium nitrite (300 mg/10 mL), sodium thiosulfate (12.5 g/50 mL).

NOTES - Risk of excessive methemoglobinemia with both nitrite components; monitor closely.

deferasirox (*Exjade*) ▶L ♀B ▶? $$$$$

ADULT - Chronic iron overload: 20 mg/kg PO daily; adjust dose q3-6 months based on ferritin trends. Max 30 mg/kg/day.

PEDS - Chronic iron overload, ≥2 yo: 20 mg/kg PO daily; adjust dose q3-6 months based on ferritin trends. Max 30 mg/kg/day.

FORMS - Trade only: Tabs for dissolving into oral suspension 125, 250, 500 mg.

NOTES - Assess creatinine in duplicate before therapy & monthly thereafter; renal failure has been reported. Monitor LFTs monthly during treatment; consider modification of dose if elevation. Perform auditory & ophthalmic testing before initiation and yearly thereafter. Do not take with aluminum-containing antacids.

deferoxamine (*Desferal*) ▶K ♀C ▶? $$$$$

ADULT - Chronic iron overload: 500 mg- 1000 mg IM daily and 2 g IV infusion (≤15 mg/kg/hr) with each unit of blood or 1-2 g SC daily (20-40 mg/kg/day) over 8-24 h via continuous infusion pump. Acute iron toxicity: IV infusion up to 15 mg/kg/hr (consult poison center).

PEDS - Acute iron toxicity: IV infusion up to 15 mg/kg/hr (consult poison center).

NOTES - Contraindicated in renal failure/anuria unless undergoing dialysis.

dimercaprol (*BAL in oil*) ▶KL ♀C ▶? $$$$$

ADULT - Specialized dosing for arsenic, mercury, gold, lead toxicity. Consult poison center. Mild arsenic or gold toxicity: 2.5 mg/kg IM qid x 2 days, then bid x 1 day, then daily x 10 days. Severe arsenic or gold toxicity: 3 mg/kg IM q4h x 2 days, then qid x 1 day, then bid x 10 days.

Mercury toxicity: 5 mg/kg IM initially, then 2.5 mg/kg daily-bid x 10 days. Begin therapy within 1-2 h of toxicity. Acute lead encephalopathy: 4 mg/kg IM initially, then q4h in combination (separate syringe) with calcium edetate x 2-7 days. May reduce dose to 3 mg/kg IM for less severe toxicity. Deep IM injection needed.

PEDS - Not approved in children.

UNAPPROVED PEDS - Adult dosing.

Duodote *(atropine + pralidoxime)* ▶K♀C▶?$

ADULT - Organophosphate insecticide / nerve agent poisoning, mild symptoms: 1 injection in thigh. Severe symptoms: 3 injections in rapid succession (may administer through clothes).

PEDS - Not approved in children.

FORMS - Each auto-injector dose delivers atropine 2.1 mg + pralidoxime 600 mg.

edetate *(EDTA, Endrate, versenate)* ▶K♀C ▶- $$$

WARNING - Beware of elevated intracranial pressure in lead encephalopathy.

ADULT - Consult poison center. Use calcium disodium form only for lead indications. Non-calcium form (eg, *Endrate*) is not interchangeable and is rarely used anymore. Lead toxicity: 1000 mg/m^2/day IM (divided into equal doses q8-12h) or IV (infuse total dose over 8-12h) x 5 days. Stop therapy for 2-4 days, then repeat same regimen. Two courses of therapy are usually necessary. Acute lead encephalopathy: edetate alone or in combination with dimercaprol. Lead nephropathy: 500 mg/m^2/dose q24h x 5 doses (creat 2-3 mg/dl), q48h x 3 doses (creat 3-4 mg/dl), or once weekly (creat >4 mg/dl). May repeat at one month intervals.

PEDS - Adult dosing.

ethanol *(alcohol)* ▶L♀D▶+ $

PEDS - Not approved in children.

UNAPPROVED ADULT - Consult poison center. Specialized dosing for methanol, ethylene glycol toxicity if fomepizole unavailable/delayed: 1000 mg/kg (10 mL/kg) of 10% ethanol (100 mg/mL) IV over 1-2h then 100 mg/kg (1 mL/kg/h) to keep level approximately 100 mg/dl.

flumazenil *(Romazicon)* ▶LK♀C▶? $$$

WARNING - Do not use in chronic benzodiazepine use or acute overdose with tricyclic antidepressants due to seizure risk.

ADULT - Benzodiazepine sedation reversal: 0.2 mg IV over 15 sec, then 0.2 mg q1 min prn up to 1 mg total dose. Usual dose is 0.6- 1 mg. Benzodiazepine overdose reversal: 0.2 mg IV over 30 sec, then 0.3-0.5 mg q30 sec prn up to 3 mg total dose.

PEDS - Benzodiazepine sedation reversal: 0.01 mg/kg up to 0.2 mg IV over 15 sec; repeat q minute to max 4 additional doses.

UNAPPROVED PEDS - Benzodiazepine overdose reversal: 0.01 mg/kg IV. Benzodiazepine sedation reversal: 0.01 mg/kg IV initially (max 0.2 mg), then 0.005-0.01 mg/kg (max 0.2 mg) q1 min to max total dose 1 mg. May repeat doses in 20 min, max 3 mg in 1 hour.

NOTES - Onset of action 1-3 min, peak effect 6-10 min. For IV use only, preferably through an IV infusion line into a large vein. Local irritation may occur following extravasation.

fomepizole *(Antizol)* ▶L♀C▶? $$$$$

ADULT - Consult poison center. Ethylene glycol or methanol toxicity: 15 mg/kg IV (load), then 10 mg/kg IV q12h x 4 doses, then 15 mg/kg IV q12h until ethylene glycol or methanol level <20 mg/dl. Administer doses as slow IV infusions over 30 minutes. Increase frequency to q4h during hemodialysis.

PEDS - Not approved in children.

hydroxocobalamin *(Cyanokit)* ▶K♀C▶? ?

ADULT - Cyanide poisoning: 5 g IV over 15 minutes; may repeat prn.

PEDS - Not approved in children.

ipecac syrup ▶Gut♀C▶? $

ADULT - Emesis: 15- 30 mL PO, then 3-4 glasses of water.

PEDS - AAP no longer recommends using ipecac for poisoning. Emesis, <1 yo: 5-10 mL, then ½ - 1 glass of water (controversial in children <1 yo). Emesis, 1- 12 yo: 15 mL, then 1-2 glasses of water. May repeat dose (15 mL) if vomiting does not occur within 20- 30 minutes.

FORMS - Generic only (OTC): syrup.

NOTES - Many believe ipecac contraindicated in infants <6 mo. Do not use if any potential for altered mental status (eg, seizure, neurotoxicity), strychnine, beta blocker, calcium channel blocker, clonidine, digitalis glycoside, corrosive, petroleum distillate ingestions, or if at risk for GI bleeding (coagulopathy).

methylene blue *(Methblue 65, Urolene blue)* ▶K♀C▶? $$

ADULT - Methemoglobinemia: 1-2 mg/kg IV over 5 minutes. Dysuria: 65-130 mg PO tid after meals with liberal water.

PEDS - Not approved in children.

UNAPPROVED PEDS - Methemoglobinemia: 1-2 mg/kg/dose IV over 5 minutes; may repeat in 1 hour prn.

FORMS - Trade only: Tab 65 mg.

NOTES - Avoid in G6PD deficiency. May turn

urine, stool, skin, contact lenses, and undergarments blue-green.

penicillamine (*Cuprimine, Depen*) ▶K ♀D ▶- $$$$

WARNING - Fatal drug-related adverse events have occurred, caution if penicillin allergy.

ADULT - Consult poison center: Specialized dosing for copper toxicity: 750 mg- 1.5 g/day PO x 3 months based on 24-hour urinary copper excretion, max 2 g/day. May start 250 mg/ day PO in patients unable to tolerate.

PEDS - Specialized dosing for copper toxicity.

FORMS - Trade only: Caps 125, 250 mg; Tabs 250 mg.

NOTES - Patients may require supplemental pyridoxine 25-50 mg/day PO. Promotes excretion of heavy metals in urine.

physostigmine (*Antilirium*) ▶LK ♀D ▶? $

WARNING - Discontinue if excessive salivation, emesis, frequent urination, or diarrhea. Rapid administration can cause bradycardia, hypersalivation, respiratory difficulties and seizures. Atropine should be available as an antagonist.

ADULT - Life-threatening anticholinergic toxicity: 2 mg IV/IM, administer IV slowly, ≤1 mg/min. May repeat q 10-30 min for severe toxicity.

PEDS - Life-threatening anticholinergic toxicity: 0.02 mg/kg IM/IV injection, administer IV slowly, ≤0.5 mg/min. May repeat q15-30 min until a therapeutic effect or max 2 mg dose.

UNAPPROVED ADULT - Postanesthesia reversal of neuromuscular blockade: 0.5-1 mg IV/IM, administer IV slowly, ≤1mg/min. May repeat q 10-30 min prn.

FORMS - Generic/Trade: 1mg/mL, 2ml ampules

pralidoxime (*Protopam, 2-PAM*) ▶K ♀C ▶? $$$

ADULT - Consult poison center: Specialized dosing for organophosphate toxicity: 1-2 g IV infusion over 15-30 min or slow IV injection ≥5 min (max rate 200 mg/min). May repeat dose after 1 h if muscle weakness persists.

PEDS - Not approved in children.

UNAPPROVED ADULT - Consult poison center: 20-40 mg/kg/dose IV infusion over 15-30 min.

UNAPPROVED PEDS - Consult poison center. 25 mg/kg load then 10-20 mg/kg/hr or 25-50 mg/kg load followed by repeat dose in 1-2 hours then q10-12h.

NOTES - Administer <36h of exposure when possible. Rapid administration may worsen cholinergic symptoms. Give in conjunction with atropine. IM or SC may be used if IV access is not available.

succimer (*Chemet*) ▶K ♀C ▶? $$$$$

PEDS - Lead toxicity ≥1 yo: Start 10 mg/kg PO or 350 mg/m^2 q8h x 5 days, then reduce the frequency to q12h x 2 weeks. Not approved in children <12 mo.

FORMS - Trade only: Caps 100 mg.

NOTES - Manufacturer recommends doses of 100 mg (8-15 kg), 200 mg (16-23 kg), 300 mg (24-34 kg), 400 mg (35-44 kg), and 500 mg (≥45 kg). Can open cap and sprinkle medicated beads over food, or give them in a spoon and follow with fruit drink. Indicated for lead levels >45 mcg/dl. Allow ≥4 weeks between edetate disodium and succimer treatment.

ANTIDOTES

Toxin	Antidote/Treatment	Toxin	Antidote/Treatment
acetaminophen	N-acetylcysteine	ethylene glycol	fomepizole
antidepressants, cyclic	bicarbonate	heparin	protamine
arsenic, mercury	dimercaprol (BAL)	iron	deferoxamine
benzodiazepine	flumazenil	lead	EDTA, succimer
beta blockers	glucagon	methanol	fomepizole
calcium channel blockers	calcium chloride, glucagon	methemoglobin	methylene blue
cyanide	hydroxocobalamin	opioids	naloxone
digoxin	dig immune Fab	organophosphates	atropine + pralidoxime
		warfarin	vitamin K, FFP

UROLOGY: Benign Prostatic Hyperplasia

alfuzosin (*UroXatral*, ♣*Xatral*) ▶KL ♀B ▶- $$$

WARNING - Postural hypotension with or without symptoms may develop within a few hours after administration. Avoid in moderate or severe hepatic insufficiency. Avoid co-administration with potent CYP3A4 inhibitors.

ADULT - BPH: 10 mg PO daily after a meal.

PEDS - Not approved in children.
UNAPPROVED ADULT - Promote spontaneous passage of ureteral calculi: 10 mg PO daily usually combined with an NSAID, antiemetic and opioid of choice.
FORMS - Trade: extended-release tab 10 mg
NOTES - Do not use in moderate to severe hepatic insufficiency. Caution in congenital or acquired QT prolongation & severe renal insufficiency. Intraoperative floppy iris syndrome has been observed during cataract surgery.

dutasteride (Avodart) ▶L ♀X ▶- $$$
ADULT - BPH: 0.5 mg PO daily.
PEDS - Not approved in children.
FORMS - Trade only: Cap 0.5 mg.
NOTES - 6 months' therapy may be needed to assess effectiveness. Pregnant or potentially pregnant women should not handle capsules due to fetal risk from absorption. Caution in hepatic insufficiency. Dutasteride will decrease PSA by 50%; new baseline PSA should be established after 3-6 months to assess potentially cancer-related PSA changes.

finasteride (Proscar) ▶L ♀X ▶- $$$
ADULT - 5 mg PO daily alone or in combination with doxazosin to reduce the risk of symptomatic progression of BPH.
PEDS - Not approved in children.
FORMS - Generic/Trade: Tab 5 mg.

NOTES - 6-12 months may be needed to assess effectiveness. Pregnant or potentially pregnant women should not handle crushed tabs because of possible absorption and fetal risk. Use with caution in hepatic insufficiency. Monitor PSA before therapy; finasteride will decrease PSA by 50% with BPH, even with prostate cancer. Does not appear to alter detection of prostate cancer.

tamsulosin (Flomax) ▶LK ♀B ▶- $$$
ADULT - BPH: 0.4 mg PO daily 30 min after the same meal each day. If an adequate response is not seen after 2-4 wks, may increase dose to 0.8 mg PO daily. If therapy is interrupted for several days, restart at the 0.4 mg dose.
PEDS - Not approved in children.
UNAPPROVED ADULT - Promote spontaneous passage of ureteral calculi: 0.4 mg PO daily usually combined with an NSAID, antiemetic and opioid of choice.
FORMS - Trade only: Cap 0.4 mg.
NOTES - Dizziness, headache, abnormal ejaculation. Alpha blockers are generally considered to be first line treatment in men with more than minimal symptoms. Caution in serious sulfa allergy; rare allergy reported. Intraoperative floppy iris syndrome with cataract surgery reported. Caution with strong inhibitors of CYP450 2D6 (fluoxetine) or 3A4 (ketoconazole).

UROLOGY: Bladder Agents – Anticholinergics & Combinations

B&O Supprettes (belladonna + opium) ▶L ♀C ▶? ©II $$$
ADULT - Bladder spasm: 1 suppository PR daily-bid, max 4 doses/day.
PEDS - Not approved in children <12 yo.
FORMS - Generic/Trade: suppositories 30 mg opium (15A), 60 mg opium (16A).
NOTES - Store at room temperature. Contraindicated in narrow-angle glaucoma, obstructive conditions (eg, pyloric, duodenal or other intestinal obstructive lesions, ileus, achalasia, and obstructive uropathies).

darifenacin (Enablex) ▶LK ♀C ▶- $$$$
ADULT - Overactive bladder with symptoms of urinary urgency, frequency and urge incontinence 7.5 mg PO daily. May increase to max dose 15 mg PO daily in 2 weeks. Max dose 7.5 mg PO daily with moderate liver impairment or when coadministered with potent CYP3A4 inhibitors (ketoconazole, itraconazole, ritonavir, nelfinavir, clarithromycin & nefazodone).

PEDS - Not approved in children.
FORMS - Trade only: Extended-release tabs 7.5, 15 mg.
NOTES - Contraindicated with uncontrolled narrow-angle glaucoma, urinary & gastric retention. Avoid use in severe hepatic impairment. May increase concentration of medications metabolized by CYP2D6.

flavoxate (Urispas) ▶K ♀B ▶? $$$$
ADULT - Bladder spasm: 100 or 200 mg PO tid-qid. Reduce dose when improved.
PEDS - Not approved in children <12 yo.
FORMS - Trade only: Tab 100 mg.
NOTES - May cause dizziness, drowsiness, blurred vision, dry mouth, N/V, urinary retention. Contraindicated in glaucoma, obstructive conditions (eg, pyloric, duodenal or other intestinal obstructive lesions, ileus, achalasia, GI hemorrhage, and obstructive uropathies).

oxybutynin (Ditropan, Ditropan XL, Oxytrol, ✦Oxybutyn, Uromax) ▶LK ♀B ▶? $

ADULT - Bladder instability: 2.5-5 mg PO bid-tid, max 5 mg PO qid. Ext'd release tabs: 5-10 mg PO daily same time each day, increase 5 mg/day q week to 30 mg/day. Oxytrol: 1 patch twice weekly on abdomen, hips or buttocks.

PEDS - Bladder instability >5 yo: 5 mg PO bid, max dose: 5 mg PO tid. Extended release, >6 yo: 5 mg PO daily, max 20 mg/day. Transdermal patch not approved in children.

UNAPPROVED PEDS - Bladder instability ≤5 yo: 0.2 mg/kg/dose PO bid-qid.

FORMS - Generic/Trade: Tab 5 mg. Syrup 5 mg/5 mL Extended release tabs 5, 10, 15 mg. Trade only: Transdermal (Oxytrol) 3.9 mg/day.

NOTES - May cause dizziness, drowsiness, blurred vision, dry mouth, urinary retention. Contraindicated with glaucoma, obstructive GU or GI disease, unstable cardiovascular status, and myasthenia gravis. Transdermal patch causes less dry mouth than oral form; avoid dose reduction by cutting.

Prosed/DS (methenamine + phenyl salicylate + methylene blue + benzoic acid + hyoscyamine) ▶KL ♀C ▶? $$$

ADULT - Bladder spasm: 1 tab PO qid with liberal fluids.

PEDS - Not approved in children

FORMS - Trade: Tab (methenamine 81.6 mg/phenyl salicylate 36.2 mg/methylene blue 10.8 mg/benzoic acid 9.0 mg/hyoscyamine sulfate 0.12 mg). Prosed EC = enteric coated form.

NOTES - May cause dizziness, drowsiness, blurred vision, dry mouth, N/V, urinary retention. May turn urine/contact lenses blue.

solifenacin (*VESIcare*) ▶LK ♀C ▶- $$$$

ADULT - Overactive bladder with symptoms of urinary urgency, frequency or urge incontinence: 5 mg PO daily. Max dose: 10 mg PO daily (5 mg PO daily if CrCl<30 mL/min, moderate hepatic impairment, or concurrent ketoconazole or other potent CYP3A4 inhibitors).

PEDS - Not approved in children.

FORMS - Trade only: Tabs 5,10 mg

NOTES - Contraindicated with uncontrolled narrow-angle glaucoma, urinary & gastric retention. Avoid use in severe hepatic impairment. Hallucinations have been reported.

tolterodine (*Detrol, Detrol LA, ✦Unidet*) ▶L ♀C ▶- $$$$

ADULT - Overactive bladder: 2 mg PO bid (Detrol) or 4 mg PO daily (Detrol LA). Decrease dose to 1 mg bid (Detrol) or 2 mg daily (Detrol LA) if adverse symptoms, hepatic insufficiency or specific coadministered drugs (see notes).

PEDS - Not approved in children.

FORMS - Trade only: Tabs 1, 2 mg. Caps, extended release 2, 4 mg.

NOTES - Contraindicated with urinary or gastric retention, uncontrolled glaucoma. High doses may prolong the QT interval. Drug interactions with CYP3A4 inhibitors (e.g. erythromycin, ketoconazole, itraconazole); decrease dose to 1 mg PO bid or 2 mg PO daily (Detrol LA).

trospium (*Sanctura, ✦Trosec*) ▶LK ♀C ▶? $$$

ADULT - Overactive bladder with urge incontinence: 20 mg PO bid. Renal impairment (CrCl <30 mL/min): 20 mg PO qhs. If ≥75 yo may taper down to 20 mg daily.

PEDS - Not approved in children.

FORMS - Trade only: Tab 20 mg

NOTES - Contraindicated with uncontrolled narrow-angle glaucoma, urinary retention, gastroparesis. May cause heat stroke due to decreased sweating. Take on an empty stomach. Improvement may be seen in a week. Causes minimum CNS side effects.

Urised (methenamine + phenyl salicylate + atropine + hyoscyamine + benzoic acid + methylene blue, *Usept*) ▶K ♀C ▶? $$$$

ADULT - Dysuria: 2 Tabs PO qid.

PEDS - Dysuria >6 yo: reduce dose based on age and weight. Not recommended if <6 yo.

FORMS - Trade only: Tab (methenamine 40.8 mg/phenyl salicylate 18.1 mg/atropine 0.03 mg/hyoscyamine 0.03 mg/4.5 mg benzoic acid/5.4 mg methylene blue).

NOTES - Take with food to minimize GI upset. May precipitate urate crystals in urine. Avoid with sulfas. May turn urine/contact lenses blue.

UTA (methenamine + sodium phosphate + phenyl salicylate + methylene blue + hyoscyamine) ▶KL ♀C ▶? $$$

ADULT - Treatment of irritative voiding/relief of inflammation, hypermotility & pain with lower urinary tract infection/relief of urinary tract symptoms caused by diagnostic procedures: 1 cap PO qid with liberal fluids.

PEDS - <6 yo: not recommended. >6 yo: dosing must be individualized by physician.

FORMS - Trade: Cap (methenamine 120 mg/Na phosphate 40.8 mg/phenyl salicylate 36 mg/methylene blue 10 mg/hyoscyamine 0.12 mg).

NOTES - May turn urine/feces blue to blue-green. Take 2 hours apart from ketoconazole. May decrease thiazide absorption. Antacids and antidiarrheals may decrease effectiveness.

UROLOGY: Bladder Agents – Other

bethanechol (*Urecholine, Duvoid, ♣Myotonachol*) ▶L ♀C ▶? $
ADULT - Urinary retention: 10-50 mg PO tid-qid or 2.5-5 mg SC tid-qid. Take 1 hour before or 2 h after meals to avoid N/V. Determine the minimum effective dose by giving 5-10 mg PO initially and repeat at hourly intervals until response or to a maximum of 50 mg.
PEDS - Not approved in children.
UNAPPROVED PEDS - Urinary retention/abdominal distention: 0.6 mg/kg/day PO divided q6-8h or 0.12-0.2 mg/kg/day SC divided q6-8h.
FORMS - Generic/Trade: Tabs 5, 10, 25, 50 mg.
NOTES - May cause drowsiness, lightheadedness, and fainting. Not for obstructive urinary retention. Avoid with cardiac disease, hyperthyroidism, parkinsonism, peptic ulcer disease, and epilepsy.

dimethyl sulfoxide (*DMSO, Rimso-50*) ▶KL ♀C ▶? $$$
ADULT - Interstitial cystitis: Instill 50 mL solution into bladder by catheter & allow to remain for 15 min; expelled by spontaneous voiding. Repeat q2 weeks until symptomatic relief is obtained; thereafter, may increase time intervals between treatments.
PEDS - Not approved in children.
NOTES - Apply analgesic lubricant gel to urethra prior to inserting the catheter to avoid spasm. May administer oral analgesics or suppositories containing belladonna & opium prior to instillation to reduce spasms. May give anesthesia in patients with severe interstitial cystitis and very sensitive bladders during the 1st, 2nd & 3rd treatment. May cause lens opacities & changes in refractive index; perform eye exams before & periodically during treatment. May cause a hypersensitivity reaction by liberating histamine. Monitor liver & renal function tests & CBC q6 months. May be harmful in patients with urinary tract malignancy; can cause DMSO-induced vasodilation. Peripheral neuropathy may occur when used with sulindac. Garlic-like taste may occur within a few minutes of administration; odor on breath & skin may be present & remain for up to 72 h.

pentosan (*Elmiron*) ▶LK ♀B ▶? $$$$
ADULT - Interstitial cystitis: 100 mg PO tid 1h before or 2h after a meal.
PEDS - Not approved in children.
FORMS - Trade only: Caps 100 mg.
NOTES - Pain relief usually occurs at 2-4 months and decreased urinary frequency takes 6 months. May increase risk of bleeding, especially with NSAIDs. Use with caution in hepatic or splenic dysfunction.

phenazopyridine (*Pyridium, Azo-Standard, Urogesic, Prodium, Pyridiate, Urodol, Baridium, UTI Relief, ♣Phenazo*) ▶K ♀B ▶? $
ADULT - Dysuria: 200 mg PO tid after meals x 2 days.
PEDS - Dysuria in children 6-12 yo: 12 mg/kg/day PO divided tid x 2 days.
FORMS - OTC Generic/Trade: Tabs 95, 97.2 mg. Rx Generic/Trade: Tabs 100, 200 mg.
NOTES - May turn urine/contact lenses orange. Contraindicated with hepatitis or renal insufficiency.

UROLOGY: Erectile Dysfunction

alprostadil (*Muse, Caverject, Caverject Impulse, Edex, Prostin VR Pediatric, prostaglandin E1, ♣Prostin VR*) ▶L ♀- ▶- $$$$
ADULT - Erectile dysfunction: 1.25-2.5 mcg intracavernosal injection over 5-10 seconds initially using a ½ inch, 27 or 30 gauge needle. If no response, may give next higher dose after 1 hour, max 2 doses/day. May increase by 2.5 mcg and then 5-10 mcg incrementally on separate occasions. Dose range= 1-40 mcg. Alternative: 125-250 mcg intraurethral pellet (Muse). Increase or decrease dose on separate occasions until erection achieved. Maximum intraurethral dose 2 pellets/24h. The lowest possible dose to produce an acceptable erection should be used.
PEDS - Temporary maintenance of patent ductus arteriosus in neonates: Start 0.1 mcg/kg/min IV infusion. Reduce dose to minimal amount that maintains therapeutic response. Max dose 0.4 mcg/kg/min.
UNAPPROVED ADULT - Erectile dysfunction intracorporeal injection: Specially formulated mixtures of alprostadil, papaverine and phentolamine. 0.10-0.50 mL injection.
FORMS - Trade only: Syringe system (Edex)

10, 20, 40 mcg. (Caverject) 5, 10, 20 mcg. (Caverject Impulse) 10, 20 mcg. Pellet (Muse) 125, 250, 500, 1000 mcg. Intracorporeal injection of locally-compounded combination agents (many variations): "Bi-mix" can be 30 mg/mL papaverine + 0.5 to 1 mg/mL phentolamine, or 30 mg/mL papaverine + 20 mcg/mL alprostadil in 10 mL vials. "Tri-mix" can be 30 mg/mL papaverine + 1 mg/mL phentolamine + 10 mcg/mL alprostadil in 5, 10 or 20 mL vials.

NOTES - Contraindicated in patients at risk for priapism, with penile fibrosis (Peyronie's disease), with penile implants, in women or children, in men for whom sexual activity is inadvisable, and for intercourse with a pregnant woman. Onset of effect is 5-20 minutes.

sildenafil (*Viagra, Revatio*) ▶LK ♀B ▶- $$$

WARNING - Contraindicated in patients taking nitrates within prior/subsequent 24 hours. Caution with alpha blockers due to potential for symptomatic hypotension. There have been a few reports of sudden vision loss due to non-arteritic ischemic optic neuropathy (NAION). Patients with prior NAION are at higher risk.

ADULT - Erectile dysfunction: 50 mg PO approximately 1h (range 0.5-4h) before sexual activity. Usual effective dose range: 25-100 mg. Maximum 1 dose/day. Use lower dose (25 mg) if >65 yo, hepatic/renal impairment, or certain coadministered drugs (see notes). Pulmonary hypertension: 20 mg PO tid.

PEDS - Not approved in children.

UNAPPROVED ADULT - Antidepressant-associated sexual dysfunction: Dosing as above.

FORMS - Trade only (Viagra): Tabs 25, 50, 100 mg. Unscored tab but can be cut in half. Revatio: Tabs 20 mg.

NOTES - Interactions with cimetidine, erythromycin, ketoconazole, itraconazole, saquinavir, ritonavir, other CYP3A4 inhibitors; use 25 mg dose. Do not exceed 25 mg/48 h with ritonavir. Doses >25 mg should not be taken <4h after an alpha-blocker. Caution if stroke, MI or other cardiovascular event within last 6 months.

tadalafil (*Cialis*) ▶L ♀B ▶- $$$$

WARNING - Contraindicated with nitrates. Caution with alpha blockers due to potential for symptomatic hypotension. There have been a few reports of sudden vision loss due to non-arteritic ischemic optic neuropathy (NAION). Patients with prior NAION are at higher risk. Retinal artery occlusion has been reported.

ADULT - Erectile dysfunction: 10 mg PO prior to sexual activity. Optimal timing of administration

unclear, but should be ≥30-45 min before sexual activity. May increase to 20 mg or decrease to 5 mg. Max 1 dose/day. Start 5 mg (max 1 dose/day) if CrCl 31-50 mL/min. Max 5 mg/day if CrCl <30 mL/min on dialysis. Max 10 mg/day if mild to moderate hepatic impairment; avoid in severe hepatic impairment. Max 10 mg once in 72 hours if concurrent potent CYP3A4 inhibitors.

PEDS - Not approved in children.

FORMS - Trade only: Tabs 5, 10, 20 mg.

NOTES - If nitrates needed give ≥48 hours after the last tadalafil dose. Improves erectile function for up to 36 hours. Not FDA-approved for women. Not recommended if MI in prior 90 days, angina during sexual activity, NYHA Class ≥II in prior 6 months, hypotension (<90/50), HTN (>170/100) or stroke in prior 6 months. Rare reports of prolonged erections.

vardenafil (*Levitra*) ▶LK ♀B ▶- $$$

WARNING - Contraindicated with nitrates (time interval for safe administration unknown). Caution with alpha blockers due to potential for symptomatic hypotension. There have been a few reports of sudden vision loss due to non-arteritic ischemic optic neuropathy (NAION). Patients with prior NAION are at higher risk.

ADULT - Erectile dysfunction: 10 mg PO 1 h before sexual activity. Usual effective dose range: 5-20 mg. Maximum 1 dose/day. Use lower dose (5 mg) if ≥65 yo or moderate hepatic impairment (max 10 mg); 2.5 mg when coadministered with certain drugs (see notes). Not FDA-approved in women.

PEDS - Not approved in children.

FORMS - Trade only: Tabs 2.5, 5, 10, 20 mg.

NOTES - See the following parenthetical vardenafil dose adjustments when taken with ritonavir (max 2.5 mg/72 hr); indinavir, saquinavir, atazanavir, clarithromycin, ketoconazole 400 mg daily, or itraconazole 400 mg daily (max 2.5mg/24 hr); ketoconazole 200 mg daily, itraconazole 200 mg daily, or erythromycin (max 5 mg/24 hr). Avoid with alpha blockers & antiarrhythmics, and in congenital QT prolongation. Caution if stroke, MI or other cardiovascular event within last 6 months, unstable angina, severe liver impairment, end stage renal disease or retinitis pigmentosa.

yohimbine (*Yocon, Yohimex*) ▶L ♀- ▶- $

ADULT - No approved indications.

PEDS - No approved indications.

UNAPPROVED ADULT - Erectile dysfunction: 1 tab PO tid. If side effects (eg, tremor, tachycar-

dia, nervousness) occur, reduce to ½ tab tid, followed by gradual increases to 1 tab tid.
FORMS - Generic/Trade: Tab 5.4 mg.
NOTES - Prescription yohimbine and yohimbine bark extract (see Herbal section) are not interchangeable. Contraindicated with renal dis-

ease. Avoid with antidepressant use, psychiatric disorders, the elderly, women, or ulcer history. Efficacy of therapy >10 weeks unclear. American Urological Association does not recommend as a standard treatment due to unproven efficacy.

UROLOGY: Nephrolithiasis

acetohydroxamic acid (*Lithostat*) ▶K ♀X ▶?
$$$
ADULT - Chronic UTI, adjunctive therapy: 250 mg PO tid-qid for a total dose of 10-15 mg/kg/day. Maximum dose is 1.5 g/day. Decrease dose in patients with renal impairment to no more than 1 g/day.
PEDS - Adjunctive therapy in chronic urea-splitting UTI (eg, Proteus): 10 mg/kg/day PO divided bid-tid.
FORMS - Trade only: Tab 250 mg.
NOTES - Do not use if CrCl <20 mL/min. Administer on an empty stomach.

cellulose sodium phosphate (*Calcibind*) ▶Fecal ♀C ▶+ $$$$
WARNING - Avoid in heart failure or ascites due to high sodium content.
ADULT - Absorptive hypercalciuria Type 1 (>16 yo): Initial dose with urinary calcium >300 mg/day (on moderate calcium-restricted diet): 5 g with each meal. Decrease dose to 5 g with supper, 2.5 g with each remaining meal when calcium declines to <150 mg/day. Initial dose with urinary calcium 200-300 mg/day (controlled calcium-restricted diet): 5 g with supper, 2.5 g with each remaining meal. Mix with water, soft drink or fruit juice. Ingest within 30 min of meal.
PEDS - Do not use if <16 yo.
FORMS - Trade only: bulk powder 300 mg
NOTES - Give concomitant supplement of 1.5 g magnesium gluconate with 15 g/day. 1 g magnesium gluconate with 10 g/day. Take magnesium supplement ≥1h before or after each dose to avoid binding. May cause hyperpara-

thyroidism. Long-term use may cause hypomagnesemia, hyperoxaluria, hypomagnesuria, depletion of trace metals (copper, zinc, iron); monitor calcium, magnesium, trace metals and CBC q3-6 months; monitor parathyroid hormone once between the first 2 weeks and 3 months, then q3-6 months thereafter. Adjust or stop treatment if PTH rises above normal. Stop when inadequate hypocalciuric response (urinary calcium of <30 mg/5 g of cellulose sodium phosphate) occurs while patient is on moderate calcium restriction. Avoid Vitamin C supplementation since metabolized to oxalate.

citrate (*Polycitra-K, Urocit-K, Bicitra, Oracit, Polycitra, Polycitra-LC*) ▶K ♀C ▶? $$$
ADULT - Prevention of calcium and urate kidney stones: 1 packet in water/juice PO tid-qid with meals. 15-30 mL PO solution tid-qid with meals. Tabs 10-20 mEq PO tid-qid with meals. Max 100 mEq/day.
PEDS - Urinary alkalinization: 5-15 mL PO qid with meals.
FORMS - Trade only: Polycitra-K packet (potassium citrate): 3300 mg. Oracit oral solution: 5 mL = sodium citrate 490 mg. Generic/Trade: Urocit-K wax (potassium citrate) Tabs 5, 10 mEq. Generic only: Polycitra-K oral solution (5 mL = potassium citrate 1100 mg), Bicitra oral solution (5 mL = sodium citrate 500 mg), Polycitra-LC oral solution (5 mL = potassium citrate 550 mg/sodium citrate 500 mg), Polycitra oral syrup (5 mL = potassium citrate 550 mg/sodium citrate 550 mg).
NOTES - Contraindicated in renal insufficiency, PUD, UTI, and hyperkalemia.

UROLOGY: Other

aminohippurate (*PAH*) ▶K ♀C ▶? $$$$
ADULT - Estimation of effective renal plasma flow & measurement of functional capacity of renal tubular secretory mechanism: Specialized infusion dosing available.
PEDS - Not approved in children.

NOTES - May precipitate heart failure. Patients receiving sulfonamides, procaine or thiazolsulfone may interfere with chemical color development essential for analysis. Concomitant use of probenecid my result in erroneously low effective renal plasma flow.

Index

Although the PDA software edition of the *Tarascon Pocket Pharmacopoeia* contains >6,000 drugs and drug names, it is physically impossible to include all of this information in pocket-sized manuals. Accordingly, a number of rarely used or highly specialized drugs appear only in our PDA edition (noted as "**pda**").

S

Page left blank for notes

Page left blank for notes

Page left blank for notes

ADULT EMERGENCY DRUGS (selected)

ALLERGY	diphenhydramine (*Benadryl*): 50 mg IV/IM. epinephrine: 0.1-0.5 mg IM (1:1000 solution), may repeat after 20 minutes. methylprednisolone (*Solu-Medrol*): 125 mg IV/IM.
HYPERTENSION	esmolol (*Brevibloc*): 500 mcg/kg IV over 1 minute, then titrate 50-200 mcg/kg/minute fenoldopam (*Corlopam*): Start 0.1 mcg/kg/min, titrate up to 1.6 mcg/kg/min labetalol (*Normodyne*): Start 20 mg slow IV, then 40-80 mg IV q10 min prn up to 300 mg total cumulative dose nitroglycerin (*Tridil*): Start 10-20 mcg/min IV infusion, then titrate prn up to 100 mcg/minute nitroprusside (*Nipride*): Start 0.3 mcg/kg/min IV infusion, then titrate prn up to 10 mcg/kg/minute
DYSRHYTHMIAS / ARREST	adenosine (*Adenocard*): PSVT (not A-fib): 6 mg rapid IV & flush, preferably through a central line or proximal IV. If no response after 1-2 minutes then 12 mg. A third dose of 12 mg may be given prn. amiodarone (*Cordarone, Pacerone*): V-fib or pulseless V-tach: 300 mg IV/IO; may repeat 150 mg just once. Life-threatening ventricular arrhythmia: Load 150 mg IV over 10 min, then 1 mg/min x 6h, then 0.5 mg/min x 18h. atropine: 0.5 mg IV, repeat prn to maximum of 3 mg. diltiazem (*Cardizem*): Rapid A-fib: bolus 0.25 mg/kg or 20 mg IV over 2 min. May repeat 0.35 mg/kg or 25 mg 15 min after 1st dose. Infusion 5-15 mg/h. epinephrine: 1 mg IV/IO q3-5 minutes for cardiac arrest. [1:10,000 solution] lidocaine (*Xylocaine*): Load 1 mg/kg IV, then 0.5 mg/kg q8-10min prn to max 3 mg/kg. Maintenance 2g in 250ml D5W (8 mg/ml) at 1-4 mg/min drip (7-30 ml/h).
PRESSORS	dobutamine (*Dobutrex*): 2-20 mcg/kg/min. 70 kg: 5 mcg/kg/min with 1 mg/mL concentration (eg, 250 mg in 250 mL D5W) = 21 mL/h. dopamine (*Intropin*): Pressor: Start at 5 mcg/kg/min, increase prn by 5-10 mcg/kg/min increments at 10 min intervals, max 50 mcg/kg/min. 70 kg: 5 mcg/kg/min with 1600 mcg/mL concentration (eg, 400 mg in 250 ml D5W) = 13 mL/h. Doses in mcg/kg/min: 2-4 = (traditional renal dose, apparently ineffective) dopaminergic receptors; 5-10 = (cardiac dose) dopaminergic and beta1 receptors; >10 = dopaminergic, beta1, and alpha1 receptors. norepinephrine (*Levophed*): 4 mg in 500 ml D5W (8 mcg/ml) at 2-4 mcg/min. 22.5 ml/h = 3 mcg/min. phenylephrine (*Neo-Synephrine*): 50 mcg boluses IV. Infusion for hypotension: 20 mg in 250ml D5W (80 mcg/ml) at 40-180 mcg/min (35-160ml/h).
INTUBATION	etomidate (*Amidate*): 0.3 mg/kg IV. methohexital (*Brevital*): 1-1.5 mg/kg IV. propofol (*Diprivan*): 2.0-2.5 mg/kg IV. rocuronium (*Zemuron*): 0.6-1.2 mg/kg IV. succinylcholine (*Anectine*): 1 mg/kg IV. Peds (<5 yo): 2 mg/kg IV. thiopental (*Pentothal*): 3-5 mg/kg IV.
SEIZURES	diazepam (*Valium*): 5-10 mg IV, or 0.2-0.5 mg/kg rectal gel up to 20 mg PR. fosphenytoin (*Cerebyx*): Load 15-20 "phenytoin equivalents" per kg either IM, or IV no faster than 100-150 mg/min. lorazepam (*Ativan*): 0.05-0.15 mg/kg up to 3-4 mg IV/IM. phenobarbital: 200-600 mg IV at rate ≤60 mg/min; titrate prn up to 20 mg/kg phenytoin (*Dilantin*): 15-20 mg/kg up to 1000 mg IV no faster than 50 mg/min.

CARDIAC DYSRHYTHMIA PROTOCOLS (for adults and adolescents)

Chest compressions ~100/minute. Ventilations 8-10/minute if intubated; otherwise 30:2 compression/ventilation ratio. Drugs that can be administered down ET tube (use 2-2.5 x usual dose): epinephrine, atropine, lidocaine, vasopressin, naloxone.

V-Fib, Pulseless V-Tach
Airway, oxygen, CPR until defibrillator ready
Defibrillate 360 J (old monophasic), 120-200 J (biphasic), or with AED
Resume CPR x 2 minutes (5 cycles)
Repeat defibrillation if no response
Vasopressor during CPR:
- Epinephrine 1 mg IV/IO q3-5 minutes, or
- Vasopressin 40 units IV to replace 1st or 2nd dose of epinephrine

Rhythm/pulse check every ~2 minutes
Consider antiarrhythmic during CPR:
- Amiodarone 300 mg IV/IO; may repeat 150 mg just once
- Lidocaine 1.0-1.5 mg/kg IV/IO, then repeat 0.5-0.75 mg/kg to max 3 doses or 3 mg/kg
- Magnesium 1-2 g IV/IO if suspect torsade de pointes

Asystole or Pulseless Electrical Activity (PEA)
Airway, oxygen, CPR
Vasopressor (when IV/IO access):
- Epinephrine 1 mg IV/IO q3-5 minutes, or
- Vasopressin 40 units IV/IO to replace 1st or 2nd dose of epinephrine

Consider atropine 1 mg IV/IO for asystole or slow PEA. Repeat q3-5 min up to 3 doses.
Rhythm/pulse check every ~2 minutes
Consider 6 H's: hypovolemia, hypoxia, H+ acidosis, hyper / hypokalemia, hypoglycemia, hypothermia
Consider 5 T's: Toxins, tamponade-cardiac, tension pneumothorax, thrombosis (coronary or pulmonary), trauma

Bradycardia, <60 bpm and Inadequate Perfusion
Airway, oxygen, IV
Prepare for transcutaneous pacing; don't delay if advanced heart block
Consider atropine 0.5 mg IV; may repeat to max 3 mg
Consider epinephrine (2-10 mcg/min) or dopamine (2-10 mcg/kg/min)
Prepare for transvenous pacing

Tachycardia with Pulses
Airway, oxygen, IV
If unstable and heart rate >150 bpm, then synchronized cardioversion
If stable narrow-QRS (<120 ms):
- Regular: Attempt vagal maneuvers. If no success, then adenosine 6 mg IV, then 12 mg prn up to twice.
- Irregular: Control rate with diltiazem or beta blocker (caution in CHF or pulmonary disease).

If stable wide-QRS (>120 ms):
- Regular and suspect V-tach: Amiodarone 150 mg IV over 10 min; repeat prn to max 2.2 g/24h. Prepare for elective synchronized cardioversion.
- Regular and suspect SVT with aberrancy: adenosine as per narrow-QRS above.
- Irregular and A-fib: Control rate with diltiazem or beta blocker (caution in CHF/pulmonary disease).
- Irregular and A-fib with pre-excitation (WPW): Avoid AV nodal blocking agents; consider amiodarone 150 mg IV over 10 minutes.
- Irregular and torsade de pointes: magnesium 1-2 g IV load over 5-60 minutes, then infusion.

bpm=beats per minute; CPR=cardiopulmonary resuscitation; ET=endotracheal; IO=intraosseous; J=Joules; ms=milliseconds; WPW=Wolf-Parkinson-White. Source *Circulation* 2005; 112, suppl IV.

Tarascon Publishing Order Form on Next Page

Price per Copy by Number of Copies Ordered				
Total # of each ordered →	1–9	10–49	50–99	≥100
Tarascon Pocket Pharmacopoeia				
• *Classic shirt pocket edition*	$11.95	$10.95	$9.95	$8.95
• *Deluxe lab coat pocket edition*	$19.95	$16.95	$14.95	$13.95
• *PDA edition on CD, 12 month subscription*	$32.95	$28.00	$26.36	$24.70
Other Tarascon Pocketbooks				
• *Tarascon Pediatric Outpatient Pocketbook*	$14.95	$13.45	$11.94	$10.44
• *Tarascon Internal Med & Critical Care Pocketbook*	$14.95	$13.45	$11.94	$10.44
• *Tarascon Primary Care Pocketbook*	$14.95	$13.45	$11.94	$10.44
• *Tarascon Pediatric Emergency Pocketbook*	$14.95	$13.45	$11.94	$10.44
• *Tarascon Adult Emergency Pocketbook*	$14.95	$13.45	$11.94	$10.44
• *Tarascon Pocket Orthopaedica*	$14.95	$13.45	$11.94	$10.44
• *How to be a Truly Excellent Junior Med Student*	$9.95	$8.25	$7.45	$6.95
Tarascon Rapid Reference Cards & Magnifier				
• *Tarascon Quick P450 Enzyme Reference Card*	$1.95	$1.85	$1.75	$1.65
• *Tarascon Quick Cardiac Arrest / Emergency*	$1.95	$1.85	$1.75	$1.65
• *Tarascon Quick Pediatric Reference Card*	$1.95	$1.85	$1.75	$1.65
• *Tarascon Quick HTN/LDL Reference Card*	$1.95	$1.85	$1.75	$1.65
• *Tarascon Fresnel Magnifying Lens and Ruler*	$1.00	$0.89	$0.78	$0.66
Other Recommended Pocketbooks				
• *Managing Contraception*	$10.00	$9.75	$9.50	$9.25
• *OB/GYN & Infertility*	$19.95	$19.55	$19.25	$18.80
• *Airway Cam Pocket Guide to Intubation*	$14.95	$14.55	$14.25	$13.80
• *Thompson's Rheumatology Pocket Reference*	$14.95	$14.55	$14.25	$13.80
• *Reproductive Endocrinology/Infertility-Pocket*	$14.95	$14.55	$14.25	$13.80
• *Reproductive Endocrinology/Infertility-Desk*	$24.95	$24.55	$24.20	$23.80

Shipping & Handling (based on subtotal on next page order form)					
If subtotal is →	≤$12	$13-29.99	$30-75.99	$76-200	$201-700
Standard shipping	$1.50	$2.75	$6.25	$8.00	$16.00
UPS 2-day air *(no PO boxes)*	$13.00	$15.00	$17.00	$20.00	$40.00

Tarascon Pocket Pharmacopoeia® Deluxe PDA Edition

Features
- Palm / Pocket PC / BlackBerry versions
- Meticulously peer-reviewed drug information
- Multiple drug interaction checking
- Continuous internet auto-updates
- Multiple tables & formulas
- Complete customer privacy

Download a FREE 30-day trial version at www.tarascon.com
Subscriptions thereafter priced at $2.50/month

Ordering Books From Tarascon Publishing

INTERNET	**MAIL**	**FAX**	**PHONE**
Order through our OnLine store with your credit card at **www.tarascon.com**	Mail order & check to: **Tarascon Publishing PO Box 517 Lompoc, CA 93438**	Fax credit card orders 24 hrs/day toll free to **877.929.9926**	For phone orders or customer service, call **800.929.9926**

Name	Company name (if applicable)		
Address			
City	State	Zip	Residential ☐ Business ☐
Phone	Email		

TARASCON POCKET PHARMACOPOEIA®		Quantity	Price*
Classic Shirt-Pocket Edition			$
Deluxe Labcoat Pocket Edition			$
PDA software on CD-ROM, 12 month subscription‡			$
OTHER TARASCON POCKETBOOKS			
Tarascon Pediatric Outpatient Pocketbook			$
Tarascon Internal Medicine & Critical Care Pocketbook			$
Tarascon Primary Care Pocketbook			$
Tarascon Pediatric Emergency Pocketbook			$
Tarascon Adult Emergency Pocketbook			$
Tarascon Pocket Orthopaedica®			$
How to be a Truly Excellent Junior Medical Student			$
TARASCON RAPID REFERENCE CARDS & MAGNIFIER			
Tarascon Quick P450 Enzyme Reference Card			$
Tarascon Quick Cardiac Arrest / Emergency Card			$
Tarascon Quick Pediatric Reference Card			$
Tarascon Quick HTN & LDL Reference Card			$
Tarascon Fresnel Magnifying Lens and Ruler			$
OTHER RECOMMENDED POCKETBOOKS			
Managing Contraception			$
OB/GYN & Infertility			$
Airway Cam Pocket Guide to Intubation			$
Thompson's Rheumatology Pocket Reference			$
Reproductive Endocrinology/Infertility Pocket edition			$
Reproductive Endocrinology/Infertility Desk edition			$

See prior page for prices / shipping. ‡Or download today at www.tarascon.com

☐ VISA ☐ Mastercard ☐ American Express ☐ Discover		**Subtotal**	$
Card number		CA only add 7.25% sales tax	$
Exp date	CID code number	Shipping / handling*	$
Signature		**TOTAL**	$